ENGINEERING THE SYSTEM OF HEALTHCARE DELIVERY

Tennenbaum Institute Series on Enterprise Systems

The mission of the Tennenbaum Institute is creation and dissemination of information, knowledge and skills to enable fundamental change of complex organizational systems. The IOS Press book series on Enterprise Systems is one of the ways that the Institute facilitates this dissemination of knowledge created by our many partners in academia, industry, and government as well as the Institute's faculty and staff.

The goal of each volume in the series is to bring together multi-disciplinary and transdisciplinary perspectives, empirical and axiomatic research, and design methods and tools within focus areas of particular importance to enable fundamental enterprise transformation in both private and public sectors. Focus areas of interest range from value creation and work processes to management decision making and social networks, all in the context of fundamental enterprise and organizational change. The objective is to address enterprise systems at all levels, ranging from technological systems to human and organizational systems.

The Institute is committed to attracting thought leaders from a wide range of disciplines, challenging them to communicate broadly, and helping them create works that can truly help those entrusted with transforming their enterprises. We intend these volumes to enable people to enhance value for all of their enterprise's stakeholders, ranging from shareholders and employees, to customers and other constituencies.

The Tennenbaum Institute is a unit of the Georgia Institute of Technology, Atlanta, Georgia, 30332, USA. For further information, please visit www.ti.gatech.edu.

Volume 3

Recently published in this series:

Vol. 2. R.C. Basole (Ed.), Enterprise Mobility: Applications, Technologies and Strategies
Vol. 1. W.B. Rouse and A.P. Sage (Eds.), Work, Workflow and Information Systems

ISSN 1874-737X

Engineering the System of Healthcare Delivery

Edited by

Dr. W.B. Rouse

Tennenbaum Institute, Georgia Institute of Technology, Atlanta, GA 30332 USA

and

Dr. D.A. Cortese

Mayo Clinic, 200 1st. Street, SW, Rochester, MN 55905, USA

IOS
Press

Amsterdam • Berlin • Tokyo • Washington, DC

ISBN 978-1-60750-531-0

Published previously in the journal *Information Knowledge Systems Management* 8 (1–4) 2009.

This book is also available as Volume 153 in the Studies in Health Technology and Informatics series,
ISBN 978-1-60750-532-7.

Publisher
IOS Press BV
Nieuwe Hemweg 6B
1013 BG Amsterdam
The Netherlands
fax: +31 20 687 0019
e-mail: order@iospress.nl

Distributor in the USA and Canada
IOS Press, Inc.
4502 Rachael Manor Drive
Fairfax, VA 22032
USA
fax: +1 703 323 3668
e-mail: iosbooks@iospress.com

PRINTED IN THE NETHERLANDS

Dedication

The editors are pleased to dedicate this book to Dr. Jerome H. Grossman, MD, a friend and colleague who stimulated and cultivated our mutual interest in the intersection of systems engineering and the science of healthcare delivery that has resulted in this book.

William B. Rouse and Denis A. Cortese

Contents

Section 4: Engineering Approaches

Section 5: Perspectives

Section 6: Conclusions

Information Knowledge Systems Management 8 (2009) 1–2
DOI 10.3233/IKS-2009-0153
IOS Press

Foreword

Introduction to Engineering Healthcare

In October, 1957, western countries were stunned when the Soviet Union launched Sputnik, the first human-made satellite to orbit the earth. Subsequently, the United States worked feverishly to launch a satellite into space using a Vanguard Missile. Unfortunately, each time the Vanguard began to lift from the launch pad, it fizzled and exploded. It was very embarrassing. The Vanguard was assembled from components, each of which was well designed and performed its function with near perfection. The problem was that the designers had concentrated on the components and had failed to think through all the ways in which they interacted with each other. So, some parts were overheated by a neighboring part, others were disturbed by vibrations of a third component, etc. The system as a whole failed, injuring our national pride, and undoubtedly amusing Soviet Premier Nikita Khrushchev.

Today, the U.S. healthcare system has many wonderful parts: an amazingly strong input of fundamental life science; extraordinary technology for diagnosis and treatment; dedicated doctors, nurses, and technicians; many fine hospital facilities; emergency transport units; widely distributed pharmacies; and a great deal of useful information available on the World Wide Web. But like the Vanguard, the many interactions of these and other components with each other, and with our populace, have not been carefully thought through; the healthcare system has evolved rather haphazardly over time. The system has not failed entirely, but it has left us with an obesity epidemic, scant attention to wellness and disease prevention, disparities in access and outcomes, persistent deficiencies in safety and quality, and the highest costs in the world – while dozens of other countries boast lower infant mortality and longer life expectancy. If this has not injured our national pride, it should.

The Vanguard Missile went back to the drawing board, and was carefully rethought from a systems perspective, i.e. all the interactions of the components were understood, and they were modified to meet the end goal of launching a satellite effectively, and without failure. We could say that the system was "engineered." As a result, the U.S. moved rapidly to become the greatest space-faring nation.

This is what must now be done with our healthcare system, and William B. Rouse and Denis A. Cortese, together with a team of highly-experienced experts, show us how to go about it. Engineering healthcare is a much more complex process than engineering a missile, because the healthcare system includes people, as individuals, as a society, and as a body politic. Healthcare depends on a myriad of organizations working in concert, including hospitals, specialty clinics, insurers, drug and device manufacturers, pharmacies, regulatory bodies, educational institutions, and more. The healthcare system must obey the laws of economics as well as those of biology, chemistry, and physics, and it must meet human aspirations, and respond appropriately to human needs and foibles. In the first instance, the framework of the system must align the incentives to each person and organization involved, from patient to care provider, to pharmaceutical company, to public health officials, to basic scientist with the goal of healthy, high-quality lives throughout the lifespan.

But a future system that will provide quality and affordable care for everyone can be designed and established. The principles are understood. An engineering approach, as espoused in this book, takes account of the system as a whole and each of its parts, their interactions and interdependencies. An engineering approach enables one to work on making each component of the health care system do its job without losing sight of the whole, and thus enable the health system as a whole to produce high-value care.

New models of care delivery have the potential to add value in caring for people with chronic diseases, keeping them out of hospitals and as well as possible. Value can be realized through primary care and the use of non-traditional providers in non-traditional settings. In these and other instances, achieving high value in health care requires that payment reforms align incentives with the goals of individuals, organizations, and society. A systematic approach to gathering, analyzing, and acting on errors – at individual hospitals and clinics and at an aggregate level – can increase safety and enhance the quality of care. More generally, an engineered health system that is efficient and effective depends on information capture, access, and use. And finally, as most modern industries have demonstrated, an engineered approach can drive out substantial waste, reduce costs, and slow the rise of spending.

As this book goes to press, the nation is engaged in a vigorous political debate about reforming healthcare. Most of the debate focuses on expanding insurance coverage and who will pay for it. This is important, as far as it goes, but it does not go far enough. Beyond additional health insurance, the American people need and deserve a health system that is dramatically improved in its operation, cost, and outcomes. This book tells how to make a high-value health system a reality.

Charles M. Vest
President of the National Academy of Engineering and
former President of the Massachusetts Institute of Technology
E-mail: Cvest@ nae.edu

Harvey V. Fineberg
President of the Institute of Medicine and
former Provost of Harvard University
E-mail: Fineberg@nas.edu

Information Knowledge Systems Management 8 (2009) 3–14
DOI 10.3233/IKS-2009-0157
IOS Press

Chapter 1

Introduction

William B. Rouse and Denis A. Cortese
E-mail: bill.rouse@ti.gatech.edu

Breakthroughs in medical science and innovations in clinical practices offer enormous opportunities for impressive improvements in the health and well being of society. Returns on investments in these endeavors can be impressive. However, we will not realize the greatest returns unless we also better engineer the system of healthcare delivery [4].

1. The enterprise of healthcare

Consider the architecture of the enterprise of healthcare delivery shown below [5]. The efficiencies that can be gained at the lowest level (clinical practices) are limited by nature of the next level (delivery operations). For example, functionally organized practices are much less efficient than delivery organized around processes.

Similarly, the efficiencies that can be gained in operations are limited by the level above (system structure). Functional operations are driven by organizations structured around specialties, e.g., anesthesiology and radiology. And, of course, efficiencies in system structure are limited by the healthcare ecosystem in which organizations operate. Differing experiences of other countries provide ample evidence of this.

The fee-for-service model central to healthcare in the United States assures that provider income is linked to activities rather than outcomes. The focus on disease and restoration of health rather than wellness and productivity assures that healthcare expenditures will be viewed as costs rather than investments. Recasting of "the problem" in terms of outcomes characterized by wellness and productivity may enable identification and pursuit of efficiencies that could not be imagined within our current frame of reference.

2. Defining value

There is currently much commentary on two things in healthcare – universal availability and cost control. However, we do not think that people want the lowest cost, universally available healthcare system. We think the central issue should really be the creation of a healthcare system that provides the highest value.

Value is often defined in terms of the benefits of the outcomes of an expenditure, divided by the costs of the expenditure. The benefits of healthcare – from a patient's perspective – include the quality of health outcomes, the safety of the process of delivery, and the services associated with the delivery process [3].

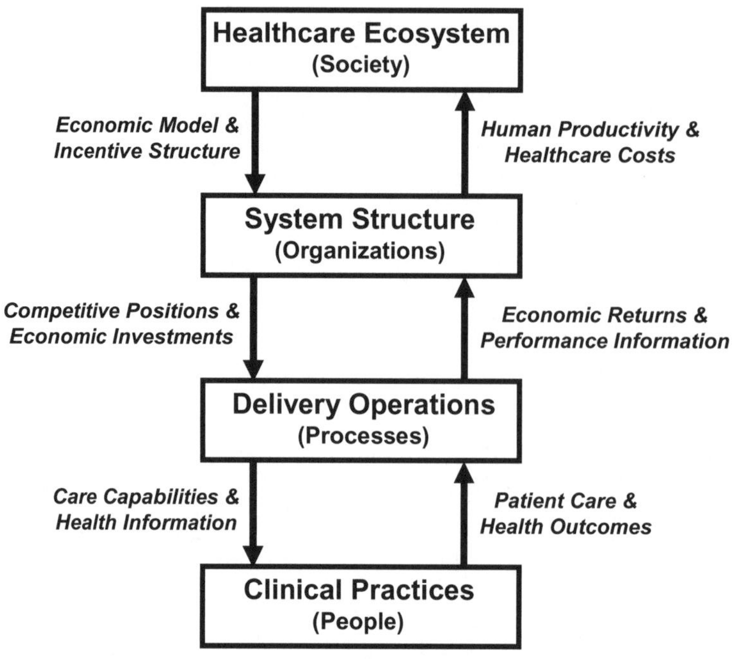

The Enterprise of Healthcare Delivery

The benefits from the perspective of society also include the availability of healthy, productive people who contribute to society in a wealth of ways. When people are not healthy, these contributions are diminished. A recent study found that the cost of the lost productivity far exceeds the cost of the healthcare [2].

For many reasons it is likely people will remain in the workforce longer than in the past. In 1960's, before Medicare got started, the average age of death was 67; the average age at retirement was 65–66. By 2005, the average age of death had reached 75 and the average age of retirement was 62. We are now seeing some people planning on working longer, perhaps up to 70. Even Social Security has delayed the eligibility age for benefits, with the retirement age for people born after 1937 increasing to 66 if born before 1955 and up to 67 if born later.

If people who do not retire at the usual Social Security retirement age stay on employers' insurance, then employers will even have an increased interest in keeping people healthy for as long as possible and doing productive work for as long as possible until the worker retires and goes onto Medicare. Employer insurance companies are glad to see the older employees roll into Medicare for the same reasons; when the greater costs are incurred it is the government's problem.

Indeed, this is the exact reason some have proposed that people enroll in and own an insurance product and keep it even after they retire. That way the insurance company will now have an interest in keeping you as well as possible even after you retire, in other words, sun setting Medicare. A Federal Employees Health Care Plan model would facilitate this option.

Thus, there will be an increasing need to keep older people healthy because they will need to remain productive longer. More pervasive, due to the "flat world" [1], will be the need to keep everyone healthy and productive. Part of the value equation, therefore, should include the productivity in the future of all the workers that do not get diabetes or have heart attacks or cancer. For this to work, our value equation will have to account for future returns from today's investments.

This broader perspective emphasizes the importance of a healthy, educated, and productive population to well-being and competitiveness of a society. Of course, a central debate in the U.S concerns who pays for this value. Regardless of how this debate is resolved, however, it is difficult to make the case for an unhealthy, uneducated, and unproductive country.

3. Delivering value

Value is delivered by value streams – the sequences of activities that create quality health outcomes safely with excellent service. Some activities create more value than others. These activities tend to involve direct patient-clinician interaction. Other activities such as billing, payroll and procurement are enablers. They should be done efficiently, and with good service, but should not divert resources from higher value activities.

Value streams are enabled by work processes, e.g., patient in processing and out processing or, perhaps more compelling, diabetes management. It has been found that value can be increased simply by thinking of an organization in terms of work processes. Such thinking fairly quickly leads to identifying, and hopefully eliminating, activities that do not add value. By thinking in terms of work processes rather than departments, for example, one can better allocate resources across activities to maximize the total value of the service to the patient and/or society rather than "suboptimizing" to maximize the financial value provided by or to each department.

Note that process-oriented thinking can have substantial implications for healthcare business models. For the process of diabetes management, for instance, one can imagine charging patients, or third party payers, for the health outcome of quality management of this disease rather than sundry fees for each of the departments and people involved in this process. This then would enable the provider to allocate resources across this process to maximize the value provided. Whether or not each department was "profitable" would no longer be central to decision making. Of course, this could remain a major issue for single specialty practices, which suggests a need for another level of rethinking of business models.

3.1. Information

There are two critical aspects of maximizing value by thinking in terms of value streams and work processes. First, information is required to understand and control the state of the system to achieve effective operations. A lack of understanding of the state of the system, as well as a lack of feedback of the current state of the system relative to intentions, severely limits the effectiveness of the system.

It is also very important to have information on what works and does not work. Randomized clinical trials are the "gold standard" for clinical evidence. However, we can also learn from the millions of patient transactions each day by mining this wealth of data for trends, insights, and new hypotheses. Such information may be the primary means for assessing the efficacy of large-scale organizational changes.

3.2. Incentives

Second, Incentives have to be aligned with the goal of maximizing value. If service revenue is driven by cost reimbursement for activities, then rational providers will maximize the number of activities. On the other hand, if service revenue is driven by health outcomes of services, then rational providers will attempt to maximize health outcomes for every dollar they expend.

Our sense is that providers that are good at proving quality health outcomes will make higher profits than they do currently. This requires that the initial conditions of the population of people for which a provider is responsible are taken into account so that funding available will enable the best providers to be able to realize a reward for keeping people well. Also, more providers are starting their own insurance products so they are closer to the first dollar and any efficiencies they attain translate into retained earnings that they can reinvest, use as salary, or pass on as reduced premiums to attract more business.

Incentives also drive how investment dollars are allocated. If better margins can be earned from addressing "lifestyle" diseases, e.g., restless legs, then investments in treatments for those diseases will diminish investments in more pervasive diseases, e.g., malaria. Further, enormous resources will be invested in convincing people that they have such lifestyle diseases.

3.3. Evaluation

Analytics can provide the means to process information to make it useful, as well as devise and evaluate incentive systems. We cannot evaluate all good ideas by deploying them in the healthcare system and assessing their impact. Instead, we should use analytical methods, including simulation, to model and evaluate a wide range of possibilities, the most promising of which can then be deployed and empirically evaluated.

4. Implementing change

As we consider implementing ideas that make it through the analytical filters, we should ask several questions:

- Who are the key stakeholders in this change?
- How will each type of stakeholder react to this change?
- What would cause them to support the change?
- Who has to act to enable both the change and support for the change?
- What political and financial resources are needed for success?

In general, these questions are focused on how to incentivize key players to change business models that they have finely tuned to the status quo. It seems like crises are often needed to prompt such changes. Perhaps this will arise in healthcare when costs preclude even the insured from receiving care, e.g., the patient's portion of the bill is so high that people avoid getting care.

These five questions relate to barriers that will have to be addressed and overcome if we are really to foster a high value system of healthcare. The stakeholders include providers; patients, private payers, employers, government, unions, associations (e.g., AARP), pharmaceutical companies, and device manufacturers and, to a lesser extent, the bodies that are now working to generate evidence to be used in medical decision making (AHRQ, IOM, Leapfrog Group, NQF, University Hospital Consortium).

5. Overview of book

This book reflects the experiences and perspectives of a rather amazing group of thought leaders in healthcare delivery. Charles Vest and Harvey Fineberg, presidents of the National Academy of Engineering and Institute of Medicine, respectively, set the stage. They lay out why the healthcare system in the United States performs so poorly relative to healthcare expenditures, as well as how the perspectives provided in this book can contribute to engineering a system to provide affordable, quality care for everyone.

Following this introductory chapter, this book is organized into sections that systematically map out the central issues, consider how information and incentives affect healthcare delivery, elaborate perspectives of major stakeholders, and discuss why change is so difficult, as well as the prospects for change.

Section 1: Issues

In Chapter 2, "Seeking Care as a System," Donald Berwick and Eva Luo of the Institute for Healthcare Improvement provide a compelling vignette of the great difficulty our current "system" has behaving like a system. The capability, audacity, and complexity of medical care have grown steadily over the past two decades. They argue that so, too, have its hazards and costs. They note how the landmark Institute of Medicine reports, *To Err Is Human* and *Crossing the Quality Chasm*, brought health care defects and the potential for improvement to the foreground, with threats to patients' safety the most charismatic and understandable of all those defects. In 2009, a socially urgent trio – cost, quality, and coverage – now dominate a loud national conversation, with the potential to lead, maybe at last, to health system reform. But, they ask, what "system" are we talking about that is to be "reformed"? As their opening vignette portrayed a patient's dependence on a vast network of interacting elements, so do almost all of the performance characteristics that reform may purport to improve. The idea of a system is neither a frill nor fine point if we are to get reform right. They argue that it lies at the very center of the scientific and political challenges that stand between us and the care we seek. They conclude that with a proper understanding of systems, authentic health care redesign is feasible and socially productive. Without that understanding, they assert, "reform" will likely do more harm than good.

Chapter 3, "Patient Safety," by Pascale Carayon and Kenneth E. Wood of the University of Wisconsin, argues that patient safety is a global challenge that requires knowledge and skills in multiple areas, including human factors and systems engineering. In this chapter, numerous conceptual approaches and methods for analyzing, preventing and mitigating medical errors are described. Given the complexity of healthcare work systems and processes, the authors emphasize the need for increasing partnerships between the health sciences and human factors and systems engineering to improve patient safety. Those partnerships, they argue, will be able to develop and implement the system redesigns that are necessary to improve healthcare work systems and processes for patient safety.

In Chapter 4, "Aging: Adding Complexity, Requiring Skill," Christine Cassel, Michelle Johnston-Fleece, and Siddhartha Reddy, of the American Board of Internal Medicine, note that the role of systems in addressing the needs of elderly and chronically ill populations remains a far from universal way of thinking, much less practice, in healthcare. Re-engineering the current fragmented system to align providers, patients and payment models to facilitate proactive management of conditions associated with advanced age and/or one or more chronic diseases – rather than respond to costly consequences of a health care system optimized for acute care conditions – will be a major challenge for all stakeholders. There are, however, promising success stories that are taking place in the United States today that may provide a model for improvement. The authors define the issues faced by the healthcare providers and payers providing care for the elderly and those with chronic conditions, which threaten to overwhelm the financial and human healthcare resources that exist to serve these populations. They define innovative ways of thinking about systems of care, and provide examples of unique systems that have applied theory into practice. These successful leaders may offer lessons in proactively managing complex health conditions, overcoming communication barriers and using technology to complement the necessary human touch that is essential to healthcare delivery.

Chapter 5, "Palliative & End of Life Care," by Robert Stroebel and Timothy Moynihan of the Mayo Clinic, indicates that health care provided in the final year of life is typically costly and often delivers unintended outcomes. However, high value can be defined for end of life care. High value clinical practices exist for end of life care and a common set of high value processes can be identified. The current system structure of healthcare delivery does not consistently support those high value processes. An improved organizational schema could foster sustained delivery of high value delivery operations. They conclude that healthcare ecosystem needs to evolve to provide appropriate incentives and support for an appropriately designed care system.

In Chapter 6, "US Healthcare Costs: The Crushing Burden," Helen Darling of the National Business Group on Health provides an overview of health care costs in the United States, including trends, sources and uses of funds, employers' role, and factors driving costs. It also reviews what analysts believe are cost drivers especially compared to other countries that have significantly lower health care costs and, often, better health outcomes. *Within* the US, there are also important differences by geography, further demonstrating that higher US costs do not reflect higher quality and greater patient and physician satisfaction. In fact, the opposite is often the case.

Section 2: Information

Chapter 7, "Engineering Information Technology for Actionable Information and Better Health," by Don Detmer of the American Medical Informatics Association and the University of Virginia, reports that information technology in health care (HIT) is getting a major boost in the United States through the passage of the American Recovery and Reinvestment Act (ARRA) of 2009. The portion of the Act that relates to health information technology (HITECH) seeks to achieve widespread implementation of electronic health records (EHRs) across the land and assure that these EHRs achieve sufficient levels of 'meaningful use' to improve care, reduce costs, and result in better outcomes. The author reviews current thinking about how HIT will facilitate collection, dissemination, and evaluation of information throughout the system. Further, it discusses the role and potential for HIT to support a learning organization. Finally, it outlines the current widely identified barriers to progress, e.g., standards development, lack of interoperability and connectivity, and limited decision support that uses evidence-based guidelines created and maintained explicitly to be actionable through computer-based records and systems.

In Chapter 8, "Electronic Health Records," William Stead of Vanderbilt University asserts that a radical change in technical approach is needed to achieve electronic health records suitable to support an engineered system of healthcare. This chapter suggests a redefinition of interoperable health information. It provides examples of how to break the electronic health record challenge into component parts to match computational technique to the scale of the problem handled by a component.

Chapter 9, "Evidence-Based Medicine," by Michael McGinnis of the Institute of Medicine, notes that whether for the generation or application of evidence to guide healthcare decisions, the success of evidence-based medicine is grounded in principles common to engineering. In the Learning Healthcare System envisioned by the Institute of Medicine's (IOM) Roundtable on Evidence-Based Medicine, evidence emerges as a natural by-product of care delivery which is thoroughly documented, pooled for continuous monitoring and analysis, integrated with insights from related studies, and fed back seamlessly to improve the consistency and appropriateness of care decisions by clinicians and their patients. Drawing from lessons shared at the IOM/NAE symposium, *Engineering a Learning Healthcare System*, this chapter provides an overview of the state-of-play in health care today, some of its key challenges, the vision and features of a learning healthcare system, applicable commonalties and principles from engineering, and potential collaborative opportunities moving forward to the benefit of both fields.

In Chapter 10, "Transforming Healthcare Through Patient Empowerment," Leslie Lenert of the Centers for Disease Control and Prevention begins with a discussion of the great illusion of American healthcare, namely, that it is an altruistic service not a business. It is easy see why medical care appears to be altruistic. "Beneficent" payers such as insurance companies, paid by employers, cover much of the costs of care for those with employment related coverage. But healthcare is a business and for every healthcare decision there are at least three perspectives: that of the patient, that of the physician and that of the payer. While physicians are sworn to advance patients' interests, over all else, the interests of physician and patient are not parallel and often diverge. Sometimes the divergence is due to physicians over estimating the benefit of procedures they offer. Other times it may be due to them underestimating the risk. However, there is no section of the Hippocratic Oath that requires physicians to deliver healthcare to the benefit of payers in the most cost-effective manner. In the current model, physicians largely share decision authority with payers, resulting in a dynamic tension where each tries to limit the financial gain of the other, while trying to do no harm to the patient. This has resulted in a complex, inefficient, and poorly performing healthcare system. This chapter examines the prospects of what would happen if we put patients rather than doctors or insurance companies in charge of decision making using a variety of technologies, strategies and other decision support methods. Results suggest that for many therapies, particularly therapies that have upfront risks for survival and quality of life benefits, allowing patients to lead decision making would lower costs, due to patients' natural risk aversion. Therapies with few up front risks are not impacted or might even be used more heavily if patients led decision making. Aligning patient decisions with payers' values on costs of care may enable approaches that allow individuals to benefit by conserving societal resources.

Section 3: Incentives

In Chapter 11, "Health Economics," Gail Wilenski of Project Hope notes that health care spending and more importantly, health care spending growth rates, are unsustainable. Past strategies of price controls, reliance on administered pricing for Medicare and the dominance of a la carte fee for service reimbursement have been part of the problem and do not represent promising strategies for the future. Too much time has been spent debating whether Medicare has done better or worse than the private sector since neither represents an acceptable path going forward. Understanding the effects of innovative payment strategies – including those that affect the patient – will be an important part in learning how to "bend the curve". Making sure that there are strategies to implement the results of successful pilots and demonstrations will also be important.

Chapter 12, "Pay for Value," by Robert Smoldt of the Mayo Clinic begins by quoting Texas Bix Bender who is not a known health economist. In fact, he's not an economist at all. He is the author of "Don't Squat with Yer Spurs On! The Cowboy's Guide to Life", and in that book he provides some insight into the issues that affect improving healthcare effectiveness and efficiency. One of his guides to life is as follows: "If you find yourself in a hole, the first thing to do is stop digging." In healthcare, the author asserts, we find ourselves in a hole. For many years, we have been expounding that our healthcare system does not provide the quality we desire and that it is too expensive. Indeed, back in the 1970's, President Richard Nixon declared that healthcare in the United States was in a crisis. Since that time, many people have made similar pronouncements. But what have we done? Basically, we have continued to dig, even though we were finding ourselves in a hole. It is time for a different approach. The author builds upon the early assertion that people do not want the lowest cost, universally available healthcare system. The central issue should really be the creation of a healthcare system that provides the highest value. This chapter outlines a path forward to this goal.

In Chapter 13, "Reform Incentives To Create A Demand For Health System Reengineering," Alain Enthoven of Stanford University, makes the argument that America needs a far more efficient health care financing and delivery system than the one we have. Our present system is a serious threat to public finances and is pricing itself out of reach. At the root of the problem are incentives and organization. The present fragmented fee-for-service small practice model is filled with cost-increasing incentives. There are some relatively efficient organized delivery systems, mostly based on large multi-specialty group practices. Unfortunately, most consumers are not offered the opportunity to save money and get better care by choosing such a system. This situation presents great opportunities for improvement in performance by re-engineering the system. However, for this to happen, incentives must be fundamentally changed so that everyone is cost conscious and care is organized in accountable care systems seeking improvement.

Section 4: Engineering Approaches

Chapter 14, "Systems Engineering and Management," by William Rouse of Georgia Tech and Dale Compton of Purdue University offers a systems view of healthcare delivery and outlines a wide range of concepts, principles, models, methods and tools from systems engineering and management that can enable the transformation of the dysfunctional "as is" healthcare system to an agreed-upon "to be" system that will provide quality, affordable care for everyone. Topics discussed include systems definition, design, analysis, and control, as well as the data and information needed to support these functions. Barriers to implementation are also considered.

In Chapter 15, "Operations Research," William Pierskalla of the University of California at Los Angeles begins by noting that in *Evita*, Andrew Lloyd Webber and Tim Rice wrote: *Politics, the Art of the Possible*. Those in the operations research community postulate: *Operations Research, the Science of Better* – (i.e. better processes, better systems and better decisions). Using their own and other scientific, engineering, mathematical, and social sciences methodologies, operations researchers help decision makers make better decisions; decisions leading to improvements: greater quality, lower costs, greater revenues, better access, better scheduling, lower risks, more satisfaction – with the goal of always striving for the best or optimal decisions.

Chapter 16, "Engineering Healthcare as a Service System, " by James Tien and Pascal Goldschmidt-Clermont of the University of Miami, argues that engineering has and will continue to have a critical impact on healthcare. They propose that the application of technology-based techniques to biological problems can be defined to be technobiology applications. This chapter is primarily focused on applying the technobiology approach of systems engineering to the development of a healthcare service system that is both integrated and adaptive. In general, healthcare services are carried out with knowledge-intensive agents or components which work together as providers and consumers to create or co-produce value. Indeed, the engineering design of a healthcare system must recognize the fact that it is actually a complex integration of human-centered activities that is increasingly dependent on information technology and knowledge. Like any service system, healthcare can be considered to be a combination or recombination of three essential components – people (characterized by behaviors, values, knowledge, etc.), processes (characterized by collaboration, customization, etc.) and products (characterized by software, hardware, infrastructures, etc.). Thus, a healthcare system is an integrated and adaptive set of people, processes and products. It is, in essence, a system of systems with objectives to enhance efficiency (leading to greater interdependency) and effectiveness (leading to improved health). Integration occurs over the physical, temporal, organizational and functional dimensions, while adaptation occurs over the monitoring, feedback, cybernetic and learning dimensions. In sum, such service systems as healthcare are indeed complex, especially due to the uncertainties associated with the human-centered aspects of these systems. Moreover, the system complexities can only be dealt with by using methods that enhance system integration and adaptation.

In Chapter 17, "Process Engineering: A Necessary Step to a Better Public Health System, " David Ross of Emory University notes that with its primary focus on community health, the public health system focuses on intervention and prevention of disease and injury to protect entire populations. As a federation of city, county and state entities operating independently under a complicated array of local, state and federal laws, public health can best be understood as a complex adaptive system. The dynamic nature of this system and the need for public health agencies to relate and respond to numerous stimuli in terms of new regulations, changing health status, emerging threats and shifting policy, can mask the commonality of underlying business processes performed within the public health sector. Heightened demand for interoperable, adaptive information systems across the broader U.S. health system necessitates the recognition of this commonality and highlights the need for comprehensive analysis and understanding of these core business processes. In turn, this analysis paves the way for public health to apply proven systems engineering techniques to streamline, automate and facilitate those processes. Here, we look at the nature of the public health system and the evolution of a purpose-built methodology for process engineering within public health. The authors present a case study based on the application of the methodology to develop requirements for public health laboratory information management systems.

Chapter 18, "Engineering Responses to Pandemics," by Richard Larson and Karima Nigmatulina of MIT, focuses on pandemic influenza and approaches the planning for and response to such a major worldwide health event as a complex engineering systems problem. Action-oriented analysis of pandemics requires a broad inclusion of academic disciplines since no one specialty can cover a significant fraction of the problem. Numerous research papers and action plans have treated pandemics as purely medical happenings, focusing on hospitals, health care professionals, creation and distribution of vaccines and anti-virals, etc. But human behavior with regard to hygiene and social distancing constitutes a first-order partial brake or control of the spread and intensity of infection. Such behavioral options are "non-pharmaceutical interventions." The chapter employs simple mathematical models to study alternative controls of infection, addressing a well-known parameter in epidemiology, R_0, the "reproductive number," defined as the mean number of new infections generated by an index case. Values of R_0 greater than 1.0 usually indicate that the infection begins with exponential growth, the generation-to-generation growth rate being R_0. R_0 is broken down into constituent parts related to the frequency and intensity of human contacts, both partially under our control. It is suggested that any numerical value for R_0 has little meaning outside the social context to which it pertains. Difference equation models are then employed to study the effects of heterogeneity of population social contact rates, the analysis showing that the disease tends to be driven by high frequency individuals. Related analyses show the futility of trying geographically to isolate the disease. Finally, the models are operated under a variety of assumptions related to social distancing and changes in hygienic behavior. The results are promising in terms of potentially reducing the total impact of the pandemic.

In Chapter 19, "Understanding and Enhancing the Dental Delivery System," Paul Griffin of Penn State reports that dental decay is the most prevalent chronic disease among both children and adults in the

U.S. The Surgeon General's Report on Oral Health found that there had been marked improvement in oral health in many Americans over the last 50 years and that good oral health could be achieved by all Americans largely due to the presence of safe and effective interventions to prevent and control oral disease However, recent national data suggest that several disparities in dental care exist. This chapter presents a model of the dental health system as well as key differences with the general medical health system. The author further discusses the major issues that the dental care delivery system will have to address in order to ensure that all Americans have access to effective interventions to prevent and control disease in an environment of decreasing supply of dentists per capita and potentially increasing demand. Strategies and policies to address these emerging issues in the context of this model are then discussed. This chapter concludes with suggestions on how engineering techniques could be used to improve the system.

Section 5: Perspectives

Chapter 20, "Integrated Health Systems," by Stephen Shortell and Rodney McCurdy of the University of California at Berkeley, argue that before meaningful gains in improving the value of health care in the US can be achieved, the fragmented nature in which health care is financed and delivered must be addressed. One type of healthcare organization, the Integrated Delivery System (IDS), is poised to play a pivotal role in reform efforts. What are these systems? What is the current evidence regarding their performance? What are the current barriers to their establishment and how can these barriers be removed? This chapter addresses these important questions. Although there are many types of IDS' in the US healthcare landscape, the chapter begins by identifying the necessary healthcare components that encompass an IDS and discusses the levels of integration that are important to improving health care quality and value. Next, it explores the recent evidence regarding IDS performance which while generally positive is less than what it could be if there was greater focus on clinical integration. To highlight, the chapter discusses the efficacy of system engineering initiatives in two examples of large, fully integrated systems: Kaiser-Permanente and the Veterans Health Administration. The evidence here is strong that the impact of system engineering methods is enhanced through the integration of processes, goals and outcomes. Reforms necessary to encourage the development of IDS' include: 1) the development of payment mechanisms designed to increase greater inter-dependency of hospitals and physicians; 2) the modification or removal of several regulatory barriers to greater clinical integration; and 3) the establishment of a more robust data collection and reporting system to increase transparency and accountability. The chapter concludes with a framework for considering these reforms across strategic, structural, cultural, and technical dimensions.

In Chapter 21, "Academic Health Centers," Fred Sanfilippo of Emory University discusses how Academic Health Centers (AHCs) are composed of academic, hospital, and clinical practice components that play a key role in healthcare delivery by their special ability to identify and implement improvements in outcomes, safety, cost-benefit, and satisfaction. They do this by utilizing a wide range of academic and clinical health professionals and disciplines to provide cutting-edge, highly specialized patient care as well as disproportionate uncompensated care in communities nationwide; to identify the effectiveness of different diagnostic and therapeutic approaches through clinical research; to foster new discoveries in biomedical science and technology and their clinical application; and to educate future generations of health professionals who apply these improvements. As the traditional homes of innovation in health and healthcare through research, and as the major sites of implementing change through education, AHCs have been at the forefront of improving healthcare. To successfully improve the effectiveness and efficiency of healthcare delivery, it is critical that AHCs continue to serve as uniquely integrated models for improving quality and value through novel approaches in education, research, and service.

Chapter 22, “Government, Health And System Transformation,” by Jonathan Perlin and Kelvin Baggett of the Hospital Corporation of America, begins by noting that all levels of government have an economic and social interest in health. In the United States, Federal, State and local government are involved in the development of health policy, funding health care, and maintaining or improving public health. Federal, State and most municipalities also engage in delivery of health services. As with the private sector, government is grappling with accelerating health care costs, increasing service demands generated by an aging and more chronically ill society, and accumulating evidence that American health outcomes are not commensurate with the resources invested. Unlike the private sector, attempts to improve value in health care – whether through legislation in Congress or regulation or program design in the Executive branch – are subject to the full intensity of the partisan political process. In order to engage effectively with government in health system transformation, an understanding of both the civic processes and the political dynamics is necessary. This chapter provides an overview of the major governmental roles in health care as formally structured and identifies points of influence in the political process.

Sections 6: Conclusions

In Chapter 23, “Barriers to Change in Engineering the System of Health Care Delivery,” Jon Saxton and Michael Johns of Emory University argue that significant reform of the health care system sufficient to achieve universal coverage, a value-driven system and administrative simplification faces enormous barriers at the level of our societal ecosystem – barriers as large as any that can be faced in public policy. These barriers exist within the health system itself as a complex adaptive system, and are structured by our economic, legal, cultural and political systems. Because there are so many barriers, significant reform is a relatively rare occurrence. Yet it does happen and there are some important examples of major health care reforms. There are a number of lessons to be learned from the successful enactment of the Medicare and Medicaid programs that appear relevant to current and future reform efforts. First, a necessary condition for achieving significant reform is the existence of large and sufficiently enduring social forces sufficient to disrupt legislative and policy stasis and drive the necessary political solutions. Second, public sentiment and electoral “mandates” might be necessary to significant reform, but they are not sufficient. Third, assuming the theoretical capacity to manage the constellation of systemic, economic, legal, cultural and legislative barriers, there remains a political “tipping point” political threshold must be crossed and translated into a Congressional super-majority in order to enact significant nationwide reform.

Chapter 24, “Prospects for Change,” by Denis Cortese of Mayo Clinic and William Rouse of Georgia Tech addresses the prospects for change in health care delivery. The focus is on value – high quality, affordable care for everyone. They consider three domains that participate in the flow of value and the nature of the interfaces among these domains. They also discuss strategic priorities that should align in various ways with these domains. Finally, they address the business transformations needed to enable the provision of value by enterprises that are viable and successful.

6. Conclusions

This summary of the chapters in this book presents a panorama of important issues, roles of information and incentives, engineering approaches, the perspectives of major stakeholder organizations in healthcare delivery, and barriers and prospects for change. This panorama is sufficiently rich to preclude a succinct summary of the nature of the system and needed changes. We leave these ideas and insights to the authors that follow.

References

[1] T.L. Friedman, *The World is Flat: A Brief History of the Twenty-First Century*, New York: Picador, 2007.
[2] R. DeVol, A. Bedroussian, A. Charuworn, A. Chatterjee, I. Kim, S. Kim and K. Klowden, *An Unhealthy America: The Economic Burden of Chronic Disease*, Santa Monica, Calif.: Milken Institute, 2007.
[3] M.E. Porter and E.O. Teisberg, *Redefining Health Care: Creating Value-Based Competition on Results*, Boston: Harvard Business School Press, 2006.
[4] W.B. Rouse, Healthcare as a complex adaptive system, *The Bridge* **38**(1) (2008), 17–25.
[5] W.B. Rouse, Engineering Perspectives on Healthcare Delivery: Can We Afford Technological Innovation in Healthcare? *Journal of Systems Research and Behavioral Science* **26** (2009), 1–10.

William B. Rouse, PhD, is the Executive Director of the Tennenbaum Institute at the Georgia Institute of Technology. He is also a professor in the College of Computing and School of Industrial and Systems Engineering. His research focuses on understanding and managing complex public-private systems such as healthcare and defense, with emphasis on mathematical and computational modeling of these systems for the purpose of policy design and analysis. Rouse has written hundreds of articles and book chapters, and has authored many books, including most recently *People and Organizations: Explorations of Human-Centered Design* (Wiley, 2007), *Essential Challenges of Strategic Management* (Wiley, 2001) and the award-winning *Don't Jump to Solutions* (Jossey-Bass, 1998). He is editor of *Enterprise Transformation: Understanding and Enabling Fundamental Change* (Wiley, 2006), co-editor of *Organizational Simulation: From Modeling & Simulation to Games & Entertainment* (Wiley, 2005), co-editor of the best-selling *Handbook of Systems Engineering and Management* (Wiley, 1999, 2009), and editor of the eight-volume series *Human/Technology Interaction in Complex Systems* (Elsevier). Among many advisory roles, he has served as Chair of the Committee on Human Factors of the National Research Council, a member of the U.S. Air Force Scientific Advisory Board, and a member of the DoD Senior Advisory Group on Modeling and Simulation. Rouse is a member of the National Academy of Engineering, as well as a fellow of four professional societies – Institute of Electrical and Electronics Engineers (IEEE), the International Council on Systems Engineering (INCOSE), the Institute for Operations Research and Management Science (INFORMS), and the Human Factors and Ergonomics Society (HFES).

Denis A. Cortese, MD, is President and CEO of Mayo Clinic. He is a graduate of Temple University Medical School, and completed Internal Medicine and Pulmonary Diseases training at Mayo Clinic. Dr. Cortese is a professor of medicine and former director of pulmonary disease training program. He served in U.S. Navy Medical Corp during 1974–1976. His major research interests focus on interventional bronchoscopy including appropriate use of photodynamic therapy, endobronchial laser therapy and endobronchial stents. He is a former president of the International Photodynamic Association. Cortese's memberships include The Institute of Medicine of the National Academies (US) and chair of the Roundtable on Evidence Based Medicine; Healthcare Leadership Council, chair for 2007–2009; Harvard/Kennedy Healthcare Policy Group; Academia Nacional de Medicina (Mexico); the Royal College of Physicians (London); Division on Engineering and Physical Science (DEPS), and National Research Council. He received the 2007 Ellis Island Award, the Medal of Merit Award in 2008, and the National Healthcare Leadership Award in November, 2009.

Section 1: Issues

Information Knowledge Systems Management 8 (2009) 17–21
DOI 10.3233/IKS-2009-0131
IOS Press

Chapter 2

Seeking care as a system

Donald M. Berwick and Eva Luo
E-mail: dberwick@ini.org

Abstract: Kim, aged 3 years, lies asleep, waiting for a miracle. Outside her room, the nurses on the night shift pad softly through the half-lighted corridors, stopping to count breaths, take pulses, or check the intravenous pumps. In the morning, Kim will have her heart fixed. She will be medicated and wheeled into the operating suite. Machines will take on the functions of her body: breathing and circulating blood. The surgeons will place a small patch over a hole within her heart, closing off a shunt between her ventricles that would, if left open, slowly kill her.

Kim will be fine if the decision to operate on her was correct; if the surgeon is competent; if that competent surgeon happens to be trained to deal with the particular anatomic wrinkle that is hidden inside Kim's heart; if the blood bank cross-matched her blood accurately and delivered it to the right place; if the blood gas analysis machine works properly and on time; if the suture does not snap; if the plastic tubing of the heart-lung machine does not suddenly spring loose; if the recovery room nurses know that she is allergic to penicillin; if the "oxygen" and "nitrogen" lines in the anesthesia machine have not been reversed by mistake; if the sterilizer temperature gauge is calibrated so that the instruments are in fact sterile; if the pharmacy does not mix up two labels; and if when the surgeon says urgently, "Clamp, right now," there is a clamp on the tray.

If all goes well, if ten thousand "ifs" go well, then Kim may sing her grandchildren to sleep some day. If not, she will be dead by noon tomorrow.

If Kim were an astronaut, strapped into her seat at the top of some throbbing rocket, the crowd assembled would hold their breath in the morning Florida sun. "How can it possibly work?" they would whisper. "How many parts are there in that machine? A million? What if one fails? My toaster fails. Please let it all work right." The machine would bellow smoke, the gantry fall away, and slowly the monster would rise, Kim on top.

If it worked, they would cheer. "A miracle," they would shout, in awe that the millions of tiny lines of effort, the millions of tiny lines of cause and effect, from job shops in Ohio and laboratories in Pasadena, criss-crossing through time and space, could converge so magnificently in a massive, gleaming rocket launched exactly right. Perfect.

If it failed, they would cry. So would the rocket's makers, who had done their very best. No one wanted it to end this way. Poor Kim. What was the trouble? What went wrong? Why?

The lines of cause will converge around Kim in the morning as she wheels toward the operating room. Thousands upon thousands of elements weaving a basket to hold her safely, all hope. No crowd holds its breath tonight; but wouldn't they if they knew?

From: Berwick DM. Controlling variation in health care: a consultation from Walter Shewhart. Medical Care 1991; 29: 1212–1225.

1. Introduction

In the two decades since those words were written, the capability, audacity, and complexity of medical care have grown steadily. So, too, have its hazards and costs. The landmark Institute of Medicine reports, *To Err Is Human* and *Crossing the Quality Chasm*, brought health care defects and the potential for improvement to the foreground, with threats to patients safety the most charismatic and understandable of all those defects. In 2009, a socially urgent trio – cost, quality, and coverage – now dominate a loud national conversation, with the potential to lead, maybe at last, to health system reform.

But, what "system" are we talking about that is to be "reformed"? As Kim's fate depended on a vast network of interacting elements, so do almost all of the performance characteristics that reform may purport to improve. The idea of a system is neither a frill nor fine point if we are to get reform right. It lies at the very center of the scientific and political challenges that stand between us and the care we seek. With a proper understanding of systems, authentic health care redesign is feasible and socially productive. Without that understanding, "reform" will likely do more harm than good.

"System" is a technical idea. It denotes a set of elements interacting to produce some shared – hopefully intended – result. An automobile is a system whose intent is transport with certain qualities, like safety, speed, fun, fuel economy, and reliability. Its capability – its quality – depends both on how each part functions (a flat tire is a problem) and on how the parts work together (the tire has to fit the wheel). Removing a part affects the rest; try driving your car without a brake shoe or a battery. And "the rest" – the whole – affects each part; try putting Porsche brakes in your Ford sedan. When it comes to a system, "the whole is more than the sum of the parts" isn't a trite phrase; it is exactly correct.

Anyone who understands systems will know immediately that optimizing parts is not a good route to systemic excellence. The great systems theorist, Russell Ackoff, suggested trying to build "the world's greatest car" by assembling and connecting "the world's greatest car parts." We will use the engine from a Ferrari, the brakes from a Porsche, the suspension from a BMW, and the body of a Volvo. What we get, of course, is nothing close to a great car; we get a pile of very expensive junk. The reason is as above: the performance of a system – its achievement of its aims – depends as much on the *interactions* among elements as on the elements, themselves.

So, how can it be that medical care is so obsessed with the performance of elements, and so often insouciant about their interactions? Why do most medical students never train formally for a day in the company of the nurses with whom they will work for the rest of their lives? Why do most residents stay up nights memorizing differential diagnoses, and spend not an hour of daylight learning, formally, about teamwork and communication? Why do departments and specialities jealously guard their prerogatives and resources, and meet so rarely to discover how they could help each other more? Why do doctors, nurses, therapists, and managers pledge different oaths to different disciplines with different heritages and uncoordinated goals?

In 1910, Dr. William Mayo's commencement speech to the Rush Medical School class included this sentence: "The best interest of the patient is the only interest to be considered, and, in order to bring advancing knowledge to the benefit of the patient, a union of forces is necessary." There, in a single phrase, are the essential elements of an effective system: shared aim ("The best interest of the patient") and carefully designed interactions ("a union of forces").

Health care reform without attention to the nature and nurture of health care as a system is doomed. It will at best simply feed the beast of suboptimization – pouring precious resources into the overdevelopment of parts, and never attending to the whole that *is* the care as our patients, their families, and their communities experience us. We will try to build, in Ackoff's image, the "best care in the world" by assembling a pile of the "best parts in the world" and the thing will never work.

In *Crossing the Quality Chasm*, the IOM designated six aims for improvement: safety, effectiveness, patient-centeredness, timeliness, efficiency, and equity. Each depends on systemness for its achievement.

- Injuries to patients happen far more at intersections and handoffs than in the deeds of single actors. Teamwork, communication, and organizational resilience – all properties of interaction – are keys to breakthrough in patient safety.
- Reliable use of scientifically grounded care, the avoidance of overuse and underuse that the *Chasm* report calls "effectiveness," requires the proper management and exchange of knowledge, not simply individual brains full of endless lists of facts. Modernization of information technologies,

a fundamental matter of system design, can support unprecedented reliability, a precondition to unprecedented effectiveness.
- Patient-centeredness depends on relationships, communication, and shared values, and also can benefit from better information systems, including shared decision-making technologies.
- Timeliness rests on the art and science of flow and mastery of some of the royal sciences of modern systems – operations research, industrial engineering, queuing theory, and the like.
- Efficiency – better thought of as "waste reduction" – devolves from system designs, as well, such as are embedded in the Toyota production system and "lean production," which are earning well-deserved attention in progressive health care organizations.
- And even the pursuit of equity, the quality goal with the highest moral urgency, requires thorough re-thinking about the boundaries and goals of health care, itself, as we learn our way into appropriate adaptations to cultural diversity and grapple, as we must, with the consequences of racism and poverty as they directly impinge on the interactions between the system of care and the beneficiaries of care.

In short, the improvement of health and health care depends on systems thinking and systemic redesign. "Reform" without that isn't reform at all.

2. Challenges

Fitness for that challenge cannot be taken for granted. Those who lead, fund, and work in American health care were not trained to think in systems terms; indeed, they were in some cases trained specifically *not* to. For that reason, between us and effective health care redesign lie a gantlet of changes in culture, belief, and norms. Success is not assured; these changes are hard ones.

A few of the big challenges are these:

1. *Placing Renewed Emphasis on Interdependence:* Romantic views of professionalism, especially in medical care, emphasize personal responsibility, hierarchy, specialization, and professional autonomy. This is evident, for example, in architecture (many hospitals have separate, designated conference rooms for nurses and for doctors), training (schools for different health professions interact poorly if at all), ethics statements (each discipline pledges to its own oath), lack of compensation for coordinative mechanisms (few insurance schemes reimburse for multidisciplinary patient care conferences), institutional boundaries (hospitals do not take responsibility for mortality measurement across the continuum; handoffs in chronic care management are notoriously defective), and in our language (we use terms like "discharge" and "admission" that encode fragmented responsibilities). Those who truly understand and value systems thinking in health care will place interdependency and its management at the top of the hierarchy of professional deeds.
2. *Making Care Processes Visible from the Viewpoint of the Patient.* Health care shackled by professional fragmentation and institutional boundaries tends to see processes from the supply side. We describe our work as we perform it, not as patients and their loved ones experience it. One immediate effect is that we expect patients to adjust to our process, instead of molding our processes to their needs. The cycle is vicious: the more we force patients into processes that do not fit them, the more we experience their expectations as unreasonable and our capacities as constrained. Possibility derives less from effort than from redesign. The first step is to make process visible from the viewpoint of those served. In the world of energy, such a viewpoint leads to what Amory Lovins calls "end use efficiency." To achieve end use efficiency requires an understanding of a system as a

whole. Health care "unreformed" has trouble doing that; we lack the mechanisms of coordination and commitment to make process visible. When a hospital "discharges" a patient, that patient is largely out of sight and out of mind to the hospital, which becomes blind to the experience of the patient over further time and space.

3. *Understanding the Importance and Value of Dynamic Learning and Local Adaptation.* The non-linearity of systems dynamics weakens the learning power of many formal, classical methods of evaluation and inquiry. These tend to be insensitive to context, mechanisms, and meaningful segmentation of patients. The same classical methods also weaken the contributions of local knowledge in an effort to protect against bias. Health care lacks habits and norms that capitalize on processes of knowledge growth in non-linear contexts. A side-effect is a schism between pragmatic engineering sciences and systems improvement methods, on the one hand, and current hierarchies of evaluation, on the other. Journals have not opened up sufficiently to the former (pragmatic sciences and experiences in improvement); their restrictiveness further impedes understanding and the shared growth of knowledge.
4. *Understanding and Taking Action on Waste.* One early harvest of systems views is knowledge of the presence, degree, and protean forms of waste. Often, waste is the manifestation of system failure and systems illiteracy. In the non-systemic view, waste feels protective and necessary, and attacks on waste (even to avoid sub-optimization) feel ill-motivated. For example, in systems-illiterate cultures, the following can feel risky and even assaultive: using someone else's laboratory findings, trying not to repeat the work of others, eliminating inventories that buffer poor flow, using capital fully, avoiding ring-fencing resources (such as operating rooms or days reserved to particular specialties), automating processes, and more. Forms of waste are many: rework, scrap, inventory, queues, motion, unused space and equipment, excess information, records of no value, loss of ideas, demotivating people through insult, and more. The economics of health care today are largely founded on waste – waste means jobs, income, profit, and preserving comfortable habits. Waste levels in US health care (defined as non-value-added activities and expenses) certainly exceed 30% and may exceed 60% if we were to use formal value-chain analyses. A proper attack on health care waste would also lead to a major, as-yet-unexplored research agenda – process analyses and experiments to reveal where waste, and its opposite, effective help, lie.
5. *Creating and Supporting Platforms for Multidisciplinary Research and Development.* Intersections are insufficient and dignity too low for the most valuable forms of collaborative research and development among engineering sciences, systems sciences, and health care yet to flourish. The barrier is dyadic, and symptomatic of the historical distance: engineers, for example, can feel unfamiliar, intimidated, and unwelcome in health care (as, in an earlier time, most statisticians did); health care leaders are not aware of the disciplines related to system sciences or suspicious about their applicability (as, in an earlier time, even academic physicians had little time for statisticians). Bridge-building is expensive and takes time. Successful examples recently, showing the promise, are Professor Eugene Litvak's work and Steven Spear's insights.
6. *Addressing Implications for Professional Development.* The health care workforce lacks training in system sciences. Most physicians and nurses escape professional education with little or no instruction on as basic a system concern as safety and its origins. No wonder then that practice does not reflect mastery of those sciences. Medical schools are only just starting to map system subjects into training – topics like safety, communication, teamwork, and operations research. We would not think of a physician emerging from medical school today who never heard of Osler, Watson and Crick, or the Krebs cycle. Yet yearly we graduate thousands who never heard of James Reason,

W. Edwards Deming, Karl Weick, or even Bob Brook or Jack Wennberg. Nor, probably, have their teachers. The academic preparation of professionals dismisses systems sciences through silence. Moreover, the siloing of professional preparation, itself, de-emphasizes the role of interdependency in the work of patient care.

7. *Redesigning Institutional Arrangements.* If we increased process literacy, knowledge, and redesign, institutions created to serve fragments would become visibly inadequate and the spaces between them would appear larger and larger. Systems knowledge leads to the desire for integrated design. It is not at all clear that we would emerge from this exploration needing hospitals, offices, insurers, or professions in anything close to their current forms. This, not political or financing rearrangements, would be the true manifestation of "health care reform." It would be "care reform," not "financing reform" or "coverage reform." Perhaps we lack the political or social will to go there – yet. But, if we ever did, then current problems of financing, coverage, and cost would begin to melt.

3. Conclusions

Kim is not alone. Sooner or later, most of us will be there, too, astronauts strapped into our high-tech capsules at the top of the throbbing health care machine. The physicians, nurses, engineers, researchers, architects, technicians, therapists, and managers who maintain that machine are, with full justice, proud of it, and wish nothing more than to put it at our service – to heal us and lighten our burden. But, fragmented, unmindful of the system in which they serve, they will fail far more often than they or we wish, and they will be party to the waste of resources we have neither the wealth nor the right to tolerate.

"Reform," if it is to reduce the chances of failure, will have to mean change of the care, itself. Changing contexts can help, such as removing the toxicity of fragmented payment, assuring universal access to care, ending senseless regulatory bars and administrative nonsense, and improving transparency about performance. But, these just set the stage. The patient depends not on the context but on the care. And it is how we build and shape that care that will determine who will see the morning, and who will not.

Donald M. Berwick, MD, MPP, FRCP, President and CEO, Institute for Healthcare Improvement (IHI), is one of the nation's leading authorities on health care quality and improvement. He is also clinical professor of pediatrics and health care policy at the Harvard Medical School and Professor in the Department of Health Policy and Management at the Harvard School of Public Health. Dr. Berwick has served as vice chair of the U.S. Preventive Services Task Force, the first "Independent Member" of the Board of Trustees of the American Hospital Association, and chair of the National Advisory Council of the Agency for Healthcare Research and Quality. An elected member of the Institute of Medicine (IOM), Dr. Berwick served two terms on the IOM's governing Council and was a member of the IOM's Global Health Board. He served on President Clinton's Advisory Commission on Consumer Protection and Quality in the Healthcare Industry. He is a recipient of numerous awards, including the 1999 Joint Commission's Ernest Amory Codman Award, the 2002 American Hospital Association's Award of Honor, the 2006 John M. Eisenberg Patient Safety and Quality Award for Individual Achievement from the National Quality Forum and the Joint Commission on Accreditation of Healthcare Organizations, the 2007 William B. Graham Prize for Health Services Research, and the 2007 Heinz Award for Public Policy from the Heinz Family Foundation. In 2005, he was appointed "Honorary Knight Commander of the British Empire" by the Queen of England in honor of his work with the British National Health Service.

Eva Luo is a medical school student at the University of Michigan Medical School. After graduating from Harvard College in June 2008 majoring in biochemical sciences, Eva joined the Institute for Healthcare Improvement (IHI) as Special Assistant to the President and CEO, Dr. Don Berwick. She worked primarily to support Dr. Berwick's presentations, speeches, correspondences, and manage special projects. Eva also worked with the Research and Development team as a research assistant and the IHI Open School for Health Professions team providing assistance in recruiting health professions students to the program and contributing to the IHI Open School blog (www.ihiopenschool.blogspot.com). Her primary interests are in maternal health, systems engineering, management, global health, medical education, cultural competency and patient-centered care, and health policy.

Information Knowledge Systems Management 8 (2009) 23–46
DOI 10.3233/IKS-2009-0134
IOS Press

Chapter 3

Patient safety

The role of human factors and systems engineering

Pascale Carayon and Kenneth E. Wood
E-mail: carayon@engr.wisc.edu

Abstract: Patient safety is a global challenge that requires knowledge and skills in multiple areas, including human factors and systems engineering. In this chapter, numerous conceptual approaches and methods for analyzing, preventing and mitigating medical errors are described. Given the complexity of healthcare work systems and processes, we emphasize the need for increasing partnerships between the health sciences and human factors and systems engineering to improve patient safety. Those partnerships will be able to develop and implement the system redesigns that are necessary to improve healthcare work systems and processes for patient safety.

1. Patient safety

A 1999 Institute of Medicine report brought medical errors to the forefront of healthcare and the American public [74]. Based on studies conducted in Colorado, Utah and New York, the IOM estimated that between 44,000 and 98,000 Americans die each year as a result of medical errors, which by definition can be prevented or mitigated. The Colorado and Utah study shows that adverse events occurred in 2.9% of the hospitalizations [127]. In the New York study, adverse events occurred in 3.7% of the hospitalizations [15]. The 2001 report by the Institute of Medicine on "Crossing the Quality Chasm" emphasizes the need to improve the design of healthcare systems and processes for patient safety. The report proposes six aims for improvement in the healthcare system: (1) safe, (2) effective, (3) patient-centered, (4) timely, (5) efficient, and (6) equitable [65]. This chapter focuses on the safety aim, i.e. how to avoid injuries to patients from the care that is intended to help them. However, the improvement aims can be related to each other. For instance, safety, timeliness and efficient can be related: inefficient processes can create delays in care and, therefore, injuries to patients that could have been prevented.

Knowledge that healthcare systems and processes may be unreliable and produce medical errors and harm patients is not new. Using the critical incident technique, Safren and Chapanis [113,114] collected information from nurses and identified 178 medication errors over 7 months in one hospital. The most common medication errors were: drug to wrong patient, wrong dose of medication, drug overdose, omitted drug, wrong drug and wrong administration time. The most commonly reported causes for these errors were: failure to follow checking procedures, written miscommunication, transcription errors, prescriptions misfiled and calculation errors. We have known for a long time that preventable errors occur in health care; however, it is only recently that patient safety has received adequate attention. This increased attention has been fueled by tragic medical errors.

1389-1995/09/$17.00

Josie King was 18 months old. In January of 2001 Josie was admitted to Johns Hopkins after suffering first and second degree burns from climbing into a hot bath. She healed well and within weeks was scheduled for release. Two days before she was to return home she died of severe dehydration and misused narcotics. The death of Josie King has been attributed primarily to lack of communication between the different healthcare providers involved in her care and lack of consideration for her parents' concerns [73].

On February 7, 2003, surgeons put the wrong organs into a teenager, Jesica Santillan, at Duke University Hospital. The organs were from a donor with blood Type A; Jesica Santillán had Type O, and people with Type O can accept transfusions or tissues only from Type O donors. Jesica Santillan died two weeks after she received the wrong heart and lungs in one transplant operation and then suffered brain damage and complications after a second transplant operation. A root cause analysis of the error showed that lack of redundancy for checking ABO compatibility was a key factor in the error [107]. Soon after this error, Duke Medical Center implemented a new organ transplantation procedure that required the transplant surgeon, the transplant coordinator, and the procuring surgeon to each validate ABO compatibility and other key data [107].

These tragedies of medical errors emphasize the most important point made by the Institute of Medicine in its various reports on patient safety [65,74]: systems and processes of care need to be redesigned to prevent medical errors and mitigate their impact.

A major area of patient safety is medication errors and adverse drug events [64]. A series of studies by Leape, Bates and colleagues showed that medication errors and adverse drug events are frequent [4], that only about 1% of medication errors lead to adverse drug events [2], that various system factors contribute to medication safety such as inadequate availability of patient information [83], and that medication errors and adverse drug events are more frequent in intensive care units primarily because of the volume of medications prescribed and administered [40]. Medication safety is a worldwide problem. For instance, a Canadian study of medication errors and adverse drug events (ADEs) found that 7.5% of hospital admissions resulted in ADEs; about 37% of the ADEs were preventable and 21% resulted in death [1].

Patient safety has received attention by international health organizations. In 2004, the World Health Organization launched the World Alliance for Patient Safety. The World Alliance for Patient Safety has targeted the following patient safety issues: prevention of healthcare-associated infections, hand hygiene, surgical safety, and patient engagement [http://www.who.int/patientsafety/en/]. For instance, the WHO issued guidelines to ensure the safety of surgical patients. The implementation of these guidelines was tested in an international study of 8 hospitals located in Jordan, India, the US, Tanzania, the Philippines, Canada, England, and New Zealand [57]. Each of the 8 hospitals used a surgical safety checklist that identified best practices during the following surgery stages: sign in (e.g., verifying patient identify and surgical site and procedure), time out (e.g., confirming patient identity) and sign out (e.g., review of key concerns for the recovery and care of the patient). Overall results showed that the intervention was successful as the death rate decreased from 1.5% to 0.8% and the complications rate decreased from 11% of patients to 7% of patients after introduction of the checklist. However, the effectiveness of the intervention varied significantly across the hospitals: 4 of the 8 hospitals displayed significant decreases in complications; 3 of these 4 hospitals also had decreases in death rates. To completely assess the actual implementation of this patient safety intervention and its effectiveness, one would have to understand the specific context or system in which the intervention was implemented, as well as the specific processes that were redesigned because of the intervention. This type of analysis would call for expertise in the area of human factors and systems engineering.

Some care settings or care situations are particularly prone to hazards, errors and system failures. For instance, in intensive care units (ICUs), patients are vulnerable, their care is complex and involves multiple disciplines and varied sources of information, and numerous activities are performed in patient care; all of these factors contribute to increasing the likelihood and impact of medical errors. A study of medical errors in a medical ICU and a coronary care unit shows that about 20% of the patients admitted in the units experienced an adverse event and 45% of the adverse events were preventable [111]. The most common errors involved in preventable adverse events were: prevention and diagnostic errors, medication errors, and preventable nosocomial infections. Various work system factors are related to patient safety problems in ICUs, such as not having daily rounds by an ICU physician [98] and inadequate ICU nursing staffing and workload [24,98]. Bracco et al. [13] found a total of 777 critical incidents in an ICU over a 1-year period: 31% were human-related incidents (human errors) that were evenly distributed between planning, execution, and surveillance. Planning errors had more severe consequences than other problems. The authors recommended timely, appropriate care to avoid planning and execution mishaps. CPOE may greatly enhance the timeliness of medication delivery by increasing the efficiency of the medication process and shortening the time between prescribing and administration.

Several studies have examined types of error in ICUs. Giraud et al. [51] conducted a prospective, observational study to examine iatrogenic complications. Thirty-one percent of the admissions had iatrogenic complications, and human errors were involved in 67% of those complications. The risk of ICU mortality was about two-fold higher for patients with complications. Donchin et al. [44] estimated a rate of 1.7 errors per ICU patient per day. A human factors analysis showed that most errors could be attributed to poor communication between physicians and nurses. Cullen and colleagues [40] compared the frequency of ADEs and potential ADEs in ICUs and non-ICUs. Incidents were reported directly by nurses and pharmacists and were also detected by daily review of medical records. The rate of preventable ADEs and potential ADEs in ICUs was 19 events per 1,000 patient days, nearly twice the rate in non-ICUs. However, when adjusting for the number of drugs used, no differences were found between ICUs and non-ICUs. In the ICUs, ADEs and potential ADEs occurred mostly at the prescribing stage (28% to 48% of the errors) and at the administration stage (27% to 56%). The rate of preventable and potential ADEs (calculated over 1,000 patient-days) was actually significantly higher in the medical ICU (2.5%) than in the surgical ICU (1.4%) [39,40]. In a systems analysis of the causes of these ADEs, Leape et al. [83] found that the majority of systems failures (representing 78% of the errors) were due to impaired access to information, e.g., availability of patient information and order transcription. Cimino et al. [30] examined medication prescribing errors in nine pediatric ICUs. Before the implementation of various interventions, 11.1% of the orders had at least one prescribing error. After the implementation of the interventions (dosing assists, communication/education, and floor stocks), the rate of prescribing errors went down to 7.6% (68% decrease). The research on patient safety in ICUs shows that errors are frequent in ICUs. However, this may be due to the volume of activities and tasks [40]. ICU patients receive about twice as many drugs as those on general care units [39]. System-related human errors seem to be particularly prevalent in ICUs. Suggestions for reducing errors in ICUs are multiple, such as improving communication between nurses and physicians [44]; improving access to information [83]; providing timely appropriate care [13]; and integrating various types of computer technology, including CPOE [128].

Another high-risk care process is transition of care. In today's healthcare system, patients are experiencing an increasing number of transitions of care. Transitions occur when patients are transferred from one care setting to another, from one level or department to another within a care setting, or from one care provider to another [31]. This time of transition is considered an interruption in the continuity of care for patients and has been defined as a gap, or a discontinuity, in care [6,35]. Each transition requires the transfer of all relevant information from one entity to the next, as well as the transfer of authority and responsibility [97,134,135]. Concerns for patient safety arise when any or all of these elements are not effectively transferred during the transition (e.g., incorrect or incomplete information is transferred or confusion exists regarding responsibility for patients or orders) [135]. Transitions may be influenced by poor communication and inconsistency in care [118], both of which have been identified as factors threatening the quality and safety of care that patients receive [6,67]. Poor transitions can have a negative impact on patient care, such as delays in treatment and adverse events.

Several studies have documented possible associations between transitions and increased risks of patients experiencing an adverse event, particularly in patient transitions from the hospital to home or long-term care [12,32,50,92] or at admission to hospital [125]. Associations have been found between medical errors and increased risk for re-hospitalization resulting from poor transitions between the inpatient and outpatient settings [92]. Transitions involving medication changes from hospital to long-term care have been shown to be a likely cause of adverse drug events [12]. Patients prescribed long-term medication therapy with warfarin were found at higher risk for discontinuation of their medication after elective surgical procedures [7]. Although transitions have been shown to be critical points at which failure may occur, they may also be considered as critical points for potential recovery from failure [31, 38]. If reevaluations take place on the receiving end, certain information that was not revealed or addressed previously may be discovered or errors may be caught at this point [97,135].

Despite the increased attention towards patient safety, it is unclear whether we are actually making any progress in improving patient safety [130]. Several reasons for this lack of progress or lack of measurable progress include: lack of reliable data on patient safety at the national level [84,130] or at the organizational level [49,119,130], difficulty in engaging clinicians in patient safety improvement activities [62, 130], and challenges in redesigning and improving complex healthcare systems and processes [84,138]. The latter reason for limited improvement in patient safety is directly related to the discipline of human factors and systems engineering. The 2005 report by the National Academy of Engineering and the Institute of Medicine clearly articulated the need for increased involvement of human factors and systems engineering to improve healthcare delivery [106]. In the rest of the chapter, we will examine various conceptual frameworks and approaches to patient safety; this knowledge is important as we need to understand the "basics" of patient safety in order to implement effective solutions that do not have negative unintended consequences. We then discuss system redesign and related issues, including the role of health information technology in patient safety. The final section of the chapter describes various human factors and systems engineering tools that can be used for improving patient safety.

2. Conceptual approaches to patient safety

Different approaches to patient safety have been proposed. In this section, we describe conceptual frameworks based on models and theories of human error and organizational accidents, focus on patient care process and system interactions, and models that link healthcare professionals' performance to patient safety. In the last part of this section, we describe the SEIPS [Systems Engineering Initiative for Patient Safety] model of work system and patient safety that integrates many elements of these other models [26].

2.1. Human errors and organizational accidents

The 1999 report by the IOM on "To Err is Human: Building a Safer Health System" highlighted the role of human errors in patient safety [74]. There is a rich literature on human error and its role in accidents. The human error literature has been very much inspired by the work of Rasmussen [99, 101] and Reason [104], which distinguishes between latent and active failures. Latent conditions are the inevitable "resident pathogens" within the system that arise from decisions made by managers, engineers, designers and others [105, p. 769]. Active failures are actions and behaviors that are directly involved in an accident: (1) action slips or lapses (e.g., picking up the wrong medication), (2) mistakes (e.g., because of lack of medication knowledge, selecting the wrong medication for the patient), and (3) violations or work-arounds (e.g., not checking patient identification before medication administration). In the context of health care and patient safety, the distinction is made between the "sharp" end (i.e. work of practitioners and other people who are in direct contact with patient) and the "blunt" end (i.e. work by healthcare management and other organizational staff) [36], which is roughly similar to the distinction between active failures and latent conditions.

Vincent and colleagues [131,132] have proposed an organizational accident model based on the research by Reason [103,104]. According to this model, accidents or adverse events happen as a consequence of latent failures (i.e. management decision, organizational processes) that create conditions of work (i.e. workload, supervision, communication, equipment, knowledge/skill), which in turn produce active failures. Barriers or defenses may prevent the active failures from turning into adverse events. This model defines seven categories of system factors that can influence clinical practice and may result in patient safety problems: (1) institutional context, (2) organizational and management factors, (3) work environment, (4) team factors, (5) individual (staff) factors, (6) task factors, and (7) patient characteristics.

Another application of Rasmussen's conceptualization of human errors and organizational accidents focuses on the temporal process by which accidents may occur. Cook and Rasmussen [33] describe how safety may be compromised when healthcare systems operate at almost maximum capacity. Under such circumstances operations tend to migrate towards the marginal boundary of safety, therefore putting the system at greater risk for accidents. This migration is influenced by management pressure towards efficiency and the gradient towards least effort, which result from the need to operate at maximum capacity.

An extension of the human error and organizational accidents approach is illustrated by the work done by the World Alliance for Patient Safety to develop an international classification and a conceptual framework for patient safety. The International Classification for Patient Safety of the World Health Organization's World Alliance for Patient Safety is a major effort at standardizing the terminology used in patient safety [112,126]. The conceptual framework for the international classification can be found in Fig. 1 [126]. Patient safety incidents are at the core of the conceptual framework; incidents can be categorized into healthcare-associated infection, medication and blood/blood products, for instance [112]. The conceptual framework shows that contributing factors or hazards can lead to incidents; incidents can be detected, mitigated (i.e. preventing or moderating patient harm), or ameliorated (i.e. actions occurring after the incident to improve or compensate for harm).

These different models of human errors and organizational accidents are important in highlighting (1) different types of errors and failures (e.g., active errors versus latent failures; sharp end versus blunt end), (2) the key role of latent factors (e.g., management and organizational issues) in patient safety [101, 104], (3) error recovery mechanisms [112,126], and (4) temporal deterioration over time that can lead to accidents [33]. These models are important to unveil the basic mechanisms and pathways that lead to patient safety incidents. It is also important to examine patient care processes and the various interactions that occur along the patient journey that can create the hazards leading to patient safety incidents.

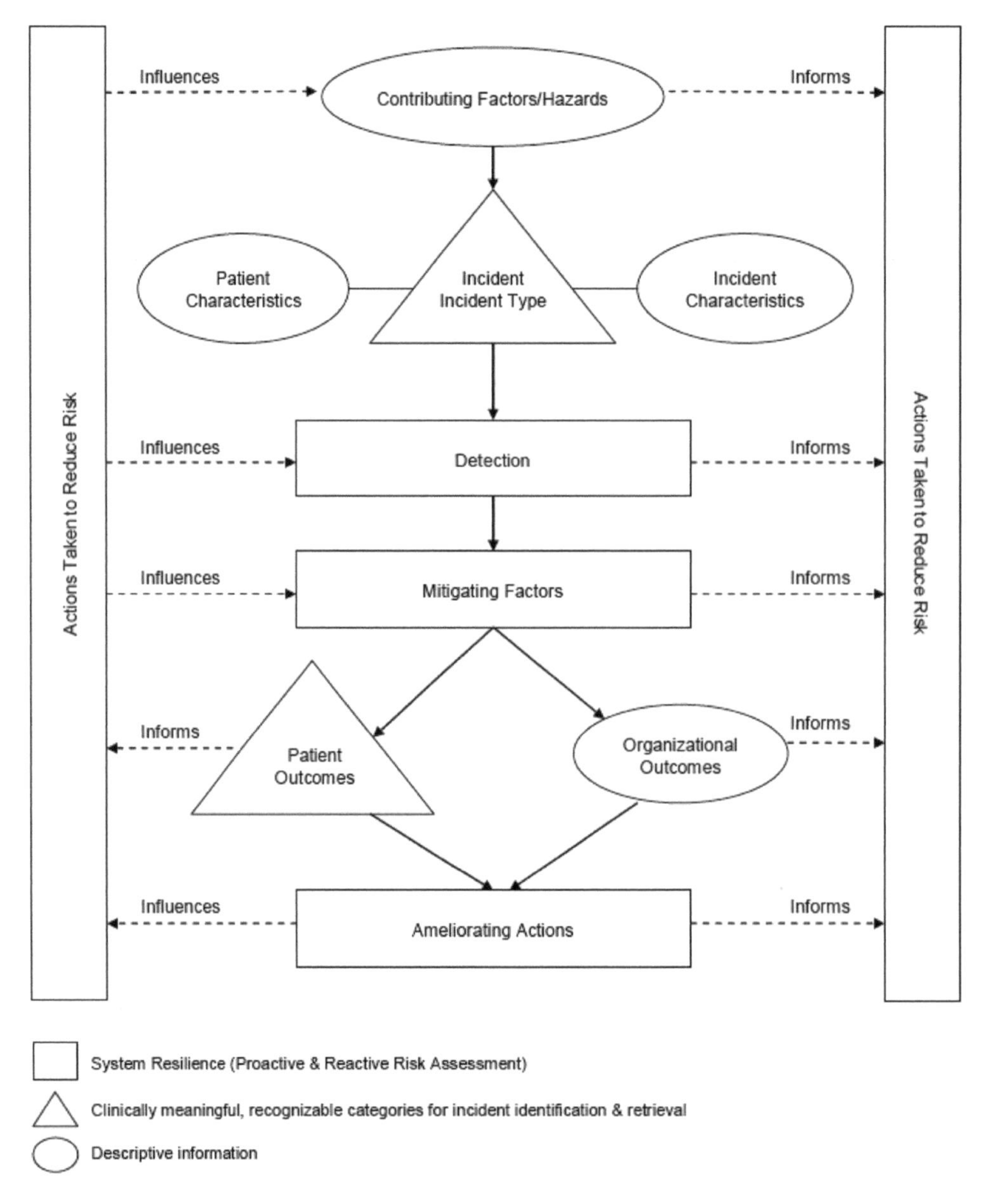

Fig. 1. Conceptual framework for the international classification for patient safety of the world health organization's world alliance for patient safety [126].

2.2. Patient journey and system interactions

Patient safety is about the patient after all [14]. Patient centeredness is one of the six improvement aims of the Institute of Medicine [65]: patient-centered care is "care that is respectful of and responsive to individual and patient preferences, needs, and values" and care that ensures "that patient values guide all clinical decisions" (page 6). Patient-centered care is very much related to patient safety. For instance, to optimize information flow and communication, experts recommend families be engaged in a relationship with physicians and nurses that fosters exchange of information as well as decision making that considers

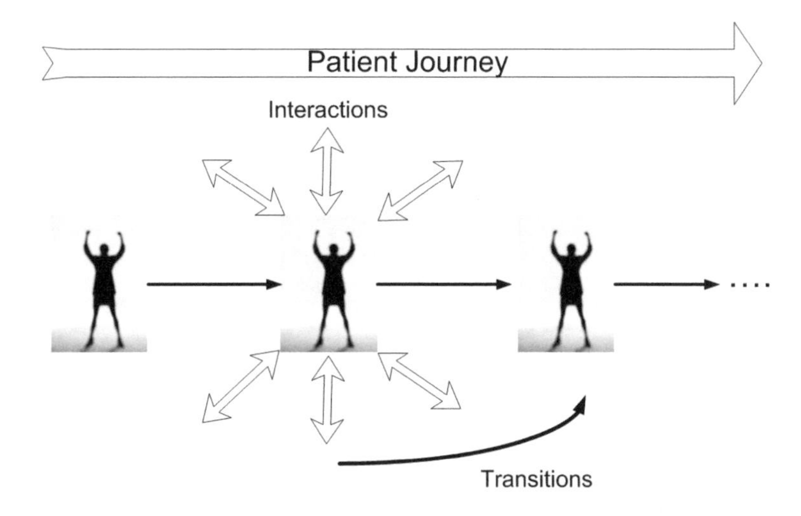

Fig. 2. Patient journey or patient care process.

family preferences and needs [124]. Patient-centered care may actually be safer care.

Care to patients is provided through a myriad of interactions between various individuals: the patients themselves, their families and friends, healthcare providers, and various other staff. These interactions involve a multitude of organizations, such as hospitals, large clinical practices, physician offices, nursing homes, pharmacies, home care agencies, and ambulatory surgery centers. These interactions among various individuals and organizations are a unique feature of 'production' within healthcare. As explained by Gaba, health care is a system of complex interactions and tight coupling that make it vulnerable to normal accidents. Care is 'produced' during a myriad of interactions with varying levels of success, i.e. with various levels of quality and safety. These interactions occur over time, and therefore produce transitions of care that influence each other and accumulate over the journey of the patient care process. Figure 2 depicts a picture of the patient journey, showing various interactions occurring at each step of the patient care process and the transitions of care or patient handoffs happening over time. A patient handoff occurs when patient care requires a change in care setting or provider. Each handoff in the patient journey involves various interactions of the patient and the healthcare provider with a task (typically information sharing), other people, tools and technologies, and a physical, social and organizational context (see Fig. 3). The growing number of transitions of care, due in part to an increasing number of shift changes and increased fragmentation of care, along with a heightened focus on patient safety, demonstrate the obvious need for safe and effective interactions to achieve successful patient handoffs.

2.2.1. Example

Let us examine an example of a patient care process to illustrate various interactions and the patient journey. See Table 1 for a description of a patient care process that shows several instances of interactions:

- Task interactions: result of pulmonary function test faxed to clinic, midlevel provider communication with patient's cardiologist
- Interpersonal interactions between the midlevel provider, the pulmonary department and the patient and his family in order to coordinate the pulmonary function test
- Interactions between the midlevel provider and several tools and technologies, such as the fax machine used to receive test results and the patient's online record

Table 1
Example of a patient care process

*A 68-year-old male with a history of COPD (Chronic Obstructive Pulmonary Disease) and poor pulmonary function is scheduled to have surgery to remove a lesion from his liver. Prior to coming to the work-up clinic located at the hospital for his pre-operative work-up, the patient was to have a pulmonary function test, but due to a bad cough, had to reschedule. There was some confusion as to whether he should have the test done at the facility near his home or have it done the day of his work-up visit. Several calls were made between the midlevel provider *, the facility's pulmonary department, the patient, and the patient's family to coordinate the test, which was then conducted the day before the work-up visit. The results from this test were faxed to the work-up clinic. However, the patient also had an appointment with his cardiologist back home prior to the work-up and the records from the cardiologist were not sent to the hospital by the day of the work-up.*
The midlevel provider begins by contacting the patient's cardiologist to request that his records be sent as soon as possible. The midlevel provider is concerned about the patient's pulmonary status and would like someone from the hospital's pulmonary department to review the patient's test results and evaluate his condition for surgery. After some searching, the midlevel determines the number to call and pages pulmonary. In the meantime, the midlevel provider checks the patient's online record, discovering that the patient did not have labs done this morning as instructed, and informs the patient that he must have his labs done before he leaves the hospital. Late in the day and after several pages, the midlevel provider hears back from the pulmonary department stating that they cannot fit the patient in yet today, but can schedule him for the following morning. Since the patient is from out of town, he would prefer to see his regular pulmonary physician back home. The midlevel provider will arrange for this appointment and be in touch with the patient and his family about the appointment and whether or not they will be able to go ahead with the surgery as planned in less than two weeks.

* A midlevel provider is a medical provider who is not a physician but is licensed to diagnose and treat patients under the supervision of a physician; it is typically a physician's assistant or a nurse practitioners (The American Heritage Stedman's Medical Dictionary, 2nd Edition, 2004, Published by Houghton Mifflin Company).

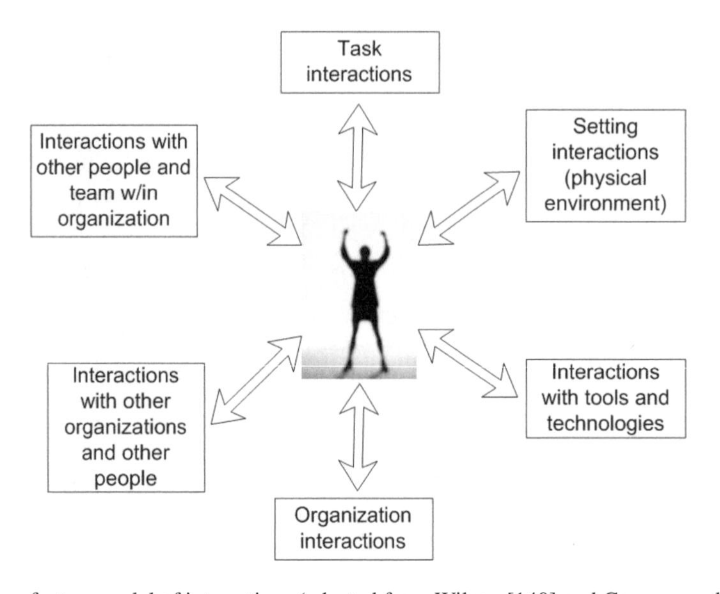

Fig. 3. Human factors model of interactions (adapted from Wilson [140] and Carayon and Smith [27].

- Interactions between the midlevel provider and outside organizations, such as the patient's cardiologist.

This example also shows several types of patient handoffs:

- Handoff from the patient's cardiologist to the midlevel provider
- Handoff between the midlevel provider and the pulmonary department
- Handoff between the midlevel provider and the patient's own pulmonary physician.

The High Reliability Organizing (HRO) approach developed by the Berkeley group [108,109] and the Michigan group [137] emphasizes the need for mindful interactions. Throughout the patient journey, we need to build systems and processes that allow various process owners and stakeholders to enhance mindfulness. Five HRO principles influence mindfulness: (1) tracking small failures, (2) resisting oversimplification, (3) sensitivity to operations, (4) resilience, and (5) deference to expertise [137]. First, patient safety may be enhanced in an organizational culture and structure that is continuously preoccupied with failures. This would encourage reporting of errors and near misses, and learning from these failures. Second, understanding the complex, changing and uncertain work systems and processes in health care would allow healthcare organizations to have a more nuanced realistic understanding of their operations and to begin to anticipate potential failures by designing better systems and processes. Third, patient safety can be enhanced by developing a deep understanding of both the sharp and blunt ends of healthcare organizations. Fourth, since errors are inevitable, patient safety needs to allow people to detect, correct and recover from those errors. Finally, because healthcare work systems and processes are complex, the application of the requisite variety principle would lead to diversity and 'migration' to expertise. These five HRO principles can enhance transitions of care and interactions throughout the patient journey.

Examining the patient journey and the various vulnerabilities that may occur throughout the interactions of the patient care process provides important insights regarding patient safety. Another important view on patient safety focuses on the healthcare professionals and their performance.

2.3. *Performance of healthcare professionals*

Patient safety is about the patient, but requires that healthcare professionals have the right tools and environment to perform their tasks and coordinate their effort. Therefore, it is important to examine patient safety models that focus on the performance of healthcare professionals.

Bogner [9] proposed the "Artichoke" model of systems factors that influence behavior. The interactions between providers and patients are the core of the system and represent the means of providing care. Several system layers influence these interactions: ambient conditions, physical environment, social environment, organizational factors, and the larger environment (e.g., legal-regulatory-reimbursement). Karsh et al. [70] have proposed a model of patient safety that defines various characteristics of performance of the healthcare professional who delivers care. The performance of the healthcare professional can be categorized into (1) physical performance (e.g., carrying, injecting, charting), (2) cognitive performance (e.g., perceiving, communicating, analyzing, awareness) and (3) social/behavioral performance (e.g., motivation, decision-making). Performance can be influenced by various characteristics of the work system, including characteristics of the 'worker' and his/her patients and their organization, as well as the external environment.

Efforts targeted at improving patient safety, therefore, need to consider the performance of healthcare providers and the various work system factors that hinder their ability to do their work, i.e. performance obstacles [25,54,55].

2.4. *SEIPS model of work system and patient safety*

The various models reviewed in previous sections emphasize specific aspects such as human error, patient care process and performance of healthcare professionals. In this section, we describe the SEIPS [Systems Engineering Initiative for Patient Safety] model of work system and patient safety as a

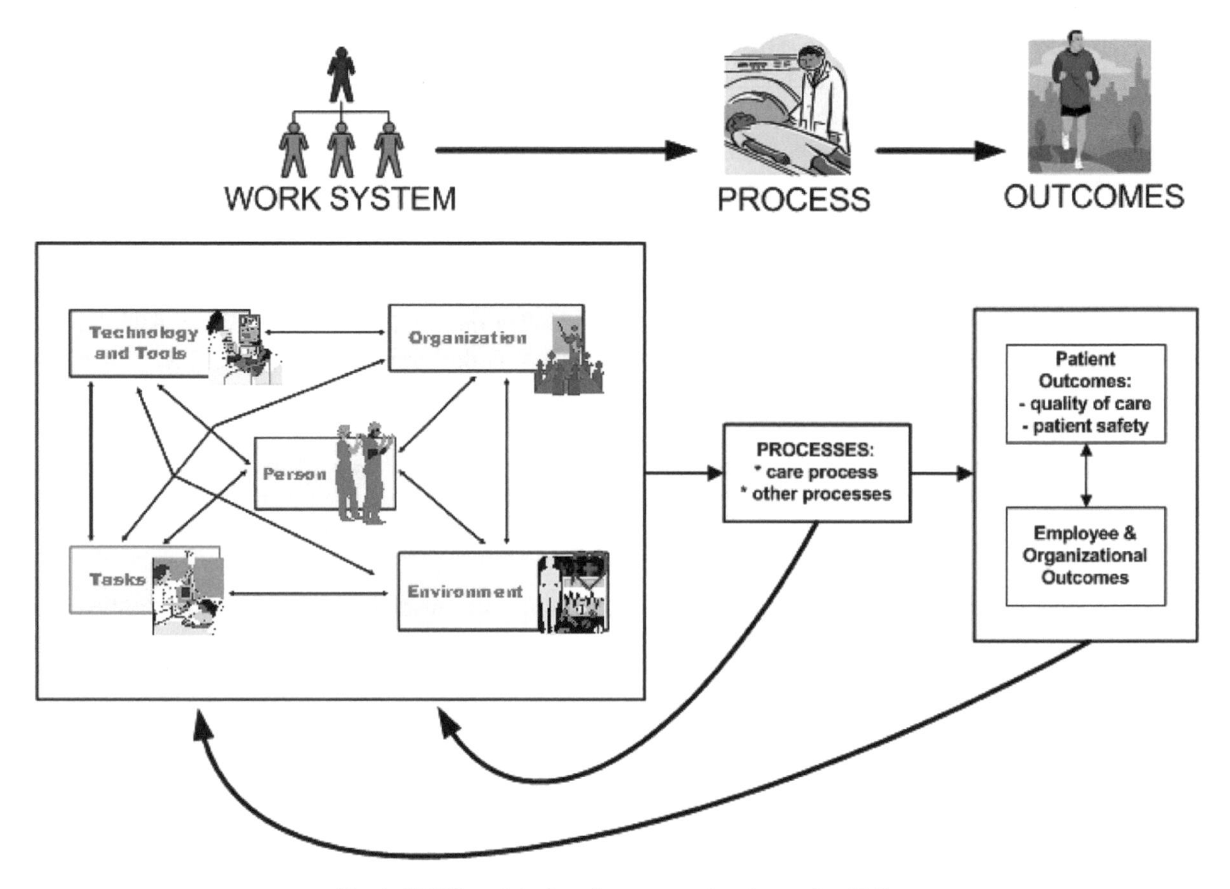

Fig. 4. SEIPS model of work system and patient safety [26].

conceptual framework that integrates many of the aspects described in other models [26]. See Fig. 4 for a graphical representation of the SEIPS model of work system and patient safety.

The SEIPS model is based on the Donabedian's [42] model of quality. According to Donabedian [42], quality can be conceptualized with regard to structure, process or outcome. Structure is defined as the setting in which care occurs and has been described as including material resources (e.g., facilities, equipment, money), human resources (e.g., staff and their qualifications) and organizational structure (e.g., methods of peer review, methods of reimbursement) [43]. Process is "what is actually done in giving and receiving care" [43, p. 1745]. Patient outcomes are measured as the effects on health status of patients and populations [43]. The SEIPS model is organized around the Structure-Process-Outcome model of Donabedian; it expands the 'structure' element by proposing the work system model of Smith and Carayon [27,121] as a way of describing the structure or system that can influence processes of care and outcomes. The SEIPS model also expands the outcomes by considering not only patient outcomes (e.g., patient safety) but also employee and organizational outcomes. In light of the importance of performance of healthcare professionals (see previous section), it is important to consider the impact of the work system on both patients and healthcare workers, as well as the potential linkage between patient safety and employee safety.

According to the SEIPS model of work system and patient safety (see Fig. 4), patient safety is an outcome that results from the design of work systems and processes. Therefore, in order to improve patient safety, one needs to examine the specific processes involved and the work system factors that

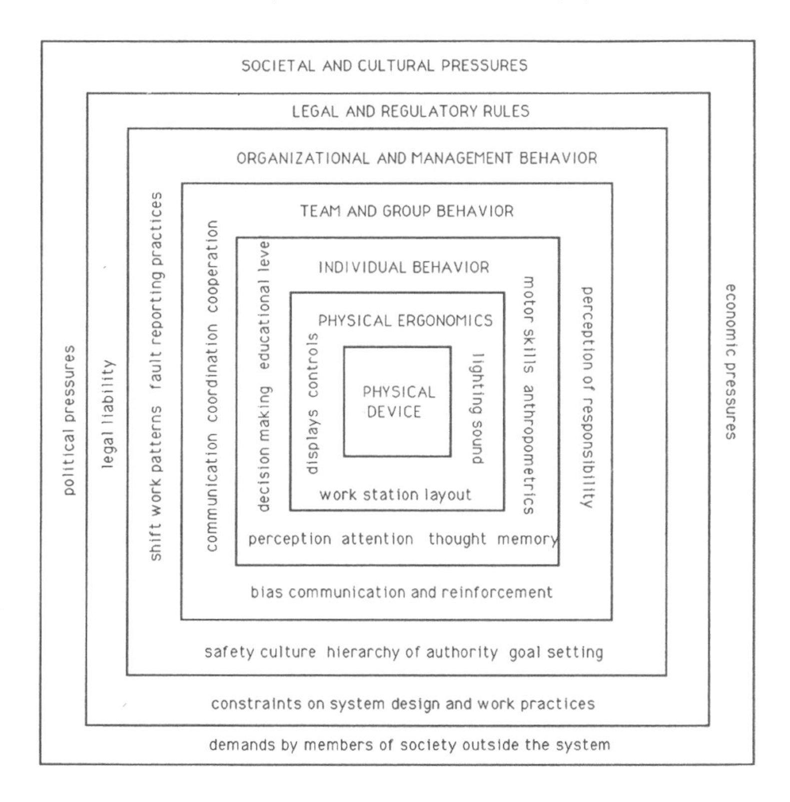

Fig. 5. Hierarchical model of human-system interaction [93].

contribute either positively or negatively to processes and outcomes. In addition, patient safety is related to numerous individual and organizational outcomes. 'Healthy' healthcare organizations focus on both the health and safety of their patients, but also the health and safety of their employees [94,116].

3. Patient safety and system redesign

As emphasized throughout this chapter, medical errors and preventable patient harm can be avoided by a renewed focus on the design of work systems and processes. This type of system redesign effort requires competencies in engineering and health sciences. Redesigning a system can be challenging, especially in healthcare organizations that have limited technical infrastructure and technical expertise in human factors and systems engineering [106].

3.1. Levels of system design

There is increasing recognition in the human factors literature of the different levels of factors that can contribute to human errors and accidents [71,100]. If the various factors are aligned 'appropriately' like 'slices of Swiss cheese', accidents can occur [103]. Table 2 summarizes different approaches to the levels of factors contributing to human error. For instance, Moray [93] has proposed a hierarchical systems model that defines multiple levels of human-system interaction (see Fig. 5). The levels of system design are organized hierarchically as follows: physical devices, physical ergonomics, individual

Table 2
Levels of system design

Authors	System factors contributing to human error
Rasmussen [100]: levels of a complex socio-technical system	Work Staff Management Company Regulators/associations Government
Moray [93]: hierarchical systems approach that includes several layers	Physical device Physical ergonomics Individual behavior Team and group behavior Organizational and management behavior Legal and regulatory rules Societal and cultural pressures
Johnson [68]: four levels of causal factors that can contribute to human error in healthcare	Level 1 factors that influence the behavior of individual clinicians (e.g., poor equipment design, poor ergonomics, technical complexity, multiple competing tasks) Level 2 factors that affect team-based performance (e.g., problems of coordination and communication, acceptance of inappropriate norms, operation of different procedures for the same tasks) Level 3 factors that relate to the management of healthcare applications (e.g., poor safety culture, inadequate resource allocation, inadequate staffing, inadequate risk assessment and clinical audit) Level 4 factors that involve regulatory and government organizations (e.g., lack of national structures to support clinical information exchange and risk management).
For comparison, levels of factors contribution to quality and safety of patient care	
(Berwick [8]; The Institute of Medicine Committee on Quality of Health Care in America [65])	Level A – experience of patients and communities Level B – microsystems of care, i.e. the small units of work that actually give the care that the patient experiences Level C – health care organizations Level D – health care environment

behavior, team and group behavior, organizational and management behavior, legal and regulatory rules, and societal and cultural pressures.

It is interesting to make a parallel between the different levels of factors contributing to human error and the levels identified to deal with quality and safety of care [8,65]. The 2001 IOM report on *Crossing the Quality Chasm* [65] defines four levels at which interventions are needed in order to improve the quality and safety of care in the United States: Level A-experience of patients and communities, Level B-microsystems of care, i.e. the small units of work that actually give the care that the patient experiences, Level C-health care organizations, and Level D-health care environment. These levels are similar to the hierarchy of levels of factors contributing to human error (see Table 1). Models and methods of human factors engineering can be particularly useful because of their underlying systems approach and capacity to integrate variables at various levels [58,88,141]. Hendrick [59] has defined a number of 'levels' of human factors or ergonomics:

- Human-machine: hardware ergonomics
- Human-environment: environmental ergonomics
- Human-software: cognitive ergonomics
- Human-job: work design ergonomics

– Human-organization: macroergonomics

Research at the first three levels has been performed in the context of quality of care and patient safety. Much still needs to be done at the levels of work design and at the macroergonomic level in order to design healthcare systems that produce high-quality safe patient care.

The levels of system design are interdependent and related to each other. In order to implement changes toward patient safety, it may be necessary to align incentives and motivation between the different levels. The case study of a radical change in a medical device manufacturer described by Vicente [129] shows how improvements in the design of a medical device for patient safety did not occur until incentives between the different levels were aligned. A medical device manufacturer implemented a human factors approach after a number of events occurred and various pressures were put on the company. The events included several programming errors with a patient-controlled analgesia (PCA) pump sold by the company; some of the errors led to over-deliveries of analgesic and patient deaths. After multiple pressures from the FDA, various professional associations (e.g., ISMP), the government (e.g., Department of Justice) and the public opinion (e.g., coverage in the lay press), in 2001, the company finally established a human factors program. This case study shows that at what happens at one level (e.g., manufacturer of the medical device) was related to other lower (e.g., patient deaths related to pump programming errors) and higher (e.g., regulatory agency) levels.

Patient safety improvement efforts should be targeted at all levels of system design. In addition, we need to ensure that incentives at various levels are aligned to encourage and support safe care.

3.2. Competencies for system redesign

System redesign for patient safety required competencies in (1) health sciences and (2) human factors and systems engineering.

As an example of the application of human factors and systems engineering to patient safety, Jack and colleagues [66] developed, implemented and tested a methodology for the redesign of hospital discharge process. As was discussed earlier, transitions of care (e.g., patient discharge) are particularly vulnerable and have been related to numerous patient safety problems. Therefore, a team at Boston Medical Center redesigned the hospital discharge process by improving information flow and coordination. Three components of the discharge process were changed: (1) in-hospital discharge process, (2) care plan post-hospital discharge, and (3) follow up with patient by pharmacist. Changes in the in-hospital discharge process included: communication with the patient (i.e. patient education and information about follow up care), organization of post-discharge services and appointments for follow-up care, review of medication plan and other elements of the discharge plan, and transmission of discharge summary to appropriate parties (e.g., primary care provider of the patient). At the time of discharge, the patient was provided with a comprehensive written discharge plan. Post-discharge, a pharmacist followed up with the patient. This system redesign effort considers all important steps of the discharge process involved in the transition of care and the many interactions that occur in the discharge process (see Fig. 3).

Patients who received the 'intervention' were less likely to be re-admitted or to visit the emergency department 30 days post-discharge. They were also more likely to visit their primary care provider. Survey data showed that patients involved in the redesigned discharge process felt more prepared for the discharge.

The study by Jack et al. [66] is an interesting example of how system and process redesign can lead to benefits in quality and safety of care. It also shows that system redesign for patient safety requires knowledge in health sciences and human factors and systems engineering. In the Boston Medical Center study, the expertise in these various domains was distributed across members of the research team.

3.3. Challenges of system redesign

It is important to emphasize that achieving patient safety is a constant process, similar to continuous quality improvement [120]. Safety cannot be 'stored'; safety is an emergent system property that is created dynamically through various interactions between people and the system during the patient journey (see Figs 2 and 3). Some anticipatory system design can be performed using human factors knowledge [23,26]. Much is already known about various types of person/system interactions (e.g., usability of technology, appropriate task workload, teamwork) that can produce positive individual and organizational outcomes. However, health care is a dynamic complex system where people and system elements continuously change, therefore requiring constant vigilance and monitoring of the various system interactions and transitions.

When changes are implemented in healthcare organizations, opportunities are created to improve and recreate awareness and learning in order to foster mindfulness in interactions. Potentially adverse consequences to patients can occur when system interactions are faulty, inconsistent, error-laden or unclear between providers and those receiving or managing care [10,21,132]. In order to maintain patient safety in healthcare organizations, healthcare providers, managers and other staff need to continuously learn [110], while reiterating or reinforcing their understanding as well as their expectations of the system of care being provided, a system that is highly dependent on ongoing interactions between countless individuals and, sometimes, organizations.

3.4. Role of health information technology in patient safety

In he alth care, technologies are often seen as an important solution to improve quality of care and reduce or eliminate medical errors [3,74]. These technologies include organizational and work technologies aimed at improving the efficiency and effectiveness of information and communication processes (e.g., computerized order entry provider and electronic medical record) and patient care technologies that are directly involved in the care processes (e.g., bar coding medication administration). For instance, the 1999 IOM report recommended adoption of new technology, like bar code administration technology, to reduce medication errors [74]. However, implementation of new technologies in health care has not been without troubles or work-arounds (see, for example, the studies by Patterson et al. [96] and Koppel et al. [76] on potential negative effects of bar coding medication administration technology). Technologies change the way work is performed [122] and because healthcare work and processes are complex, negative consequences of new technologies are possible [5,34].

When looking for solutions to improving patient safety, technology may or may not be the only solution. For instance, a study of the implementation of nursing information computer systems in 17 New Jersey hospitals showed many problems experienced by hospitals, such as delays, and lack of software customization [61]. On the other hand, at least initially, nursing staff reported positive perceptions, in particular with regard to documentation (more readable, complete and timely). However, a more rigorous evaluation of the quality of nursing documentation following the implementation of bedside terminals did not confirm those initial impressions [89]. This later result was due to the low use of bedside terminals by the nurses. This technology implementation may have ignored the impact of the technology on the tasks performed by the nurses. Nurses may have needed time away from the patient's bedside in order to organize their thoughts and collaborate with colleagues [89]. This study demonstrates the need for a systems approach to understand the impact of technology (see Fig. 4). For instance, instead of using the "leftover" approach to function and task allocation, a human-centered approach to function and task allocation should be used [60]. This approach considers the simultaneous design of the technology and the work system in order to achieve a balanced work system. One possible outcome of this allocation approach would be to rely on human and organizational characteristics that can foster safety (e.g., autonomy provided at the source of the variance; human capacity for error recovery), instead of completely 'trusting' the technology to achieve high quality and safety of care.

Whenever implementing a technology, one should examine the potential positive and negative influences of the technology on the other work system elements [5,81,121]. In a study of the implementation of an Electronic Medical Record (EMR) system in a small family medicine clinic, a number of issues were examined: impact of the EMR technology on work patterns, employee perceptions related to the EMR technology and its potential/actual effect on work, and the EMR implementation process [28]. Employee questionnaire data showed the following impact of the EMR technology on work: increased dependence on computers was found, as well as an increase in quantitative workload and a perceived negative influence on performance occurring at least in part from the introduction of the EMR [63]. It is important to examine for what tasks technology can be useful to provide better, safer care [56].

The human factors characteristics of the new technologies' design (e.g., usability) should also be studied carefully [5]. An experimental study by Lin et al. [86] showed the application of human factors engineering principles to the design of the interface of an analgesia device. Results showed that the new interface led to the elimination of drug concentration errors, and to the reduction of other errors. A study by Effken et al. [47] shows the application of a human factors engineering model, i.e. the ecological approach to interface design, to the design of a haemodynamic monitoring device.

The new technology may also bring its own 'forms of failure' [5,34,75,103]. For instance, bar coding medication administration technology can prevent patient misidentifications, but the possibility exists that an error during patient registration may be disseminated throughout the information system and may be more difficult to detect and correct than with conventional systems [133]. A study by Koppel et al. [75] describes how the design and implementation of computerized provider order entry in a hospital contributed to 22 types of medication errors that were categorized into: (1) information errors due to fragmentation and systems integration failure (e.g., failure to renew antibiotics because of delays in re-approval), and (2) human-machine interface flaws (e.g., wrong patient selection or wrong medication selection).

In addition, the manner in which a new technology is implemented is as critical to its success as its technological capabilities [46,122]. End user involvement in the design and implementation of a new technology is a good way to help ensure a successful technological investment. Korunka and his colleagues [77–79] have empirically demonstrated the crucial importance of end user involvement in the implementation of technology to the health and well-being of end users. The implementation of technology in an organization has both positive and negative effects on the job characteristics that ultimately affect individual outcomes (quality of working life, such as job satisfaction and stress; and perceived quality of care delivered or self-rated performance) [18]. Inadequate planning when introducing a new technology designed to decrease medical errors has led to technology falling short of achieving its patient safety goal [72,96]. The most common reason for failure of technology implementations is that the implementation process is treated as a technological problem, and the human and organizational issues are ignored or not recognized [45]. When a technology is implemented, several human and organizational issues are important to consider [17,122]. According to the SEIPS model of work system and patient safety [26], the implementation of a new technology will have impact on the entire work system, which will result in changes in processes of care and will therefore affect both patient and staff outcomes (see Fig. 4).

3.5. Link between efficiency and patient safety

System redesign for patient safety should not be achieved at the expense of efficiency. On the contrary, it is important to recognize the possible synergies that can be obtained by patient safety and efficiency improvement efforts.

Efficiency issues related to access to intensive care services and crowding in emergency departments have been studied by Litvak and colleagues [91,102]. Patients are often refused a bed in an intensive care unit; ICUs are well-known bottlenecks to patient flow. A study by McManus et al. [91] shows that scheduled surgeries (as opposed to unscheduled surgeries and emergencies) can have a significant impact on rejections to the ICU. Although counterintuitive, this result demonstrates how scheduled surgeries can contribute to erratic patient flow and intermittent periods of extreme overload and have a negative impact on ICUs. This clearly outlines the relationship between efficiency of scheduling process and workload experienced by the ICU staff, which is a well-known contributor to patient safety [22,24]. More broadly, Litvak et al. [87] propose that unnecessary variability in healthcare processes contribute to nursing stress and patient safety problems. System redesign efforts aimed at removing or reducing unnecessary variability can improve both efficiency and patient safety.

Improving the efficiency of care processes can have very direct impact on patient safety. For instance, the delay between prescription of an antibiotic medication and its administration to septic shock patients is clearly related to patient outcomes [82]: each hour of delay in administration of antibiotic medication is associated with an average increase in mortality of 7.6%. Therefore, improving the efficiency and timeliness of the medication process can improve quality and safety of care.

4. Human factors and systems engineering tools for patient safety

The need for human factors and systems engineering expertise is pervasive throughout healthcare organizations. For instance, knowledge about work system and physical ergonomics can be used for understanding the relationship between employee safety and patient safety. This knowledge will be important for the employee health department of healthcare organizations. Purchasing departments of healthcare organizations need to have knowledge about usability and user-centered design in order to ensure that the equipment and devices are ergonomically designed. Given the major stress and workload problems experienced by many nurses, nursing managers need to know about job stress and workload management. Risk management represents the front-line of patient safety accidents; they need to understand human errors and other mechanisms involved in accidents. With the push toward health information technology, issues of technology design and implementation are receiving increasing attention. People involved in the design and implementation of those technologies need to have basic knowledge about interface design and usability, as well as sociotechnical system design. Biomedical engineers in healthcare organizations and medical device manufacturers design, purchase and maintain various equipment and technologies and, therefore, need to know about usability and user-centered design. The operating room is an example of a healthcare setting in which teamwork coordination and collaboration are critical for patient safety; human factors principles of team training are very relevant for this type of care setting.

We believe that improvements in the quality and safety of health care can be achieved by better integrating human factors and systems engineering expertise throughout the various layers and units of healthcare organizations. Some of the barriers to the widespread dissemination of this knowledge in healthcare organizations include: lack of recognition of the importance of systems design in various aspects of healthcare, technical jargon and terminology of human factors and systems engineering, and need for development of knowledge regarding the application of human factors and systems engineering in healthcare [20].

Numerous books provide information on human factors methods [117,123,140]. Human factors methods can be classified as: (1) general methods (e.g., direct observation of work), (2) collection of information about people (e.g., physical measurement of anthropometric dimensions), (3) analysis and design (e.g., task analysis, time study), (4) evaluation of human-machine system performance (e.g., usability, performance measures, error analysis, accident reporting), (5) evaluation of demands on people (e.g., mental workload), and (6) management and implementation of ergonomics (e.g., participative methods). This shows the diversity of human factors methods to address various patient safety problems. In this section, we describe selected human factors methods that have been used to evaluate high-risk care processes and technologies.

4.1. Human factors evaluation of high-risk processes

Numerous methods can be used to evaluate high-risk processes in health care. FMEA (Failure Modes and Effects Analysis) is one method that can be used to analyze, redesign and improve healthcare processes to meet the Joint Commission's National Patient Safety Goals. The National Patient Safety Center of the VA has adapted the industrial FMEA method to healthcare [41]. FMEA or other proactive risk assessment techniques have been applied to a range of healthcare processes, such as blood transfusion [16], organ transplant [37], medication administration with implementation of smart infusion pump technology [139], and use of computerized provider order entry [11].

Proactive risk analysis of healthcare processes needs to begin with a good understanding of the actual process. This often involves extensive data collection and analysis about the process. For instance, Carayon and colleagues [29] used direct observations and interviews to analyze the vulnerabilities in the medication administration process and the use of bar coding medication administration technology by nurses. Such data collection and process analysis was guided and informed by the SEIPS model of work system and patient safety [26] (see Fig. 4) in order to ensure that all system characteristics were adequately addressed in the process analysis.

The actual healthcare process may actually be different from organizational procedures for numerous reasons. For instance, a procedure may not have been updated after some technological or organizational change or the procedure may have been written by people who did not have a full understanding of the work and its context. A key concept in human factors engineering is the difference between the 'prescribed' work and the 'real' work [53,85]. Therefore, whenever analyzing a healthcare process, one needs to gather information about the 'real' process and the associated work system characteristics in its actual context.

4.2. Human factors evaluation of technologies

As discussed in a previous section, technologies are often presented as solutions to improve patient safety and prevent medical errors [74]. Technologies can lead to patient safety improvements only if they are designed, implemented and used according to human factors and systems engineering principles [115, 117].

At the design stage, a number of human factors tools are available to ensure that technologies fit human characteristics and are usable [90,95]. Usability evaluation and testing methods are increasingly used by manufacturers and vendors of healthcare technologies. Healthcare organizations are also more likely to request information about the usability of technologies they purchase. Fairbanks and Caplan [48] describe examples of how poor interface design of technologies used by paramedics can lead to medical errors. Gosbee and Gosbee [52] provide practical information about usability evaluation and testing at the stage of technology design.

At the implementation stage, it is important to consider the rich literature on technological and organizational change that list principles for 'good' technology implementation [77,79,122,115]. For instance, a review of literature by Karsh [69] highlights the following principles for technology implementation to promote patient safety:

- Top management commitment to the change
- Responsibility and accountability structure for the change
- Structured approach to the change
- Training
- Pilot testing
- Communication
- Feedback
- Simulation
- End user participation.

Even after a technology has been implemented, it is important to continue to monitor its use in the 'real' context and to identify potential problems and work-arounds. About 2–3 years after the implementation of bar coding medication administration (BCMA) technology in a large academic medical center, a study of nurses' use of the technology shows a range of work-arounds [29]. For instance, nurses had developed work-arounds to be able to administer medications to patients in isolation rooms: it was very difficult for nurses to use the BCMA handheld device wrapped in a plastic bag; therefore, often the medication was scanned and documented as administered before the nurse would enter the patient room and administer the medication. This type of work-around results from a lack of fit between the context (i.e. patient in isolation room), the technology (i.e. BCMA handheld device) and the nurses' task (i.e. medication administration). Some of these interactions may not be anticipated at the stage of designing the technology and may be 'visible' only after the technology is in use in the real context. This emphasizes the need to adopt a 'continuous' technology change approach that identifies problems associated with the technology's use [19,136].

5. Conclusion

Improving patient safety involves major system redesign of healthcare work systems and processes [26]. This chapter has outlined important conceptual approaches to patient safety; we have also discussed issues about system redesign and presented examples of human factors and systems engineering tools that can be used to improve patient safety. Additional information about human factors and systems engineering in patient safety is available elsewhere (see, for example, Carayon [21] and Bogner [10]).

Improving patient safety requires knowledge and skills in a range of disciplines, in particular health sciences and human factors and systems engineering. This is in line with the main recommendation by the NAE/IOM report on "*Building a Better Delivery System. A New Engineering/Health Care Partnership*" [106]. A number of partnerships between engineering and health care have grown and emerged since the publication of the NAE/IOM report. However, more progress is required, in particular in the area of patient safety. We need to train clinicians in human factors and systems engineering and to train engineers in health systems engineering; this major education and training effort should promote collaboration between the health sciences and human factors and systems engineering in various patient safety improvement projects. An example of this educational effort is the yearly week-long course on human factors engineering and patient safety taught by the SEIPS [Systems Engineering Initiative for Patient Safety] group at the University of Wisconsin-Madison [http://cqpi.engr.wisc.edu/seips_home/]. Similar efforts and more extensive educational offerings are necessary to train future healthcare leaders, professionals and engineers.

Acknowledgments

This publication was partially supported by grant 1UL1RR025011 from the Clinical & Translational Science Award (CTSA) program of the National Center for Research Resources National Institutes of Health (PI: M. Drezner) and by grant 1R01 HS015274-01 from the Agency for Healthcare Research and Quality (PI: P. Carayon, co-PI: K. Wood).

References

[1] G.R. Baker, P.G. Norton, V. Flintoft, R. Blais, A. Brown, J. Cox et al., The Canadian adverse events study: The incidence of adverse events among hospital patients in Canada, *Journal of the Canadian Medical Association* **170**(11) (2004), 1678–1686.

[2] D.W. Bates, D.L. Boyle, M.B. Vander Vliet al, e., Relationship between medication errors and adverse drug events, *Journal of General Internal Medicine* **10**(4) (1995), 199–205.

[3] D.W. Bates and A.A. Gawande, Improving safety with information technology, *The New England Journal of Medicine* **348**(25) (2003), 2526–2534.

[4] D.W. Bates, L.L. Leape and S. Petrycki, Incidence and preventability of adverse drug events in hospitalized adults. *Journal of General Internal Medicine* **8**(6) (1993), 289–294.

[5] J.B. Battles and M.A. Keyes, Technology and patient safety: A two-edged sword, *Biomedical Instrumentation & Technology* **36**(2) (2002), 84–88.

[6] C. Beach, P. Croskerry and M. Shapiro, Profiles in patient safety: emergency care transitions, *Academic Emergency Medicine* **10**(4) (2003), 364–367.

[7] C.M. Bell, J. Bajcar, A.S. Bierman, P. Li, M.M. Mamdani and D.R. Urbach, Potentially unintended discontinuation of long-term medication use after elective surgical procedures, *Archives of Internal Medicine* **166**(22) (2006), 2525–2531.

[8] D.M. Berwick, A user's manual for the IOM's 'Quality Chasm' report, *Health Affairs* **21**(3) (2002), 80–90.

[9] M.S. Bogner, The artichoke systems approach for identifying the why of error, in: *Handbook of Human Factors in Health Care and Patient Safety*, P. Carayon, ed., Mahwah, NJ: Lawrence Erlbaum, 2007, pp. 109–126.

[10] M.S. Bogner, ed., *Human Error in Medicine*, Hillsdale, NJ: Lawrence Erlbaum Associates, 1994.

[11] P. Bonnabry, C. Despont-Gros, D. Grauser, P. Casez, M. Despond, D. Pugin et al., A risk analysis method to evaluate the impact of a computerized provider order entry system on patient safety. *Journal of the American Medical Informatics Association* **15**(4) (2008), 453–460.

[12] K. Boockvar, E. Fishman, C.K. Kyriacou, A. Monias, S. Gavi and T. Cortes, Adverse events due to discontinuations in drug use and dose changes in patients transferred between acute and long-term care facilities. [Original Investigation], *Archives of Internal Medicine* **164**(5) (2004), 545–550.

[13] D. Bracco, J.-B. Favre, B. Bissonnette, J.-B. Wasserfallen, J.-P. Revelly, P. Ravussin et al., Human errors in a multidisciplinary intensive care unit: a 1-year prospective study, *Intensive Care Medicine* **27**(1) (2000), 137–145.

[14] P.F. Brennan and C. Safran, Patient safety. Remember who it's really for, *International Journal of Medical Informatics* **73**(7–8) (2004), 547–550.

[15] T.A. Brennan, L.L. Leape, N.M. Laird, L. Hebert, A.R. Localio, A.G. Lawthers et al., Incidence of adverse events and negligence in hospitalized patients, Results of the Harvard Medical Practice Study I, *New England Journal of Medicine* **324**(6) (1991), 370–376.

[16] J. Burgmeier, Failure mode and effect analysis: An application in reducing risk in blood transfusion, *The Joint Commission Journal on Quality Improvement* **28**(6) (2002), 331–339.

[17] P. Carayon-Sainfort, The use of computers in offices: Impact on task characteristics and worker stress, *International Journal of Human Computer Interaction* **4**(3) (1992), 245–261.
[18] P. Carayon and M.C. Haims, Information and communication technology and work organization: Achieving a balanced system, in: *Humans on the Net-Information and Communication Technology (ICT)*, G. Bradley, ed., Work Organization and Human Beings, Sweden: Prevent, 2001, pp. 119–138.
[19] P. Carayon, Human factors of complex sociotechnical systems, *Applied Ergonomics* **37** (2006), 525–535.
[20] P. Carayon, Human factors in patient safety as an innovation, *Applied Ergonomics, to be published* (2009).
[21] P. Carayon, ed., *Handbook of Human Factors in Health Care and Patient Safety*, Mahwah, New Jersey: Lawrence Erlbaum Associates, 2007.
[22] P. Carayon and C. Alvarado, Workload and patient safety among critical care nurses, *Critical Care Nursing Clinics* **8**(5) (2007), 395–428.
[23] P. Carayon, C. Alvarado and A.S. Hundt, *Reducing Workload and Increasing Patient Safety Through Work and Workspace Design*, Washington, DC: Institute of Medicine, 2003.
[24] P. Carayon and A. Gurses, Nursing workload and patient safety in intensive care units: A human factors engineering evaluation of the literature, *Intensive and Critical Care Nursing* **21** (2005), 284–301.
[25] P. Carayon, A.P. Gurses, A.S. Hundt, P. Ayoub and C.J. Alvarado, Performance obstacles and facilitators of healthcare providers, in: *Change and Quality in Human Service Work*, (Vol. 4), C. Korunka and P. Hoffmann, eds, Munchen, Germany: Hampp Publishers, 2005, pp. 257–276.
[26] P. Carayon, A.S. Hundt, B.-T. Karsh, A.P. Gurses, C.J. Alvarado, M. Smith et al., Work system design for patient safety: The SEIPS model, *Quality & Safety in Health Care* **15**(Supplement I) (2006), i50–i58.
[27] P. Carayon and M.J. Smith, Work organization and ergonomics, *Applied Ergonomics* **31** (2000), 649–662.
[28] P. Carayon, P. Smith, A.S. Hundt, V. Kuruchittham and Q. Li, Implementation of an Electronic Health Records system in a small clinic, *Behaviour and Information Technology* **28**(1) (2009), 5–20.
[29] P. Carayon, T.B. Wetterneck, A.S. Hundt, M. Ozkaynak, J. DeSilvey, B. Ludwig et al., Evaluation of nurse interaction with bar code medication administration technology in the work environment, *Journal of Patient Safety* **3**(1) (2007), 34–42.
[30] M.A. Cimino, M.S. Kirschbaum, L. Brodsky and S.H. Shaha, Assessing medication prescribing errors in pediatric intensive care units, *Pediatric Critical Care Medicine* **5**(2) (2004), 124–132.
[31] C.M. Clancy, Care transitions: A threat and an opportunity for patient safety, *American Journal of Medical Quality* **21**(6) (2006), 415–417.
[32] E.A. Coleman, J.D. Smith, D. Raha and S.-J. Min, Posthospital medication discrepancies – Prevalence and contributing factors, *Archives of Internal Medicine* **165** (2005), 1842–1847.
[33] R. Cook and J. Rasmussen, "Going solid": A model of system dynamics and consequences for patient safety, *Quality & Safety in Health Care* **14** (2005), 130–134.
[34] R.I. Cook, Safety technology: Solutions or experiments? *Nursing Economic* **20**(2) (2002), 80–82.
[35] R.I. Cook, M. Render andD.D. Woods, Gaps in the continuity of care and progress on patient safety, *British Medical Journal* **320** (2000), 791–794.
[36] R.I. Cook, D.D. Woods andC. Miller, *A Tale of Two Stories: Contrasting Views of Patient Safety*, Chicago, IL: National Patient Safety Foundation, 1998.
[37] R.I. Cook, J. Wreathall, A. Smith, D.C. Cronin, O. Rivero, R.C. Harland et al., Probabilistic risk assessment of accidental ABO-incompatible thoracic organ transplantation before and after 2003, *Transplantation* **84**(12) (2007), 1602–1609.
[38] J.B. Cooper, Do short breaks increase or decrease anesthetic risk? *Journal of Clinical Anesthesiology* **1**(3) (1989), 228–231.
[39] D.J. Cullen, D.W. Bates, L.L. Leape and The Adverse Drug Even Prevention Study Group, Prevention of adverse drug events: A decade of progress in patient safety, *Journal of Clinical Anesthesia* **12** (2001), 600–614.
[40] D.J. Cullen, B.J. Sweitzer, D.W. Bates, E. Burdick, A. Edmondson and L.L. Leape, Preventable adverse drug events in hospitalized patients: A comparative study of intensive care and general care units, *Critical Care Medicine* **25**(8) (1997), 1289–1297.
[41] J. DeRosier, E. Stalhandske, J.P. Bagian and T. Nudell, Using health care Failure Mode and Effect Analysis: The VA National Center for Patient Safety's prospective risk analysis system, *Joint Commission Journal on Quality Improvement* **28**(5) (2002), 248–267, 209.
[42] A. Donabedian, The quality of medical care, *Science* **200** (1978), 856–864.
[43] A. Donabedian, The quality of care. How can it be assessed? *Journal of the American Medical Association* **260**(12) (1988), 1743–1748.
[44] Y. Donchin, D. Gopher, M. Olin, Y. Badihi, M. Biesky, C.L. Sprung et al., A look into the nature and causes of human errors in the intensive care unit, *Critical Care Medicine* **23**(2) (1995), 294–300.
[45] K. Eason, *Information Technology and Organizational Change*, London: Taylor & Francis, 1988.

[46] K.D. Eason, The process of introducing information technology, *Behaviour and Information Technology* **1**(2) (1982), 197–213.
[47] J.A. Effken, M.-G. Kim and R.E. Shaw, Making the constraints visible: Testing the ecological approach to interface design, *Ergonomics* **40**(1) (1997), 1–27.
[48] R.J. Fairbanks and S. Caplan, Poor interface design and lack of usability testing facilitate medical error, *Joint Commission Journal on Quality and Safety* **30**(10) (2004), 579–584.
[49] D.O. Farley, A. Haviland, S. Champagne, A.K. Jain, J.B. Battles, W.B. Munier et al., Adverse-event-reporting practices by us hospitals: Results of a national survey, *Quality & Safety in Health Care* **17**(6) (2008), 416–423.
[50] A.J. Forster, H.D. Clark, A. Menard, N. Dupuis, R. Chernish, N. Chandok et al., Adverse events among medical patients after discharge from hospital, *Canadian Medical Association Journal* **170**(3) (2004), 345–349.
[51] T. Giraud, J.-F. Dhainaut, J.-F. Vaxelaire, T. Joseph, D. Journois, G. Bleichner et al., Iatrogenic complications in adult intensive care units: A prospective two-center study, *Critical Care Medicine* **21**(1) (1993), 40–51.
[52] J.W. Gosbeee and L.L. Gosbee, eds, *Using Human Factors Engineering to Improve Patient Safety*, Oakbrook Terrrace, Illinois: Joint Commission Resources, 2005.
[53] F. Guerin, A. Laville, F. Daniellou, J. Duraffourg and A. Kerguelen, *Understanding and Transforming Work – The Practice of Ergonomics Lyon*, France: ANACT, 2006.
[54] A. Gurses, P. Carayon and M. Wall, Impact of performance obstacles on intensive care nurses workload, perceived quality and safety of care, and quality of working life, *Health Services Research* (2009), 422–443.
[55] A.P. Gurses and P. Carayon, Performance obstacles of intensive care nurses, *Nursing Research* **56**(3) (2007), 185–194.
[56] J. Hahnel, W. Friesdorf, B. Schwilk, T. Marx and S. Blessing, Can a clinician predict the technical equipment a patient will need during intensive care unit treatment? An approach to standardize and redesign the intensive care unit workstation, *Journal of Clinical Monitoring* **8**(1) (1992), 1–6.
[57] A.B. Haynes, T.G. Weiser, W.R. Berry, S.R. Lipsitz, A.H. Breizat, E.P. Dellinger et al., A surgical safety checklist to reduce morbidity and mortality in a global population, *New England Journal of Medicine* **360**(5) (2009), 491–499.
[58] H.W. Hendrick, Human factors in organizational design and management, *Ergonomics* **34** (1991), 743–756.
[59] H.W. Hendrick, Organizational design and macroergonomics, in: *Handbook of Human Factors and Ergonomics*, G. Salvendy, ed., New York: John Wiley & Sons (1997), pp. 594–636.
[60] H.W. Hendrick and B.M. Kleiner, *Macroergonomics – An Introduction to Work System Design*. Santa Monica, CA: The Human Factors and Ergonomics Society (2001).
[61] G. Hendrickson, C.T. Kovner, J.R. Knickman and S.A. Finkler, Implementation of a variety of computerized bedside nursing information systems in 17 New Jersey hospitals, *Computers in Nursing* **13**(3) (1995), 96–102.
[62] T.J. Hoff, How work context shapes physician approach to safety and error, *Quality Management in Health Care April/June* **17**(2) (2008), 140–153.
[63] A.S. Hundt, P. Carayon, P.D. Smith and V. Kuruchittham, A macroergonomic case study assessing Electronic Medical Record implementation in a small clinic, The Human Factors and Ergonomics Society (Ed.), in: *Proceedings of the Human Factors and Ergonomics Society 46th Annual Meeting* Santa Monica, CA, 2002, pp. 1385–1388.
[64] Institute of Medicine, *Preventing Medication Errors*, Washington, DC: The National Academies Press, 2006.
[65] Institute of Medicine Committee on Quality of Health Care in America, *Crossing the Quality Chasm: A New Health System for the 21st Century*. Washington, DC: National Academy Press, 2001.
[66] B.W. Jack, V.K. Chetty, D. Anthony, J.L. Greenwald, G.M. Sanchez, A.E. Johnson et al., A reengineered hospital discharge program to decrease rehospitalization: A randomized trial, *Annals of Internal Medicine* **150**(3) (2009), 178–187.
[67] JCAHO, Delays in Treatment, *Sentinel Event Alert* (26) (2002).
[68] C. Johnson, The causes of human error in medicine. *Cognition, Technology & Work* **4** (2002), 65–70.
[69] B.-T. Karsh, Beyond usability: Designing effective technology implementation systems to promote patient safety, *Quality and Safety in Health Care* **13** (2004), 388–394.
[70] B.-T. Karsh, R. J. Holden, S.J. Alper and C.K.L. Or, A human factors engineering paradigm for patient safety: Designing to support the performance of the healthcare professional, *Quality & Safety in Health Care* **15**(i6) (2006), i59–i65.
[71] B. Karsh and R. Brown, Macroergonomics and patient safety: The impact of levels on theory, measurement, analysis and intervention in medical error research, *Applied Ergonomics* (2009) to be published.
[72] R. Kaushal and D.W. Bates, Computerized Physician Order Entry (CPOE) with Clinical Decision Support Systems (CDSSs), in: *Making Health Care Safer: A Critical Analysis of Patient Safety Practices*, K.G. Shojania, B.W. Duncan, K.M. McDonald and R.M. Wachter, eds, (Vol. Evidence Report/Technology Assessment), AHRQ, 2001, pp. 59–69.
[73] S. King, Our story, *Pediatric Radiology* **36**(4) (2006), 284–286.
[74] L.T. Kohn, J.M. Corrigan and M.S. Donaldson, eds, *To Err is Human: Building a Safer Health System*, Washington, D.C.: National Academy Press, 1999.
[75] R. Koppel, J.P. Metlay, A. Cohen, B. Abaluck, A.R. Localio, S.E. Kimmel et al., Role of computerized physician order entry systems in facilitating medications errors, *Journal of the American Medical Association* **293**(10) (2005), 1197–

1203.
[76] R. Koppel, T. Wetterneck, J.L. Telles and B.-T. Karsh, Workarounds to barcode medication administration systems: Their occurrences, causes, and threats to patient safety, *Journal of the American Medical Informatics Association* **15**(M2616) (2008), 408–423.
[77] C. Korunka and P. Carayon, Continuous implementations of information technology: The development of an interview guide and a cross-national comparison of Austrian and American organizations, *The International Journal of Human Factors in Manufacturing* **9**(2) (1999), 165–183.
[78] C. Korunka, A. Weiss and B. Karetta, Effects of new technologies with special regard for the implementation process per se, *Journal of Organizational Behavior* **14**(4) (1993), 331–348.
[79] C. Korunka, A. Weiss and S. Zauchner, An interview study of "continuous" implementations of information technologies, *Behaviour and Information Technology* **16**(1) (1997), 3–16.
[80] C. Korunka, S. Zauchner and A. Weiss, New information technologies, job profiles, and external workload as predictors of subjectively experienced stress and dissatisfaction at work, *International Journal of Human-Computer Interaction* **9**(4) (1997), 407–424.
[81] C.T. Kovner, G. Hendrickson, J.R. Knickman and S.A. Finkler, Changing the delivery of nursing care – Implementation issues and qualitative findings, *Journal of Nursing Administration* **23**(11) (1993), 24–34.
[82] A. Kumar, D. Roberts, K.E. Wood, B. Light, J.E. Parrillo, S. Sharma et al., Duration of hypotension before initiation of effective antimicrobial therapy is the critical determinant of survival in human septic shock, *Critical Care Medicine* **34**(6) (2006), 1589–1596.
[83] L.L. Leape, D.W. Bates, D.J. Cullen, J. Cooper, H.J. Demonaco, T. Gallivan et al., Systems analysis of adverse drug events, *Journal of the American Medical Association* **274**(1) (1995), 35–43.
[84] L.L. Leape and D.M. Berwick, Five years after To Err Is Human: What have we learned? *Journal of the American Medical Association* **293**(19) (2005), 2384–2390.
[85] J. Leplat, Error analysis, instrument and object of task analysis, *Ergonomics* **32**(7) (1989), 813–822.
[86] L. Lin, K.J. Vicente and D.J. Doyle, Patient safety, potential adverse drug events, and medical device design: A human factors engineering approach, *Journal of Biomedical Informatics* **34**(4) (2001), 274–284.
[87] E. Litvak, P.I. Buerhaus, F. Davidoff, M.C. Long, M.L. McManus and D.M. Berwick, Managing unnecessary variability in patient demand to reduce nursing stress and improve patient safety, *Joint Commission Journal on Quality and Patient Safety* **31**(6) (2005), 330–338.
[88] H. Luczak, Task analysis, in: *Handbook of Human Factors and Ergonomics*, (Second ed.), G. Salvendy, ed., New York: John Wiley & Sons, 1997, pp. 340–416.
[89] P.B. Marr, E. Duthie, K.S. Glassman, D.M. Janovas, J.B. Kelly, E. Graham et al., Bedside terminals and quality of nursing documentation, *Computers in Nursing* **11**(4) (1993), 176–182.
[90] D.J. Mayhew, *The Usability Engineering Lifecycle*. San Francisco, CA: Morgan Kaufmann Publisher Inc, 1999.
[91] M.L. McManus, M.C. Long, A. Cooper, J. Mandell, D.M. Berwick, M. Pagano et al., Variability in surgical caseload and access to intensive care services, *Anesthesiology* **98**(6) (2003), 1491–1496.
[92] C. Moore, J. Wisnivesky, S. Williams and T. McGinn, Medical errors related to discontinuity of care from an inpatient to an outpatient setting, *Journal of General Internal Medicine* **18**(8) (2003), 646–651.
[93] N. Moray, Error reduction as a systems problem, in: *Human Error in Medicine*, M.S. Bogner, ed., Hillsdale, NJ: Lawrence Erlbaum Associates, 1994, pp. 67–91.
[94] L.R. Murphy and C.L. Cooper, eds, *Healthy and Productive Work: An International Perspective*, London: Taylor and Francis, 2000.
[95] J. Nielsen, *Usability Engineering*, Morgan Kaufmann: Amsterdam, The Netherlands, 1993.
[96] E.S. Patterson, R.I. Cook and M.L. Render, Improving patient safety by identifying side effects from introducing bar coding in medication administration, *Journal of the American Medial Informatics Association* **9** (2002), 540–553.
[97] S. Perry, Transitions in care: studying safety in emergency department signovers, *Focus on Patient Safety* **7**(2) (2004), 1–3.
[98] P.J. Pronovost, M.W. Jenckes, T. Dorman, E. Garrett, M.J. Breslow, B.A. Rosenfeld et al., Organizational characteristics of intensive care units related to outcomes of abdominal aortic surgery, *Journal of the American Medical Association* **281**(14) (1999), 1310–1317.
[99] J. Rasmussen, The role of error in organizing behaviour, *Ergonomics* **33**(10/11) (1990), 1185–1199.
[100] J. Rasmussen, Human factors in a dynamic information society: Where are we heading? *Ergonomics* **43**(7) (2000), 869–879.
[101] J. Rasmussen, A.M. Pejtersen and L.P. Goodstein, *Cognitive Systems Engineering*, New York: Wiley, 1994.
[102] N.K. Rathlev, J. Chessare, J. Olshaker, D. Obendorfer, S.D. Mehta, T. Rothenhaus et al., Time series analysis of variables associated with daily mean emergency department length of stay, *Annals of Emergency Medicine* **49**(3) (2007), 265–271.
[103] J. Reason, *Human Error*, Cambridge: Cambridge University Press, 1990.
[104] J. Reason, *Managing the Risks of Organizational Accidents*, Burlington, Vermont: Ashgate, 1997.

[105] J. Reason, Human error: Models and management, *BMJ* **320**(7237) (2000), 768–770.
[106] P.R. Reid, W.D. Compton, J.H. Grossman and G. Fanjiang, *Building a Better Delivery System. A New Engineering/Health Care Partnership*. Washington, D.C.: The National Academies Press, 2005.
[107] D. Resnick, The Jesica Santillan tragedy: Lessons learned, *The Hastings Center Report* **33**(4) (2003), 15–20.
[108] K.H. Roberts and R. Bea, Must accidents happen? Lessons from high-reliability organizations, *Academy of Management Executive* **15**(3) (2001), 70–78.
[109] K.H. Roberts and R.G. Bea, When systems fail. *Organizational Dynamics* **29**(3) (2001), 179–191.
[110] G.I. Rochlin, Safe operation as a social construct, *Ergonomics* **42**(11) (1999), 1549–1560.
[111] J.M. Rothschild, C.P. Landrigan, J.W. Cronin, R. Kaushal, S.W. Lockley, E. Burdick et al., The Critical Care Safety Study: The incidence and nature of adverse events and serious medical errors in intensive care, *Critical Care Medicine* **33** (2005), 1694–1700.
[112] W. Runciman, P. Hibbert, R. Thomson, T. Van Der Schaaf, H. Sherman and P. Lewalle, Towards an international classification for patient safety: Key concepts and terms, *International Journal for Quality in Health Care* **21**(1) (2009), 18–26.
[113] M.A. Safren and A. Chapanis, A critical incident study of hospital medication errors – Part 1, *Hospitals* **34** (1960), 32–34; 57–66.
[114] M.A. Safren and A. Chapanis, A critical incident study of hospital medication errors – Part 2, *Hospitals* **34** (1960), 53; 65–68.
[115] A.P. Sage and W.B. Rouse, eds, *Handbook of Systems Engineering and Management*, New York: John Wiley & Sons, 1999.
[116] F. Sainfort, B. Karsh, B.C. Booske and M.J. Smith, Applying quality improvement principles to achieve healthy work organizations, *Journal on Quality Improvement* **27**(9) (2001), 469–483.
[117] G. Salvendy, ed., *Handbook of Human Factors and Ergonomics*, (Third ed.), New York, NY: John Wiley & Sons, 2006.
[118] K. Schultz, P. Carayon, A.S. Hundt and S. Springman, Care transitions in the outpatient surgery preoperative process: Facilitators and obstacles to information flow and their consequences, *Cognition, Technology & Work* **9**(4) (2007), 219–231.
[119] K.G. Shojania, The frustrating case of incident-reporting systems, *Quality & Safety in Health Care* **17**(6) (2008), 400–402.
[120] S.M. Shortell, J.E. Zimmerman, R.R. Gillies, J. Duffy, K.J. Devers, D.M. Rousseau et al., Continuously improving patient care: Practical lessons and an assessment tool from the National ICU study, *Quality Review Bulletin* **18**(5) (1992), 150–155.
[121] M.J. Smith and P. Carayon-Sainfort, A balance theory of job design for stress reduction, *International Journal of Industrial Ergonomics* **4**(1) (1989), 67–79.
[122] M.J. Smith and P. Carayon, New technology, automation, and work organization: Stress problems and improved technology implementation strategies, *The International Journal of Human Factors in Manufacturing* **5**(1) (1995), 99–116.
[123] N. Stanton, A. Hedge, K. Brookhuis, E. Salas and H.W. Hendrick, eds, *Handbook of Human Factors and Ergonomics Methods*, Boca Raton, FL: CRC Press, 2004.
[124] E.R. Stucky, Prevention of medication errors in the pediatric inpatient setting, *Pediatrics* **112** (2003), 431–436.
[125] V.C. Tam, S.R. Knowles, P.L. Cornish, N. Fine, R. Marchesano and E.E. Etchells, Frequency, type and clinical importance of medication history errors at admission to hospital: A systematic review, *Canadian Medical Association Journal* **173**(5) (2005), 510–515.
[126] The World Alliance For Patient Safety Drafting Group, H. Sherman, G. Castro, M. Fletcher, on behalf of The World Alliance for Patient Safety, M. Hatlie et al., Towards an international classification for patient safety: The conceptual framework, *International Journal for Quality in Health Care* **21**(1) (2009), 2–8.
[127] E.J. Thomas, D.M. Studdert, H.R. Burstin, E.J. Orav, T. Zeena, E.J. Williams et al., Incidence and types of adverse events and negligent care in Utah and Colorado, *Medical Care* **38**(3) (2000), 261–271.
[128] J. Varon and P.E. Marik, Clinical information systems and the electronic medical record in the intensive care unit, *Current Opinion in Critical Care* **8** (2002), 616–624.
[129] K.J. Vicente, What does it take? A case study of radical change toward patient safety, *Joint Commission Journal on Quality and Safety* **29**(11) (2003), 598–609.
[130] C. Vincent, P. Aylin, B.D. Franklin, A. Holmes, S. Iskander, A. Jacklin et al., Is health care getting safer? *British Medical Journal* **337**(7680) (2008), 1205–1207.
[131] C. Vincent, S. Taylor-Adams, E.J. Chapman, D. Hewett, S. Prior, P. Strange et al., How to investigate and analyse clinical incidents: Clinical risk unit and association of litigation and risk management protocol, *BMJ, 320* (2000), 777–781.
[132] C. Vincent, S. Taylor-Adams and N. Stanhope, Framework for analysing risk and safety in clinical medicine, *BMJ* **316**(7138) (1998), 1154–1157.

[133] H. Wald and K. Shojania, Prevention of misidentifications, in: *Making Health Care Safer: A Critical Analysis of Patient Safety Practices*, D.G. Shojania, B.W. Duncan, K.M. McDonald and R.M. Wachter, eds, Washington, DC: Agency for Healthcare Research and Quality, AHRQ publication 01-E058, 2001, pp. 491–503.
[134] R.L. Wears, S.J. Perry, E. Eisenberg, L. Murphy, M. Shapiro, C. Beach et al., *Transitions in care: signovers in the emergency department,* Paper presented at the Human Factors and Ergonomics Society 48th Annual Meeting, New Orleans, LA, 2004.
[135] R.L. Wears, S.J. Perry, M. Shapiro, C. Beach, P. Croskerry and R. Behara, *Shift changes among emergency physicians: best of times, worst of times,* Paper presented at the Human Factors and Ergonomics Society 47th Annual Meeting, Denver, CO, 2003.
[136] K.E. Weick and R.E. Quinn, Organizational change and development, *Annual Review of Psychology* **50** (1999), 361–386.
[137] K.E. Weick and K.M. Sutcliffe, *Managing the Unexpected: Assuring High Performance in an Age of Complexity*, San Francisco, CA: Jossey-Bass, 2001.
[138] C.R. Weinert and H.J. Mann, The science of implementation: Changing the practice of critical care, *Current Opinion in Critical Care* **14**(4) (2008), 460–465.
[139] T.B. Wetterneck, K.A. Skibinski, T.L. Roberts, S.M. Kleppin, M. Schroeder, M. Enloe et al., Using failure mode and effects analysis to plan implementation of Smart intravenous pump technology, *American Journal of Health-System Pharmacy* **63** (2006), 1528–1538.
[140] J.R. Wilson and N. Corlett, eds, *Evaluation of Human Work*, (Third ed.), Boca Raton, FL: CRC Press, 2005.
[141] K. Zink, Ergonomics in the past and the future: From a German perspective to an international one, *Ergonomics, 43*(7) (2000), 920–930.

Pascale Carayon is Procter & Gamble Bascom Professor in Total Quality and Associate Chair in the Department of Industrial and Systems Engineering and the Director of the Center for Quality and Productivity Improvement (CQPI) at the University of Wisconsin-Madison. She received her Engineer diploma from the Ecole Centrale de Paris, France, in 1984 and her Ph.D. in Industrial Engineering from the University of Wisconsin-Madison in 1988. Her research examines systems engineering, human factors and ergonomics, sociotechnical engineering and occupational health and safety, and has been funded by the Agency for Healthcare Research and Quality, the National Science Foundation, the National Institutes for Health (NIH), the National Institute for Occupational Safety and Health, the Department of Defense, various foundations and private industry. Dr. Carayon leads the Systems Engineering Initiative for Patient Safety (SEIPS) at the University of Wisconsin-Madison (http://cqpi.engr.wisc.edu/seips_home).

Dr. Kenneth Wood is a Professor of Medicine and Anesthesiology at the University of Wisconsin School of Medicine and Public Health where he is the Senior Director of Medical Affairs, Director of Critical Care Medicine/Respiratory Care and The Trauma and Life Support Center at University Hospital. He received his undergraduate degree from Lehigh University in 1979, medical degree from the Philadelphia College of Osteopathic Medicine in 1983, and completed training/certification in Internal Medicine and Critical Care Medicine. In addition to his administrative responsibilities and actively staffing as an Intensivist in the Trauma and Life Support Unit, Dr. Wood's research interests are related to Critical Care outcomes, the impact of technology on quality, patient safety and cost-effectiveness and have been funded by the Agency for Healthcare Research and Quality.

Information Knowledge Systems Management 8 (2009) 47–69
DOI 10.3233/IKS-2009-0135
IOS Press

Chapter 4

Aging: Adding complexity, requiring skills

Christine K. Cassel, Michelle Johnston-Fleece and Siddharta Reddy
E-mail: ccassel@abim.org

Abstract: The role of systems in addressing the needs of elderly and chronically ill populations remains a far from universal way of thinking, much less practice, in health care. Re-engineering the current fragmented system to align providers, patients and payment models to facilitate proactive management of conditions associated with advanced age and/or one or more chronic diseases – rather than responding to costly consequences of a health care system optimized for acute care conditions – will be a major challenge for all stakeholders. There are, however, promising success stories that are taking place in the United States today that may provide a model for improvement. The authors define the issues faced by the health care providers and payers that arise when providing care for the elderly and those with chronic conditions – issues that threaten to overwhelm the financial and human health care resources that exist to serve these populations. They define innovative ways of thinking about systems of care, and provide examples of unique systems that have applied theory into practice. These successful leaders may offer lessons in proactively managing complex health conditions, overcoming communication barriers and using technology to complement the necessary human touch that is essential to health care delivery.

1. Introduction

The term "system" can refer to many different things. In the arena of chronic illness and an aging population a system can mean information transmittal, shared accountability or human systems. Walker Percy, a physician who never practiced medicine because he contracted tuberculosis soon after graduating from medical school in 1941, spent years in a sanatorium where he read deeply in philosophy and literature, and became a visionary novelist. He lived out the rest of his life in New Orleans writing novels, including a futuristic apocalyptic vision titled *Love in the Ruins*. In it he imagined an electronic tool called "More's Qualitative Quantitative Ontological Lapsometer." The lapsometer would be waved over the head of a patient who had a complex mental illness and reveal the diagnosis [58]. If we had such a lapsometer for physical illness in the contemporary age we might drastically reduce unnecessary hospitalizations, painful and risky laboratory tests, adverse consequences of medications and medical complications for the elderly and chronically ill. The lapsometer cannot be imitated by our contemporary technology, however advanced; it must be replaced by expertise and human interaction. But that expertise and that human interaction can indeed be better linked by information systems and by highly functioning, well-engineered systems of human expectations, team role function and effective feedback processes. These types of systems are the most vitally important to providing better and more cost-effective care for an aging population.

Chronic illness is the biggest challenge to the health care system in the United States and in all developed countries, as well as many developing countries where public health advances have prevented early deaths and modern medicine is available to some. The lives that have been extended often are people who live with chronic illness. Research shows that access to modern medical technology has made

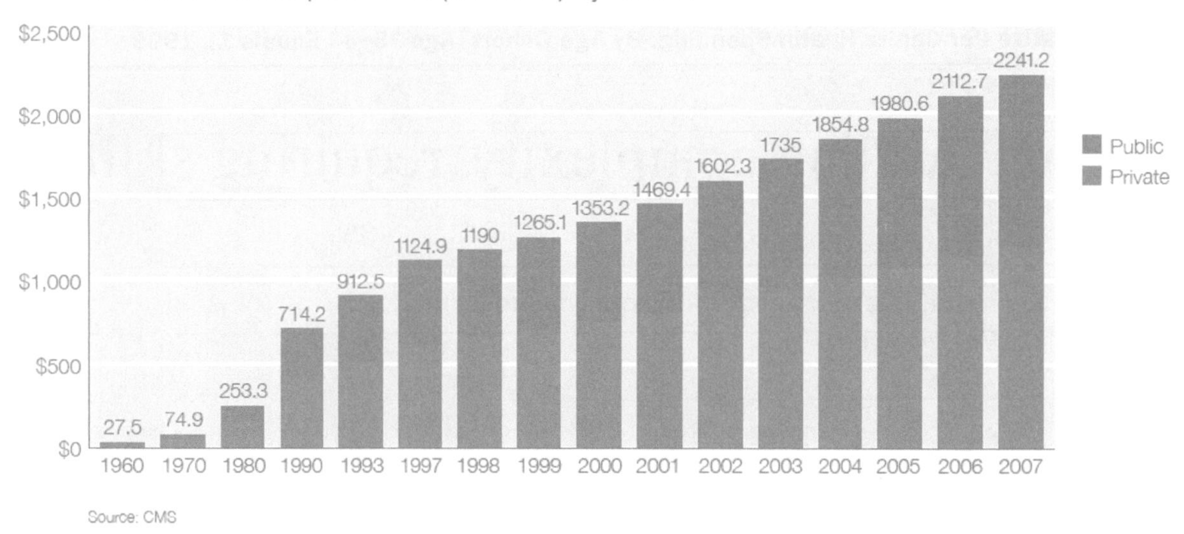

Fig. 1. Source: Partnership to Fight Chronic Disease. (2009). *2009 almanac of chronic disease*. Retrieved May 19, 2009, from http://www.fightchronicdisease.org/pdfs/2009_PFCDAlmanac.pdf.

actually only a small contribution to the increased longevity of modern civilization [10]. Environmental and social factors have much more powerful effects on healthy aging than do medical treatments. The MacArthur Foundation Research Network on Successful Aging, an international and interdisciplinary group, worked from 1984–1994 developing evidence for the framework of "successful aging" [65]. They estimated that 70 percent of healthy aging is related to socio-economic status, education, lifestyle behaviors and other characteristics of civilized society, with only 30 percent due to a combination of genetics and medical treatment. While modern medicine is not the primary cause of increased longevity, the success stories of longer life spans result, however, in dramatic increases in medical costs. Here too there are some counter-intuitive realities resulting from health services research. The dramatically rising cost of health care in the United States (see Fig. 1) is not primarily due to demographic factors, such as the aging of society, but much more directly related to the increasing use of specialists and the intensity of medical care per person [3].

While it is true that cost of health care per capita increases as individuals age (see Fig. 2), the costs of care increase more dramatically with the number of chronic conditions per individual (see Fig. 3) [14]. Nearly all of the growth in Medicare spending is due to beneficiaries with five or more chronic illnesses rather than simply the aging of the population, which, as baby boomers age, will have a relatively modest effect on rising costs [20,25,75]. In Medicare's budget, more than 92 percent of costs are attributable to beneficiaries with three or more chronic conditions [75]; in fact, 61.5 percent of Medicare's costs are related to only 10 percent of beneficiaries [20]. Chronic conditions are costly in the private insurance market as well. In a recent analysis of the 8.5 million members of Kaiser Permanente it appears that 80 percent of the costs are related to 10 percent of patients and 75 percent of costs are associated with chronic conditions [34]. So the tremendous costs and intensity of care largely relate to a small but significant number of people who have enormous health care needs. As we look at the advances in systems of care, a major question is: to what degree can systems of care reduce these costs and produce better outcomes?

The United States is moving to an emphasis on measurement of quality of care, linked to both public reporting and payment rewards for higher quality, sometimes called value-based purchasing [30]. The

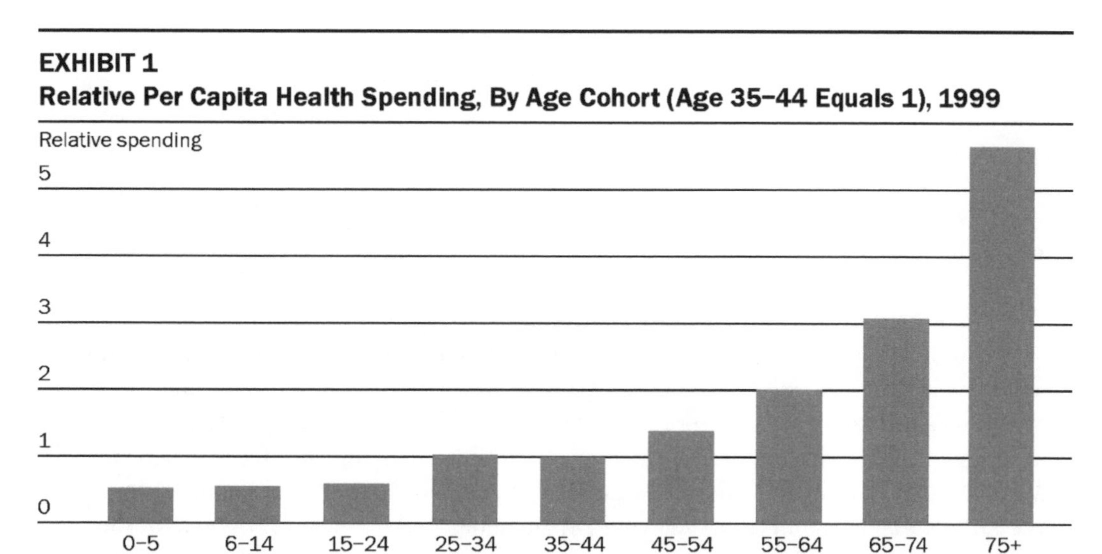

Fig. 2. Source: Reinhardt, U. E. (2003). Does The Aging Of The Population Really Drive The Demand For Health Care? *Health Affairs, 22*(6), 27–39.

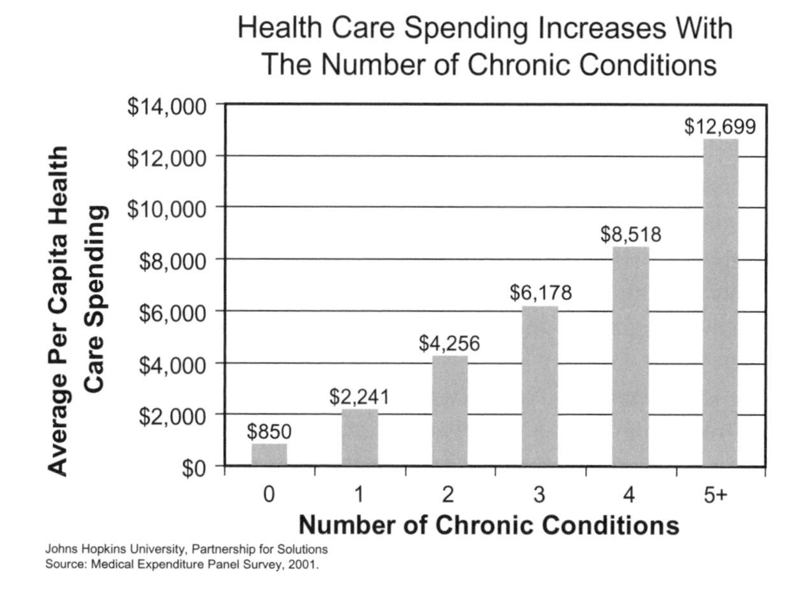

Fig. 3. Source: Partnership for Solutions. (2001). *Chronic Conditions: Making the Case for Ongoing Care.* Retrieved July 1, 2009, from: http://www.partnershipforsolutions.org/DMS/files/chronicbook2004.pdf.

combination of public reporting and financial incentives is hoped to advance both lower costs and better quality of care. The world of measurement, however, still is too often limited to process and outcome measures related to specific diseases and not to the overall function and quality of life for patients. This focus is important for a number of reasons. Management of individual conditions, such as diabetes, hypertension and heart failure, have specific markers that can and should be used to advance the clinician's understanding of what needs to be done for a patient. But what is often most important is not chasing lab values, but rather understanding the impact of the multiple conditions, plus their treatments, on the patient's life and function. This is a key principle from geriatric medicine that has yet to be truly integrated into the chronic disease model as it is applied to modern assessment of quality of care.

2. Systems thinking in health care

Systems thinking can make extraordinary contributions to improving health care, as has already been demonstrated in hospital safety and medication management. Rouse has aptly described health care as a "complex adaptive system" that includes many different players and forces, and therefore cannot be thought of as a hierarchical function [64]. This observation is vividly true in the arena of geriatric care and chronic illness, where focusing on single conditions can neglect others, where focusing only on known conditions can lead to missed diagnoses, where patients and families need to be viewed as integral to the care management team, and where financial incentives – especially fee for service, that is, volume-oriented rather than value-oriented payments – can lead to very poor outcomes and higher costs. Among the "independent agents" in Rouse's portrait of the health care landscape are patients, families and communities. Also included are the multiple specialist physicians and multiple non-physician providers who will come in contact with the patient. How to organize these agents for the best possible quality and affordability is a big challenge in the fragmented "non-system" we currently have.

Systems have much promise in the challenge of aging and chronic illness, but must be seen hand-in-hand with the attributes of individuals and their expertise in geriatrics. However, systems thinking cannot describe all aspects of the real world exactly because its goal is to develop "mental models" that attempt to describe the real world through different perspectives. In the field of health care, individual output and personal responsibility are the most common markers of a successful system, so systems thinking in this context presents the following challenges [69]:

- Systems are designed to produce a certain amount of output. That is, whatever the system outputs, is what it was designed to produce.
- Systems are composed of several different people, processes and things that interact with one another and affect the functioning of one another, as well as the entire system. This may be conscious and intentional, or not.
- Systems are designed to maximize output of the system, not of the individual components. (This is why an individual "working harder" does not actually change output or improve safety.)
- Systems have many dimensions of output (e.g. safety, patient-centeredness, efficiency, etc.), but in health care it is not possible to maximize all dimensions. Instead, one can optimize a dimension based on the needs and capacity of individual stakeholders.
- Systems are usually open and are affected by or dependent upon external factors. Systems may also feed other or larger systems. Systems exist within subsystems and are a part of micro-, macro- and mega-systems.
- Systems are complex and will produce unintended consequences.

2.1. Clinical microsystems

One system theory that has been useful in terms of health care is that of clinical microsystems (www.clinicalmicrosystems.org), which are defined as the frontline units that provide most health care to the most people. The microsystem is composed of the smallest replicable unit that provides safe, efficient care to a patient, who is at the center of every clinical microsystem. For instance, the microsystem includes the patient, family, care team, the building or structure where the care team and patient meet and the technology that supports the provision of care. The microsystem changes from the perspective of the patient as he or she moves from one setting to the next, for example, when receiving care from a specialist. Since the microsystem serves as the building block of larger systems, such as hospitals, the quality of care can not be greater than the inherent quality of the microsystem, akin to strength of a chain being dependent upon its weakest link. Quality improvement is built in to microsystems. That is, the purpose of staff is to provide and improve care, which is accomplished through measurement of processes and outcomes and implementing rapid cycle improvements [52].

2.2. Care transitions

An area in which important system functions are needed is within the delivery network. With few exceptions, the United States health care system is fragmented into silos of care delivery by different sources of reimbursement, different kinds of expertise and often missing connections between different components of the care system. These missing connections often lead to medical errors of many sorts, so much so that the term "care transitions" has become a technical term for health services researchers who have tried through research demonstration projects to identify additional health professionals to bridge these gaps [15,17,49–51].

A growing body of scholarship has identified these care transitions as high risk events for medical errors including missing needed checkups and performing redundant, unindicated, or contraindicated tests or treatments [17,50]. Transitions are events in the trajectory of patient care where the responsibility for the patient transfers from one set of providers to another (called "hand-offs" when this occurs within one setting, such as shift changes among nurses or doctors in the hospital) or between care settings, such as discharge from hospital to a home, rehabilitation facility or nursing home. To think about the delivery network, one has to first imagine the acute care setting, the hospital and then all of the physician specialists who have some connection to a patient with multiple complex illnesses. Most of these physicians do not have any information or coordination function with one another and many of them do not have any connection with the hospital in which a patient may experience a hospitalization [50]. Physician specialists have even less interaction with residential or non-residential rehabilitation centers, nursing homes, assisted living centers and home care within the community [16].

The risk of error is related to gaps in information as well as lapses in accountability. Patients admitted to hospitals through ERs or discharged to nursing homes all too often are not accompanied by complete records of medical conditions, medications, allergies, personal preferences and family situations. Without stored electronic data systems, even a written "transfer note" or "discharge summary" is likely to be incomplete, especially for older patients with multiple conditions and multiple clinical specialists.

In all of these settings, services are reimbursed by different sources (the closer one gets to the home or community setting the more likely there is no reimbursement) and hospitals have no consistent way of communicating all of the information about a patient who is transferred from a hospital to a nursing home [16]. Similarly, when patients become ill at a nursing home and the staff dials 911 to summon an ambulance, the information that accompanies that patient to the hospital is very limited. What is missing could include vitally important medication and historical information; information about the patient's family and personal physician where important information could be gained; and very importantly, it could include advance directives and other personal information about that patient's preference for aggressive or non-aggressive care in the event of a life-threatening illness. Most often, such information is not available as a patient moves from silo to silo or specialist to specialist.

It is important in this context to consider not only that information transfer is needed, but accountability transfer is also needed. How to establish this accountability transfer is a major challenge for health policy. Information technology can create the conditions under which the accountability for the care of an individual patient can be established but that accountability does not happen automatically just with the transfer of information.

2.3. Chronic Care Model

Edward Wagner developed the Chronic Care Model in 1998 to address the health care needs of individuals and families dealing with chronic illness. Wagner contends that traditional primary care is suited to populations with acute care needs where care is sought due to symptoms of illness that can be addressed in short visits. The visit is supported by information from laboratory tests, and the patient follows up on any additional care. Such an organization is ill equipped to accommodate continuous health needs of the chronically ill who need the focus to be placed on prevention and worsening of conditions. Wagner thus proposed a comprehensive system change that emphasizes high quality care rather than simply relying on cost reduction as an indicator of better care. The components of the model include *self-management support* so that patients gain the skills and confidence to maintain their own health; *decision support* based on proven guidelines that providers can use to plan care; *delivery system design* to ensure that all providers have clear roles in the care of patients and have the information needed to carry out and follow-up on those processes; *clinical information systems*, such as a registry, that allow providers to track individuals or populations; *organization of health care* to coordinate providers and help ensure the creation of an efficient care delivery environment; and finally, a *community* of aligned providers, patients and policies to ensure a well-functioning system of care. This model in itself has been a major breakthrough and is a key component of the contemporary patient-centered medical home movement (to be discussed later) [81].

2.4. Patches on the fragmented non-system: Building bridges across the gaps

Recognizing the need for better coordination of care has led to a number of different approaches toward providing information transfer at key junctures or specifically trained professionals to fill a missing role making needed connections.

These approaches are partial fixes to the problem, but they cannot create "patches" to cover every transition. The best context for minimizing transition-related errors and waste have been integrated health systems – with care settings that include home care, community facilities and acute care hospitals linked by a single electronic data system. All providers seeing a patient have concurrent access to accurate data and the patient and family would also be able to see this information to ensure they are as well informed as possible. Integrated systems do exist in the United States (such as Mayo Clinic, Health Partners, Group Health and Kaiser Permanente) but are far from common.

The systems that have the greatest capability to respond to the complexity of the needs of an aging population are those who explicitly see themselves as systems, usually including employed or contracted multispecialty physician workforce, other health professionals as part of the team, one or more hospitals, nursing homes, rehabilitation centers and homecare programs. The largest of these systems, Kaiser Permanente, has excellent outcomes in quality measures for chronic illness in their Medicare population.

They employ multidisciplinary geriatric expert teams, have a unitary medical record throughout the system and innovative approaches to engaging patients, families, non-physician providers and communities in the process of care. Geisinger Health System is much smaller, and has less direct oversight of the long term care sector, but as the dominant system in a large region of Pennsylvania it has been able to work closely with both its employed physicians and community providers to achieve outstanding improvements in safety, quality and reduction of unnecessary hospitalizations and – especially – readmissions. Denver Health is a public health – oriented care system that has a large Medicaid and dual-eligible population. They have re-engineered care using the "lean" model of Toyota to make optimal use of limited resources. They have in common with other successful systems a shared, unitary electronic record with meaningful decision-support tools, salaried physicians, interdisciplinary teams and significant roots in the communities they serve. Intermountain Healthcare shares these same attributes, and has engineered care delivery in non-traditional ways, relying on care mostly provided by non-physician providers, but overseen by physicians with expertise in chronic care management. Mayo Clinic has a long tradition of salaried physicians and an explicit culture of patient-centeredness that leads to communication and coordination for the complex patients who receive continuing care there. Their commitment extends to using their electronic data to inform ongoing research for evidence based care, and continuous maintenance of provider knowledge and skills.

But these large systems, and a few others like them, are not the primary context for medical care in the United States. If they were, the challenge of improving quality and affordability in care for an aging population would be easier to envision. But the vast majority of care in our country is provided by small practices. Patients have no one who is responsible for coordinating care between different specialists or with community resources and long term care providers, which leads to both underuse and overuse problems, risk of errors because of missing information and the risk of worse outcomes for the patient.

Our challenge is how to create the advantages of such integrated systems with the nearly 50 percent of U.S. physicians in small practices with one or two physicians [43] whose patients are seen by multiple specialists who do not communicate with one another or with community resources such as home care, nursing homes, social service agencies and the patient and family.

3. What does it take? Critical components of a system for effective care of complex chronic illness

3.1. Community engagement as health care

Building on and parallel to the MacArthur Network on Successful Aging, Linda Fried, a geriatrician at John Hopkins University, established an extensive research network to examine the predictors and correlations with frailty and advanced age. "Frailty" has become a specific biomedical/social term for a condition of elderly patients that reduces resilience, increases risk of disabling events, such as falls and fractures, and is significantly associated with the need for assistive services, long-term care and mortality. There is now extensive research evidence that activity of all kinds is associated with reduced risk of developing frailty [5,11,24,60,66]. Physical activity, including moderate walking and other kinds of physical activity is what we most commonly think of as related to successful aging and indeed it even seems to correlate with reducing the likelihood of developing cognitive impairment and Alzheimer's disease [37,79]. It has also been shown that modest resistance training with even three to five pound free weights can increase postural stability, as well as muscle strength [61,84]. One of the conditions that occur with frailty is referred to as sarcopenia, which is quite literally a reduction in the size and number of muscle cells. As elderly people become frailer, they become less able to exercise physically as muscles actually shrink and weaken; even with an active older person, bed rest for even a few days can decrease muscle strength. This observation is the source of the approaches of the Acute Care for the Elderly (ACE) units, which work with older people when they are hospitalized to maintain muscle strength, balance and postural stability even while being treated for significant illnesses such as pneumonia, heart failure or post-operative care [55,56]. This approach has been applied with success to surgical interventions in elderly patients, such as hip fracture treatment [22,42].

In addition to physical activity, mental and social activities have also been linked to reducing risk for frailty. It has become a truism now that doing crossword puzzles is good for the aging brain. This is not specific to crossword puzzles, but is applied to any problem-solving activity or new learning [79]. Passive activities, such as watching television, do not engage the brain in problem solving, while activities such as crossword or Sudoku puzzles, learning a new language, playing bridge or chess, are linked with reduced risk of cognitive impairment and frailty [67].

The most difficult to measure and yet equally important is social activity and engagement. It has been found that social isolation also increases one's risk of frailty and early mortality [4,6]. Thus, senior centers, volunteering and other such activities are not just ways for seniors to "give back to society," but are also actually good for their health. This insight was the most striking finding that emerged from the work of Fried and her group in Baltimore in the development of the "Experience Corps" of older people who engage in organized volunteer activity in troubled public schools and other kinds of socially worthy activities [12,27,28,31,39,73].

What does all this community activity have to do with systems of health care? As the focus on health care for older people, and both the reduction of incidents and consequences of multiple chronic illnesses becomes more and more of a challenge for our nation, the health care system will need to find a way to take advantage of these extremely important but non-medical observations.

First, ambulatory and primary care organizations that care for older people who live in the community (such as the newly proposed patient-centered medical home) will need to find ways to engage with community resources to promote physical, mental and social activity among their patients. The data show that these interventions can be every bit as important as the correct medical management of these conditions [26,38,78,79].

Second, for patients who are in nursing homes, the nursing homes should be connected similarly with community resources to offer nursing home residents opportunities for physical, mental and social engagement to the degree that they are capable.

Third, in hospitals interdisciplinary teams all need greater awareness of the factors related to risk of complications for older people. Several of these concepts are derived from the patient safety world – systems are important to reduce the risk of medication errors, but as important are the concerted multiple daily events that could help or hinder the recovery of an older person. When an independent, 85-year-old woman develops pneumonia and a cough, that dramatic cough could lead to a vertebral crush fracture causing extreme pain and inability for her to move around and care for herself. She will now need a combination of antibiotic and pulmonary therapy, as well as stabilization and pain treatment for her back pain. A strong temptation is to hospitalize this woman and restrict her to bed rest. Yet, if the pain is treated adequately and she can be helped out of bed and into a chair and simply walked up and down the hospital corridor once, or optimally twice, each day, that could mean the difference between her discharge to home or her discharge to a nursing home. Nursing home placement would mean ultimately losing her independence, causing a dramatic reduction in her quality of life and much greater cost to society. Furthermore, adequate pain treatment for this older woman requires geriatric and palliative care expertise to understand, not only how to treat the pain, but to do so without reducing her ability to manage and avoid serious complications, such as constipation, which can lead to fecal impaction and the need for acute abdominal surgery.

3.2. Teams

The most important thing this type of care takes is more than one clinician. This approach cannot be managed by a physician alone, or even by physician and nurse alone, in the traditional medical model. It goes beyond the conventional concept of the "physician extender." The issue is not that the physician is too busy and therefore his or her skills need to be extended. Different team members have different kinds of expertise, which are as important to the patient management as medical expertise. Teams need the essential expertise of multiple medical specialties, including a geriatrician or generalist physician with comprehensive care and team skills, but there will inevitably be need for deep knowledge in surgical specialties, physical medicine and rehabilitation, psychiatry and neurology and others. Interaction, information exchange and shared decision making must also occur among all of these physicians. Here is one place where health care in the United States desperately needs better systems.

Secondly, nursing is essential. The nurse is trained to be a patient educator and to evaluate patients' experience of illness, a key component of the patient-centered approach outlined in Wagner's Chronic Care Model [82], In addition, as advanced illness leads to disability, it impacts function and social vulnerability; therefore, social work expertise is essential.

Pharmacy is another essential expertise, since even the best-trained physician cannot be in total command of the ever changing knowledge base of pharmaceutical therapies. Experts in pharmacy are needed for patients with multiple chronic conditions who take multiple medications in order to identify and highlight risks of medication interactions and adverse events. Information systems can dramatically increase the accuracy of these interactions.

Finally, patients and their families need to be linked to multiple providers of care at the community level, including those we usually consider health care workers, such as rehabilitation centers, physical and occupational therapy, etc.; but also those we may not think of as health care providers, such as local centers on aging, faith-based organizations and community centers, or even neighborhood groups.

3.3. Systems in support of expertise

Not every graduate of every training program in primary care, nursing and social work is well equipped to deal with the specific challenges presented by an aging population. Scientific research in aging – called gerontology – has dramatically advanced in the biological, medical, social and psychological arenas. Much more is known about intrinsic factors related to the aging process and how they interact with illness. Older people are more vulnerable to age-related conditions (heart disease, cancer, arthritis and osteoporosis, etc.). These conditions, and their treatments, interact with each other and with underlying biological declines related to aging itself. A patient's ability to continue functioning with these illnesses may also depend on underlying biological factors, social situations and mental or emotional conditions related to aging [63,71].

This work is a specialty also requiring extensive knowledge in a broad range of areas. It also requires generalist expertise, and contrasts vividly with the tendency of medicine to become ever more specialized. Physician specialists, who know a great deal about a narrow topic, are needed. But management of older patients with multiple conditions requires the ability to understand complex interacting realities, to manage decision-making in the face of uncertainty and high level communication skills to include patient and family empowerment in the care process. This knowledge is the core of the curriculum of those who specialize in geriatric health care. In medicine, these specialists are geriatricians, but there are also specialists in geriatric psychiatry, nursing and social work. Even some subspecialties, such as oncology, are now developing geriatric subspecialties and some surgical specialists are beginning to focus on geriatrics as an area of special expertise – cancer treatment and surgery need to be different for an 80-year old as compared to a 50-year old [74]. Integrating what is known about inherent changes that occur with the aging process with what is known about the prevalence of illness as one ages, assessing the interaction of acute and chronic illness can dramatically increase the accuracy of diagnosis when changes occur in a patient with chronic illness. Classically, these changes are manifested in what are known as geriatric syndromes [2,32]. Patients suffer from dizziness, cognitive impairment, urinary incontinence, falls and postural instability. These are symptoms, not diseases. These syndromes may be irreversible consequences of an underlying illness, such as Alzheimer's disease or Parkinson's disease. But they also may be treatable manifestations of medication toxicity or even if disease-related, may be ameliorated by appropriate physical therapy, dietary interventions and/or medication. It is not enough to have a simple primary care check-up to make the most accurate diagnosis of these sometimes subtle conditions. It is also not enough to look at "report cards" of "measures of quality" related only to one disease or condition. These are skills of human understanding and system navigation.

Health professionals need to keep up to date, but a given physician or nurse cannot possibly know everything there is to know. Modern systems can support clinician expertise. The best example of systems supporting clinical expertise is decision supports for analyzing difficult situations – ideally at the point of care – in patient interactions. Electronic information systems and health records can be used to identify trends and patterns within an individual patient's care that provide recent and updated evidence to physicians as they make decisions on behalf of that patient's care. Decision support brings electronic research capability to the physician to expand his or her expertise. Decision support has not been a major focus of much of the conversation about electronic medical records and yet needs to be built in to every physician's office practice, and to the expectation of every patient as they interact with the physician. We need to see a time when it is the norm for a patient or a family member to say, "Well, doctor, have you checked the other alternatives online?" This will take a major transition in patients' expectations of physicians and physicians' willingness to acknowledge that it is impossible to be completely knowledgeable about every new advance in medicine. Faced with a difficult challenge in sorting out patients' symptoms, checking an online decision support tool could be a way of adding extraordinary efficiency to the process and reducing the burden of unnecessary testing or errors. Online resources also offer ways to help patients make decisions, with patient-centered decision support, such as that provided by Health Dialog (www.healthdialog.com). Through video interviews and online guided information tours, patients facing difficult decisions about whether to pursue surgery or other medical treatments where evidence is equivocal, can hear from other patients who have been through similar situations and find ways to understand existing evidence so it relates to them and their personal situation.

3.4. Systems in support of patient empowerment

Electronic health records ideally provide extensive information to be shared by all of the physicians involved in a patient's care, but also can be enabled for that information to be provided to the patient in what is sometimes called a Personal Health Record. Here the patient has access to the same information as the physician – all of the medical information in the clinical record, but ideally, translated into actionable data for patient use, such as trend line graphs for blood pressure, blood sugar and other kinds of key personal health information. Electronic health systems, such as the EpicCare EMR model now widely used around the country and most visibly within the Kaiser Permanente system, allow patients to communicate via secure email with their physicians to ask about their symptoms or medications and to schedule themselves appointments for tests or clinician visits. This functionality enables patients with chronic illness to get out of the "illness model" and into a more empowered model, which is exactly what Edward Wagner was seeking in the Chronic Care Model that he described. The patient feels the illness is theirs, they have responsibility to take care of it and with online resources they have tools and information that allows them to feel more able to do that.

3.5. Systems in support of coordination between specialists

Links with other caregivers are essential, and in integrated health systems are an automatic part of an electronic information exchange. But most Americans do not receive care in integrated health systems. More than two-thirds of U.S. physicians practice in groups of five or fewer, and nearly 37 percent are still in solo practice [43]. For all the logic in quality and efficiency demonstrated by large integrated multi-specialty groups – especially if they control or manage their own hospitals and health plans – the culture of American medicine has been dominated by the "small business" model. Patients often see these smaller practices as "more personal," but do not realize that they lack the advantage of care coordination, access and efficiency. The combined challenge of quality measurement and the growing pressure for managing costs more efficiently will be a real challenge to the concept of virtual integrated systems that can take shared accountability for patients. A virtual integrated system is one in which the disparate caregivers who provide any kind of care to a patient share information in a reciprocal fashion with the other caregivers in terms which are actionable and understandable and in which accountability is shared. Policymakers and insurance companies are considering if it is possible to create financing mechanisms that will lead to virtual integration of the "small business" [84]. Reciprocal, actionable and accountable information sharing remain the major challenges for the fragmented small-practice model that still represents more than 75 percent of patient visits in the United States [36]. In addition, the culture of medicine has to expand in ways that geriatric medicine already understands and implements; that is, it needs to link with community resources and other provider information that affect each patient. It is very difficult for a physician in a small practice to find ways to get meaningful information from the nursing home, the rehab center or the homecare service that is caring for a patient who may show up in his or her office one day. Much more likely is a scenario in which the patient shows up in the office and the physician has no way of accessing any external care information. This scenario represents an important challenge in the next stage in improving quality of care – not only providing the tools, but educating providers about the capabilities of these other care systems in order to enlist them in care coordination for patients.

4. Innovative models: What have we learned?

4.1. Program for All-encompassing Care for the Elderly (PACE)

The Program for All-encompassing Care for the Elderly (PACE) model, now supported by Medicare, evolved from a program called On Lok in Chinatown in San Francisco. The first Chinatown On Lok program began in 1971 as a long term care solution that would allow elderly people to remain in their homes, with friends or family, and receive medical care; the idea being to avoid institutionalized care for as long as possible. The term On Lok is a Cantonese phrase meaning "peaceful, happy abode." The program was first funded by Medicaid and Medicare waivers, grants from the Administration on Aging and California's Department of Health Services. Two years later the program was launched, and by 1986 was considered a success and led to the development of the Program for All-encompassing

Elderly (PACE), which is based on the principles of On Lok. Demonstration sites began nationwide in 1986 and care for the 20 sites were operational by the early 1990s. When evaluation of the PACE sites proved successful in terms of cost-effectiveness and meeting the long-term care needs of its residents, the program was made permanent and vastly expanded under the Balanced Budget Act of 1997 [18,19].

PACE operating expenses come from Medicare and Medicaid prepayment for each resident. If a resident is not Medicaid-eligible, then he or she is responsible for that portion. In return, the program provides complete health care services for residents, including home health visits, care management for all chronic care and disabling conditions and a wide range of expenditures that aim to keep residents healthy, independent and out of costly hospital-based care. Residents bear no additional cost for any utilization of needed services [18].

The central tenet of the PACE program is regular clinical care team visits with enrollees at a care center, which occur an average of 10 days each month. The care team includes physicians, nurse practitioners, nurses – an average of 15 interdisciplinary members – who rely on these routine visits to become familiar with residents. In addition to providing necessary services, the team is also able to recognize subtle changes that would otherwise be missed in less frequent ambulatory visits with a primary care provider. It is these early signs that enable proactive measures to be taken that either minimize exacerbations that would otherwise lead to costly hospitalizations as a result of reactive approaches [18].

It has been found that elderly residents who lived without a caregiver did better in PACE than in the general population, suggesting that the PACE staff may be meeting the needs of the elderly and taking the place of caregivers [29]. A study evaluating process and outcome measures among eight PACE sites found that while care was generally above community standards, despite high variability across sites [54].

The concept of seeing a patient's complex set of interrelated conditions, including the social determinants of health, grew out of frustration with attempts at cost containment that focused on managing single diseases. The disease management model would entail, for instance, one care provider managing a panel of patients with diabetes. However, a number of those patients may also have other chronic diseases that are either not addressed, or addressed by another disease management program. These different care providers will likely not communicate with each other or with the primary care provider. Thus there is no one centrally managing all aspects of the patients health needs.

4.2. Green House

The Green House is a group home concept that aims to replace the structure and culture of a traditional nursing home with one that promotes a sense of community, independence and improved quality of life for residents. These goals are achieved, most noticeably, by creating a physically smaller space where 8–12 elderly individuals live and receive care from certified nursing assistants, known as *Shahbazim*, who are supervised by a *guide* (or administrator). In fact, many of the terms and clinical features associated with institutions have been renamed, minimized, or removed to provide residents with a more home-like feel. For instance, builders are directed to use residential fixtures instead of those seen in nursing homes. Residents, family and staff make interior design decisions together and residents are encouraged to bring their own furniture. Meals are served at a dining table rather than in a dining hall, and meal times themselves are completely flexible. The Shahbazim are also responsible for cooking, cleaning, laundry, shopping for household supplies and being available as a resource for the residents. Green Houses also seek to prevent boredom and loneliness by encouraging residents to participate in daily activities, such as preparing meals, caring for pets and gardening; but also by involving residents in decisions concerning their care. Multiple Green Houses situated near one another comprise a nursing home equivalent. They must also meet minimum data sets (MDS) that ensure quality of care. An extended care team makes regular visits to support the residents' health care needs, but do not reside there, which again reinforces the sense of a home instead of an institution. The first site was established in Tupelo, Mississippi in 2002 by Mississippi Methodist Senior Services. The site consisted of four Green Houses with a total of 40 residents from nursing facilities or assisted living centers. The residents who volunteered to participate were similar in terms of disability, gender, levels of activities of daily living and other respects, to residents who remained at the traditional nursing facilities [62].

A two-year, quasi-experimental (non-randomized) study compared the Tupelo, Mississippi Green House with two traditional nursing home sites in the area, and measured 11 areas including resident quality of life and satisfaction, health and functional status and quality of care. The Green House residents fared better than the comparison residents with statistically significant self-reported quality of life in nine of 11 domains, such as privacy, dignity, autonomy, food enjoyment, individuality and satisfaction. Furthermore, the Green House group had lower incidence of decline in activities of daily living. Green House resident quality of care was equal to traditional nursing home care [35].

4.3. Veterans Affairs innovation

The U.S. Department of Veterans Affairs (VA) has also trialed variations of all-inclusive care, including PACE, among its nursing home eligible veteran population. A three year study, with 386 veterans enrolled, compared three models of care: VA as sole provider; a VA-community PACE partnership where PACE managed care; and VA as care manager with PACE as the care provider. It was found that 53 percent of veterans in the model where VA was sole provider used adult day health care (ADHC) while patients in the other two models all used ADHC. This is obvious given that regular health visits are central to the operation of the PACE program. Routine interaction with staff drives information to other providers should additional care be needed, regardless of who acts as the manager. Hospital or outpatient utilization did not differ six months prior to and six months after enrollment in any model of all-inclusive care. While nursing home use was increased, permanent placement remained low, and 92 percent of enrollees still in all-inclusive care remained in the community [83].

Another VA program that targets frail and elderly veterans by bringing care providers directly into the home is known as Home-based Primary Care. The program specifically targets chronically ill patients who can benefit from in-home geriatric care, but where such care is not covered by either Medicare or Medicaid. An interdisciplinary care team addresses the medical, social and rehabilitation needs of the population and ensures that care maintains continuity, is coordinated with other providers and utilizes a wide range of services to meet the patients' needs. This care is provided until the end of life, does not require the patient's condition to improve, and does not provide intensive care. However, a patient may leave the program due to nursing home placement or if he moves from the limited geographic area served by the program. While home-based care is a primary goal, reducing length of stay for needed hospitalizations is a complimentary goal. In fact, patients enrolled in this program experienced 27 percent fewer hospital admissions and 69 percent fewer inpatient days. The program must follow clinical guidelines for disease management, meeting MDS standards, and assess caregiver stress. A random sample of patient satisfaction with the program showed that 98 percent rated their care as excellent or very good [21].

The similarities between the successes of these models of elderly care are significant. The Shahbazim in the Green Houses and care teams in the PACE and VA Home-based Care programs engage in regular contact with residents and are thus able to recognize subtle changes in physical or mental status, as well as other issues that arise, and call on appropriate experts early, avoiding costly hospitalizations that would occur if conditions worsened due to neglect. Furthermore, all of these models share the goal of avoiding institutionalized care. That individuals are able to remain in a community setting, and are encouraged to be independent, carry on with daily activities that give them meaning and avoid boredom, improves their overall quality of life. While a cost-saving component is apparent in each of these models, cost does not appear to be the driving force. The underlying philosophy centers around respect for residents, quality of care and radically challenging how care is delivered under the current health care framework.

4.4. Chronic Care Model (CCM) programs

Premier Health Partners in Ohio has focused on diabetes in their implementation of the CCM, with support from the Robert Wood Johnson Improving Chronic Illness Care (ICIC) program and the Institute for Healthcare Improvement (IHI). Using practice guidelines, academic detailing and decision support materials for their clinical staff to use with patients, they increased their patient population with a glycosylated hemoglobin (HbA_{1c}) of 7 percent or lower from 42 percent to 70 percent within three years, among other positive outcomes. Furthermore, they instituted self-management support (patient education); delivery system redesign (practice teams of physicians and nurses) to monitor diabetes flowsheets; and clinical information systems (medical record review) to inform physicians on patients with poor control. Finally, recognition of outcomes (annual bonuses for diabetes exceeding performance measures) by an insurer provided support for continued efforts and improvement [7].

HealthPartners Medical Group (HPMG) in Minneapolis also joined with support from ICIC-IHI and implemented four of the six components of the CCM. They managed diabetes with self-management support (training from diabetic resource nurses), decision support (guidelines, education updates and support teams), clinical information systems (registry to generate reminders and quarterly reports) and delivery system design (practice teams, group visits and case management). As a result of these efforts, in one year HPMG diabetic patients lowered their average HbA_{1c} from 7.86 percent to 7.47 percent, which was statistically significant. Also, patients with HbA_{1c} levels below 8 percent increased 13 percent and those 10 percent or above fell 30 percent [8].

Clinica Campensina in Denver operates community health centers that serve a primarily uninsured Hispanic population. They instituted several components of the CCM: delivery system design (primary care team with division of labor); clinical information systems (diabetes registry and physician reminders); and patient self-management support (diabetes group visits and education). Clinica Campensina was able reduce mean HbA_{1c} from 10.5 percent to 8.6 percent and increase rates of semiannual diabetic testing from 11 percent to 72 percent in less than three years. In less than 6 months patients with self-management goals increased from 3 percent to 65 percent, eye exams increased from 7 percent to 51 percent and foot exams increased from 15 percent to 76 percent [7].

Kaiser Permanente Northern California (KPNC) serves 3 million people in the area and is managing several chronic diseases using the CCM. Implementing a delivery system design, KPNC divided their chronic care population into three groups: level 1 patients are able to manage their own disease and receive care from a primary care team; level 2 patients, who have difficulty managing their conditions indicated by outcome measures, are assisted by a disease-specific care manager who works with a small group over time to advance them into a level 1 category; level 3 patients are high-users with often complex and multiple chronic diseases that require the use of a comprehensive care manager since multiple conditions are involved. Care managers – a multidisciplinary group of nurses, health educators, pharmacists and others – emphasize education towards self-management and use clinical information systems (registry) to track patients and exchange patient data with primary care teams to also ensure level 1 or 2 patients do not escalate into higher levels [7].

The Chronic Care Model stops short of explicit engagement of geriatric syndromes and outcomes, but the principles are suitable to geriatric care goals. A patient who is struggling with multiple chronic conditions, taking multiple medications and dealing with multiple specialists, diagnostic tests and intermittent treatments does so to improve quality of life, function and – especially in very advanced illness – reduce suffering. It may be that compromises need to be made around the intensity of evaluation or treatment of specific conditions in order to maximize function and those decisions need to be made with patients and sometimes family deeply engaged. Thus the Wagner model is correct in that patients need to be involved in their own care, but not just to empower them in staying as healthy as they can, but also to understand their values in setting limits to health care interventions. The systems question this presents us with is: what kind of systems best empower this sort of management and what kind of health professional training is best suited to successfully manage this kind of system?

4.5. Physician's Orders for Life-Sustaining Treatment (POLST)

An innovative approach to one narrow but important part of this problem – end-of-life care – occurred in Oregon. A unique instrument called a Physician's Orders for Life-Sustaining Treatment (POLST) was developed and tested by internist/ethicist Susan Tolle and her colleagues at the Oregon Health & Science University. The POLST Paradigm is a program that facilitates communication among health care professionals, from emergency medical technicians to hospital staff. It utilizes a bright pink form that communicates more types of medical information, such as antibiotic use, than simple do not resuscitate (DNR) forms. The POLST form is a legally recognized document, considered as physician orders, and is transferable from home to nursing home to rehab center to hospital throughout the entire state, which means states must agree to adopt the program in order for it to be effective. This ensures that if a patient is transferred by hospital in one direction or another, consistent advance directives follow that patient [76].

The National POLST Program Initiative Task Force allows states to operate under one of two POLST programs: *Developing* and *Endorsed*. An *Endorsed* program must meet certain requirements set forth by the task force, including recognition of the form and process by health care professionals, understanding of the patient population, condition and situations for which it is best suited, training for those health care professionals, and that the form itself is easily identifiable and consistent throughout the state. Until those and other requirements have been met, states may adopt elements of the POLST form and program and be considered a *Developing* program. In both cases, states must register with the POLST program online (www.polst.org) and submit regular updates [13].

POLST has been fully implemented by a few states (Oregon, Washington, California, New York, West Virginia, North Carolina and portions of Wisconsin), and is limited to end-of-life decisions such as advance directives, but it illustrates the importance of information systems linked to clinical and legal accountability. Several other states have been recognized as *Developing* programs (Alaska, Hawaii, Montana, Idaho, Utah, Colorado, Texas, Louisiana, Florida, Tennessee, Ohio, Michigan, Missouri, Iowa, Maine, New Hampshire, Georgia, Washington, D.C. and portions of Nevada, North Dakota, Minnesota, Pennsylvania, Wisconsin and Wyoming) [13].

5. Emerging models

5.1. "Disease management" and "care management"

A major and costly Medicare demonstration evaluated the use of commercial care management and disease management companies to achieve the goal of reduced costs and better outcomes through adding professionals (mostly nurses) to help patients negotiate all their specialists and coordinate their care. In a recent study, the fifteen Medicare-funded care coordination demonstration programs that addressed the needs of chronically ill populations were evaluated for reducing total Medicare expenditures or improving the quality of health care services provided and satisfaction of beneficiaries without increasing expenditures. The demonstration, which began in 2002, allowed the chosen programs to define their own treatment and control groups from among their populations covered by Medicare fee-for-service with at least one chronic condition. Eligible conditions included coronary artery disease, congestive heart failure, diabetes and chronic pulmonary disease [59].

Thirteen of the fifteen sites exhibited no significant reductions in hospitalizations and none of the programs reduced Medicare expenditures overall. Only two programs were able to reduce hospitalizations, with only one program achieving statistical significance. Patient surveys of quality of care showed that treatment groups were more likely to remember receiving information about diet and exercise, as well as education to recognize warning signs of their health getting worse. However, surveys of outcomes of care revealed that treatment groups understood the information no better than control groups, and treatment groups reported only a small improvement in functional status, health related quality of life and activities of daily living. Physicians surveyed were overall positive about the intervention, but were mixed on the roles of care coordinators, and did not think it improved patients' self-management skills.

At an estimated cost of $64 million over four years [40], the demonstration was distinctly less than successful. Only two of 15 programs improved care and lowered costs. A closer examination of the two programs that were successful found that their care coordinators had more frequent contact with patients (approaching one coordinator visit per month per patient), than did comparable programs that did not succeed. Patients in these programs were also more likely to receive education on medication use. Coordinators in these programs were able to better manage care transitions and have fewer readmissions by working with local hospitals, which notified programs when their patients were hospitalized. Finally, coordinators in these programs had frequent contact with physicians that established stronger relationships; most other programs lacked this component. When possible, the same coordinator managed all patients from a given physician's practice. These human success factors illustrate the importance of communication in health care programs to manage chronic illness care that made similar programs like PACE successful. That is, frequent interaction with patients in order to establish trust, support patient education and understand patient needs, establishing a communication link with hospitals that is patient-centered and strengthening physician relationships to ensure that patients receive the best coordination assistance.

5.2. Patient-centered medical home

Examining systems of care for chronic illness and aging requires a look at the patient-centered medical home (PCMH). The United States has awakened once again to the fact that primary care services are undervalued and, as of 2009, dramatically reduced in availability to the American public. Physicians, undercompensated and under-supported, are abandoning the field. Young physicians are choosing more lucrative and more highly respected specialties, while primary care, which in many ways is much more difficult and challenging, is perceived as the work of nurses. Indeed, the nursing profession has stepped up in many ways to fill the void in primary care by developing retail clinics in shopping areas, acute centers within the workplace and other such opportunities for the treatment of simple, acute illness. But the primary care that is most sorely needed is not for the easy, treatable, acute condition, but is the ongoing management of multiple chronic conditions, which characterize the aging of the population. The patient-centered medical home model could be a response to this need for complex care management, and at the same time could drive increasing value for geriatrician specialists. There are now numerous demonstrations supported by private payers and by Medicare to promote the idea of the patient-centered medical home. It is unclear at this point whether they will focus specifically on geriatric, high risk and/or high needs populations.

Four primary care specialty societies – American Academy of Family Physicians (AAFP), American Academy of Pediatrics (AAP), American College of Physicians (ACP) and American Osteopathic Association (AOA) – worked together to develop "Joint Principles" for the PCMH in 2007. These principles define the medical home as "a health care setting that facilitates partnerships between individual patients and their personal physicians, and when appropriate, the patient's family" and lay out the key characteristics of a medical home, which are: access to a personal physician; a practice that is physician-directed; whole person orientation of care; integration and/or coordination of care; a focus on quality and safety; enhanced access (i.e., expanded hours and new modes of communication with physicians such as email); and a payment structure that reimburses physician work outside the face-to-face visit, care coordination and health information technology investment, takes into account case mix differences and allows physicians to share in cost savings from reduced hospitalizations and receive bonuses for continuous, measurable quality improvement [1].

Since the Joint Principles were developed, the PCMH concept has gained momentum as a proposed model to increase patient-centeredness and quality of care, as well as to revitalize primary care and improve care for the chronically ill. Driving this momentum is the Patient-Centered Primary Care Collaborative, a coalition of major health care stakeholder groups – including employers, consumer groups, patient quality organizations, health plans, labor unions, hospitals, physicians and others – who have joined together to develop and advance the patient-centered medical home model. Among the over 400 members of the multi-stakeholder collaborative are: IBM, General Motors, FedEx Corporation, AARP, Health Dialog, the American Board of Medical Specialties, CIGNA, Aetna, Kaiser Permanente, the Mayo Clinic's Center for Innovation, Pfizer, the National Committee for Quality Assurance, Alliance for Children and Families, National Association of Community Health Centers, Novartis, UnitedHealthcare, Wal-mart, Society of General Internal Medicine, the National Partnership for Women & Families, WellPoint, the American Academy of Pediatrics and WebMD [57].

The challenge for the PCMH model will be in determining its cost-effectiveness and ensuring that physicians, nurses and other team members have the expertise and the internal systems to actually deliver improved care, support care coordination and reduce costs.

Understanding that systems of care are important, the current qualifying measure set being used to accredit medical practices as "medical homes" that will receive increased payments within most demonstration projects is the National Committee for Quality Assurance (NCQA) "Physician Practice Connections – Patient Centered Medical Home." This tool evaluates an office system, not the performance of the providers, and accreditation can be achieved in one of three tiers based on the level of a practice's alignment with the standards established in the tool [46]. This measure is an update to an earlier version known as the Physician Practice Connections Readiness Survey (PPC-RS), which was also developed by NCQA and based on the concepts of the Chronic Care Model to measure certain components and score them along a 100 point scale [44,45]. The areas that the PPC-PCMH assesses are: access and communication; patient tracking and registry functions; care management; patient self-management support; electronic prescribing; test tracking; referral tracking; performance reporting and improvement; and advanced electronic communications. The PPC-PCMH has been endorsed by the developers of the Joint Principles for the PCMH, other medical specialties groups and the PCPCC for use in medical home demonstration projects. It was also endorsed in September 2008 by the National Quality Forum as medical home system survey [77] and a modified version of the PPC-PCMH is being considered for potential multi-state Medicare PCMH demonstration projects [47].

It is worth noting that the current areas measured by the PPC-PCMH are addressed by different numbers of items and weighted differently in scoring. A substantial portion of the total score relies upon the presence of electronic systems to manage patient information, prescriptions and test results. Practices that meet minimum score and "must-pass element" requirements have also been eligible in pay for performance programs, such as the Bridges to Excellence program [9,48].

Research has shown, however, that physician and office staff self-reported responses on the PPC-PCMH varied in overall agreement, as well as by survey section, with an on-site auditor. Agreement was lowest for care management practices, which play a critical role in ensuring that chronic disease and geriatric populations receive consistent and evidence-based care. Average agreement between physicians and office staff about what they could do was very poor in this area. Also, it was found that physicians and staff tended to under-report the capabilities of their practice systems [68]. These findings suggest a knowledge gap of a practice's system capabilities among staff. Research has also shown that an electronic health record (EHR) may not be needed to have the functioning components of a practice system, such as for care management, but practices with an EHR tend to have more comprehensive practice systems and higher scores on the PPC-PCMH (as a result of the survey components) [70]. According to NCQA, upcoming versions of the PPC-PCMH will address some of the shortcomings of the current version, including more focus on care coordination between primary and specialist care providers [53].

The leaders of the PCMH movement make it clear that these systems are essential if the promise of the medical home is to be achieved. At this time, however, there remain a lot of unanswered questions about whether the PPC-PCMH survey alone can describe what is needed for an adequate medical home. In particular, two dimensions of effective primary care for advanced chronic illness are missing from this picture: the first is physician expertise. Managing complex chronic illness in an aging population requires extensive knowledge in multiple medical, as well as other, disciplines. This is why geriatrics, which is even more difficult and challenging than traditional primary care and yet undervalued and underpaid, is attracting even fewer medical students to its ranks [33]. And yet that is the knowledge base that is necessary to make appropriate diagnostic judgments of the multiple functional complaints and symptoms in older people, as well as to know effectively how to work with a team and how to make use of electronic information systems. This set of skills, considered part of "systems-based practice" and "practice-based learning and improvement," are two of the six core competencies currently required of U.S. medical training programs, specialty board certification and maintenance of certification. Yet it is clear that many physicians do not have these skills. We see this even with the advance of EHRs. Only four percent of U.S. practices have fully functioning EHRs, which allow for improved clinical decision making by facilitating registry development or denominator-based clinical information systems, for example [23].

In addition to physician expertise, the second component, which as of yet has been poorly and incompletely described in the PCMH movement, is the degree to which physician, nurse and other medical professionals' role definitions will change. The Ambulatory ICU model developed for the

Hotel Employees and Restaurant Employees International Union and Welfare Fund (HEREIU) union demonstrations, are perhaps the most extreme and well-described version of this, where patients with simple, uncomplicated acute illnesses can be managed by nurses and other health professionals, while more complex problems or patients with multiple complex illnesses are managed by physicians with special expertise in that area [41]. On the face of it this appears to be the most cost – effective use of services and can provide true care coordination if the electronic information system, such as medical records and personal health records, are available to all of the members of the team that are caring for the population. Unanswered questions remain about whether small practices that have neither these extensive inter-disciplinary teams nor physicians who demonstrate these advanced skills will be successful in implementing the PCMH model of care for elderly patients with multiple chronic illnesses.

6. Conclusion

This is a time of challenge for the American health care system. As experts have said, we have the best of care in some places – but far from everywhere – and this care is increasingly unaffordable. Each of these models has aspects of the changes that must occur to increase quality and reduce complications for the highest risk patients. The opportunity for leadership now is to extend these learnings broadly so everyone, old and young alike, will benefit.

Acknowledgements

The authors wish to acknowledge the capable editing assistance of Beth Cote.

References

[1] American Academy of Family Physicians, American Academy of Pediatrics, American College of Physicians, & American Osteopathic Association. (2007). Joint Principles of the Patient-Centered Medical Home. Retrieved May 17, 2009, from http://www.aafp.org/online/etc/medialib/aafp_org/documents/policy/fed/jointprinciplespcmh0207.Par.0001.File.tmp/022107medicalhome.pdf.

[2] American Geriatrics Society, & AGS Foundation. (2007). The AGS Foundation for Health in Aging Guide to Geriatric Syndromes – Parts 1 & 2. Retrieved May 17, 2009, from http://www.healthinaging.org/public_education/geriatric_syndromes.php.

[3] G.F. Anderson, U.E. Reinhardt, P.S. Hussey and V. Petrosyan, It's the prices, stupid: why the United States is so different from other countries, *Health Affairs* **22**(3) (2003), 89–105. In: *Slowing the Growth of U.S. Health Care Expenditures: What are the Options?* K. Davis, C. Schoen, S. Guterman, T. Shih, S.C. Schoenbaum and I. Weinbaum, eds, (January 2007). Prepared for: 2007 Bipartisan Congressional Health Policy Conference. Miami, Florida: The Commonwealth Fund.

[4] S.S. Bassuk, T.A. Glass and L.F. Berkman, Social disengagement and incident cognitive decline in community-dwelling elderly persons, *Annals of Internal Medicine* **131**(3) (1999), 165–173.

[5] E.F. Binder, K.B. Schechtman, A.A. Ehsani, K. Steger-May, M. Brown, D.R. Sinacore et al., Effects of exercise training on frailty in community-dwelling older adults: results of a randomized, controlled trial, *Journal of the American Geriatrics Society* **50**(12) (2002), 1921–1928.

[6] D.G. Blazer, Social support and mortality in an elderly community population, *American Journal of Epidemiology* **115**(5) (1982), 684–694.

[7] T. Bodenheimer, E.H. Wagner and K. Grumbach, Improving primary care for patients with chronic illness, *JAMA: Journal of the American Medical Association* **288**(14) (2002), 1775.

[8] T. Bodenheimer, E.H. Wagner and K. Grumbach, Improving primary care for patients with chronic illness: The Chronic Care Model, Part 2, *JAMA: Journal of the American Medical Association* **288**(15) (2002), 1909.

[9] Bridges to Excellence. (2009). *BTE Medical Home*. Retrieved May 12, 2009, from http://www.bridgestoexcellence.org/Content/ContentDisplay.aspx?ContentID=124.
[10] J.P. Bunker, H.S. Frazier and F. Mosteller, Improving health: measuring effects of medical care, *Milbank Quarterly* **72**(2) (1994), 225.
[11] A.J. Campbell, M.C. Robertson, M.M. Gardner, R.N. Norton, M.W. Tilyard and D.M. Buchner, Randomised controlled trial of a general practice programme of home based exercise to prevent falls in elderly women, *BMJ* (*British Medical Journal*) **315**(7115) (1997), 1065–1069.
[12] M.C. Carlson, J.S. Saczynski, G.W. Rebok, T. Seeman, T.A. Glass, S. McGill et al., Exploring the Effects of an "Everyday" Activity Program on Executive Function and Memory in Older Adults: Experience Corps, *Gerontologist* **48**(6) (2008), 793–801.
[13] Center for Ethics in Health Care, & Oregon Health & Science University. (2009), *Physician orders for life-sustaining treatment paradigm*. Retrieved May 17, 2009, from http://www.ohsu.edu/polst/.
[14] M. Charlson, R.F. Charlson, W. Briggs and J. Hollenberg, Can disease management target patients most likely to generate high costs? The impact of comorbidity, *Journal of General Internal Medicine* **22**(4) (2007), 464–469.
[15] E. Coleman, J. Smith, J. Frank, T. Eilertsen, J. Thiare and A. Kramer, Development and testing of a measure designed to assess the quality of care transitions, *International Journal of Integrated Care* **2** (2002), e02.
[16] E.A. Coleman and R.A. Berenson, Lost in transition: challenges and opportunities for improving the quality of transitional care, *Annals of Internal Medicine* **141**(7) (2004), 533–W–599.
[17] E.A. Coleman, C. Parry, S. Chalmers and S. Min, The care transitions intervention, *Archives of Internal Medicine* **166**(17) (2006), 1822–1828.
[18] J. Coleman, PACE programs. Part 1, *The Case Manager* **11**(3) (2000), 35–41.
[19] J. Coleman, PACE programs. Part II, *The Case Manager* **11**(4) (2000), 34–37.
[20] Congressional Budget Office, *The long-term outlook for health care spending*. (CBO Publication No. 3085). Washington, D.C.: The Congress of the United States, 2007.
[21] D.F. Cooper, O.R. Granadillo and C.M. Stacey, Home-based primary care: the care of the veteran at home, *Home Healthcare Nurse* **25**(5) (2007), 315–322.
[22] M. Creditor, Hazards of hospitalization of the elderly, *Annals of Internal Medicine* **118**(3) (1993), 219–223.
[23] C.M. DesRoches, E.G. Campbell, S.R. Rao, K. Donelan, T.G. Ferris, A. Jha et al., Electronic health records in ambulatory care: a national survey of physicians, *New England Journal of Medicine* **359**(1) (2008), 50–60.
[24] M.A. Fiatarone, E.F. O'Neill, N.D. Ryan, K.M. Clements, G.R. Solares, M.E. Nelson et al., Exercise training and nutritional supplementation for physical frailty in very elderly people, *New England Journal of Medicine* **330**(25) (1994), 1769–1775.
[25] R.W. Fogel, Forecasting the costs of U.S. health care in 2040. National Bureau of Economic Research Working Paper 14361. Retrieved February 10, 2009 from http://www.nber.org/papers/w14361, 2008.
[26] L. Fratiglioni, S. Paillard-Borg and B. Winblad, An active and socially integrated lifestyle in late life might protect against dementia, *Lancet Neurology* **3**(6) (2004), 343–353.
[27] L. Fried, M. Carlson, M. Freedman, K. Frick, T. Glass, J. Hill et al., A social model for health promotion for an aging population: Initial evidence on the experience corps model, *Journal of Urban Health* **81**(1) (2004), 64–78.
[28] L. Fried, (2009). *Experience Corps: The Difference for Members*. Retrieved May 17, 2009, from http://www.experiencecorps.org/impact/for_members.cfm
[29] S.M. Friedman, D.M. Steinwachs, H. Temkin-Greener and D.B. Mukamel, Informal caregivers and the risk of nursing home admission among individuals enrolled in the Program of All-Inclusive Care for the Elderly, *Gerontologist* **46**(4) (2006), 456–463.
[30] R.S. Galvin, S. Delbanco, A. Milstein and G. Belden, Has The Leapfrog Group had an impact on the health care market? *Health Affairs* **24**(1) (2005), 228–233.
[31] T. Glass, M. Freedman, M. Carlson, J. Hill, K. Frick, N. Ialongo et al., Experience Corps: design of an intergenerational program to boost social capital and promote the health of an aging society, *Journal of Urban Health* **81**(1) (2004), 94–105.
[32] S.K. Inouye, S. Studenski, M.E. Tinetti and G.A. Kuchel, Geriatric syndromes: clinical, research, and policy implications of a core geriatric concept, *Journal of the American Geriatrics Society* **55**(5) (2007), 780–791.
[33] Institute of Medicine. (2008). *Retooling for an aging America: building the health care workforce*. Retrieved May 19, 2009, from http://www.nap.edu/catalog/12089.html.
[34] Kaiser Permanente. (2009). *Case study: collaborative cardiac care service – collaborative teams improve cardiac care with health information technology*. Retrieved May 12, 2009, from http://xnet.kp.org/future/ahrstudy/032709cardiac.html.
[35] R.A. Kane, T.Y. Lum, L.J. Cutler, H.B. Degenholtz and T.-C. Yu, Resident outcomes in small-house nursing homes: a longitudinal evaluation of the initial Green House Program, *Journal of the American Geriatrics Society* **55**(6) (2007), 832–839.
[36] B.E. Landon and S.L. Normand, Performance measurement in the small office practice: challenges and potential solutions, *Annals of Internal Medicine* **148**(5) (2008), 353–357.

[37] D. Laurin, R. Verreault, J. Lindsay, K. MacPherson and K. Rockwood, Physical activity and risk of cognitive impairment and dementia in elderly persons, *Archives of Neurology* **58**(3) (2001), 498–504.

[38] C. Lennartsson and M. Silverstein, Does engagement with life enhance survival of elderly people in Sweden? The role of social and leisure activities, *The Journals of Gerontology. Series B, Psychological Sciences and Social Sciences* **56**(6) (2001), S335–342.

[39] I. Martinez, K. Frick, T. Glass, M. Carlson, E. Tanner, M. Ricks et al., Engaging older adults in high impact volunteering that enhances health: recruitment and retention in The Experience Corps Baltimore, *Journal of Urban Health* **83**(5) (2006), 941–953.

[40] C.K. Mason, Medicare Care Coordination Demonstration Cost. In S. Reddy (Ed.), Washington DC, 2009.

[41] Mercer Human Resource Consulting, *Redesigning primary care for breakthrough in health insurance affordability. Model I: the ambulatory intensive caring unit*. Report to the California HealthCare Foundation. [unpublished], 2005.

[42] R.S. Morrison, S. Flanagan, D. Fischberg, A. Cintron and A.L. Siu, A Novel Interdisciplinary Analgesic Program Reduces Pain and Improves Function in Older Adults After Orthopedic Surgery, *Journal of the American Geriatrics Society* **57**(1) (2009), 1–10.

[43] National Center for Health Statistics *Characteristics of office-based physicians and their practices: United States, 2005–2006*. (DHHS Publication No. PHS 2008–1737). Washington, DC: U.S. Government Printing Office, 2008.

[44] National Committee for Quality Assurance (NCQA). (2001). *Patient-Centered Medical Home™ Bridges to Excellence*. Retrieved May 12, 2009, from http://www.ncqa.org/Portals/0/Programs/Recognition/BTE_Doc_Insert.pdf.

[45] NCQA. (2001). *Patient-Centered Medical Home™ PPC Fact Sheet*. Retrieved May 12, 2009, from http://www.ncqa.org/tabid/631/Default.aspx.

[46] NCQA. (2008). *Standards and guidelines for Physician Practice Connections – Patient-Centered Medical Home (PPC-PCMH)*. Washington, D.C.: National Committee for Quality Assurance.

[47] NCQA. (2009). *National Committee for Quality Assurance 2009 Programs and Initiatives Case Statement*. Retrieved May 12, 2009, 2009, from http://www.ncqa.org/Portals/0/Sponsor/2009_Case_Statement.pdf.

[48] NCQA. (2009). *Physician Practice Connections®-Patient-Centered Medical Home™ Bridges to Excellence*. Retrieved May 12, 2009, from http://www.ncqa.org/Portals/0/Programs/Recognition/BTE_Doc_Insert.pdf.

[49] M. Naylor and S. Keating, Transitional care, *The American Journal of Nursing* **108**(9) (2008), 58.

[50] M.D. Naylor, A decade of transitional care research with vulnerable elders, *Journal of Cardiovascular Nursing* **14**(3) (2000), 1–14.

[51] M.D. Naylor, D.A. Brooten, R.L. Campbell, G. Maislin, K.M. McCauley and J.S. Schwartz, Transitional care of older adults hospitalized with heart failure: a randomized, controlled trial, *Journal of the American Geriatrics Society* **52**(5) (2004), 675–684.

[52] E.C. Nelson, M.M. Godfrey, P.B. Batalden, S.A. Berry, A.E. Bothe Jr., K.E. McKinley et al., Clinical microsystems, part 1. The building blocks of health systems, *Joint Commission Journal on Quality and Patient Safety* **34**(7) (2008), 367–378.

[53] A. O'Malley and P. Cunningham, Patient experiences with coordination of care: the benefit of continuity and primary care physician as referral source, *Journal of General Internal Medicine* **24**(2) (2009), 170–177.

[54] J.T. Pacala, R.L. Kane, A.J. Atherly and M.A. Smith, Using structured implicit review to assess quality of care in the Program of All-Inclusive Care for the Elderly (PACE), *Journal of the American Geriatrics Society* **48**(8) (2000), 903–910.

[55] R.M. Palmer, S.R. Counsell and C. Landefeld, Acute care for elders units: practical considerations for optimizing health outcomes, *Disease Management and Health Outcomes* **11**(8) (2003), 507–517.

[56] R.M. Palmer, C. Landefeld, D. Kresevic and J. Kowal, A medical unit for the acute care of the elderly, *Journal of the American Geriatrics Society* **42**(5) (1994), 545–552.

[57] Patient-Centered Primary Care Collaborative. (2009). *Patient-Centered Primary Care Collaborative*. Retrieved May 12, 2009, from http://www.pcpcc.net/content/about-collaborative.

[58] W. Percy, *Love in the ruins*. New York: Farrar, Straus and Giroux, 1971.

[59] D. Peikes, A. Chen, J. Schore and R. Brown, Effects of care coordination on hospitalization, quality of care, and health care expenditures among Medicare beneficiaries, *JAMA: Journal of the American Medical Association* **301**(6) (2009), 603–618.

[60] M.A. Province, E.C. Hadley, M.C. Hornbrook, L.A. Lipsitz, J.P. Miller, C.D. Mulrow et al., The effects of exercise on falls in elderly patients. A preplanned meta-analysis of the FICSIT Trials. Frailty and Injuries: Cooperative Studies of Intervention Techniques, *JAMA: Journal of the American Medical Association* **273**(17) (1995), 1341–1347.

[61] G. Pyka and E. Lindenberger, Muscle strength and fiber adaptations to a year-long resistance training program in elderly men, *Journal of Gerontology* **49**(1) (1994), M22.

[62] J. Rabig, W. Thomas, R.A. Kane, L.J. Cutler and S. McAlilly, Radical redesign of nursing homes: applying the Green House concept in Tupelo, Mississippi, *Gerontologist* **46**(4) (2006), 533–539.

[63] D. Reed, D. Foley, L. White, H. Heimovitz, C. Burchfiel and K. Masaki, Predictors of healthy aging in men with high life expectancies, *American Journal of Public Health* **88**(10) (1998), 1463–1468.

[64] W.B. Rouse, Health care as a complex adaptive system: implications for design and management, *The Bridge* **38**(1) (2008), 17–25.

[65] J.W. Rowe and R.L. Kahn, *Successful Aging*. New York: Dell, 1999.

[66] L.Z. Rubenstein, K.R. Josephson, P.R. Trueblood, S. Loy, J.O. Harker, F.M. Pietruszka et al., Effects of a group exercise program on strength, mobility, and falls among fall-prone elderly men, *The Journals of Gerontology. Series A, Biological Sciences and Medical Sciences* **55**(6) (2000), M317–M321.

[67] T. Rundek and D. Bennett, Cognitive leisure activities, but not watching TV, for future brain benefits, *Neurology* **66**(6) (2006), 794–795.

[68] S.H. Scholle, L.G. Pawlson, L.I. Solberg, S.C. Shih, S.E. Asche, A.F. Chou et al., Measuring practice systems for chronic illness care: accuracy of self-reports from clinical personnel, *Joint Commission Journal on Quality and Patient Safety* **34**(7) (2008), 407–416.

[69] P.M. Schyve, Microsystems, macrosystems, and kernicterus, *Joint Commission Journal on Quality and Safety* **30**(11) (2004), 591–592.

[70] L.I. Solberg, S.H. Scholle, S.E. Asche, S.C. Shih, L.G. Pawlson, M.J. Thoele et al., Practice systems for chronic care: frequency and dependence on an electronic medical record, *The American Journal of Managed Care* **11**(12) (2005), 789–796.

[71] W. Strawbridge, R. Cohen, S. Shema and G. Kaplan, Successful aging: predictors and associated activities, *American Journal of Epidemiology* **144**(2) (1996), 135–141.

[72] E. Tan, Q. Xue, T. Li, M. Carlson and L. Fried, Volunteering: a physical activity intervention for older adults – The Experience Corps program in Baltimore, *Journal of Urban Health* **83**(5) (2006), 954–969.

[73] C. Terret, G.B. Zulian, A. Naiem and G. Albrand, Multidisciplinary approach to the geriatric oncology patient, *Journal of Clinical Oncology* **25**(14) (2007), 1876–1881.

[74] K. Thorpe and D. Howard, The rise in spending among Medicare beneficiaries: the role of chronic disease prevalence and changes in treatment intensity, *Health Affairs* **25**(5) (2006), w378–w388.

[75] S.W. Tolle, V.P. Tilden, C.A. Nelson and P.M. Dunn, A prospective study of the efficacy of the physician order form for life-sustaining treatment, *Journal of the American Geriatrics Society* **46**(9) (1998), 1097–1102.

[76] P. Torda and J. Channin, (2009). Update: patient-centered medical home [Powerpoint slides]. Presented at: Patient-Centered Primary Care Collaborative webinar, February 17, 2009.

[77] J. Verghese, A. LeValley, C. Derby, G. Kuslansky, M. Katz, C. Hall et al., Leisure activities and the risk of amnestic mild cognitive impairment in the elderly, *Neurology* **66**(6) (2006), 821–827.

[78] J. Verghese, R.B. Lipton, M.J. Katz, C.B. Hall, C.A. Derby, G. Kuslansky et al., Leisure activities and the risk of dementia in the elderly, *New England Journal of Medicine* **348**(25) (2003), 2508–2516.

[79] E.H. Wagner, Chronic disease management: what will it take to improve care for chronic illness? *Effective Clinical Practice: ECP* **1**(1) (1998), 2–4.

[80] E.H. Wagner, The role of patient care teams in chronic disease management, *BMJ* (*British Medical Journal*) **320**(7234) (2000), 569–572.

[81] E.H. Wagner, B.T. Austin, C. Davis, M. Hindmarsh, J. Schaefer and A. Bonomi, Improving chronic illness care: translating evidence into action, *Health Affairs* **20**(6) (2001), 64.

[82] F.M. Weaver, E.C. Hickey, S.L. Hughes, V. Parker, D. Fortunato, J. Rose et al., Providing all-inclusive care for frail elderly veterans: evaluation of three models of care, *Journal of the American Geriatrics Society* **56**(2) (2008), 345–353.

[83] L. Wolfson, R. Whipple, C. Derby, J. Judge, M. King, P. Amerman et al., Balance and strength training in older adults: intervention gains and Tai Chi maintenance, *Journal of the American Geriatrics Society* **44**(5) (1996), 498–506.

[84] D.M. Zimba, (1998). *Vertical versus virtual integration*. Retrieved May 17, 2009, from http://www.physiciansnews.com/business/198zimba.html.

Christine Cassel, MD, MACP, is President and CEO of the American Board of Internal Medicine and the ABIM Foundation, and a leading expert in geriatric medicine, medical ethics and quality of care. Dr. Cassel, board certified in both internal medicine and geriatric medicine, has achieved a number of firsts for women in medicine – she was the first female board chair of the American Board of Internal Medicine from 1995–1996, the first female President of the American College of Physicians from 1996–1997 and the first female dean of Oregon Health & Science University, Portland, Oregon in 2002.

In April 2009, Dr. Cassel was chosen by President Obama as one of 20 scientists to serve on the President's Council of Advisors on Science and Technology (PCAST), which advises the President in areas where an understanding of science, technology, and innovation is key to forming responsible and effective policy. In addition, having chaired influential IOM reports on end-of-life care and public health, Dr. Cassel also serves on the IOM's Comparative Effective Research Committee mandated by Congress to set priorities for the national CER effort. An active scholar and lecturer, she is the author or co-author of 14 books and more than 150 journal articles on geriatric medicine, aging, bioethics and health policy. Her most recent book is *Medicare Matters: What Geriatric Medicine Can Teach American Health Care*.

Dr. Cassel is a representative to the National Quality Forum's National Priorities Partnership, a member of the Commonwealth Fund's Commission on a High Performance Health System and is a former member of the Institute of Medicine's Governing

Council. She also sits on the board of directors of the Greenwall Foundation, Kaiser Permanente, Premier Inc. and other organizations with quality health care agendas. She was appointed by President Clinton to serve on the President's Advisory Commission on Consumer Protection and Quality in the Health Care Industry, and has been central to other national leadership efforts to inspire quality of care.

Dr. Cassel has served as the President of the American Federation for Aging Research, dean of the School of Medicine and vice president for medical affairs at Oregon Health and Science University, and chair of the Department of Geriatrics and Adult Development at Mount Sinai School of Medicine in New York, where she was also professor of geriatrics and medicine. She spent a decade at the University of Chicago Pritzker School of Medicine, as chief of General Internal Medicine and a founding Health Policy Director of the Harris School of Public Policy.

Dr. Cassel received her bachelor's degree from the University of Chicago and her medical degree from the University of Massachusetts Medical School. She is the recipient of numerous honorary degrees and is an Honorary Fellow of the Royal Colleges of Medicine of the U.K. and Canada and the European Federation of Internal Medicine, and was elected a master of the American College of Physicians in 1997.

Michelle Johnston-Fleece is Policy and Research Analyst at the American Board of Internal Medicine and ABIM Foundation. She is responsible for providing research support for numerous ABIM and ABIM Foundation policy initiatives, with particular interest in issues surrounding chronic illness, palliative care and consumer engagement in health care.

She received a bachelor's degree in sociology and media studies from New York University and a Master of Public Health in health systems and policy from the University of Medicine and Dentistry of New Jersey (UMDNJ).

Siddharta Reddy is a Research Associate at the American Board of Internal Medicine with experience in clinical, public health and quality improvement research, including survey design and data collection, quantitative and qualitative analysis, and manuscript development. He has managed evaluative and exploratory research projects in the areas of physician quality improvement, graduate medical education, and systems of care. He has a Master of Public Health from the University of Texas-Houston Health Science Center (Houston, Texas) and has previously worked for the Department of Veterans Affairs providing web-based psychometric information on measures and surveys used by VA health services researchers.

Information Knowledge Systems Management 8 (2009) 71–86
DOI 10.3233/IKS-2009-0136
IOS Press

Chapter 5

Palliative and end of life care

Robert Stroebel and Timothy Moynihan
E-mail: Stroebel.Robert@mayo.edu

Abstract: Health care provided in the final year of life is typically costly and often delivers unintended outcomes. High value can be defined for end of life care. High value clinical practices exist for end of life care and a common set of high value processes can be identified. The current system structure of healthcare delivery does not consistently support those high value processes. An improved organizational schema could foster sustained delivery of high value delivery operations. The healthcare ecosystem needs to evolve to provide appropriate incentives and support for an appropriately designed care system.

1. Statement of the problem

1.1. A case

At 3:30 a.m. Mrs. M. died in her hospital bed. She was alone at the time of her death. In the preceding two months she had been hospitalized four separate times, spending a total of 27 days in the hospital. Her hospitalizations included one major cardiac procedure, two extended intensive care unit stays, varying levels of discomfort and extended periods of confusion, agitation and disorientation.

The care she received was well within the standard of care in her community. Her care was delivered by highly trained specialists using the very latest medical technologies. Her case was not marked by any adverse events or significant medical errors. Our medical system provided exactly the type of care it is designed for.

Ironically, had we asked Mrs. M or her family two years earlier how she would like to spend the last two months of her life, it is almost certain that she would have not chosen the experience that befell her. It is likely she would have chosen to spend her last two months of life in her home, in relative comfort, surrounded by family and friends. The clinical practices to enable that outcome exist in Mrs. M's community and are accessible to her care providers. What is it about the healthcare system that prevented those practices from being utilized in this case?

1.2. Unresponsive care

In 1986 Medicare first implemented the hospice benefit for patients at the end of life. Since that time there has been a remarkable growth in the number and availability of hospice in the United States. Up to 39% of all deaths in the United States now occur in patients enrolled in a hospice program, with 1.4 million patients enrolled in hospice nation wide as of 2007 and approximately 900,000 deaths [39]. Most hospice programs still feel that their services are not being utilized to their fullest capacity as the median length of stay remains at 22 days and up to one third of patients die within seven days of a

1389-1995/09/$17.00

hospice referral. This does not allow adequate time to prepare the patient and family for death, nor to adequately address all physical, psychosocial and spiritual problems for the dying patient. Palliative care programs, while growing in number and utilization, are similarly underutilized. A survey of primary care practitioners in Great Britain suggest that palliative care is the area of health care in which doctors can make the greatest difference to their patients [5]. The National Quality Forum has made Palliative and End of Life care one of its nine priorities for rapid national action in its May 2008 statement on needs of the medical system [25].

1.3. Lack of education of health care professionals

Many different factors contribute to the delay in providing hospice and palliative services, chief among these is physician reluctance to communicate realistic prognostic information to families which further delays patient's ability to choose the care pathways that may be most appropriate for their own goals of care. Much of this is not done out of any ill will on the part of the health care professional, but most physicians have not been adequately instructed in how to conduct conversations with patients and their families regarding difficult or life limiting prognoses. Many health care providers are fearful of causing patients to "lose hope" by telling patients and their families' realistic information about prognosis in critical illnesses. Recent studies have shown that open and honest discussions can lead to improved decision making for the patient, decreased bereavement complications for the surviving family members and improvement in family perceptions about symptom management [54]. Unfortunately, these discussions are often the exception, rather than the rule. Several examples help to illustrate the point.

End stage renal disease has become much more manageable and less likely to cause death in the short term since the development of dialysis. However, most patients with end stage renal disease will still succumb to their illness. Many nephrologists, however, are poorly trained in providing advanced planning or palliative care to patients on dialysis. In a study of nephrology fellows, Holley and colleagues found that most (78%) were not trained in communication skills required telling patients that they are dying, and the trainees felt they were most prepared to manage hemodialysis, and least prepared to care for patients who are dying [23]. Incorporating training in end of life care for nephrologists would allow appropriate and timely withdrawal or non initiation of hemodialysis in the appropriate setting for specific patients.

While use of ventilation support can provide significant benefit to patients, in end of life care the burden of intubation and mechanical ventilation may outweigh the benefits. Many patients, once they comprehend the true nature of their terminal illness will make the decision to avoid the invasive nature of ventilatory support, that requires use of intensive care units and prefer to spend their final days at home in the company of their families, away from the noisy and impersonal intensive care unit. The most potent predictors of withdrawal of ventilatory support are physician's perceptions of prognosis, the likelihood of impaired neurologic outcome and physician's perception of patient's preference for use of life support [12]. This certainly suggests that understanding of a patient's preferences and goals may help to defer the costly and invasive procedure, leading to avoidance of significant discomfort and cost, while providing high value.

Implantable cardiac defibrillators have significantly increased in use and number of indications for insertion. While highly beneficial in many patient populations, these have created new dilemmas for patients at the end of life. As patients die from some underlying disease, be it cardiac or other illnesses, the ICD is often forgotten. Patients who may desire no longer to undergo cardiac resuscitation still receive shocks from their device, because no one considered what to do with the device, and it was never deactivated. In addition, when a patient dies the family is traumatized by seeing the patient shocked several times after death, at times injuring the family member holding the patient's hand. Discussions of what to do with the ICD when a patient approaches death should be held prior to insertion of the device. While for some patients this may be many years, perhaps even decades in the future, multiple conversations regarding the goals of care and use of the ICD will lead to decreased inappropriate cardioversion in the last days of life [2].

Many cancer patients continue to receive aggressive chemotherapy in spite of a very low likelihood of response or meaningful response [15]. Such treatments lead to substantial toxicity, clinic and hospital visits and numerous tests and other procedures. Adequate communication between physician and patient can lead to decreased use of futile chemotherapy.

2. Costly care

Delays in addressing realistic goals of care, aligned to the patient's needs and condition, leads to tremendous skewing of the expenditure of health care resources. Medicare costs in the last year of life account for approximately a quarter of the program's total budget. It is difficult to determine to what extent those dollars are spent on interventions that neither prolong survival nor enhance quality of life. Anecdotally, we are all familiar with instances among friends or family members in which neither goal was accomplished. Such unnecessary and futile care leads to complications with prolonged and repeated hospitalizations that could be avoided had the choice of pursuing primarily palliation and symptom management been offered to the patient.

Studies looking at the likelihood of receiving chemotherapy near the end of life show that in 1996 22% of all Medicare patients with cancer began a new chemotherapy regimen within one month of dying and in the last two weeks of life 18.5% began a new chemotherapy treatment, numbers that increased from 13.8% in 1993 [15]. The likelihood of initiating chemotherapy in this time frame is not proportional to chances of tumor response [16,45]. While continued use of aggressive therapies near the end of life are the patient's choice, studies have suggested that patient's perception of benefit from these therapies is much greater than what the physicians estimate [38]. Up to one out of three patients being treated for incurable, metastatic lung cancer believed that they were receiving potentially curative therapy while a similar number of patients receiving radiation therapy for metastatic disease had similar understanding of the goal for therapy [10,32].

Cost of care also shows marked variation across geographic regions. Dartmouth atlas data demonstrates that cost of care in the last two years of life is less costly when delivered at Mayo Clinic in Rochester, Minnesota, when compared to similar care at a comparable medical center in California. While both institutions are well recognized and respected as leaders in health care, differences in process and mechanisms of care seem to lead to significant differences in expenditures [53].

2.1. Fragmented care

The current health care system has developed into a highly fragmented system. No longer is the primary care physician the solitary source of direction and coordination of a patient's care. The primary care physician is typically overly busy and unable to spend adequate time communicating with the patient and family regarding prognosis and goals of care. This lack of planning for upcoming medical conditions that may be relatively predictable, removes the opportunity to allow patients and families the choice of therapeutic goals. Advanced care planning is completed by only a minority of patients [37].

While the primary care provider is often the one has the most intimate and consistent knowledge of the patient and family, when significant medical complications or conditions develop, referrals to specialists and Subspecialists often ensues. Lack of full communication between the primary care and the Subspecialists often follows and the primary care provider may loose contact with the patient and family. Lack of a uniform, readily accessible comprehensive medical record hinders the ability to keep all parties caring for the patient to see and share the same data to help guide the patient's care. Multiple Subspecialists may become involved all with different viewpoints on the patient's condition and without coordinated, dedicated time to plan what is most appropriate for the patient. Subspecalists may also pay close attention to the organ system involved without developing a whole patient assessment. Such focused care has led to tremendous developments in advancing the care of patients, however, at the cost of losing site of the overall goals and whole patient care. This leads to patients with advanced, incurable metastatic cancers with expected survival measured in weeks or months sill receiving statin therapies for hypercholesterolemia, an expensive and potentially toxic therapy that could not possibly offer the patient any meaningful benefit in this end of life setting.

Communication with nursing staff who provide the bulk of real time care to inpatients hinders patient care. Regularly scheduled team care rounds can help reduce these communication deficits and enhance goal setting appropriate for the individual patient. The nursing staff typically interact the most with the family members and they often understand the practical abilities and disabilities and challenges that patients and families face. They also often will see social situations long before a physician can detect. Thus, regular, coordinated team care conferences with communication between all parties can help shorten hospital stays and ease transitions of care to the outpatient setting.

A key part of the health care team must be the social worker. Skilled in the care needs of the families and resources available within the community, regular coordinated multi-disciplinary work rounds or conferences can facilitate placement and appropriate utilization of resources. Lack of resources for social work and lack of recognition of their role in patient care provides a significant barrier to idealized patient care.

All patients and families struggling with significant medical conditions have spiritual or existential needs that are often unmet or not addressed and left to the patients and families own resources to deal with. Incorporating chaplaincy can help to quell troubling aspects of the patient's illness and improve patients and families struggles in the end of life journey.

3. Defining value

There is a growing consensus that our delivery systems for providing care at the end of life should be improved. To achieve an improved delivery system for patients at the end of life it is useful to have a definition of high value end of life care. At first glance, the concept of value in end of life care may seem inappropriate. Wellness and productivity are not outcomes commonly associated with the dying process. Quantity of time, by definition, cannot be meaningfully increased. The value equation does apply, however, if one formulates outcomes and cost in terms appropriate to end of life care.

Multiple measures can be utilized to define value in end of life care. Included in such measures would be patient's choice of place of death, use of hospitalization or acute care services in last weeks of life, symptom control (pain, dyspnea, nausea etc.), family satisfaction with symptom control, family bereavement and decrease in likelihood of complicated bereavement, overall family satisfaction with care givers in terminal illness and finally decreased global cost of care.

3.1. Quality and service outcomes

Outcomes are primarily defined from the perspective of the patient and families, although there are also societal outcomes to be considered. Patient and family perceptions of quality at end of life vary greatly [48]. For patients, several quality of life measures have been developed to assess the patient and family experience. The measures cross several domains including symptoms, functional status, relationships, well-being and meaning [6,7,41,49]. A high value system would promote and support an end of life experience that maximizes responsiveness in each of these domains. As needs change throughout the dying experience the perception of high quality may shift. The system needs to respond to this dynamic environment.

Service parameters for the dying patient include provision of services well beyond the clinic or hospital. As suggested in the quality of life measures, the needs of the dying patient necessarily involve other settings including the work site, home, assisted living facility or skilled nursing facility. The range of services needed also extends beyond the traditional provision of medical testing, treatments and management. Social services, spiritual support, medical equipment, and transportation needs all require attention.

Perceptions of quality at the end of life can also be considered from the perspective of the community or society. In the traditional model of health care rapid access to emergency care, intensive care units, high tech imaging, invasive procedures and powerful medications conveys the image of high quality care. However, high intensity, painful and de-personalized care delivered in the hospital environment in the last days or weeks of life may create a perception of isolation and futility. Similarly, the perception of elderly patients languishing for years in under-funded, poorly staffed long term care facilities is not an attractive vision for our society.

An alternative perception of quality for care delivered at the end of life is emerging. Systems of care delivery designed to respond to patient and family needs are gaining in recognition and acceptance [33]. Enrollment in hospice has increased steadily over the past several years. Palliative care program growth has occurred linearly this decade [35]. The increasing utilization of hospice and palliative care programs reflects the development of a new paradigm for high quality care during the dying process. Ideally, our society will have a high level of comfort with the quality of palliative or hospice care delivered in the final years of our lives.

3.2. Costs

Cost of care for the dying patient can be considered in terms of direct and indirect expenditures. The direct costs of care in final two years of life are staggering. These dollars, largely paid through Medicare or Medicaid consume approximately 26% of these program's budgets [30].

Indirect cost savings to families and communities may be also be considered. The traditional medical model of end of life care often can defer time and opportunity costs on to families and communities. As a patient's functional status deteriorates at the end of life, activities of daily living, financial, social and spiritual needs may be inadequately met. A consideration of direct care costs does not recognize this significant burden incurred at the end of life. Indirect costs should be considered as we consider the societal burdens of end of life care.

The value equation does apply at the end of our lives and we can use the concept to define what high value end of life care would look like.

High value end of life care would addresses patient and family needs across several domains and would be responsive to changing needs through the dying process. High value end of life care would instill a high degree of confidence in our communities that the dying process was a time of supportive, considerate care, not isolation and suffering. High value end of life care could potentially, reduce direct care costs and limit the burden of indirect costs to our communities in support of dying family or community members.

4. High value clinical practices

4.1. Advanced directives

A core group of clinical practices are emerging and gaining support and acceptance in our healthcare delivery system. There is a growing body of evidence and perception that these practices do offer high healthcare value. Extensive descriptions of these programs are widely available elsewhere. We will briefly describe these practices in this chapter, focusing primarily on the processes and structures required to support and promote these practices.

One of the simplest high value clinical practices, precisely because of the limited cost of implementation, is the use of advanced directives. Completion of such documents can help guide the care of patients who find themselves in a position where they can no longer speak for themselves. This removes the burden of decision making from family members who are often at a loss as to what their loved one desired in the circumstances, and this is often viewed by the family as a great gift.

Advanced directives alone, however are not sufficient for many clinical scenarios that arise in the end of life. A more comprehensive document, the Physician Orders for Life-Sustaining Treatment (POLST) provides guidance for a multitude of use or avoidance of advanced and aggressive technologies that can be matched to patient's personal preferences and goals of care [4,22]. Avoidance of undesired interventions that have the potential to lead to increased suffering, and offer little long term benefit clearly can add significant value to a patient's care.

4.2. Hospice

In the hospice model supportive care is provided to people in the final phase of a terminal illness or condition. The focus of care is on comfort and quality of life, rather than cure. Patients who have been referred to hospice have been shown to be more likely to die in the location of the patient's choosing when compared to those who are not referred to hospice. This does not mean that all patients need to die in a hospice setting, but it does reflect that patient and families choices are more likely to be respected. This may also include the patient's desire to die in an intensive care setting, and while this is typically avoided in hospice care, if that is the patient's choice, it still is meeting their needs. Most hospice personnel will relate that having time to work with patients and families is the best tool available to try and avoid aggressive and dramatic, oftentimes painful and dangerous medical interventions. Assuring the patients and families that you will not abandon them if they wish to forgo aggressive medical interventions and that you will always treat them, even when you no longer treat the underlying illness, often leads to a welcomed acceptance of the inevitability of death. This acceptance may also come as a relief, by giving the patient permission to not have to take any more burdensome treatments that may carry more risk of harm than any realistic benefits.

4.3. Palliative care

While the hospice benefit has provided significant improvements in the care for patients nearing the end of life and their families, dramatic limitations to the restrictions of the defined benefit plan have become manifest. Due to the funding structure and inability to pay for expensive potentially life prolonging therapies, many patients have had to choose between continuing with aggressive, therapy and hospice care. Thus many patients delay enrolling in hospice until very late in their course when they and their families can not derive full benefit of hospice services. This has prompted the development of the specialty of palliative care where the same multidisciplinary team care used in the hospice model is applied at an earlier stage in the patient's course, without limitations on estimated survival. In this model, curative and life prolonging, even experimental medications or therapies are utilized in addition to meticulous symptom management, psychosocial, spiritual and emotional support. A large focus does remain on communication and delineating goals of care and future projections for the patient and family. When situations develop that signify a significant decline, the palliative care team can rapidly transition the patient to hospice care and utilize the medicare hospice benefit. If curative therapy has intervened, then the role of the palliative care team may fade into the background, until such time as symptoms and clinical situation warrants.

Improved symptom management is seen in patients receiving palliative care along with standard cancer therapy. A study by Rabow and colleagues demonstrated that palliative care consultation led to statistically significant improvement in pain, anxiety, depression, relationship problems, overall well-being, and being at peace over the course of the study. No difference was seen in patient's report of fatigue [43].

Patients referred to hospice and palliative are programs are less likely to undergo hospitalization or admission to ICU in the last weeks to months of life. Cassel and Kerr reviewed 14 published randomized trials looking at the ability of palliative care consultations to effect length of stay in both the hospital setting as well as the ICU. Eleven of fourteen published studies do demonstrate a shortened length of stay in the ICU when palliative care consultations are obtained, but no alteration was noted in overall hospital length of stay [9].

It is unclear if increased enrollment in hospice and or palliative care would necessarily reduce total costs. The evidence to date is mixed [8,36]. This picture may reflect the relatively immature systems that exist to support high value end of life care. For example, many patients may be enrolled in hospice or palliative care programs too late in the course of their illness to substantially alter costs. End of life programs likely need to be tailored to fit the specific needs for different groups of patients. One size programs may not fit all. Support systems may not be coordinated enough to provide a truly integrated system of care between the clinic and home care services that is able to avoid potentially unnecessary hospitalizations. As systems become more sophisticated and responsive to the vastly differing needs of dying patients additional cost savings may be realized.

5. High value delivery operations (Processes)

A number of core operations or processes are essential to support the delivery of high value end of life care as exemplified by highly functioning palliative care and hospice programs. Necessary characteristics include team-based delivery models, seamless interaction with the community and integrated and coordinated processes. Information systems must enable integration; facilitate concurrent and prospective patient identification, easy enrollment and comprehensive care planning. Above all, systems must be responsive and flexible to meet the changing needs of the dying patient and their family. Care delivery models with these capabilities are more likely to support and promote effective end of life programs [26, 31].

5.1. Teams

A team-based approach is a necessary condition for the delivery of high value care. A majority of in-patient palliative care programs have adopted a multi-specialty team approach. This approach would seem to have high face validity. The needs of end of life patients extend well beyond the immediate medical issues. Diverse professional and non-professional skill sets are required to address the needs. Anecdotal and retrospective data would seem to endorse this approach. A recent multi-site randomized trial in the U.S. conducted among five hundred patients demonstrated improved patient satisfaction and lowered health care costs. In this study the intervention team included physicians, nurses, chaplains and social workers [18].

As palliative care extends to the outpatient setting the requirements for service diversifies. Additional skills and capabilities need to be accounted for, thus necessitating broader team membership. A recent prospective randomized trial enrolled patients in a care program managed by a Comprehensive Care Team. Members of the team included physicians, nurses, chaplains, social workers, volunteer coordinators, pharmacists, psychologists and art therapists. Outcomes of this intervention suggest that outpatient team based intervention resulted in improved patient outcomes. It was not clear if significant cost savings were realized [42,44].

Enhanced communication skills are essential to highly functioning teams. Unfortunately, team training has not been a prominent component of most graduate level medical education to date. Good data exists that shows communication skills can be taught [17], and multiple regulatory agencies such as ACGME now require physicians demonstrate competence in patient communication [3]. Traditional physician training in medical school and the post graduate setting did not include instruction in end of life care until recently. So, while the current generation of medical students and recent graduates have had end of life care incorporated into their curriculum, physicians in practice have not received such instruction. Fortunately, organizations and programs such as the Center to Advance Palliative Care (CAPC) and the Education in Palliative and End of Life Care (EPEC) provide instruction as well as resources for practicing physicians to acquire the skill set needed.

5.2. Community

The aforementioned examples are teams based out of hospitals and medical clinics. A delivery process with the potential to encompass a broader team is based on a community model. Some of the over 3000 hospice care programs in the United States are run by not for profit community organizations. For profit hospice organizations exist as well. In Great Britain there is a model of community centered palliative care. In this model the health care system is one facet of a multi-faceted web in which the patient is in the center. Other contributors to care in this model include family, friends, volunteers, community nurses, social workers, mental health workers and spiritual support [19]. The community based programs offer the advantage of supporting patients and families in their home environments. The disadvantage is the coordination and management of care across a diverse array of resources and services.

5.3. Information technology

Readily available information regarding a patient's status, care plan, goals and contacts is a crucial component of a high value delivery process. The hospital record or clinic chart is inadequate to cover the scope of management required over the end of life process and neither is readily available beyond the healthcare setting. Sharing of information between providers, hospitals, specialists, home health agencies and social service providers remains a significant challenge. Studies of the use of IT in palliative care and hospice programs suggest that use of information technology is emerging, but that significant work and study remains to be done [14,29].

The personal health record may prove to be a useful tool for the end-of – life patient as they transition across numerous care settings and interact with multi-disciplinary teams [28]. Limited work with personal health records in hospice or palliative care programs has been completed to date. The potential benefits of a central repository for a patient's medical history, medications, active issues, contacts, plan of care, goals and preferences is apparent.

5.4. Integration and coordination

Regardless of the tools used, integration and coordination of care is essential. As we have discussed, patients at the end of life often transition among a number of care settings including home, clinic, hospital, assisted living facility and skilled nursing facility. Care integration is critical to insure continuity. Similarly, numerous individuals or entities will provide services including health care workers, social workers, therapists, clergy, health aids, friends, neighbors and community groups. It is not realistic to expect a dying patient or bereaved family to coordinate the care.

Integrated health care systems offer the advantage of coordinated care between outpatient and inpatient services, diagnostic and therapeutic services, and primary and specialty care providers. It is reasonable to assume that the greater value demonstrated by integrated delivery systems in care at the end of the life would also be conferred in the palliative or hospice care modes [53].

Coordination with community resources is an additional level of complexity. The PACE program may provide an appropriate model on which to base efforts to coordinate end-of-life care between traditional medical care and community based resources [40]. This CMS program features a comprehensive service delivery system and integrated financing. The program centers on the system of acute and long term care services with a goal of allowing clients to remain at home and avoid admission to long term care facilities. This level of integrated and coordinated care delivery can be expanded to include extension of hospice or palliative care benefits.

5.5. Proactive identification

Identification and enrollment of appropriate patients into end-of life programs is a complex process. Providers or patients may initiate the process. The decision to participate in hospice or palliative care often occurs in reaction to the worsening or acute exacerbation of chronic illness. Hospice eligibility involves an established timeline for expected end of life. Palliative care enrollment is not dependent on an expected duration of time before the end of life. Identification of patients can be challenging for providers, patients and family members. Extensive lists of potential conditions exist and may be useful if considered and readily available [26]. Detailed enrollment guidelines for Hospice eligibility exist and can be helpful as well [24]. In either case, however, the process is only initiated once eligibility is recognized by providers, patients or family members and a decision is made to offer or inquire about these programs. Clinical inertia can be a barrier to this recognition.

5.6. Active enrollment

Once a patient has been identified, a variety of tools are available to facilitate enrollment and communications of status. Advanced Care Planning is a structured communication tool to introduce and facilitate the discussion between provider and patient regarding enrollment in end of life care [1]. Patients may have already established the groundwork for this communication with their own Advanced Directives document shared with their providers and families. Multiple tools exist to help primary care physicians prepare patients for future expected or unexpected events. The Physician Orders for Life-Sustaining Treatment (POLST) program was instituted in LaCrosse, Wisconsin, in 1997 in a response to legislation in the state mandating use of a wrist bracelet for advanced directives status for residents of nursing homes and long term care facilities. Area wide distribution and acceptance of the POLST forms and training of medical personnel have led to an 80% completion rate in the 5 counties where the original study began. This program has now spread to include multiple states and is gaining a national acceptance. The primary goal is to enhance the quality of care at the end of life by facilitating communication of the patients' wishes for aggressive therapy. Hickman and colleagues have shown this tool to decrease the use of aggressive life prolonging measures and admission to ICU in nursing homes where it has been implemented [22]. This is but one example of an easily used tool that may enhance care and decrease cost of care at the end of life.

Oftentimes, the decision to enter hospice programs or consider palliative care is considered during times of stress and duress. As a result, decision making is negatively impacted and eligible patients or their families often choose aggressive forms of therapy or interventions despite the futility of those options [51]. This is frustrating for providers and may lead to poor outcomes, disappointment and unnecessary suffering. In some systems, the capability exists to enable proactive identification of eligible patients through administrative data base analysis. In the identified patients it would be appropriate to initiate advanced care planning or to propose completion of advanced directives. A risk assessment tool has been utilized to identify elders at very high risk for death or skilled nursing placement within 24 months. This assessment does not require hospitalization or an office visit as it relies on administrative data available in the patient's medical record [50]. A high score on the risk assessment tool can trigger proactive contact with patients and their family members to initiate advanced care planning or to schedule an appointment with an MD or social worker. This approach provides a trigger to the health care team that can help overcome the barrier of clinical inertia.

6. System structure and organization

A unifying organization or structure is essential to appropriately foster and integrate the disparate delivery processes previously described. As we have discussed, our current system of health care delivery, with few isolated exceptions, does not provide incentives for coordination and integration of services in the end of life. A conceptual model commonly applied to the organization of chronic disease delivery could provide a framework for integrated, coordinated end of life care.

The Chronic Care Model (CCM) is a widely applied and extensively researched framework for the management of patients with chronic disease. The health care requirements of the patient and family at the end of life are similar to the patient with chronic illness. In fact, it is helpful to consider end of life care as a logical extension of the provision of high quality chronic disease care. It is extremely useful, therefore, to consider the CCM as an appropriate organizational construct for the establishment of high value end of life care. At the heart of the model is a fundamental shift from a reactive, unplanned and fragmented delivery system to a planned, proactive and integrated system for organizing and delivering care [52].

Six elements are incorporated into the basic model. The delivery system is organized to provide care that is pro-active, planned and supports patient self-management. Decision support is used to integrate evidence-based, safe, effective care into all aspects of the delivery system. Clinical information systems are used to identify and track patients. Self management is supported and encouraged. Community resources are integrated and coordinated with the delivery system. Finally, the leadership of the health system is charged with supporting and coordinating activities of the model in support of patient focused care delivery. Each individual model element is considered necessary but not sufficient to deliver the highest quality of chronic disease care. A basic tenet of the model is that all elements are required to deliver the highest possible outcomes for patients [11].

There is a high level of overlap between the organizational structure of the CCM and the high quality clinical practices and processes previously discussed in this chapter. A well coordinated multi-disciplinary care team will be at the core of an effective end-of-life delivery system. Teams are typically led by a physician. The primary care physician or hospital physician is usually in the best position to initiate the palliative care process and oversee the subsequent management. A care coordinator or care manager, often a nurse or mid-level provider, is frequently the primary contact for the patient and family. A critical role of the team will be to support self-management for the dying patient, and perhaps more importantly, for the patient's family or friends. Evidence-based order sets, protocols and clinical pathways are useful tools for integrating high value decision support into the palliative care process. The utilization of providers trained in palliative or hospice care as specialist support to the primary care team or the family is another excellent example of integrating decision support into the end-of-life process. A commonly shared and available clinical information system remains an area of pressing need in the management of the dying patient.

The importance of community involvement and integration may be a more important model component in end-of-life care than in chronic disease care. To a large degree the processes of care around the dying individual often become less medicalized as an individual nears the end of life. Financial, personal, spiritual and transportation needs increasingly become the province of the larger community outside of what we consider to be the traditional health care delivery system. Finally, the model component of leadership or organizational support is certainly critical to the palliative care or hospice system. Of course, the definition or location of leadership is not necessarily clear. As care is de-medicalized near the end of life, clinic or hospital leadership may have minimal impact on delivery of a high value end of life experience. The leadership of disparate elements in the community may be as, if not more important to the process.

A diverse group of health care organizations across our country have utilized the CCM as the framework from which to deliver their care to their populations [13]. The National Health Service in the UK has also applied this model across their primary care providers as an organizational framework for their efforts to reform their chronic disease delivery [46]. It would seem that the CCM is an apt conceptual model to support a comprehensive organizational approach to end-of-life care in our country.

7. Healthcare ecosystem and society

The current state of our health care delivery system at the end of life is a reflection of the complexity that exists in our society regarding our perceptions of health care and death. We apply our consumer mentality to healthcare. Our insurance plans, particularly Medicare, have largely insulated health care consumers from considerations of price. We have expectations for the best possible care regardless of the cost. If a little is good, more must be better. Our reimbursement system rewards delivery of units of care. The modern health care system can provide unlimited options, our seemingly rational response is to maximize our utilization of any or all care offered.

We have an infatuation with technology, yet our understanding of medical science and complexity of care is often rudimentary. Our understanding of risk and benefit is primitive. The concept of medical futility is both intellectually and philosophically difficult for us to grasp. Belief in magical thinking or the power of miracles is widespread. As we have become more urbanized, and abandoned a rural life, our experience with death has become limited. Death is no longer viewed as an extension or natural part of life. It is more commonly denied, ignored, or avoided at all possible costs [20].

As extended families have become a rarity, we have lost a support network to help provide care for our loved ones. Care for the sick or dying has become the job of clinics and hospitals. The primary focus of clinics and hospitals, however, is to cure and heal. Modern hospitals are highly effective at bringing to bear a tremendous amount of resource in an extremely rapidly pace. The momentum of the process is overwhelming. When viewed in this light it is no wonder that we have the system of end of life care that we do. Or perhaps it is more accurate to say that we have no system at all.

8. Implementing change

There is no single stake holder that will have the capacity to effect change in a vacuum. Effective change will only come about when the providers, insurers, purchasers and most importantly, the consumers of healthcare in this country all work together to achieve a common goal of high value end-of-life care.

8.1. Providers

Among providers, leadership in palliative and end of life care had been lacking, but a critical mass is being developed. National and international leaders such as Dr. Diane Meier from Mount Sinai in New York have established the Center to Advance Palliative Care, a non profit center to foster the development of independent palliative care programs throughout not only the United States, but internationally as well. Her work has recently been recognized through the awarding of a MacArthur Foundation Genius award. Similarly the Education in Palliative and End of Life care (EPEC) based at Northwestern University with Linda Emmanuel MD as principle investigator has help to disseminate education by recruiting and teaching local champions in palliative and end of life care and giving them the tools to return to their home communities and provide the necessary education to their own caregiver communities.

The field of Palliative care has now been recognized as a unique subspecialty by the American Board of Medical Specialties. Board certification within palliative care became available as of 2008. Fellowship training in Palliative care is now recognized and subject to the same rigorous standards as other medical specialty training by the ACGME. It will be important for leaders in medical education to integrate curricular elements focusing on advanced directives, care planning, palliative care and hospice care into undergraduate and graduate medical education. This is a tremendous opportunity to educate the next generation of health care providers in this country.

Providers, clinics, hospitals and health systems need to establish uniform expectations for standards of care at the end of life. The Institute of Clinical Systems Improvement (ICSI) is a regional health-care collaborative organization comprised of representatives of over 50 medical groups in Minnesota, representing 85% of Minnesota physicians. ICSI has developed a set of clinical guidelines establishing accepted standards of care for management of several medical conditions.

The second edition of the Palliative Care Guideline was published in May of 2008. The document delineates a set of priority aims, implementation recommendations ans supporting documentation. It serves to both set a standard of high value end-of-life care and provide a blueprint for practices to follow as they begin to develop programs. The model of regional collaboratives could be used by provider groups to encourage and promote wide implementation of high value care planning, palliative care and hospice programs [26].

8.2. Insurers

Unfortunately, reimbursement schemes currently utilized by insurers, including CMS, serve to fragment care delivery. The primary driving principle behind palliative and end of life care is the meticulous care of the patients and their families. However, in the current economic climate simply "doing the right thing" is insufficient to sustain the field. The overwhelming majority of reimbursement policies to date offer no remuneration for continuity of care or the coordination or integration of care at the end of life.

There are some potentially promising developments. Primary care organizations including the AAFP, ACP and AAP have developed and promoted the concept of the Patient Centered Health Care Home [27]. A fundamental tenet of this construct is that care coordination is an essential component of care delivery. In fact, proposed payment schemes in support of the medical home concept stipulate payments specifically for care coordination and continuity of care. This approach is designed to support the medical home approach within our current fee for service remuneration system. Payment for medical home provision and care coordination would need to create incentives for care providers to participate. The medical home concept would, by definition, extend to include end-of-life care for patients. Similarly, end-of-life health care homes could be developed specifically for dying patients not already cared for in an existing medical home.

In Minnesota the legislature has passed a health care reform bill that incorporates new health care reimbursement strategies. These strategies include quality based incentive payments, payment for care coordination and bundled payments for coordinated management of conditions such as coronary artery disease, diabetes and asthma. The bundled payment structure rewards effective management of a defined "baskets of care" that comprehensively addresses all relevant aspects of a condition [34]. An end-of-life bundle could be envisioned that would create incentives for a medical group or practice to provide integrated, coordinated end of life care as has been previously described. This system of bundled care begins to get to the concept of payment for the actual process of care rather than payment for units of work delivered during the overall process of care delivery.

In England, the National Health Service has recently funded sixteen organizations to pilot new models of integrated care. Three of the models focus on the elderly and end of life care. Outcomes of interest with the pilots are better experience for the patients and greater cost effectiveness. The program represents a commitment by the key insurer in England to seriously investigate the potential for integrated chronic disease and end of life care to improve value [21]. It is clear that a similar commitment on the part of insurers, including CMS, in this country will be a necessary condition of system reform.

8.3. Consumers and purchasers

Finally, the consumers and purchasers of healthcare must be fully engaged in the process of changing the system of care delivery. Patients need to become more interested in and aware of their role in their personal care planning. Every adult citizen should complete an advanced directive document and actively participate with their health care team in the development of an individualized care plan. Incentives could be created by communities, governments or employers to encourage more engagement on the part of individuals in the guidance of their own healthcare. Finally, our country needs to begin a series of honest conversations regarding our attitudes toward death and dying. This conversation can be informed, and encouraged by members of the healthcare community through extensive public education efforts. We can no longer afford as individuals, families, communities or a nation to pretend that death and dying is not part of life. Ultimately, it will be patients that determine whether the transformational efforts underway in the provider and payer communities will turn out to be a house of cards or a stable foundation upon which to build a high value healthcare delivery system for patients at the end of life.

9. Resources

As previously noted, the evidence is mixed regarding cost savings related to appropriate end-of-life care. The best data to date, however, suggests significant cost savings are achievable through implementation of effective palliative care programs. In a large, retrospective study of eight geographically and structurally diverse hospitals palliative care patients who were discharged alive had a net savings of nearly $1700 dollars per admission. Palliative care patients who died had a net savings of nearly $5000 dollars per admission [34]. Given our older and sicker population and the proportion of our health care dollars that are spent in the hospital during the last one to two years of life it is hard underestimate the implications of this potential cost savings. Further exploration of this opportunity should be of considerable interest to all stakeholders in this ongoing discussion.

10. Conclusion

In the United States our friends and family members are likely to spend their last months of life receiving costly, invasive, and often futile medical care delivered in hospital wards and intensive care units. These circumstances are inconsistent with the wishes and values most of us would espouse. This outcome is the result of a health care delivery system designed to deliver acute or emergent care with the intention of restoring health. High value clinical practices utilized by palliative care services and hospice programs deliver care specifically designed to attend to the needs of patients at the end of their lives. These programs deliver high quality end-of-life care consistent with the needs and values of a dying patient. The programs offer the potential of significant cost savings for our health care system. Unfortunately, the organization of our health care system does not consistently support these programs. Our clinical systems fail to fully utilize these programs and our reimbursement models fail to create proper incentives to do so. The chronic care model is an organizational model for health care that can be used to support appropriate end of life care delivery. Baskets of care or care coordination fees are examples of reimbursement models that could increase the likelihood that palliative care and hospice programs are utilized. Providers, insurers, purchasers and consumers must all work to reform the system to create an environment conducive to the consistent delivery of high value end of life care. It will require a coordinated effort from each sector of our health care system to produce a system that consistently delivers high value health care at the end of life.

Acknowledgment

The authors would like to thank Theresa A. Kuhn for her assistance in manuscript preparation.

References

[1] C. Arenella, Medical issues to be considered in advance care planning, *American Hospice Foundation.* (Available on line).
[2] J.M. Ballentine, Pacemaker and defibrillator deactivation in competent hospice patients: an ethical consideration, *American Journal of Hospice and Palliative Care* **22**(2) (2005), 14–19.
[3] F.A. Bock.
[4] P.A. Bomba and D. Vermilyea, Integrating POLST into palliative guidelines: a paradigm shift in advance care planning in oncology, *Journal of National Comprehensive Cancer Network* **4** (2006), 819–829.
[5] *British Medical Journal*, 5 April 2008.
[6] C. Brunelli, M. Costantini, P. Di Giulio, M. Gallucci, F. Fusco, G. Miccinesi et al., Quality-of-life evaluation: When do terminal cancer patients and health-care providers agree? *Journal of Pain and Symptom Management* **15** (1998).
[7] I. Byock and M. Merriman, Measuring quality of life for patients with terminal illness: the Missoula-VITAS quality of life index, *Palliative Medicine* **12** (1998).
[8] D.E. Campbell, J. Lynn, T.A. Louis and L.R. Shugarman, Medicare program expenditures associated with hospice use, *Annals of Internal Medicine* **140**(4) (2004), 269–277.
[9] J.B. Cassel and K. Kerr, Does PC consultation reduce hospital length of stay? *AAHPM Annual Assembly March*, Austin, Texas, 2009.
[10] E. Chow, L. Andersson and R. Wong, Patients with advanced cancer: A survey of the understanding of their illness and expectations from palliative radiotherapy for symptomatic metastases, *Clinical Oncology* **13** (2001), 204–208.
[11] The chronic care model, *Improving Chronic Care Org*. (Available on line).
[12] D. Cook, S. Rocker and J. Marshall, Withdrawal of mechanical ventilation in anticipation of death in the Intensive Care Unit, *New England Journal of Medicine* **349** (2003), 1123–1132.
[13] Curing the system: Stories of change in chronic illness care, *ACT for America's Health* (Available on line).
[14] G. Demiris, E. Wittenberg-Lyles, D. Parker-Oliver and K.L. Courtney, A survey on the use of technology to support hospice interdisciplinary team meetings, *International Journal of Electronic Healthcare* **4**(3/4) (2008), 244–256.
[15] C.C. Earle, B.A. Neville and M.B. Landrum, Trends in the aggressiveness of cancer near the end of life, *Journal of Clinical Oncology* **22** (2004), 315–321.
[16] E.J. Emmanuel, Y. Young-XU and N.G. Levinski, Chemotherapy use among Medicare beneficiaries at the end of life, *Annals of Internal Medicine* **138** (2003), 639–643.
[17] From AAHPM meeting 2009.
[18] G. Gade, I. Venohr, K. McGrady, J. Beane, R.H. Richardson, M.P. Williams et al., Impact of an inpatient palliative care team: a randomized control trial, *Journal of Palliative Medicine*, **11**(2) (2008), 180–190.
[19] The gold standards framework: A program for community palliative care. (Available on line).
[20] E. Goodman, (2009). *Boston Editorial Boston com* (Available on line).
[21] H. Hawkes, Health policy: Integrated care, *BMJ* **338** (2009).
[22] S.E. Hickman, C.A. Nelson, A.H. Moss, B.J. Hammes and S.W. Tolle, Converting treatment wishes into order at the end of life: A multi-state study of the POLST (physician's orders for life-sustaining treatment) in nursing facilities (417-C), *AAHPM annual assembly Austin Texas*, March 2009.
[23] J.L. Holley, S.S. Carmody and A.H. Moss, The need of end-of-life care training in Nephrology: National survey results of nephrology fellows, *American Journal of Kidney Disease* **42** (2003), 813–820.
[24] Hospice payment system, *CMS* (Available on line).
[25] http://www.qualityforum.org/about/NPP/. Accessed 4–5–09.
[26] ICSI healthcare guidelines: Palliative care, *ICSI* (Available on line).
[27] Joint principles of the patient-centered medical home. (2007). (Available on line).
[28] M.I. Kim and K.B. Johnson, Personal health records: Evaluation of functionality and utility, *Journal of the American Medical Informatics Association* **9** (2002), 171–180.
[29] C.E. Kuziemsky, J.H. Jahnke and F. Lau, The e-Hospice: Beyond traditional boundaries of palliative care, *Science Direct* (Available on-line), 2005.
[30] J. Lynn, Sick to death and not going to take it anymore!: Reforming health care for the last years of life. *University of California Press*, 2004.
[31] J. Lynn and D.M. Adamson, Living well at the end of life: Adapting health care to serious chronic illness in old age, *Rand Health White Paper WP-137*, 2003.

[32] W.J. Mackillop, W.E. Stewart and A.D. Gingsburg, Cancer patients' perceptions of their disease and its treatment, *British Journal of Cancer* **58** (1988), 355–358.
[33] J.E. Mathews, (2007). Access to hospice care. (Available on line).
[34] Minnesota: Payment reform and price transparency, *The Commonwealth Fund* (Available on line).
[35] R.S. Morrison, C. Maroney-Galin, P.D. Kralovec and D.E. Meier, The growth of palliative care programs in United States hospitals, *Journal of Palliative Medicine* **8**(6) (2005), 1127–1134.
[36] R.S. Morrison, J.D. Penrod, B. Cassel, M. Caust-Ellengogen, A. Litke, L. Spragens et al., Cost savings associated with US hospital palliative care consultation program, *Archives Internal Medicine* **168**(16) (2008), 1783–1790.
[37] R.S. Morrison and D. Meier, High rates of advance care planning in New York City's elderly population, *Archives Internal Medicine* **164**(22) (2004), 2421–2426.
[38] New study sheds better light on hospice use across America. *National Hospice and Palliative Care Organization*.
[39] NHPCO web site accessed 3–27–09, http://www.nhpco.org.
[40] Program for all inclusive care for the elderly (PACE) http://www.cms.hhs.gov/PACE/.
[41] T. Okon, J. Gomez and L. Blackhall, Palliative educational outcome with implementation of PEACE tool integrated clinical pathway, *Journal of Palliative Medicine* **7** (2004).
[42] M.W. Rabow, S.L. Dibble, S.Z. Pantial and S.J. McPhee, The comprehensive care team: a controlled trial of outpatient palliative medicine consultation, *Archives Internal Medicine* **164**(1) (2004), 83–91.
[43] M.W. Rabow, B.L. Miller, K. Kerr and J. Ross, CA symptom managments among patients receiving concurrent outpatient palliative and oncologic care: results fromt he symptom management service (316-A) *Presented at AAHPM annual assembly*, Austin, Texas, March 2009.
[44] M.W. Rabow, J. Petersen, K. Schanche, S. Dibble and S.J. McPhee, The comprehensive care team: A description of a controlled trial of care at the beginning of the end of life, *Journal of Palliative Medicine* **6**(3) (2003).
[45] T.D. Shanafelt, C.L. Loprinzi and R. Marks, Are chemotherapy response rates related to treatment induced survival prolongations in patients with advanced cancer, *Journal of Clinical Oncology* **22**(1966–1974) (2004).
[46] D. Singh and C. Ham, *Improving care for people with long-term conditions*, 2006.
[47] A review of UK and international frameworks.
[48] K.E. Steinhasuer, N.A. Christakis and E.C. Clipp, Factors considered important at the end of life by patients, family, phsyicains, and other care providers, *JAMA* **284** (2000), 2476.
[49] K. Steinhauser, E. Clipp, H. Bosworth, M. McNeilly, N. Christakis, C. Voils et al., Measuring quality of life at the end of life: Validation of the QUAL-E, *Palliative and Supportive Care* **2** (2004).
[50] P.Y. Takahashi, S.J. Crane, E.E. Tung, S.S. Cha and G.J. Hanson, Increased hospitalization cost in older adults with higher elderly risk assessment, *Journal of the American Geriatrics Society* **57** (2009), S99.
[51] M. Thelen, End-of-life decision making in intensive care, *Critical Care Nurse* **25** (2005), 28–37.
[52] E.H. Wagner, Chronic disease management: What will it take to improve care for chronic illness? *Eff Clin Pract* **1** (1998), 2–4.
[53] J.E. Wennberg, E.S. Fisher and S.M. Sharp, (2006). The care of patients with severe chronic illnesses: An online report of the Medicare program by the Dartmouth Atlas Project, *The Dartmouth Atlas of Healthcare*, Available on line.
[54] A.A. Wright, B. Zhang, A. Ray et al., Associations between end of life discussions, patient mental health, medical care near death, and caregiver bereavement adjustment, *JAMA* **300**(14) (8 Oct 2008), 1665–1673.

Robert Stroebel, MD, is chair of the Division of Primary Care Internal Medicine at Mayo Clinic Rochester and an Assistant Professor of Medicine, Mayo Clinic College of Medicine. He has practiced Internal Medicine for the past 17 years with a career focus in practice redesign.

Timothy J. Moynihan, MD, is education chair for the Department of Medical Oncology, Director of the Palliative Care program at Mayo Clinic Rochester, Associate Medical Director for Mayo Clinic Hospice, and an Associate Professor of Oncology, Mayo Clinic College of Medicine. He has practiced in Medical Oncology for 17 years with a focus on brain and breast cancer, symptom management, palliative and end of life care.

Information Knowledge Systems Management 8 (2009) 87–104
DOI 10.3233/IKS-2009-0137
IOS Press

Chapter 6

US health care costs: The crushing burden

Helen Darling
E-mail: darling@businessgrouphealth.org

Abstract: This chapter provides an overview of health care costs in the United States, including trends, sources and uses of funds, employers' role, and factors driving costs. It also reviews what analysts believe are cost drivers especially compared to other countries that have significantly lower health care costs and, often, better health outcomes. *Within* the US, there are also important differences by geography, further demonstrating that higher US costs do not reflect higher quality and greater patient and physician satisfaction. In fact, the opposite is often the case.

1. Introduction

The United States has the highest health care costs in the world, far higher than other countries with impressive standards of living, such as Germany, Switzerland, Netherlands, Sweden, Norway, and Denmark, enumerating just those in Europe (See Table 1). Not surprisingly, health care costs have become one of the two or three most prominent concerns cited in every report on health care and, increasingly, on the state of the US economy. Cost pressures are helping to fuel the stepped-up drive for health care reform in the US.

Costs have been a problem for a long time but the mismatch between ever rising costs, flat wages, absolute dollar amounts compared to household income, and the 2008–2009 recession have exacerbated this long-standing challenge (See Table 2). More and more, talk of solutions to the health care crisis has had to include serious ways to address the *costs* of health care, not just health insurance for all Americans, another topic under discussion for over 30 years. Even health care providers and others whose revenues would be affected have come to understand that the relentless growth in health care costs, and the unsatisfying and discouraging value proposition for the investment are not sustainable.

Already $2.5 trillion dollars in national health expenditures in 2009, costs rise roughly 6% per year. At this rate, the proportion of Gross Domestic Product (GDP) spending on health is projected to be about 20.3% by 2018 (See Exhibit 1). The growth in medical care prices is the largest influence on spending. Growth in medical care utilization is the second most important driver of expenses. Neither population growth nor age is a major factor in the increase [26].

The public sector now accounts for 56% of health spending within the civilian non-institutionalized population [24]. With the rapid growth in the federal deficit, partly due to recent wars, financial markets' collapse and federal bailouts, the United States will find it harder and harder to subsidize its profligacy, much of it for unfunded health care, which in turn will push up interest on the national debt. "Health care costs are the key to our fiscal stability," according to Peter Orszag, Director of the US Office of Management and Budget (OMB) under President Obama [19].

Table 1

Per Capita Spending on Health Care

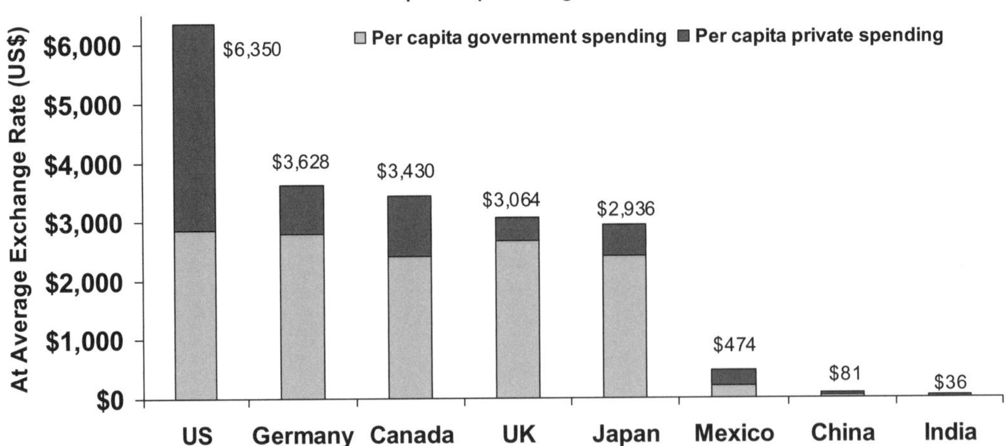

Note: Figures represent total per capita government spending plus private spending in 2005. China figure does not include Hong Kong and Macao Special Administrative Regions.
Source: 2008 World Health Organization Statistics.

3

Table 2

Percent Change in Total Private Expenditures, Workers Earnings and Inflation

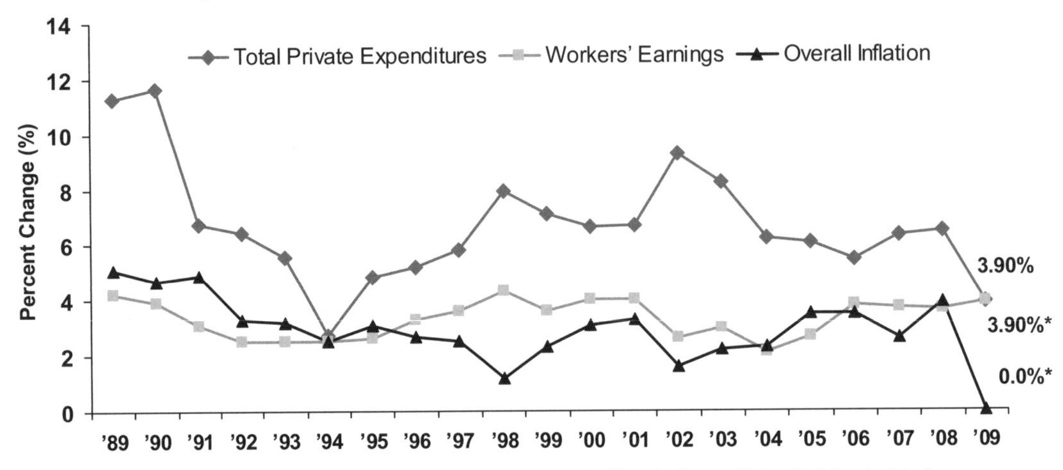

*2008-2009 (January to January) figures for workers' earnings and over all inflation were obtained from the Bureau of Labor Statistics. April-April figures are not yet available for 2009.
Source: 1989-2009 N ational Health Expenditure Data, with projections starting i n 2008 (total private expenditure constitutes private ins urance, out- of- pocket payments and other private funds); Bureau of Labor Statistics, Consumer Price Index, U .S. City Average of Annual Inflation, 1989-2008 (April to April); Bureau of Labor Statistics, Seasonally Adjusted Data from the Current Employment Statistics Survey, 1989- 2008 (April to April).

1

The deep recession in 2008–2009 resulted in a sharp drop in the GDP, negative 6.1% in the first quarter of 2009 [30] (See Fig. 1). The contraction during the 4th quarter 2008 and 1st quarter 2009 was the worst pullback since 1958, fifty years before. Not only is it a problem that national health expenditures have continued to outpace economic growth over many years, the historic pattern, but actual *decline* in the GDP means that the percentage of NHE, the numerator, and the GDP, the denominator, have made our health economy profile even worse than projected. The Congressional Budget Office reports that

EXHIBIT 1

Growth In National Health Spending Versus Gross Domestic Product (GDP), 1990–2018

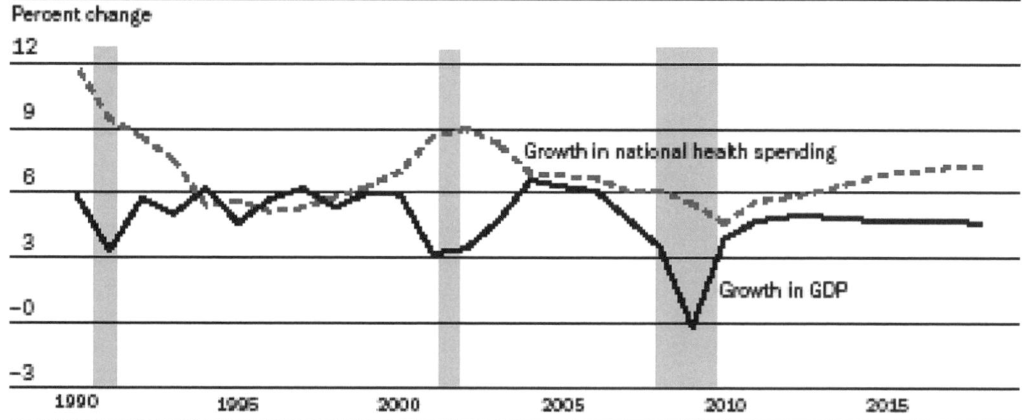

SOURCES: Centers for Medicare and Medicaid Services, Office of the Actuary, National Health Statistics Group; U.S. Department of Commerce, Bureau of Economic Analysis; and National Bureau of Economic Research.
NOTES: Historical data through 2007; projected data from 2008 to 2018. Recessions took place during July 1990–March 1991; March 2001–November 2001; and December 2007–2009 (projected) and are denoted by shading.

from 1975 and 2005, health care costs rose at least 2.2% faster than the GDP, reaching nearly 17% of the GDP in 2008. Without significant changes that will “bend the curve,” jargon for reductions in cost increases, which are not true reductions in health care spending, health care *could* consume 50% of the GDP by 2082.

The US has a fiscal crisis, not just a health care crisis. While health care can certainly not be blamed for all of the nations’ woes, the budget deficit alone is equal to 13.1% of the GDP. Deficits add each year to the already bloated national debt, which in turn has to be financed by paying interest to the bond holders. One of the fixed budget costs of the federal government then becomes interest on the national debt which has to be paid, no matter what. That essential expenditure directly limits the nation’s ability to pay for other goods and services.

The hole the US is in could become even more challenging if countries, such as China, Japan and Korea, that have been buying the debt, start demanding higher interest rates in return for greater risk. Between the interest on the national debt, costs of prior and current wars, national security, and health care, there will be little money for many other necessary services, a formula for stagnation and decline for any nation.

In terms of costs, economists, health services researchers and experts from a number of disciplines talk not just about direct expenditures but about what we get for the investment, what the society is willing to pay through direct payments and through taxes and other subsidies, what businesses have to earn to cover ever rising health costs, and what other goods and services (e.g. education) cannot be supported because of the amount of our economy that goes into health care. Again, the evidence is that the US does not get nearly as good a return on its investment as it should [8]. The US health care system gets a failing grade on all of those dimensions.

2. Lack of any health insurance is a problem

Ironically, and partly because care is so expensive, the US has nearly 46 million people without any

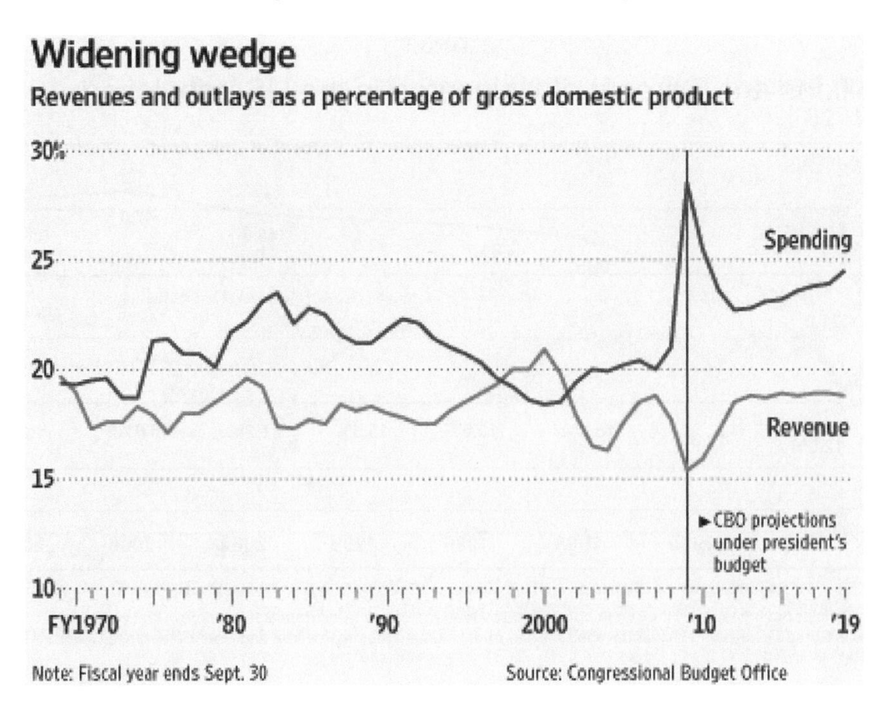

Fig. 1.

health insurance for the whole year (See Table 3). The number is even higher if people uninsured for any part of the year are included. In previous years when the nation's lawmakers tried to make health insurance universally available, unlike virtually every other advanced industrial nation, proponents often argued that the US had to cover the millions of uninsured first then work on controlling costs. But, political leaders in 2009, including President Obama and Senator Baucus, Chair of the powerful Senate Finance Committee acknowledged that the nation has to reduce what the President refers to as the "crushing burden of health care costs" [18] which is negatively affecting US families, its economy and the government's abilities to deliver on its promises. The primary emphasis on controlling costs as *central* to ensuring universal coverage was new to the national debates started in 2008.

3. Health of the population is not good

The crisis the US faces is not just about costs but how much real health, not just health care, the nation is getting for its expenditures. By virtually all measures of health, the other countries' populations cited above are healthier or just as healthy for about half or less of the investment. While there are many, complex reasons for the high costs and for the less healthy population, virtually all experts agree that there is substantial room for improvement in the US in costs, quality, safety and access to health care, as well documented by the Commonwealth Fund Commission on a High Performance Health System's "Why Not the Best? Results from the National Scorecard on US Health System Performance, 2008" [7]. As discussed later, the rapid rise in costs is not just about increased utilization, price increases and new services layered on to old, but also due to the many obese people in the US who have, as a result, an expanding number of serious, expensive chronic conditions such as diabetes and heart disease, at younger and younger ages.

Table 3

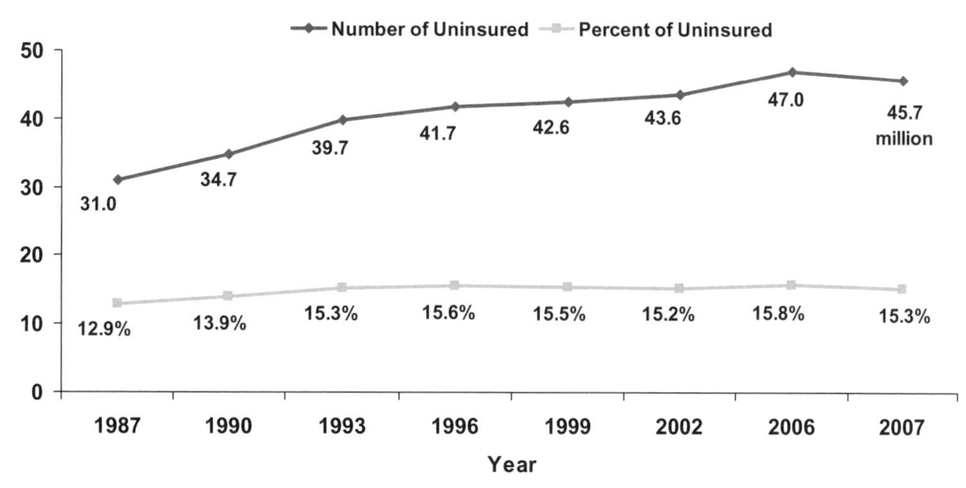

Note: People were considered uninsured if they were not covered by any type of health insurance at any time in that year.
Source: U.S. Census Bureau, Current Population Reports: Consumer Income. Income, Poverty, and Health Insurance Coverage in the United States: 2007.

4. The role of employers

In the US, employers provide health care coverage for over 60% of the adults under 65 and their children, about 160 million people. While the US has had an employer-based health insurance system since the 1930's, employers are concerned for a number of reasons about the sustainability of an employer-based method of ensuring that all residents of the country have the right kind of health insurance. Coverage tied to employment can negatively affect employees and families when they choose to change jobs or when they lose their jobs. The impact of a recession such as in 2008–2009 showed again how severe the effect can be when health benefits are terminated along with job loss.

In addition, employers and employees are finding it increasingly difficult to absorb the rising costs. Compared to just 7–8 years ago, employers are paying 100% more for health care, at an average of over $9,000 per employee for active employees, not counting retiree coverage, which a shrinking number of employers still provide. The costs of family coverage in 2009, according to Milliman's Medical Index, are $16,771 [17]. Employers are paying on average $9,947 for family coverage and employees pay $4,004 for their share of the premiums out of their pay checks. Employees and their families pay another $2,820 in out-of-pocket costs, such as, copayments, coinsurance, deductibles and other uncovered medical expenses. With a median wage of around $42,000, the proportion of total pay (wages plus benefits) to employees that goes to health care alone is way out of line with other needs. This means that many families cannot afford to take coverage they are offered or the employee takes his or her own coverage because the cost sharing is lower but cannot afford to cover family members. For every 1% increase in health care premiums an estimated 300,000 to 400,000 will lose their health care coverage, according to John Sheils, in May 9, 2007, as reported in Denny et al. [25]. Increasingly, smaller and low margin businesses have not been able to offer health benefits to their employees, adding to the number of working people who are uninsured.

In the US, federal law requires that individuals who lose health benefits due to an involuntary termination or death, disability or divorce have the right to buy their own coverage back for periods of 18 months to 36 months. Called COBRA continuation coverage, it is an option, but realistically COBRA is rarely taken. Former employees or dependents have to pay 102% of the costs of the coverage, which few can afford, especially when unemployed. With the federal stimulus bill, enacted early in 2009, Congress authorized the federal government to pay 65% of the COBRA premium for up to 9 months for employees who were involuntarily terminated between September 1, 2008 and December 31, 2009. Employers could also allow the employee to select another, presumably less expensive, plan right away.

While all employers have to struggle with paying for health insurance for their employees and dependents, businesses have a serious disadvantage in the global economy if they need to manufacture or provide other services in the US which can be done at far lower costs outside the US Not surprisingly, companies increasingly create new jobs outside the US when that is economically advantageous. The lack of affordable health insurance keeps employers, especially small employers and those in low margin businesses, from providing any benefits, reducing work hours or not filling jobs, especially during tough economic times.

Virtually all large employers (200 or more employees) provide health insurance because it is seen as an essential recruitment and retention tool and because employers want their employees and dependents to get care they need to be productive and healthy.

In general, health insurance cost increases have "slowed" to an average increase of 6% per year, which is a welcome break from some previous years, although that growth is way out of whack with virtually all other economic measures. Table 2 shows the comparisons of private health expenditures with workers earnings and overall inflation. In some respects, it could reasonably be said that the workers of the US have been giving their pay raises to the health care system for 20 years. Economists and most other policy analysts readily agree that workers, not employers, pay for their health benefits through foregone wages and other benefits. Interestingly, however, since workers themselves do not fully understand this or how much of what they spend their money for is of low value, they still report on surveys that they would be willing to give up some more wages for more health benefits [10].

5. What do national expenditures pay for

As published in a recent study by Hartman et al., in *Health Affairs*, national health spending in 2007 [12], the most recent year for which there are actual data, reached $2.2 trillion, 16.2% of the GDP, or $7,421 per person. Of that, as shown in Table 4, about 31% went to hospitals, 21% to physicians and clinics, 10% to drugs, 25% to other and 7% to administration. Total spending increased 6.1% over 2006. Hospitals increased 7.3%, but prescription drugs had a significant drop in the rate of increase to 4.9%, the lowest in 44 years, due mainly to the increased use of generics, slower price growth and "increased concerns about the safety of certain drugs" due to a larger number of "black box" warnings from the FDA in 2007. Administration and net costs also grew at the slower pace of 3.6% primarily because of the effect of the Medicare Part D drug benefit rolled out in 2006.

6. Who pays?

In the US, there are 3 primary sources of payment for health care: government programs, employers/insurers, and consumers. Of all government programs, Medicare is usually seen as the largest and most influential since it provides health insurance for 45.3 million beneficiaries who are either age 65, permanently and totally disabled, or have End Stage Renal Disease. In 2008, Medicare's outlays reached

Table 4

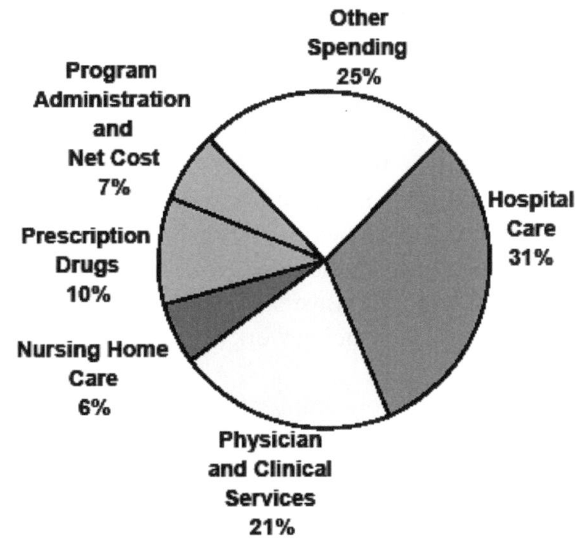

$466 billion, having increased 8.1% over 2007. It is anticipated that Medicare will grow another 8% in 2009 [26]. Medicaid, a federal-state program for low income people, including children, costs $352.1 billion and covers 59 million people (some are eligible for Medicare and Medicaid). The 2008–2009 recession increased the number of people eligible for Medicaid so its expenditures will increase even more. Private health insurance (the category that includes what employers pay) accounts for another $817.4 billion in outlays for care in 2008. CMS analysts believe that private health insurance costs will be dampened by the recession to a rate of increase close to or slightly below 6% [26]. If that is correct, it will be the lowest rate since the managed care era in the 1990's. Without other strong countervailing pressures, however, that slowdown will not last long. In fact, anecdotal evidence suggests that 2009 and 2010 may be more expensive years for employers, insurers and consumers because providers are raising their prices, possibly fearful about new fiscal constraints ahead, and payment policies continue to reward volume of services and tests and services that do not add clinical value, some of which doctors may order as potential defenses against fears of malpractice suits in the litigious US culture.

Medicare's costs have risen rapidly, so much so that together with all other health programs, health care was seen as the "pacman" of the federal budget. The rate of public spending overall has grown faster than private spending, mainly because of the passage of legislation that covered outpatient prescription drugs for all Medicare beneficiaries for the first time in its 40 year history so that the percent of national expenditures paid by public funds went from 37.6% in 1970 to 46.2% in 2007. Much of that expense had been absorbed by Medicare beneficiaries who previously had to pay for their own prescription drugs, unless they had other coverage. With Medicare Part D, prescription drug coverage, many consumers had their out of pocket reduced sharply, especially if they had no Medicare wraparound policies or employer retiree coverage which most did not. Table 5 illustrates the unsustainable federal health spending trend.

Table 5

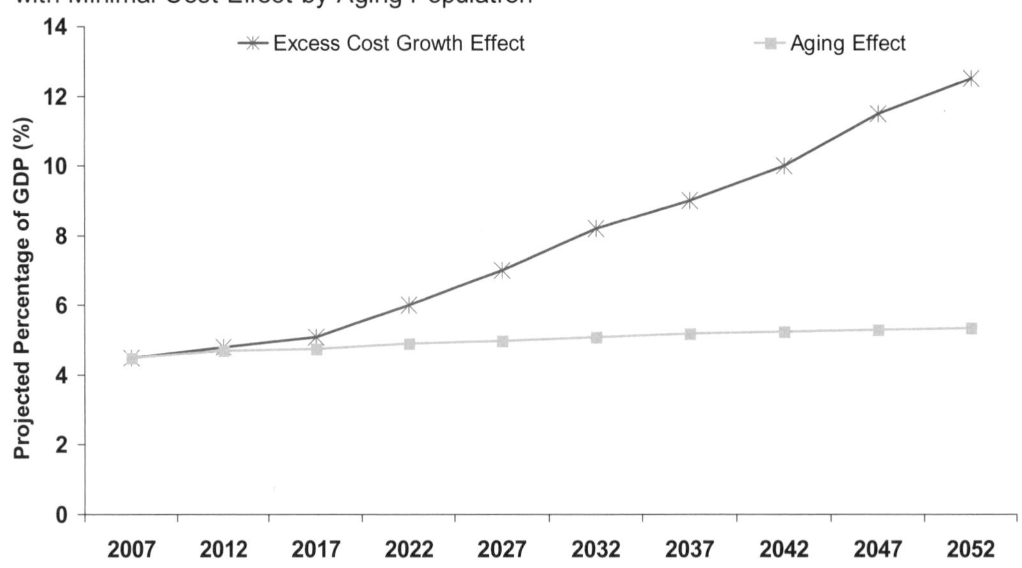

Note: Excess cost growth is the extent to which the increase in health care spending for an aver age indi vidual exceeds the growth in per capita gross domestic product (GDP).
Source: Congressional Budget Office, 2007

2

7. Why is the US so much more expensive

Anderson, Reinhardt et al. compared US expenditures with OECD countries, and concluded that the key differences are due to higher prices, not that Americans receive many more services or have substantially more resources [3]. For example, on many measures per capita, such as physicians, nurses, hospitals and measures of use, the US is actually lower than OECD countries. While US costs are currently much higher than OECD countries, their rates of growth are almost the same – 4.4% for US and 4.3% for OECD average.

Thorpe and colleagues looked at disease prevalence and treatment rates for ten of the costliest health conditions in 1976–1980 and 1999–2000 to try to explain the cost differences. They found that disease prevalence and the rates of medication use were much higher in the US. Payments per case were driven by technology. With more and more new technology, those costs rose but "changes in treated disease prevalence are caused by a rise in the population prevalence of disease, changes in clinical thresholds (and awareness) for treating and diagnosing disease and new technologies that allow treating additional patients with a particular medical condition." To give the reader a sense of the problem, in this study, according to the usually underestimated self-reporting, 33% of the adults age 50 and older were obese, compared to a 17% obesity rate in 10 European countries. Older US adults in this study were more likely to have smoked or were current smokers, 53% to 43% [28]. In turn, they attribute disease prevalence growth to more obesity in the population. (See Exhibit 2) For example, for adults ages 20–74, 14.5% were obese in 1976–1980 but 30.4% twenty years later.

In an earlier paper, Thorpe, Florence, Howard and Joski, examined the top 20 medical conditions for adults 18–64 in 1987–2002. In that research, Thorpe et al. found that for 16 of the conditions, over half of the health care spending increases was due to the increase in disease prevalence. They

EXHIBIT 2

EXHIBIT 2
Prevalence And Treated Prevalence In The United States And Ten European Countries, 2004

	United States		Europe		
	Percent	95% CI	Percent	95% CI	U.S./Europe difference
Prevalence[a]					
Heart disease	21.8	21.1, 22.4	11.4	10.7, 12.0	10.4
High blood pressure	50.0	49.2, 50.9	32.9	32.0, 33.9	17.1
High cholesterol	21.7	20.7, 22.7	19.6	18.9, 20.4	2.1
Stroke/cerebrovascular disease	5.3	4.9, 5.6	3.5	3.1, 3.9	1.8
Diabetes	16.4	15.8, 17.0	10.9	10.3, 11.5	5.5
Chronic lung disease	9.7	9.2, 10.2	5.4	4.9, 5.8	4.3
Asthma	4.4	3.9, 4.8	4.3	3.9, 4.6	0.1
Arthritis	53.8	52.9, 54.6	21.3	20.5, 22.1	32.5
Osteoporosis	5.0	4.4, 5.5	7.8	7.2, 8.3	-2.8
Cancer	12.2	11.6, 12.2	5.4	4.9, 5.9	6.8
Obese	33.1	32.3, 33.9	17.1	16.3, 17.8	16.0
Current smoker	20.9	20.2, 21.7	17.8	17.1, 18.6	3.1
Former smoker	31.7	30.9, 32.5	25.2	24.3, 26.0	6.5
Never smoked	47.3	46.5, 48.2	57.0	56.0, 58.0	9.7
Medication use[b]					
Heart disease	60.7	59.1, 62.4	54.5	51.6, 57.4	6.2
High blood pressure	88.0	87.2, 88.8	88.9	87.8, 90.0	-0.9
High cholesterol	88.1	86.4, 89.9	62.4	60.4, 64.5	25.7
Stroke/cerebrovascular disease	45.1	41.8, 48.4	44.6	39.7, 49.5	0.5
Diabetes	81.3	79.7, 82.9	81.5	79.2, 83.7	-0.2
Chronic lung disease	51.2	48.6, 53.9	28.0	24.4, 31.7	23.2
Asthma	85.5	81.7, 89.2	65.1	60.6, 69.6	20.4
Arthritis	44.9	43.8, 46.0	49.5	47.3, 51.7	-4.6
Osteoporosis	83.6	79.6, 87.7	44.2	40.7, 47.6	39.4
Cancer	–[c]		–[c]		
Treated prevalence[d]					
Heart disease	13.2	12.7, 13.7	6.2	5.7, 6.7	7.0
High blood pressure	44.0	43.2, 44.8	29.3	28.4, 30.2	14.7
High cholesterol	19.1	18.2, 20.1	12.3	11.6, 12.9	6.8
Stroke/cerebrovascular disease	2.4	2.1, 2.6	1.6	1.3, 1.8	0.8
Diabetes	13.3	12.8, 13.9	8.9	8.3, 9.5	4.4
Chronic lung disease	5.0	4.6, 5.3	1.5	1.3, 1.7	3.5
Asthma	3.7	3.3, 4.2	2.8	2.5, 3.1	0.9
Arthritis	24.1	23.4, 24.8	10.6	9.9, 11.2	13.5
Osteoporosis	4.1	3.6, 4.6	3.4	3.1, 3.8	0.7
Cancer	–[e]		–[e]		

SOURCE: Authors' analysis of data from the Survey of Health, Ageing, and Retirement in Europe (SHARE) (ten European countries); the Health and Retirement Survey (HRS); and the Medical Expenditure Panel Survey (MEPS) (the latter two: U.S. data).

NOTES: U.S. estimates for high cholesterol, asthma, and osteoporosis were obtained from MEPS. CI is confidence interval.

[a] Respondents with physician-diagnosed disease.

[b] Proportion of prevalent cases reporting medication use associated with the condition.

[c] Not available.

[d] Product of prevalence and medication use.

[e] Not applicable.

found these relationships particularly true for conditions most linked with obesity such as diabetes and hyperlipidimia. (See Exhibit 1).

In another study, using data from the National Center for Health Statistics, by Decker et al., of the use of medical care for 8 major chronic conditions, the authors found that "even after adjusting for age, ambulatory visits rose by 21 percent in the ten year period between 1995–1996 and 2005–2006. Visits for arthritis, hypertension, diabetes and depression grew by 30%. Hospital discharge rates fell 9%, especially for heart disease, cancer and cerebrovascular disease" [11].

Many years of research on health care systems across the globe, most especially work done by Barbara Starfield and by the Commonwealth Fund, have established that countries in which primary care is the foundation for their systems have much better health outcomes and more satisfied patients and physicians. As Don Berwick, the president of the Institute for Healthcare Improvement, said: "The current system is very hospital-centric; we wait for people to get sick, then we invest enormous sums to fix them up. We should build primary care as the core" [29]. While the use of hospitals may not be all that different from Europe, a difference may be that the US has more people with health problems, due to poor lifestyle choices, without a strong primary care based system and almost unlimited ways to test, screen, monitor and treat people. Most significantly, the bulk of those costs are paid for, not at the site of care, but through a labyrinthine third party payment system that baffles even those who work in it. Given those factors, the high costs are not at all surprising.

8. What are the main cost drivers?

Major contributors to the high health costs in the US include new technology, new and very expensive specialty drugs, devices and procedures [4]. New technology adds to costs, but unlike other sectors in which new technology replaces old technology, health care is different. Often new technology is additive, leading to what is called layering on of technology. The innovation does not replace the old but is just added on. Unfortunately, while the new technology may provide additional information, it may not add information that changes treatment. It almost always costs more because it costs more to produce and it may even have some additional functionality. Yet, there may be no changes in treatment because of more functionality and no difference in health outcomes.

In a study published in 2006, PricewaterhouseCoopers, calculated the factors that contributed to a 8.8% increase in health insurance premiums. They reported that general inflation accounted for 27%, price increases beyond inflation contributed another 30% and 43% was due to increase in services delivered [21].

In a 10-year study of the use of CT-scans and MRI scans, Rebecca Smith-Bindman found that they increased two-fold and three-fold, respectively, per patient in that period. The average cost per patient went from $229 to $443 [27]. Another study by the General Accountability Office (GAO) concluded that medical imaging doubled between 2000 and 2006.

In addition to new technologies being more expensive, in many instances but not always, some new technology is actually less expensive, but because it is safer and less invasive may result in many more patients being seen as suitable candidates, according to David Cutler [9] "treatment expansion" proved to be quantitatively more important than "treatment substitution."

Uwe Reinhardt, who has written extensively on this topic over many years, argues that a major reason that Americans spend so much more than other countries on health care is due to the excess spending on administration. He cites the work of the McKinsey Global Institute that estimated that excess spending

EXHIBIT 3

The Rise In Treated Disease Prevalence And Its Impact On Private Insurance Spending, 1987–2002

Medical condition	Treated prevalence per 100,000		Cost per treated case ($)		Percent contribution to total growth in spending, 1987–2002	Percent change in spending due to change in treated prevalence[a]
	1987	2002	1987	2002		
Newborn and maternity care	3,406	2,940	773	3,950	8.1	-21
Cancer	2,710	3,666	3,081	3,999	6.4	61
Pulmonary conditions	9,294	17,699	507	639	6.3	81
Arthritis	4,573	7,640	701	1,282	6.1	60
Mental disorders	4,658	10,984	1,242	972	4.9	126
Hyperlipidemia	1,383	7,427	278	618	3.7	89
Hypertension	9,372	11,988	456	664	3.7	47
Lupus	4,177	6,535	470	868	3.5	55
Back problems	4,581	8,144	1,457	1,202	3.4	138
Upper gastrointestinal	2,618	7,042	854	769	3.0	107
Diabetes	2,420	3,972	1,293	1,551	3.0	79
Kidney problems	662	1,318	3,918	4,101	2.7	96
Infectious disease	5,858	5,793	268	726	2.5	-2
Heart disease	4,610	5,002	2,734	2,753	2.3	92
Skin disorders	6,695	9,144	344	471	2.0	58
Bronchitis	13,400	11,685	146	282	1.4	-36
Endocrine disorders	6,402	7,906	389	467	1.3	58.2
Other gastrointestinal diseases	1,280	2,461	664	848	1.2	81
Bone disorders	620	2,030	555	700	1.0	91.7
Cerebrovascular disease	132	345	7,812	4,742	0.6	166.8

SOURCE: Tabulations from 1987 NMES and 2002 MEPS.

NOTE: The twenty conditions together contributed 66.8 percent to the growth in total spending.

[a] Ratio of the percentage of total spending growth linked to a rise in treated prevalence to the percentage linked to treated prevalence and cost per case combined.

on health administration and insurance accounted for as much as 21% or $150 billion in 2003. Reinhardt estimates that the figure would be $650 billion in 2008.

There has been an expanding body of evidence of the high costs of administration in the US, much of which is due to the lack of standardization for multiple payers, diverse rules, and woefully inadequate use of electronic records and digital communication. The difference between the national health expenditures (NHE) report of much lower costs of administration and these other studies is explained by what is counted. For example, NHE estimates include only data on the costs of administering government health programs and on net spending on private insurance policies (revenues from premiums minus medical payments). Those figures do not include costs the system bears for clerical work and the time providers and their staffs spend on dealing with the complex, fragmented payment system the US has. While there is a wide variation in results of studies done to quantify the excess costs of administration in the US health care system, the NHE figure is low. CMS estimates that private health insurance administrative costs per person covered was $453 in 2006.There is a robust research literature on this topic. How hard it is to assess administrative costs is summarized by Henry Aaron in "The Costs of Health Care Administration in the United States and Canada: Questionable Answers to a Questionable Question." [2].

James Hefferman tracked in great detail physician billing costs in one large physician organization and concluded that the administrative burden is approximately "11% of net patient service revenue or

$26 billion nationally" [14]. Lawrence Casalino reported on a survey of physician practices to learn how much time they spent interacting with health plans. He concluded that the total tab nationally is $25–33 billion annually or $54,000–$72,000 per physician [5].

For a very comprehensive review of the research on health care costs, see Paul Ginsburg's, High and Rising Health Care Costs: Demystifying US Health Care Spending", Robert Wood Johnson Foundation, Research Synthesis Report [15].

Researchers have also learned within the last 10 years how much of the costs are due to a number of factors in the disorganized, fragmented US health care system that result in more expensive care as well as care that is harmful or does not add any benefits. In either case, this is wasteful in a system in which there are also many unmet needs. For example, studies have shown that patients discharged from the hospital are frequently readmitted to the hospital for a variety of reasons at great expense. These are preventable with relatively simple measures. Patients who have been given clear information about their after-hospital care are 30% less likely to be readmitted or go to the emergency room and have average costs lower by $412 [1]. In addition to those readmitted are many more who have poorer recovery, pain and other problems because they lacked adequate discharge planning and information.

9. Unexplained and costly geographic variations

Over 30 years of research by Jack Wennberg, Elliott Fisher, and others at Dartmouth has documented highly variable patterns of health care use and costs *within* the US that seemingly bear little relation to quality of care and patient and physician satisfaction. Their studies have revealed over and over unexplained variation in medical practice patterns and that some areas, such as Minnesota, provide high quality care at considerably lower costs than other areas, such as Dade County, Florida. For example, Medicare spent $16,351 per person annually in Miami and $5,873 in Grand Junction, Colorado. While some of the causes of variation are not clear, differences do occur especially in procedures or treatment where there is less certainty about the right treatment. In those cases, the supply of physicians, specialists, hospitals, imaging and ambulatory facilities ("supply-sensitive services") correlate with higher use. In areas with many specialists, hospitalized Medicare patients are seen by many more specialists. Patients are hospitalized more often, have more tests and imaging, spend more time in the ICU before death, and little or no time in hospice in spite of advanced illness.

Variations in rates of certain surgical procedures include: coronary artery bypass grafting; percutaneous coronary artery angioplasty; back surgery; cholecystectomy; hip replacement surgery. Interestingly, for conditions for which there is strong evidence for best treatments and relatively little individual variability, use across geographic areas is also relatively homogeneous, such as emergency hip fracture repair or colectomy for colon cancer.

Their work suggests that the gap between high and low utilizing regions may equal about 30% of health care spending. Since survey data reveal that patients and physicians in the low use areas are generally more satisfied, and the outcomes are either the same or better, policymakers have become convinced that creating solutions that reduce unwarranted variation provide extremely promising ways to improve the productivity and quality of the health system while also saving money [31].

10. Overuse and waste

Prepared by PricewaterhouseCoopers' Health Research Institute, Table 6 provides a breakdown of estimated costs associated with activities that could be made more efficient, reduced or eliminated. In

Table 6
Per capita spending on health care

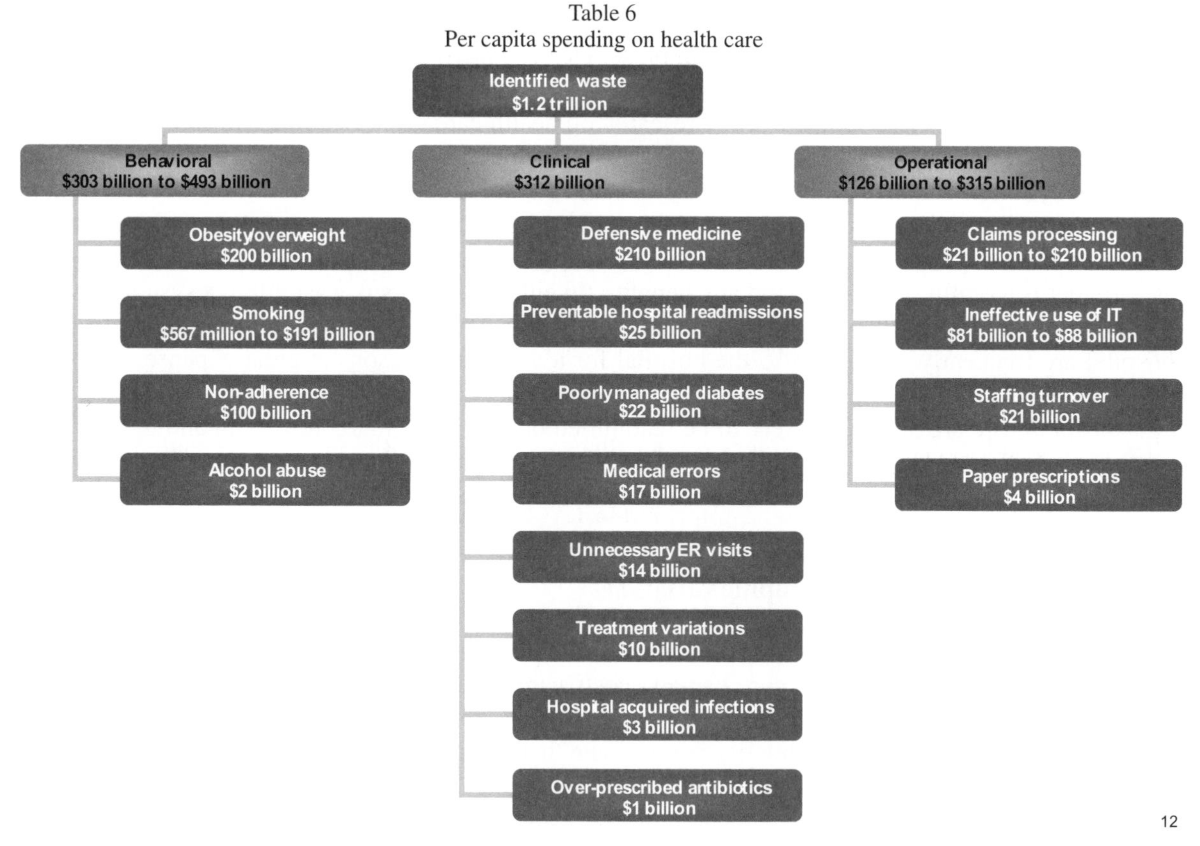

Source: PricewaterhouseCoopers Health Research Institute. The Price of Excess: Identifying waste in healthcare spending. 2008.

this chart, the total is a startling $1.2 trillion. They divided the categories into 3 types. The first are behavioral, such as obesity ($200 billion), smoking ($200 billion), non-adherence to prescription drugs ($100 billion) and other self care, and alcohol abuse ($2 billion). A review of the items suggests that it will not be easy to change the behaviors needed to achieve these reductions, but all of them are already being worked on by a variety of programs, including many using incentives and penalties to encourage people to change.

The second type includes clinical drivers of overuse and waste. At the top are defensive medical practices which are estimated to cost about $210 billion a year. As a highly litigious country, physicians, hospitals and other providers are at risk for being sued even for results over which they had no control. Providers often feel that they have to order tests and imaging, or return visits, so that they would have protection against an argument that they had not done everything possible. Waste in other clinical areas include: preventable readmissions ($25 billion); poorly managed diabetes ($22 billion), medical errors ($17 billion), unnecessary ER visits ($14 billion), unwarranted treatment variations ($10 billion), hospital acquired infections ($3 billion) and over-prescribed antibiotics ($1 billion).

The third type of examples of waste in the health care system are operational. Included are claims processing (somewhere between $21 billion and $210 billion), ineffective use of information technology ($81–88 billion), staffing turnover ($21 billion) and paper prescriptions ($4 billion.)

The CDC estimated that healthcare-associated infections alone cost $28–38 billion in excess healthcare costs each year for the 2 million patients directly infected, of which 99,000 patients died [6]. Not included is the waste due to duplicative tests, imaging and visits because a patient changes or has to change their physicians for a variety of reasons. All of these problems cause a great deal of time uselessly spent by the patient and providers because of an inefficient, paper-laden system in which data can rarely be shared among physicians.

On the operational side, a great deal is spent on claims processing. Progress will need to be made in the use of health information technology to garner those savings. Changes need to be made to payment methods, related oversight, and the required business process changes that really reduce costs. Automating wasteful practices does not produce efficiencies and higher productivity [22].

11. Obesity: Already driving costs

Obesity prevalence has doubled in just 20 years. More than 72 million Americans are already obese. They are at risk for a wide range of very serious illnesses and disabilities. In 2003, a study by Manson and Bassuk, concluded that "obesity has become pandemic in the US" Two out of every three adults were classified as obese or overweight, compared to 1 in 4 in the early 1960s [16].

As recently documented by Ken Thorpe, et al. [29], obesity alone contributed nearly 29 million additional chronic conditions in 2005 over the 1997 level. Overall obesity accounts for 27% of the increase in inflation-adjusted health expenditures among working age adults." Put another way, Thorpe et al. estimated that "if obesity levels today were the same as in 1987, health care spending would be 10% lower per person or about *$200 billion less each year.*

12. End-of-life care

It is often thought that care at the end of life is a significant driver of per capita health care costs. According to research from Dartmouth's Institute for Health Policy and Clinical Practice, there is substantial unwarranted variation in care in the last two years of life by geography. Adjusted for age, race and diagnosis, Medicare spending per patient was $93,842 at UCLA Medical Center, $85,729 at Johns Hopkins but $53,432 at the Mayo Clinic and $55,333 at the Cleveland Clinic. (See earlier discussion of geographic variations for more details.)

When care at the end of life is examined, the results are very interesting, indicating that costs of end-of-life care need to be analyzed at least by age. Interestingly, research reported in Health Affairs' found that the "costs of death are independent of age, based on data suggesting health status matters more than age. Medical spending in the last year of life falls from $32,000 for those who die young (ages 65–69) to half that amount for those who die above 90. "The diseases that older people die from are different, and the amount of medical care differs as well" [9].

In another important study, Hogan et al., found that end-of-life costs are only slightly higher for persons who died than for those who survived. Significantly, the authors reported that patients who die have "multiple (at least 4) significant medical problems in the year of death ... while the average for survivors was slightly more than one in the typical calendar year" [13]. The most interesting finding was that end-of-life costs for minorities (in this case, African-Americans) and those from high poverty areas were 28% higher than for others. "Much of what has been labeled the 'high cost of dying' is just the cost of caring for severe illness and functional impairment. Decedents' costs are, roughly speaking, not much different from those of other with similarly complex medical needs." If these differences are put together with what is known about geographic variations and the overuse that likely occurs in supply-sensitive conditions, it is not surprising that there can be very high costs in certain locations and organizations.

13. We are all in this together – 21st century version of the medical commons

Many of the problems in the US health care system derive from forces and factors that are both positive and negative, such as new technology that can certainly be life saving or enhancing but may also be expensive, used inappropriately and not add sufficient value to be worth the expense. Much of what goes on is hard to categorize as one or the other (positive or not), which is one of the reasons agreement on how to reform the healthcare system has been so elusive over many years. As Uwe Reinhardt famously said long ago: "National health expenditures are also national health incomes," so any change may be seen as a threat to those benefiting from a mostly lucrative industry.

With a predominantly fee-for-service, open-ended health care financing system, almost always paid by a third party (employer, insurer, government program) who is not a direct party in the transaction involving health care decisions, neither the patient nor the doctor has any reason to think about costs or even the possible need for tradeoffs between what is recommended to the patient and what is not, what has value for improving health or not, and under what circumstances. Many policymakers feel that being protected from costs when sick or needing acute or preventive care is exactly what patients or consumers want and need and if care isn't virtually free to the patient then the patient will not get what is needed. Health care systems outside the United States with which it is often compared, unfavorably, have not only universal coverage, but the amount that average citizens pay toward their care (at least outside taxation) is miniscule by US standards. Other policymakers and many employers believe that, without some financial stake in choice decisions and in the use of health care, consumers and patients will not pay attention to what they should be doing and thinking about. They will overuse health care services, especially if they are encouraged to overuse by providers who may have some financial incentive to order more tests, or encourage more visits. Consumers too tend to avoid changing their own behavior even where it is contributing to their own poor health and look to health care or prescription drugs to fix their health problems. Physicians frequently report how patients ask for prescriptions or tests even if the doctor does not believe they are needed. Consumers sometimes have whole body scans because a doctor or imaging center has advertised it at a discount rate and to be "reassured" that the patient is not suffering from cancer or heart disease.

There is certainly evidence that having their own money at stake does affect use of health services and prescription drugs. But, opponents of consumerism or consumer-directed health care believe that is exactly what they don't want to happen. They fear that low income consumers will not get needed care.

The resetting of the economy with the 2008–2009 recession exacerbated all of the challenges related to health care, leading the American public to be open to new approaches to universal coverage. The Presidential and Congressional elections of 2008 reflected the growing discontent with public policies that were not solving problems, such as the health care cost crisis, and enabled a much more ambitious agenda for action, led by the President and powerful Congressional leaders, who are as committed to national health care reform as the President.

President Obama, in his first 100 days, made health care one of his top 3 initiatives to reform before the end of his first year in office. His language and commitment were strong. With the economy almost on its knees in late 2008 and early 2009, he said the nation could not have a lasting recovery and a strong economy unless the US reins in health care costs. He also reminded everyone that the nation had not only to control costs but also seek long-term deficit reduction by controlling expenditures for Medicare, Medicaid and Social Security. The head of the Congressional Budget Office, Peter Orszag, moved to head the Office of Management and Budget, taking with him his strong analytical and negotiating skills which helped ensure his prominent role in health care and fiscal reform under President Obama.

14. What is the outlook for controlling costs?

If the best predictor is past behavior, there is little reason for optimism about the degree to which health care costs will be controlled especially in the short term. In fact, the operative term among policy people in Washington became "bending the curve," which clearly reflected how hard it will be to reduce costs. While the US has avoided many cost control methods used by other nations, if all residents of the US under one kind of health plan or another are covered and high proportions of people are covered by governmental programs, no matter what types, far more public funds will be needed. US policymakers will have to find new approaches to "bend the curve."

The rate of increase did level off in 2007 at a relatively modest amount – 6% – though on a higher base. But cost drivers are as strong as ever or worse, starting with the number and prevalence of obese and super obese people who are not yet taking care of themselves or may already be very sick from diabetes, heart disease, depression, sleep apnea and other problems.

In 2009, hospitals and drug makers raised their prices slightly more than usual, surprising analysts since it was in the middle of a recession when many prices were either going down or holding steady. One Pharmaceutical Benefit Manager, Express Scripts reported that drug prices increased by 10% to 15% between the 1st quarter of 2008 and 2009 [19].

Specialty drugs which have been the fastest growing Rx expenses have not yet slowed down. If the pattern follows the usual one, we may see additional growth as new conditions are treated with drugs originally approved for other purposes. In addition, if the many millions of uninsured do become covered under new insurance plans or other kinds of private or public coverage, they will certainly have an impact on how many services and medications are obtained. While many of the previously uninsured typically received emergency services when needed, if private or public insurance is available, the ongoing treatment with routine primary care, screenings and low intensity acute care will increase costs. If the projected dearth of primary care physicians holds true, people will be forced to use ERs again, even though they will have health insurance.

Medicare spending will likely increase at an accelerated rate up to 8.6% (from 6.2%) under current law as the oldest baby boomers become eligible for Medicare. Outlays for prescription drugs will increase even faster at 10.2% per year [26].

In 2009, millions of Americans had their retirement plans changed by the decline in the value of their savings in the 2008–2009 recession and economic contraction, and what has been a pattern of early retirement has been slowed if not reversed. The effect of that on health care utilization is not known. There was some evidence of increased elective procedures when time was available and there were fears of losing insurance, but previous experiences with recessions have generally mixed results on health care use.

Most of the emphasis on trying to control costs has focused on trying to push down prices, of which students of health care policies are wisely skeptical if not scornful, since they believe price controls only drive up the volume of services. Other strategies include: reducing the number of obese people or smokers, through health improvement programs so there is less need for health services; shifting costs from one payer or another including the consumer; using financial incentives to change behavior; and adding more regulation. James Robinson and Mark Smith offer another approach, broadening and applying Clay Christensen's "disruptive innovation" to health care." They press for essential changes to health care that will open the system up to more cost reduction. They believe public policies should aggressively promote them, such as supporting the replacement not the layering on of new products that are cheaper. The authors provide examples such as self administered tests and over the counter medicines. They also note the "changes in processes that allow less trained yet sufficiently competent workers to substitute for more highly trained... and changes in care sites, such as ambulatory surgery centers" [23].

The balance of this book offers numerous opportunities for significant reform of health care in the US and a fresh approach to using reengineering methods to increase productivity and efficiency of the current system. The nation does not lack for opportunities to improve. There is evidence that the US has the political will and leadership for change that it needs to be successful in both improving the safety and quality of health care in the country, as well as improve its value proposition. Details matter. Most promising will be those strategies that look like the high performing, high quality integrated health care organizations, such as Geisinger Clinic, Kaiser-Permanente, Mayo Clinic, Intermountain Health Care, and others who are willing to be accountable. To succeed there will need to be dramatic payment reform, and wide use of evidence-based treatment protocols. Virtual organizations may work in locations with too dispersed a population to support single organizations.

References

[1] C. Clancy, Reengineering Hospital Discharge: A Protocol to Improve Patient Safety, Reduce Costs, and Boost Patient Satisfaction, *American Journal of Medical Quality* **24** (2009), 344–346.

[2] H. Aaron, The Costs of Health Care Administration in the United Stations and Canada – questionable answers to a questionable question, *The New England Journal of Medicine*, Bostion: (21 August 2003).

[3] G. Anderson, U. Reinhardt, P. Hussey and V. Petrosyan, It's the Prices, Stupid: Why the United States is So different from Other Countries, *Health Affairs* **22**(3) (2003), 89–105.

[4] T. Bodenheimer, High and Rising Health Care Costs, part 2: Technologic Innovation, *Ann Intern Med* **142** (2005), 932–937.

[5] L. Casalino et al., What Does It Cost Physician Practices to Interact with Health Insurance Plans? *Health Affairs* **28**(4) (2009), w533–w543. (published on line 14 May 2009;10.1377/hlthhaff.28.4.w533).

[6] C. Clancy (4/01/09) – House Appropriations Subcommittee on Labor, HHS, Education, and Related Agencies Hearing: Statement on Reducing Health-care Associated Infections.

[7] Commonwealth Fund, *High Performance Health System's "Why Not the Best? Results from the National Scorecard on US Health System Performance*, (July 2008).

[8] G. Anderson and B. Frogner, Health Spending in OECD Countries: Obtaining Value Per Dollar, *Health Affairs* **27**(6) (2008), 1718–1727.

[9] Cutler, David, The Potential for Cost Savings in Medicare's Future, *Health Affairs Web Exclusive* (26 September 2005) WR-R78.

[10] H. Darling, *"How Employees Value Their Employer-Provided Benefits,"* Press Conference, *National Press Club* (12 April 2007).

[11] S. Decker et al., Use of Medical Care for Chronic Conditions, *Health Affairs* **28**(1) (2009), 26–35.

[12] M. Hartman et al., National Health Spending In 2007: Slower Drug Spending Contributes To Lowest Rate Of Overall Growth Since 1998; *Health Affairs* **28**(1) (January/February 2009), 246–261.

[13] C. Hogan, "Medicare Beneficiaries' Costs of Care in the Last Year of Life," *Health Affairs* **20**(4) (July/August 2001), 188–195.

[14] J. Hefferman, Institute of Medicine's Workshop, The Healthcare Imperative: Lowering Costs and Improving Outcomes, May 21–22, 2009.

[15] P. Ginsburg, High and Rising Health Care Costs: Demystifying US Health Care Spending; Robert Wood Johnson Foundation, Research Synthesis Report, No. 16, October 2008.

[16] J. Manson and S. Bassuk, Obesity in the United States, *JAMA* **289**(2) (8 January 2003), 229–230.

[17] Milliman (2008), *Average Health Care Spending.*

[18] Obama, President Obama, spoken at White House Summit on Health Reform, January 2009.

[19] P. Orszag, Health Costs Are the Real Deficit Threat, *Wall Street Journal* (15 May 2009).

[20] Personal Communication with Express Scripts (4/15/09).

[21] PricewaterhouseCoopers, The Factors Fueling Rising Healthcare Costs, (2006).

[22] PricewaterhouseCoopers' Health Research Institute, *The Price of Excess: Identifying Waste in Healthcare Spending*, 2008.

[23] J. Robinson and M. Smith, Cost-Reducing Innovation in Health Care, *Health Affairs* **27**(5) (September/October 2008), 1353–1356.
[24] T. Selden and M. Sing, The Distribution of Public Spending for Health Care in the United States, 2002, *Health Affairs-Web Exclusive* (29 July 2008), w349–w359.
[25] Sheils, John (May 9, 2007), as reported in Denny et al., Denny C, Emanuel E, Pearson S, *Why well-insured patients should demand value-based insurance benefits*, *JAMA* **297** (2007), 2515–2518.
[26] A. Sisko et al., *Health Spending Projections Through 2018: Recession Effects Add Uncertainty to the Outlook*, *Health Affairs* **28**(2) (2009), w346–w357. (Published online 24 February 2009).
[27] R. Smith-Bindman, Rising Use of Diagnostic Medical Imaging in a Large Integrated Health System, *Health Affairs* **27**(6) (2008), 1491–1502.
[28] K. Thorpe et al., Difference in Disease Prevalence as a Source of the US-European Health Care Spending Gap, *Health Affairs* **26**(6) (2007), w678–w686.
[29] K. Thorpe *"Weighty Matters: How Obesity Drives Poor Health and Health Spending in the US"* (National Business Group on Health, 2009) Washington Post (30 November 2008) page: A6.
[30] Wall Street Journal (9 April 2009), Budget Reality Means Obama Can't Deliver It All.
[31] J. Wennberg, E. Fisher, T. Stukel, S. Sharp, Use of Medicare Claims Data to Monitor Provider-Specific Performance Among Patients with Severe Chronic IIlness, *Health Affairs Web Exclusive* (7 October 2004).

Helen Darling is President, National Business Group on Health, a national, non-profit, membership organization devoted exclusively to providing practical solutions to its employer members' most important health care problems and representing large employers' perspective on national health policy issues. Its 280 plus members, including 60 of the Fortune 100 in 2009, purchase health and disability benefits for over 50 million employees, retirees and dependents. Previously, Darling purchased health benefits at Xerox Corporation for 55 thousand US employees, plus their dependents and retirees. She worked in the US Senate and at the Institute of Medicine. She is a member of the IOM's Roundtable on Evidence-Based Medicine and the Board of the National Quality Forum. Darling received a master's degree in Demography/Sociology and a bachelor of science degree, cum laude, from the University of Memphis.

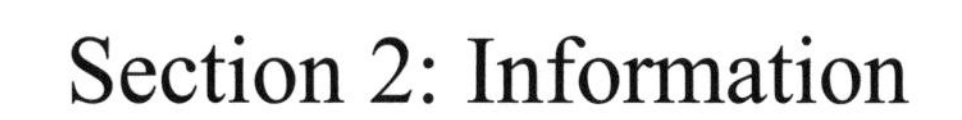

Section 2: Information

Information Knowledge Systems Management 8 (2009) 107–118
DOI 10.3233/IKS-2009-0138
IOS Press

Chapter 7

Engineering information technology for actionable information and better health

Balancing social values through desired outcomes, complementary standards and decision-support

Don E. Detmer
E-mail: d.detmer@virginia.edu

The alternative route to transforming the system sets all of its sights on the destination. (Diamond, C., and Shirky, C. (2008). Health Information Technology: A Few Years of Magical Thinking? Health Affairs. 27(5), 383–390.)

Abstract: Information technology in health care (HIT) is getting a major boost in the United States through the passage of the American Recovery and Reinvestment Act (ARRA) of 2009. The portion of the Act that relates to health information technology (HITECH) seeks to achieve widespread implementation of electronic health records (EHRs) across the land and assure that these EHRs achieve sufficient levels of 'meaningful use' to improve care, reduce costs, and result in better outcomes. This chapter sets the stage for the other chapters that follow in this section. The chapter will review current thinking about how HIT will facilitate collection, dissemination, and evaluation of information throughout the system. Further, it will discuss the role and potential for HIT to support a learning organization [7,8]. Finally, it will outline the current widely identified barriers to progress, e.g., standards development, lack of interoperability and connectivity, and limited decision support that uses evidence-based guidelines created and maintained explicitly to be actionable through computer-based records and systems. Further, with the passage of HITECH, there is a continued attention given to privacy policy at the expense of access to person-specific health information for legitimate social purposes including research and community health. More will be said about this near the end of the chapter. Finally, the chapter will end with a discussion of the difference between information and communication and it will advocate for greater attention to the use of technology as a tool for improve communications and not simply storage and transmission of information.

1. Introduction

HIT has the capacity to capture, store, and retrieve information in a number of sites and formats virtually simultaneously. Amazingly, we are just now realizing that healthcare is essentially an information industry. Perhaps this is due to the role that research is now playing in adding more insight and new treatments and technology at an ever-increasing pace. It has been abundantly clear for some time that human memory is too limited for such a world and these limitations are increasingly apparent with the growth in relevant information [26]. Care of acceptable quality is dependent on information being available to clinicians, patients, and managers in a manner that is timely, valid, complete, accurate, and secure. In such instances, the information becomes a compelling communications tool to help change behavior that is stubbornly resistant.

HIT requires a great deal of infrastructure including robust terminology and classification that capture meaning accurately and moves it without loss of fidelity. While natural language processing has made real strides, there is still a tension between data recorded as a patient's narrative and structured datasets for managing well-described clinical diseases. So, while progress has been made in promoting international adoption of standard terminology through the formation of the International Health Terminology Standards Development Organization (IHTSDO) and greater collaboration among ISO, CEN, HL7, IHTSDO, and CDISC, more remains to be done [3]. The organizations plus a few other terms and a brief description of each are included in Table 1. In general terms, this challenge is a renewed priority for the Office of the National Coordinator through the ARRA/HITECH legislation; time will tell how it is addressed by the committees on policy and standards constituted in early summer 2009 but the prospects are bright. The National Committee on Vital and Health Statistics remains interested and committed to this as well.

2. Standards

Progress has been made over the past five years in the area of HIT standards development, selection, and implementation. Among the items deserving mention are the HITSP implementation specification; structured product labels for approved drugs disseminated through DailyMed, linked to RxNorm and other knowledge sources, e.g., ClinicalTrials.gov; proactive expansion of LOINC to include genetic tests and newborn screening tests; a new version of the Surgeon General's Family Health History tool, with SNOMED HL7 standards built in; the AHIC Working Group on Personal Health Care standards matrix (test LOINC) that detect conditions (SNOMED CT) for newborn screening; and, international standards published by ISO on the EHR and on privacy and security [12]. Finally, AMIA recently launched its *Standard's Standard*, a quarterly newsletter summarizing current activities among the various global health standard setting groups [4].

The approach to the setting of HIT standards is at a historic flexion point from the past and we have to be alert to unintended consequences that may result. In the past, standards were developed through a bottom-up approach in which expert volunteers met on their own time and developed well-vetted standards prior to their adoption. There were downsides to this approach in that visions were limited to the focus of the group that led at times to too many standards. Also, this disaggregated approach slowed global harmonization. The emerging top-down approach means that actual standards will be set since approval and use by huge government agencies essentially creates *a* standard as *the* standard. There is greater potential for globalization as well as more stable funding for creation and maintenance and access to standards. Potential problems that may arise in this new structure may be that some needed standards will not be considered that would have gotten attention through expressions of concerned experts in the field, or some standards may move forward for the 'wrong' reasons, e.g., political pressure. It remains to be seen if there will be sufficient vetting of standards prior to adoption, or if other issues arise that are not discernable today. Idealism can gain the upper hand over pragmatism in either approach and must always remain a consideration.

Remaining areas for HIT standards development, selection, and implementation are in at least six areas including decision support, personalized care, population health support, semantic interoperability (tying SNOMED CT to record structures), clinical knowledge models that reflect clinical best practices, and selection challenges (device terminology and identifiers). Further, additional standards used in care processes need national adoption. RxNorm identifiers should be available with the drug at the time of approval when the SPL is released. LOINC should be on all test kits and outputs from test devices should be labeled with LOINC.

Table 1
Some international health standards bodies and related terms

CDISC CDISC is a global, multidisciplinary, non-profit organization that has established open global standards to support the acquisition, exchange, submission/reporting and archive of medical research data. The CDISC standards are freely available via the CDISC website.

CEN/TC 251 CEN/TC 251's domain is the application of information and communication technology in healthcare, social care and wellness. CEN/TC 251 is a regional (European) Standards Development Organisation (SDO) among international or domain specific SDOs and its focus is almost exclusively content technology and not communication technology.

Daily Med DailyMed provides high quality information about marketed drugs. This information includes FDA approved labels (package inserts).

HL7 HL7 is an international community of healthcare subject matter experts and information scientists who work together to create accredited standards for the exchange, management and integration of electronic healthcare information. The HL7 community is organized in the form of a global organization (Health Level Seven, Inc.) and country-specific affiliate organizations. HL7 affiliate organizations exist in over 30 countries. HL7's standards are accredited by the US ANSI organization and many HL7 standards have also been adopted as ISO standards.

I HTSDO The International Health Terminology Standards Development Organisation (**http://www.ihtsdo.org**), a not-for-profit Danish association formed in 2007, purchased SNOMED CT (Systematized Nomenclature of MEDicine – Clinical Terms) from the College of American Pathologists (CAP) in April 2007 and is now responsible for its ongoing maintenance, development, quality assurance, and distribution. The goal of the change in ownership was to promote international adoption and use of SNOMED CT. The IHTSDO recently announced that SNOMED CT licenses are now available free of charge in another 49 countries designated as low income economies by the World Bank. To oversimplify, SNOMED CT is 'bottom up' with its terminology while ICDL (International Classification of Diseases) is 'top down'.

ICD-10 ICD-10 is the 10th edition of the International Classification of Diseases. ICD-10 was endorsed by the Forty-third World Health Assembly in May 1990 and came into use in WHO Member States as from 1994. The US Department of Health and Human Services is just now beginning a transition from ICD-9 to ICD-10. The ICD-10 code sets proposed rule would concurrently adopt the International Classification of Diseases, Tenth Revision, Clinical Modification (ICD-10-CM) for diagnosis coding, and the International Classification of Diseases, Tenth Revision, Procedure Coding System (ICD-10-PCS) for inpatient hospital procedure coding. The new codes would replace the International Classification of Diseases, Ninth Revision, Clinical Modification (ICD-9-CM) Volumes 1 and 2, and the International Classification of Diseases, Ninth Revision, Clinical Modification (CM) Volume 3 for diagnosis and procedure codes, respectively.

ISO TC 215 on Health Informatics Technical Committee 215 of the International Standards Organization (ISO) on Health Informatics was formed in 1998. The parent ISO organization is non-governmental and based in Geneva. TC215 is structured into four core Working Groups: Data Structure (frameworks and models), Data Interchanges (harmonization and messaging), Semantic Content (terminology and knowledge), and Security (confidentiality, integrity, and availability).

LOINC ® (Logical Observation Identifiers Names and Codes) is a coding system for laboratory and other clinical measures and documents used in electronic transactions between independent computer systems. LOINC is used worldwide by local hospitals and laboratories, public health departments, healthcare provider networks, electronic health information exchanges, software vendors, payers and managed care organizations.

RxNorm RxNorm is a standardized nomenclature for clinical drugs and drug delivery devices produced by the National Library of Medicine (NLM). In RxNorm, the name of a clinical drug combines its ingredients, strengths, and/or form.

SPL Structured Product Labels are Health Level-7 (HL7) version 3 Structured Product Labeling (SPL) standards for representing human readable label documents with computer-processable drug knowledge. SPL descriptions agree well with RxNorm. SPL can be used as the primary source of drug information for e-prescribing systems.

UMLS According to the National Library of Medicine, the purpose of its Unified Medical Language System ® (UMLS) is to facilitate the development of computer systems that behave as if they "understand" the meaning of the language of biomedicine and health. To that end, NLM produces and distributes the UMLS Knowledge Sources (databases) and associated software tools (programs) for use by system developers. See http://www.nlm.nih.gov/research/umls/about_umls.html.

3. Workforce

Without question, there is also a need for a workforce that is more skilled with respect to the use of informatics [16]. This includes clinical informaticians, public health informaticians, translational bioinformaticians, and people employing informatics methods for research purposes, including construction of repositories of clinical and other databases, as well as data mining and data presentation. Whether these people will be 'standard' informaticians or some admixture of informatician/clinical epidemiologist is not clear yet to this writer. Among the needed sets of crucial skills are 'people' skills relating to implementing change in complex adaptive systems, how to be a successful 'team worker' who understands quality measurement and quality improvement, and how to develop systems and programs that put the patient into the center of communications as a critical member of the team. Today, too many people do not yet distinguish between an IT expert and an informatician. The differences are real, since informaticians deal specifically with both an in-depth knowledge of the topic area of focus, e.g., health sciences, as well as how human thinking and computer technology can best address specific challenges.

Beyond the workforce, there is a need for an underlying architecture that will manage information coming from three sets of communications and their related records. They include the patient record, e.g. the computer-based health record kept by clinics, hospitals, or other care facility or unit), personal health records, and public health/population records. Unless these three kinds of records are part of an integrated architecture that allows questions to be asked and solutions evaluated across all three perspectives, there will be serious limitations to the potential of such a system to evolve into a learning system for health and healthcare.

Ideally, there needs to be a set of clinicians, managers, and informaticians looking constantly at ways questions can be asked of the data in order to improve care quality, outcomes, and work processes from the perspectives of all key stakeholders. Also, there is a need for evaluation of the impact of changes in approaches to care and/or system management and having a data infrastructure that allows an array of queries. Dramatic improvements can only be expected from environments sharing these configurations. Such systems allow for 'hypothesis testing' prior to deciding to make a more formal study or implement an intervention, thereby saving a lot of time and resources.

4. Infrastructure

To assure a sufficiently robust infrastructure, or 'infostructure' as considered by the Canadian Infoway, since it will include both the technology and relevant health information, there needs to be an amalgam of computer-based standards and repositories plus organizational structures to assure appropriate change over time, as well as on-going system maintenance. Indeed, if one is to consider dimensions of 'meaningful use' as mandated in ARRA/HITECH from an informatics perspective, there is a hierarchy of functions from basic to more sophisticated in order to move toward creation of a 'learning' organization. While there is not yet a common agreement on the list of functionalities, one should continue to follow the 'meaningful use' discussions on the ONC website. Important elements and function include:

1. Data recording and results retrieval
2. The capability to move the data into a repository to track progress and outcomes
3. The creation of evidence-based workflow guidelines for decision-support
4. Implementation of workflows that assure high quality processes
5. Implementation of uniform care processes where applicable

6. Reviewing and sharing of results among key stakeholders
7. Evaluation of outcomes and further revision and/or improvement of processes
8. Engagement of patients through secure web-portals
9. Engagement of patients and/or populations (potential patients) who 'didn't show up' but need care based upon an analysis of current utilization and 'blind areas' identified through Geo-mapping.

This final step is key to moving from a value-driven care system that focuses solely on individuals who manage to find care to a value-driven care system that is committed to the health of both individuals and populations, e.g., all those who would benefit greatly from care see Blue Ridge Group reports at http://whsc.emory.edu/blueridge/reports.cfm.

Equally important is the need for electronic records (including relevant decision support) that looks at the care needs as a continuum as emphasized by Naylor of the University of Pennsylvania [20–22]. Stakeholders need relevant information but what they really need is information arrayed so that caregivers and care systems can integrate care across important dimensions. Decision support should not simply inform but be presented in ways that facilitate appropriate action by clinicians, patients, and managers.

For example, Naylor conceives of a care continuum for the elderly that tracks people across four life stages including *healthy*, *acutely ill, living with chronic illness/disability*, and *frail/coping with illness at the end of life*. Each stage has its information needs and the information needs to be transmitted in actionable language and content. At the *healthy* level, EHRs need data acquisition and decision support for tracking people at a population level and helping them assure a health environment, "healthy home". For those who have been *acutely ill*, EHRs having the same kind of actionable advice is needed to assure transitional support to avoid readmissions and avoidable setbacks. For those with *chronic illness/disability,* help is needed for chronic care management that is keyed to local resources and environments. And, finally, at the *end of life,* EHRs are needed that comprise a program for all-inclusive care of the elderly (PACE) as well as hospice care. Today, we know that billions of care dollars are spent in what prove to be the last few months of life. Further, we know that the entire domain relating to advance directives for end-of-life care are poorly managed. Finally, we know from places like the Gunderson Lutheran Hospital in La Crosse, Wisconsin that programs can and do work and achieve both better human outcomes for those involved as well as resulting in much less costly care [15]. Complimentary sets of standards are needed relating to functional aspects of care itself, and then communications among critical parties to assure that details are attended to properly.

5. Information and communication

I propose that one set of content could be seen as primarily being relevant *information* such as facts and treatment guidelines while the other set relates to the support of critical *communications* needed to meet these practice standards. Most computer-based EHRs are more information-based than communication-based in this context, even those that seek as a routine to remind a clinician to order a preventive test. In contradistinction, one might consider an e-mail or text message to be first a communication that then morphs into information stored in the record, even though information itself is passed along. Most doctors when seeing a patient are primarily interested in *communicating with* the patient, that is, working together to find words and concepts (the relevant information) that may convey a shared clear meaning between them.

The EHR ends up containing a distillate of such communications as well as related relevant information. However, simply exchanging information does not assure that the information was accurately communicated. This is most evident when language and cultural barriers intervene. Could explicitly developed *communications technologies* better align information technology with such communication technology? What one wishes to convey is meaning, caring and conviction in terms that engage the patient as a unique person can focus upon. To achieve greater effectiveness in care and enhance *learning* as a system objective, we need to focus both on information itself as well as how it is communicated for the information to become alive for the patients and clinicians so that they can and will internalize it and pursue relevant actions. An example follows.

First, we need end-of-life standards that are Health Information Technology templates to accurately express information on the personal choices of patients in a clearly understandable fashion for clinicians to use. We know that such choices can shift when one moves from a state of full health to critical illness. Thus, we need Health Communication Technology templates to support clinicians and patients working together to assess options over time and what is then involved for each of them to do justice to their decisions. For example, there could be periodic reminders scheduled for both clinicians through their EHRs and for patients (via their integrated PHR) urging them to review and refine prior wishes if shifts in health status occur that might have long-term implications for survival or major quality of life considerations. At the time of hospitalization, an alert could go to both the clinician and patient or a designated family member (depending on the level of illness) that shows the current directives so the HIT information becomes communicated among those involved. Finally, alerts to the relevant clinical teams engaged in the direct care of the patient would be communicated when the patient's clinical status either approached or crossed the decision thresholds.

While simply knowing that a directive exists (as information) may be useful but what is essential is help all along the way so that the critical information is timely and actionable and is communicated appropriately. Standards in this sense are explicit representations that reflect our view of the world, and hence, what we choose to recognize and value. Short of having such standards, we risk what Rene Dubos has noted, "That which is measured drives out that which is important." Today, our approach to clinical decision support and related directives are undervaluing our humanity and our moral attitudes and habits. HICT may be used to make us more fully human in our care. It is not clear that we should maintain the distinction between HIT and HCT for the communications. However, clinicians focused on traditional HIT are at risk of disproportionately focusing on the information rather than the communications. A patient values the personal connection that comes through clear, direct communications with their care-giver [18]. This makes the information come alive.

6. Broader perspective

The proper role of and the potential for IT and information systems is to take personal, patient, and population records, and personal health records and integrate them in such a way that a learning organization is created and supported. This means more than simply having patient or clinician alerts for such items as drug-drug interactions. Ultimately, it means that clinicians and patients collaborate in the evaluation of care guidelines to determine circumstances in which a given care protocol is adopted by all providers as the standard for that environment. Obviously, there is a great deal of science and evaluation that must stand behind such an approach and continued tracking of outcomes is needed to assure that the protocol is as rigorous as possible and also is fully compatible with appropriate actions in care environments.

It is for this reason that the American Medical Informatics Association is most enamored with personal health records that are structured within the EHR system via secure web portals that allow patients and clinicians to communicate directly with one another while viewing the same clinical data [13]. 'Integrated' personal records of this type stay up to date and are complete and audited by both patients and clinicians. At the minimum, they should include access to appointments, the problem list, medications, allergies and/or reactions, a subset of test results, demographic and insurance information, and educational materials. In addition, some actionable functions are essential including requests for appointments, medication delivery through the mails, secure messaging among those involved, and family members should be able to have access to view data with permission and within some constraints.

In sum, it is not sufficient to have simply the right information for decision-making purposes, it is also essential that the key stakeholders know how best to accomplish better care outcomes through the *use* of such information. Thomas Jefferson made this distinction years ago when he envisioned the University of Virginia to be a site and source for 'useful' knowledge. Getting the knowledge applied is central to achieving care outcomes. It is relevant that medical specialties are moving from their traditional structure of continuing education that consisted of attending lectures, etc. to a new target of actual professional performance improvement. It remains a challenge to refocus quality improvement initiatives away from measuring performance to improving actual performance. This movement within medicine toward performance improvement also takes the focus solely off the individual provider and moves the focus to achievement of clinical objectives and performance of a clinical team or unit responsible for care that works within a complex adaptive system. This shift of focus will have implications on how EHRs will be structured to report performance as well as how clinical guidelines are developed and used by teams. Further, the shift to performance improvement within the group responsible for the total care of the patient is certain to stimulate clinical decision support activities and in new directions.

7. Clinical decision support

According to the Clinical Decision Support (CDS) Roadmap report done for the Office of the National Coordinator, CDS is *"providing clinicians, patients, or individuals with knowledge and person-specific or population information, intelligently filtered or present at appropriate times, to foster better health processes, better individual patient care, and better population health*" [24]. According to this report, "the challenge is to create a national coordinated action to ensure that usable and effective clinical decision support is widely used by providers and patients to improve healthcare." Today, there are multiple aspects in which we underachieve including lack of interoperability, guidelines lacking the capability to be put into computer-usable language or precluding implementation into EHRs, wheel-reinvention, a slow path from new knowledge to widely usable knowledge and limited adoption for financial or legal reasons. To enhance health and healthcare through CDS will require activity in three domains and integration of work across them. The domains include having the best knowledge available when it is needed, high adoption and effective use, and continuous improvement of CDS methods and knowledge. To achieve these goals will require practical, standard formats for knowledge representation and interventions, standard approaches for collecting, organizing, and distributing CDS, addressing a variety of policy, financial, and legal barriers and creating additional support and enablers, compiling and disseminating best practices for usability and implementation, developing methods to collect, learn from, and share experience with CDS, and using EHR data systematically to advance knowledge. Work is progressing on many of these dimensions [25]. Certainly, the HITECH legislation will move this along as well.

Translational Bioinformatics: From Organs And Systems To Molecular medicine The transition from clinical care based upon clinical phenotype (largely organs and systems) to molecular medicine based upon one's unique biology will come slowly but it has already begun. The reports from use of the HANES database in this country and the Wellcome Trust Case Control Consortium in the UK have shown that the era of genome-wide scans is here [10,29].

Two public policy challenges that are emerging already as a result of this emerging discipline are how best to manage the implications of these developments in a consumer-driven commercial environment. The first relates to personal privacy and the second relates to getting a sound interpretation of what the data reveal about one's health and future prospects. Recent research has made it clear that it is very difficult to camouflage one's personal identify if one's genomic information is available and it is likely to be equally difficult to find a cost-effective source for data interpretation of what a genetic analysis may actually mean for one's life. The innovations are certain to generate greater public discussion in the near future as the costs continue to drop. Having said this, we are in early days since ultimately, there will be some clinical implications from structural genomics but also more from functional genomics, proteomics and other effector molecules.

Space limits what can be described here but the field of 'translational bioinformatics' is expanding rapidly through greater developments of informatics methods of data mining as well as availability of phenotypic data sets for comparison with genomic data as referenced above. Patient populations clustered for their Coumadin sensitivity based up the trial-and-error method used by clinicians to regulate Coumadin sensitivity were analyzed against their structural data. Use of this approach suggests that it is likely that only two only clinically significant single-nucleotide polymorphs (SNPs) are disease-related genes [11]. Strictly using evolving data-mining approaches are also yielding both stronger methods and interesting findings. A mix of diseases and conditions are implicated, including insights that relate to complex behaviors. For those outside this field, yet interested in keeping up with these developments, the annual year-in-review given by Russ Altman at the AMIA Translational Bioinformatics Summit held each March is strongly advised [1,2]. For insights into progress in not only translational bioinformatics but informatics in general, the annual year-in-review by Daniel Masys given at the AMIA Annual Symposium each November is equally valuable. Kindly, each puts their presentations on the web [1,2, 17].

Since most conditions are multi-factorial and include a mix of biology, environment, access to care and its quality, the manner in which this powerful rising new science will evolve and integrate into clinical and public health practice will be intrinsically complex yet powerful. Robust computer-based health records must be the norm in care settings, in the home, and in public health environments in order to carry out such work. Data interpretation will require an ongoing structured 'assessment of the knowledge base' with a combination of 'carbon- and silicon-based' intelligence akin to the comparative effectiveness studies mandated in the ARRA legislation. Among the dimensions that will be impacted by these developments include prediction of disease, more commonly susceptibility and risk for developing disease, prevention, screening, early diagnosis, and therapeutic interventions. Translational bioinformatics is transforming rapidly from a field focused on methods to a discipline that generates scientific discovery in their own right through the use of high end computing. The outcome of this work will seep into all of the domains listed above in both subtle and dramatic ways.

8. Towards success

Today, there are many barriers to achieving the right mixture of human and HIT capabilities to assure a value-driven care system that focuses on individuals and populations. Among the barriers to achieving more rapid progress through organizational adoption are dysfunctional attitudes and habits, costs, privacy policy and related issues, lack of standard definitions, lack of interconnectivity/interoperability standards, and lack of a well developed program and approach to actionable decision support equally cued to key stakeholders, including patient, clinicians, and managers. That is, some of the challenges relate to policies and procedures, others to organizational structures, rewards and incentives for key players including some that are monetary. Before speaking to issues at the institutional level, a few words are appropriately focused at federal and state policy with respect to privacy and access to person-specific health information and unique personal identifiers.

With the passage of ARRA/HITECH, privacy policy continues to crowd out efforts to meet other legitimate social goods. Policy makers who are disproportionately concerned about privacy enact more and more regulation limiting timely access to person-specific health information for totally legitimate social purposes including safety, legitimate biomedical and health services research, freedom, and personal autonomy. Policy supporting altruistic behavior is displaced by this excessive focus on privacy. And, misplaced privacy fears even result in added risks to patient safety. For example, unique health identifiers help assure that an individual patient's data is authenticated properly so that one patient does not receive data relating to another patient with the same name and/or similar demographic data.

Today, citizens are not even allowed the option of having a personal health identifier if they wish to have one. Rather, they are forced to face a higher risk of receiving another person's health information into their own EHRs, or having their information not be sent to them but to someone else's record, thereby invading yet another person's privacy. Similarly, citizens supportive of legitimate biomedical research are not allowed as a matter of national government policy, to opt to agree to have their EHR data made available to the research community. There should be a national clearinghouse that allows citizens to agree to offer access to their personal health data for legitimate biomedical and public health research.

A number of studies now confirm that legitimate biomedical and health research is being harmed in this country as a result of national privacy policy [19,28]. This includes research sponsored by the National Institutes of Health and other publically funded research. Public policy must develop and implement ways to allow individuals to offer an informed blanket approval for their data to be accessed for legitimate biomedical and health research, e.g., IRB approved research protocols. Further, citizens should be given a simple way to offer access to their own DNA data for research uses if they so desire.

The strategies for correcting these imbalances vary widely but there is little structure today to support necessary reforms. For example, the recently enacted American Recovery and Reinvestment Act of 2009 with its support for a national health information infrastructure and support for comparative effectiveness research offers a window of opportunity. Clearly, there will need to be access to data for quality control and research if we are to make progress in the area of comparative effectiveness. At the same time, within the same law, increasing privacy constraints to the "liquidity" of health information were enhanced [5]. The Booz Allen Hamilton report favors giving citizens the right to choose a unique health identifier for caregivers and researchers to use for better authentication as well as making an 'altruistic' choice that might help others while not necessarily helping themselves.

Ideally, it should be an option for those who elect to participate, to be contacted if they would meet the human subject criteria for a particular research project so they might participate or decline to do so. What this would require is both standards for dealing with the information itself in a structured manner, e.g., templates using information technology *plus* standards for contacting them with relevant information if they sought to participate, e.g., communications technology.

The value of supportive societal policies for connecting citizens and researchers is becoming ever more important as we approach the area of molecular medicine. In short, public policy should support an infrastructure to foster value-driven health care for a healthy society that is also altruistic in its public policies, including support of education and research. Only policy and standards relating to health IT and health CT to support actions that are more adaptive for continued improvement, greater sustainability and better outcomes would accomplish this end. Policy needs to orchestrate harmony and balance across the knowledge, care and payment domains. So, a greater dialogue is needed if we are to develop policy supportive of health within the broader society as well as within the healthcare delivery system and the standards to make them operational. Standards, in the sense used for electronic health records and record systems, should be benchmarked against desired outcomes and processes. Such standards would then be reformulated over time to better achieve desired social ends. Government must learn to tolerate the ongoing creative tension across policy efforts that relate to system management, care standards and related education and research.

According to the Blue Ridge Academic Health Group [6], "a value-driven health system would utilize performance-based incentives and balanced competition between the care and payment domains in achieving national health goals. It would develop incentives to improve the health outcomes of both individuals and populations, while achieving the highest possible value for the dollars invested and spent. A national health information infrastructure would allow secure communications of relevant data for diagnosis, treatment and outcomes tracking by those with a right and need to know."

As progress continues through discoveries utilizing computational biology and translational bioinformatics, we will continue to see a shift from the traditional focus on organs and organ systems to cells and molecules as the basis of human therapeutics. We will need information and communications standards that speak to these discoveries within our EHRs and the ongoing clinical and health services research agenda. Communications standards will increasingly gravitate to mobile communications technology when favored by the patient or the clinician, including wireless monitoring, etc. The focus should be on the involved patient and clinician and in some cases the community as we can derive evidence on community health from pooled clinical and other public health databases while still tending to legitimate data security needs.

Since the Institute of Medicine published the Computer-based Patient Record in 1991, the focus of nearly all of the energy and investment within the healthcare industry has been on *information* technology [14]. The focus and the resultant standards that have evolved to support EHRs and EHR systems have related heavily to documentation, e.g., preserving meaning and context while moving from paper-based to computer-based records. Certainly, functionality with respect to decision support has focused heavily on professional clinicians with little focus on supporting health related decision making of either patients or improved decision relating to the general health of citizens. Unfortunately, the acronym HITECH focuses on the technology rather than the more relevant challenge of integrating human dimensions of work processes and change with computer/communications technology. Connectivity, decision support and data mining are at least as important as automation as pointed out by the NRC [27].

9. Conclusions

Essential to making progress is having an enterprise-wide sense of mission and commitment that allows for systems to try new approaches, evaluate them and then move the best ideas into uniform practice. What this entails is ongoing education and research and an environment that is flexible and capable of change. Typically, the least of one's problems are the HIT system(s) themselves; the work comes when the interface between people and the systems is engaged. Today's systems are far from perfect and an attitude of openness and willingness to help improve the system is crucial. With a commitment to ongoing education and research, we can improve quality, safety, cost-efficiency, effectiveness, equity, patient-centered and timely care. At the same time, we must assure that public policy and environmental factors are in alignment to be supportive.

References

[1] R.B. Altman, The Translational Bioinformatics Year in Review. http://74.125.113.132/search?q=cache:3dY0xTAoHPMJ: files.me.com/russbaltman/ 6jf1pa+russ+altman+year+in+review&cd=4&hl=en&ct=clnk&gl=us, 2008.

[2] R.B. Altman, The Translational Bioinformatics Year in Review. http://74.125.113.132/search?q=cache:OucRQGGa31gJ: files.me.com/russbaltman/ 6pfvfo+russ+altman+year+in+review&cd=3&hl=en&ct=clnk&gl=us, 2009.

[3] AMIA/AHIMA, Healthcare Terminologies and Classifications: Essential Keys to Interoperability. http://www.amia.org/ files/HealthcareTerminologiesand Classifications.pdf, 2007.

[4] AMIA, Standard's Standard. http://www.amia.org/amia-standards-standard/welcome-amias-standards-standar d, 2009.

[5] BAH, Toward Health Information Liquidity: Realization of Better, More Efficient Care From the Free Flow of Information. http://www.fah.org/fahCMS/Documents/On%20The%20Record/Research/2009/Bo oz_Allen_Toward_Hlth_Info_Liquidity.pdf, 2009.

[6] Blue Ridge Academic Health Group, Converging on Consensus. Report No. 8, Available at http://www.whsc.emory.edu/ blueridge/reports.cfm], 2004.

[7] Blue Ridge Academic Health Group. Health care Quality and Safety in the Academic Health Center. Report Available at http://whsc.emory.edu/blueridge/_pdf/blue_ridge_report_11_20 07.pdf, 2007.

[8] Blue Ridge Academic Health Group. The Emerging Transformational Role of Informatics. Available at http://whsc. emory.edu/blueridge/_pdf/blue_ridge_report_12_20 08.pdf, 2007.

[9] Blue Ridge Academic Health Group. Fall 2008 Policy – oposal: A United States Health Board. http://whsc.emory.edu/ blueridge/reports.cfm, 2009.

[10] M.H. Chang, M.L. Lindegren, M.A. Butler, S.J. Chanock, N.F. Dowling, M. Gallagher, R. Moonesinghe, C.A. Moore, R.M. Ned, M.R. Reichler, C.L. Sanders, R. Welch, A. Yesupriya and M.J. Khoury, CDC/NCI NHANES III Genomics Working Group. Prevalence in the United States of selected candidate gene variants: Third National Health and Nutrition Examination Survey, 1991-1994, *Am J Epidemiol* **169**(1) (2009), 54–66.

[11] G.M. Cooper, J.A. Johnson, T.Y. Langaee, H. Feng, I.B. Stanaway, U.I. Schwarz, M.D. Ritchie, C.M. Stein, D.M. Roden, J.D. Smith, D.L. Veenstra, A.E. Rettie and M.J. Rieder, A genome-wide scan for common genetic variants with a large influence on warfarin maintenance dose, *Blood* **112**(4) (2008), 1022–1027.

[12] D.E. Detmer, *The National Healthcare Information Technology Environment*, Testimony to National Committee on Vital and Health Statistics Standards Subcommittee Hearing, Setting the Context for the Evolution of Health IT Standards. (http://www.ncvhs.hhs.gov/090224p2.pdf), 2009.

[13] D.E. Detmer, M. Bloomrosen, B. Raymond and P. Tang, Integrated personal health records: Transformative tools for consumer-centric care, *BMC Medical Informatics and Decision Making* **8** (2008), 45–72.

[14] R. Dick and E. Steen, The Computer-based Patient Record: An Essential Technology for Health Care. Washington, DC: National Academies Press, 1991.

[15] T.J. Greaney, Movement grows in planning end-of-life strategy, *Columbia Daily Tribune*, (19 April 2009). http://www.columbiatribune.com/news/2009/apr/19/movement-grows-in-planning-e nd-of-life-strategy/.

[16] W.A. Hersh, stimulus to define informatics and health information technology, *BMC Medical Informatics and Decision Making* **9** (2009), 24. http://www.biomedcentral.com/1472-6947/9/24.

[17] D.R. Masys, The Year in Review. See http://dbmichair.mc.vanderbilt.edu/amia2008/; http://dbmichair.mc.vanderbilt.edu/amia2007/; and, http://dbmichair.mc.vanderbilt.edu/amia2006/.

[18] D. Mechanic and S. Meyer, Concepts of trust among patients with serious illness, *Soc Sci Med* **51** (2000), 657–668.

[19] S.J. Nass, L.A. Levit and L.O. Gostin, eds, Beyond the HIPAA Privacy Rule: Enhancing Privacy, Improving Health Through Research. Washington, DC: Institute of Medicine, 2009.

[20] M. Naylor, Transitional Care of Older Adults, in: *Annual Review of Nursing Research*, P. Archbold and B. Stewart eds, New York: Springer, **20** (2002), pp. 127–147.

[21] M. Naylor, K. Bowles, R. Campbell and K. McCauley, Discharge planning: design and implementation, in: *Critical Care Nursing of the Elderly*, T.T. Fulmer, M.D. Foreman, M. Walker and K.S. Montgomery, eds, 2nd Edition, New York: Springer, 2001, pp. 197–212.

[22] M. Naylor and P. Roe-Prior, (1999). Transitions Between Acute and Long Term Care, in: *Advances in Long Term Care*, (Volume IV), P.R. Katz, M. Mezey and R. Kane, eds, New York: Springer, 1999, pp. 1–22.

[23] S.J. Nass, L.A. Levit and L.O. Gostin eds, Beyond the HIPAA Privacy Rule: Enhancing Privacy, Improving Health Through Research. National Academy Press, Washington, DC: Institute of Medicine, 2009.

[24] J.A. Osheroff, J.M. Teich, B.F. Middleton, E.B. Steen, A. Wright and D.E. Detmer, A Roadmap for National Action on Clinical Decision Support. Released June 13, 2006 on contract with the Office of the National Coordinator of Health Information Technology, *JAMIA* **14** (2007), 141–155.
[25] J.A. Osheroff, ed., Improving Medication Use and Outcomes with Clinical Decision Support: A Step-by-Step Guide. HIMSS, Chicago, 2009.
[26] W. Stead, The demise of expert-based practice is inevitable. Evidence-Based Medicine and The Changing Nature Of Health Care: 2007 IOM Annual Meeting Summary. Washington, DC: The National Academies Press, 2008.
[27] W. Steed and M. Lin, eds, Computational Technology for Effective Health Care: Immediate Steps and Strategic Directions. Washington, DC: National Academies Press. Available at http://www.nap.edu/catalog.php?record_id=12572, 2009.
[28] M.J. Steinberg and E.R. Rubin, The HIPPA Privacy Rule: Lacks Patient Benefit, Impedes Research Growth. Washington, DC: AAHC, 2009.
[29] The Wellcome Trust Case Control Consortium. Genome-wide association study of 14,000 cases of seven common diseases and 3,000 shared controls, *Nature* **447** (2007), 661–678.
[30] G.R. Uhl, Promise of pharmacogenomics in smoking cessation, *Pharmacogenomics* **10**(7) (2009), 1123–1125.

Don Eugene Detmer, MD, MA, is currently Professor Emeritus and Professor of Medical Education at the University of Virginia; Senior Advisor to the American Medical Informatics Association (AMIA); Visiting Professor at CHIME, University College of London; Co-chair of the Blue Ridge Academic Health Group; and Chair of MedBiquitous and the IOM Membership Committee. Dr. Detmer is a member of the Institute of Medicine, a lifetime Associate of the National Academies, and a fellow of AAAS, American College of Medical Informatics, ACS, and ACSM (emeritus). Among his past leadership positions, he is the immediate past President and CEO of AMIA, past chairman of the IOM's Board on Health Care Services, the National Committee on Vital and Health Statistics, and the Board of Regents of the National Library of Medicine. He chaired the 1991 IOM study on Computer-based Patient Records, and contributed to IOM Reports, *To Error is Human* and *Crossing the Quality Chasm*. He is a past Vice President for Health Sciences at the Universities of Virginia and Utah. His medical degree is from Kansas with subsequent vascular surgical training at NIH, the Johns Hopkins Hospital, and Duke University Medical Center. He was the first policy fellow of the Institute of Medicine. His MA is from the University of Cambridge. He was a founder of the Administrative Medicine Program at the University of Wisconsin-Madison. From 1999–2003 he was Gillings Professor of Health Management at Cambridge University. He has been a consultant to the government of England and the Hospital Authority of Hong Kong, and many agencies of the U.S. Government. Dr. Detmer's research interests include national and international health information policy, quality improvement, administrative medicine, vascular surgery, sports medicine, education of clinician-executives and informaticians, and leadership of academic health sciences centers. He has published books, book chapters and many articles relating to systems thinking in health care and health policy.

Information Knowledge Systems Management 8 (2009) 119–143
DOI 10.3233/IKS-2009-0140
IOS Press

Chapter 8

Electronic health records

William W. Stead
E-mail: Bill.stead@vanderbut.edu

Abstract: A radical change in technical approach is needed to achieve electronic health records suitable to support an engineered system of healthcare. This chapter suggests a redefinition of interoperable health information. It provides examples of how to break the electronic health record challenge into component parts to match computational technique to the scale of the problem handled by a component.

1. Introduction

President Obama has pledged $50 billion over 5 years to achieve the goal of electronic health records for every American by 2014. RAND Corporation has estimated potential savings of $81 billion per year [7]. This estimate makes common sense to anyone who has more than one doctor, and finds themselves carrying information back and forth, undergoing repeated tests, and sorting through conflicting prescriptions [1].

Electronic health records are not a new idea. Pioneers began writing programs to store and retrieve patient records in 1958 [14]. The Institute of Medicine identified the computer-based record as "an essential technology for healthcare" in 1991 [4]. However surveys conducted in 2008 report only 17% of outpatient practices [3] and 9.1% of hospitals [10] use even basic electronic health records. Recent scientific reports include examples of unintended adverse clinical consequences in healthcare settings using such systems [6] because of the mismatch between healthcare work and information system design or implementation [12].

Interoperable health information is essential to engineering the system of healthcare delivery. However, a recent National Research Council (NRC) committee found "current efforts aimed at nationwide deployment of healthcare information technology will not be sufficient to achieve the vision of 21st century healthcare, and may even set back the cause" [20].

This chapter calls for a radically different approach to achieving the goal of interoperable health information. It focuses on the challenge of creating and maintaining electronic health records, data about individuals and populations. It begins by drawing on the NRC committee's observations to summarize expectations for electronic health records suitable to support an engineered system of healthcare and to contrast those expectations to the reality of today's deployed systems. Next, it makes the case that the failure of electronic health records to deliver on their potential is rooted in a mismatch between technical approach to their implementation and the nature of the individuals those records are trying to describe and the clinical work they are trying to document. It calls for a shift in the paradigm from thinking of the electronic health record as a by-product of automating practice, to thinking of it as a visualization of signals accumulated across scales of biology, time and geography. Using examples from Vanderbilt

University Medical Center (VUMC), it shows how this shift breaks the electronic health record into its component parts. The scope of each component and computational technique are matched to the breadth of coverage and depth of function supported.

This shift in the paradigm for electronic health records makes possible the flexibility to continually adapt people's roles, process and the technology. It breaks the cycle of ripping out and replacing software to achieve data integration. It cuts the cost and time to implement electronic health records by an order of magnitude.

2. Expectations for the electronic health record

The Institute of Medicine's vision for 21st century healthcare and wellness calls for a system that is safe, effective, patient-centered, timely, efficient and equitable (IOM Comm Healthcare America, 2001). This vision calls for electronic health records as part of the information infrastructure to support a systems approach to practice. In system-supported practice, the focus is on the system's performance [19]. Teams of people, well defined processes and information technology work in concert to produce the desired result consistently. People provide compassion, pattern recognition and judgment. Well defined processes standardize and simplify workflow. Information technology tools decrease dependence on memory and force action where needed. The desired result is expected every time. Each failure feeds back to support just-in-time correction or iterative adaptive design. The system of behaviors, processes and tools makes it easy for the individual to do the right thing every time.

The NRC Committee identified several information intensive aspects of this vision [20, pp. 20–24].

- Comprehensive data on patients' conditions, treatments and outcomes.
- Cognitive support for healthcare professionals and patients to help integrate patient-specific data where possible and account for any uncertainties that remain.
- Cognitive support for healthcare professionals to help integrate evidence-based practice guidelines and research results into daily practice.
- Instruments that allow providers to manage a portfolio of patients and highlight problems as they arise within both individual patients and populations.
- Rapid integration of new instrumentation, biological knowledge, treatment modalities, etc., into a "learning" healthcare system that encourages early adoption of promising methods but also analyzes all patient experience as experimental data.
- Accommodation of growing heterogeneity of locales for provision of care, including home instrumentation for monitoring and treatment, lifestyle integration, and remote assistance.
- Empowerment of patients and their families in effective management of healthcare decisions and execution, including personal health records (as contrasted to medical records held by care providers), education about the individual's conditions and options, and support of timely and focused communication with professional healthcare providers.

3. Today's reality

The NRC Committee visited 8 health systems – sites that are leaders in use of healthcare information technology to improve quality – to assess the gap between the best of what is deployed today and what is needed. The sites represented a broad spectrum – government, for profit, not for profit – academic, community – commercial systems, home grown systems. While the Committee reported many successes, it concluded that these successes, even in aggregate, fall far short of what would be needed to achieve the IOM's vision for 21st century healthcare. Problematic aspects include [20, appendix C]:

- Patient records are fragmented; computer-based and paper records coexist; computer records are divided among task-specific transaction processing systems; users have to know where to look.
- Clinical user interfaces mimic their paper predecessors, without design to reflect human and safety factors.
- Systems are used most often to document what has been done, manually, frequently hours after the fact.
- Support for evidence-based medicine and computer-based advice is rare.
- Biomedical devices are poorly integrated.
- Care processes and outcomes are rarely documented in machine-readable form.
- Work is frequently interrupted with gaps between steps and manual handoffs at seams of the process.
- Errors and near misses are frequent and use of data to identify patterns is rare.
- Clinical research activities are not well integrated into ongoing clinical care.
- Centralization of management and reduction in the number of information systems is the predominant method for standardization; while innovation requires locally adaptable systems.
- Security and privacy compete with workflow optimization.
- Implementation time lines are long and course changes are expensive.
- Response times are variable and long down times occur.

4. Roots of the failure

The failure of electronic health records to deliver on their potential is rooted in a mismatch between the conventional technical approach to their implementation and the nature of both the individuals those records are trying to describe and the clinical work they are trying to document [15,18]. Simply put, the technical approach does not scale-up to handle the variability in biological systems and the complexity of clinical work.

4.1. Conventional approach to electronic health records

Today's predominant approach to implementing electronic health records involves purchasing an information system to automate, or script care processes. The vendor may provide a "starter set" but commonly the healthcare provider has to build its pick lists to support data capture, its decision or communication support logic, etc. As the provider uses the system, the electronic health record is created "for free" as a byproduct of using the automated care process [13]. When care takes place in an area of the practice that is not yet automated, the record catches up through "after-the-fact" data entry. The vendors often seek to increase the coverage of the record by providing a suite of applications that work together supported by a common database. Data elements are mapped into standard formats, such as Health Level 7 (HL7), for exchange with parts of the vendor's suite that are not well integrated into the database or products from other vendors. Much of that mapping is repeated practice by practice because exchange standards clarify what the data element is, such as a drug orderable, but not what it means, such as its chemical ingredients, dose-form and strength.

This automation approach is workable if the patient population and the healthcare provider are largely self-contained – and if the provider can afford IT staff to handle the setup and data mapping, and the clinical process expertise to adapt practice and systems to avoid unintended consequences. Even when all of those conditions fall into place, the provider does not obtain the quality and safety benefits of electronic records until the automation of each part of the practice is complete enough to fill out the record. Once the automation is complete, the information system makes the process rigid, providing a barrier to change over time as new business demands are experienced, as advances in biomedical science alter in substantive ways approaches to defining and confirming specific diagnoses and as communities of patients and providers alter their approach toward managing health problems.

Automation and transaction processing have their place supporting well defined, small scale work processes that can be done over and over again with little variation – when specific treatment of disorders is clearly defined for some period, e.g. hernia repair, cardiac angiography, adjuvant chemotherapy for some malignancies. However, healthcare often attempts to extend the use of automation to more complex situations that require general problem-solving and both inter-dependencies and variations in work processes to manage combinations of disorders. These more complex problems are more easily handled by other domains of information technology [20, p. 28]. Examples include: connectivity – linking people to each other and systems; decision support – making choices clear; and data mining – discovering relationships among data. This imbalance is depicted in Fig. 1. Even when healthcare uses domains other than automation, they are often bolted onto a pre-existing core of automation. This core limits the range of scale of the data, knowledge, processes and roles that can be accommodated. This

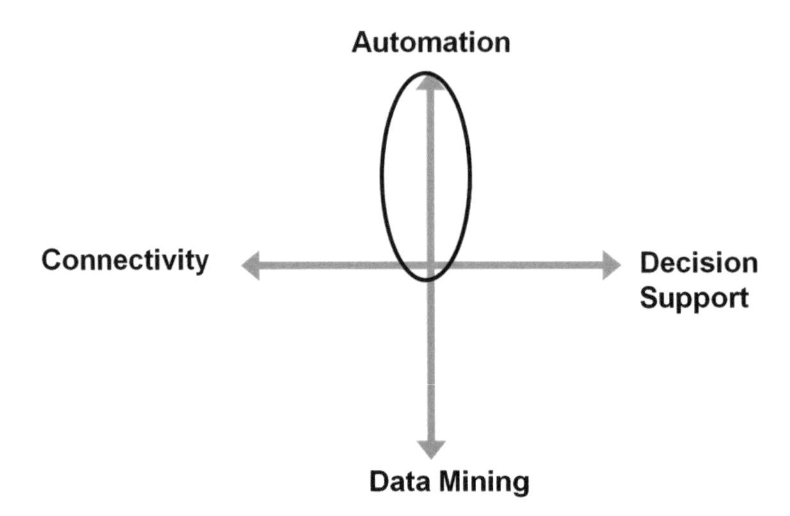

Fig. 1. Imbalance in healthcare information technology portfolio. Four domains of computational techniques are represented by the axes. Elipse shows relative use of each domain by typical electronic health record systems.

dependence upon automation, in turn, leads to other flawed industry practices. For example, healthcare information technology vendors, who sell enterprise solutions, compete on how completely their system can automate the practices that make up the enterprise instead of competing on how well their systems work with data originating outside of them. This inward focus impedes progress towards the patient-centered health care society requires. To get the benefit of a complete record, the provider must either invest in costly excessively complex interfaces or rip out and replace pre-existing systems with a single vendor system that attempts to cover every current and future aspect of care and administration – even if most aspects of their pre-existing systems are doing a satisfactory job of their primary task of automating an aspect of the practice. If the make-up of the enterprise evolves with merger or acquisition, the process starts over.

Similarly, the focus on automation leads to over-specification of coding and terminology standards. The intent is to develop a standard terminology that can be used to capture data in a form that accommodates the first system's purpose while enabling reuse of the data by other systems with other purposes without additional human intervention. This intent requires a standard that can accommodate the maximum detail anticipated. It requires synchronization of maintenance of related standards and their inter-standard mappings. Since individual components of a system change frequently, updating these complex relationships is a never-ending and costly process.

4.2. The nature of individuals

Individuals are highly variable biological systems. Each cell carries its own copy of its parent's blue print (DNA) and changes are introduced in the copying process. In addition, each cell makes decisions about what parts of the blueprint to build out or not based on its environment. Accordingly, no two individuals respond to disease or treatment in exactly the same way. Their reaction represents the sum of the interactions of their genetics, brain, environment, disease and treatment. We do not know how to capture the detail to fully represent even the simplest of biological systems.

The contrast between biological systems and the physical systems highlights the challenge. Physical systems behave according to the laws of physics. Once understood and modeled, they behave as expected every time. You can capture all of the detail of an instance of a complex physical system by recording the few parameters in the relevant models.

4.2.1. Clinical measurements rarely have precise meaning

Physiological measurements, such as a person's pulse or blood pressure, reflect not only their health conditions, but also their body's response to many factors. For example, blood pressure is higher if a person is lying down than if they are sitting or standing. It goes up if they are stressed or active. If they are obese, a larger cuff is needed to avoid artificially high readings. The reading itself has little meaning without detailed information about the context in which it was taken. Little of this context was written in paper records because it was known to the person writing and using the records. With the shift toward electronic records, the information is usually transferred among people out of context because it is too labor intensive to record all aspects of the context explicitly.

Laboratory results are equally difficult to interpret out of context. Even the most straightforward tests such as serum chemistries measure something that correlates with the substance being measured, not the substance itself. The resulting number does not have an absolute meaning. It is only meaningful when compared to the result that instrument obtained with a panel of standard control specimens. The problem is even greater with bioassays and imaging.

4.2.2. Diagnoses lack clinical detail

A diagnosis matches the constellation of findings observed in a person to patterns that have been shown to cluster in patients, respond to treatment in a comparable fashion, or have a common cause. Findings and responses are shared among diagnoses and multiple diagnoses co-exist in one individual. A diagnosis is the clinician's interpretation of their observations. The detail of those observations can not be inferred from the diagnosis.

As new knowledge is discovered about biology and disease, the diagnostic classifications change. In 1979 for example, 2 types of diabetes mellitus were recognized. By 1997, the classification of diabetes mellitus included four forms. Genomics is adding new classifications. When new diagnostic classifications are subdivisions of a prior one, a record with the prior less granular "aggregate" diagnosis is still useful. However, when new classifications map to only a part of multiple prior classifications, the information content of the record decays. For example, juvenile onset diabetes and insulin dependent diabetes were once thought to be one condition. Adult onset diabetes and non-insulin dependent diabetes were thought to be another. The current classifications are type 1 diabetes (autoimmune destruction of insulin producing beta cells) and type 2 diabetes (insulin resistance). Both occur both in children and adults, and type 2 can be insulin or non-insulin dependent.

In a time of paper records, diagnosis codes were developed to lump patients into the common causes of mortality for easy tabulation, or into groups according to likely utilization of services to support prospective reimbursement. The full record was still available when needed for clarification. With the shift to electronic records, people commonly use the codes for diagnosis as if they were a more complete record despite the lack of clinical detail.

4.3. The nature of clinical work

Clinical work is chaotic. The clinician moves from task to task, focusing on what is most important. When a more important problem surfaces, she stops what she is doing to deal with it.

4.3.1. Clinical work is an opaque ecosystem

People's roles, process and technology work together to accomplish clinical work. Each has evolved together in response to changes in capability, patient mix, administrative requirements, etc. As problems surface, situation-specific work-arounds have been added. Take the paper order sheet as an example. The clinician writes a set of orders for care, diagnosis and treatment when a patient is admitted to the hospital. Thereafter, orders are added, stopped or changed one at a time. After the patient has been in the hospital for a short time, there is no one place where anyone can see all of the active orders for the patient. As a result, it has been common to require by policy that all orders be re-written on major transitions such as transfer of a patient from intensive care to intermediate care.

The processes from the paper world are used as a starting point from which to develop requirements for new information technology. It is difficult to separate the purpose and essential steps of a work process from the related work-around. To continue the example, a system analyst is unlikely to realize that ready access to the list of active orders in the computer record accomplishes the purpose of the policy. They are likely to judge the re-writing of orders as a requirement, and design a workflow within the order entry application to allow the clinician to carry out the task as quickly as possible. Despite their best effort, the computer entry task is likely to take the clinician more time than writing on paper.

Once the system is live an unexpected consequence is noticed. To continue the example, a patient was transferred from an intensive care unit to an intermediate care unit with an order that first transports the patient to the radiology department for an imaging study. While the patient was in transit, the clinician re-wrote their orders, discontinuing the order for the imaging study because it would be complete by the time the patient reached intermediate care. When the patient arrived in radiology, the technician could not find an active order and sent the patient on without performing the study. In the paper-based world, the chart with the order sheet would have been with the patient, preventing this occurrence. A system analyst is likely to respond by requesting a change to the program to check and prevent cancellation of an imaging order once the patient is in transit for the study. Sometime later clinicians will complain that they need to be able to cancel orders in that circumstance and recall the patient before the study is completed. This cycle of problem identification, followed by addition of complexity to the system, followed by a new problem, will repeat until someone has an epiphany. In a digital world, the right approach is to change policy. Instead of requiring all orders to be re-written on change in level of care, require review and update of orders followed by entry of a single order confirming that the review is complete. The clinician saves time and the system is simplified.

4.3.2. Perspectives vary by role

Each role on the clinical team has a unique perspective. For example, physicians and nurses use the word "diagnosis" differently to achieve complimentary aims. Their use reflects their disciplinary background and their span of control. A physician is trained to think about a patient in terms of diseases, their causes and their treatments. A nurse is trained to think about a patient in terms of the problems the patient is experiencing and must reconcile care for the patient according to their own perspective as well as the physician's diagnoses and orders. Physicians and nurses may use the word diagnosis differently. A physician diagnosis reflects the cause of the problem, such as *retinal detachment*. A nursing diagnosis reflects the effect of the cause on the patient's health or ability to function, such as *visual impairment*. Although both are diagnoses, retinal detachment is but one of many causes of visual impairment. Conversely, a nurse will not make a diagnosis of visual impairment in cases with retinal detachment unless the impairment is severe enough to affect the patient's functioning. The presence of one of these diagnoses can not be taken to mean the other is present. Neither is sufficient to meet the other's purpose.

Perspectives must be coupled dynamically so that individuals with different roles on the clinical team can work together to accomplish a task. Each role works with data at a different scale or level of detail. Take treatment of a patient with a medication as an example. The person prescribing (physician, nurse practitioner, physician assistant, etc.) decides what regimen to prescribe. She considers the patient's diagnoses, efficacy of alternatives, potential interactions, adverse effects and formulary constraints. She writes an order specifying the ingredients, the dose form, the strength, the route, the frequency and the duration, for example, gentamycin 60 mg IV every 8 hours for 10 days. This order (what is to be done) is then passed to the person dispensing (pharmacist, nurse, etc) to decide what to dispense (how it is to be done). She acts within the scope or context of the order. She checks to see that it fits with what she knows about the patient, makes substitutions among equivalent products based on availability or cost, and adds detail related to the product selected. For example, she might dispense 40 mg ampules with instructions to infuse 1.5 ampules over 30 min every 8 hours. She creates a label that is then passed to the person administering the medication (nurse, patient, etc). She checks that it makes sense with what she knows about the patient and then adds detail by selecting the time for each dose adapting to meals, shift schedules, etc. Although each succeeding part of the task fits within the context established by the previous steps, it is not possible to back calculate the exact order from the administration record. If a change in the original order is required at some point in the process, the change has to be made at the level of detail and authority of the original order (the decision of what is to be done), and then flow back down through the additional levels of detail.

5. Shifting the paradigm

To summarize, today's predominant approach to implementing electronic health records involves automating clinical workflow. One person enters data so that others can access the data later. They are encouraged to record findings and impressions using standard codes or terminologies. Clinical workflow and the clinician-patient interaction are interrupted by data entry. The detailed context and observations are lost. The information content of the record decays as advances in biology and healthcare result in changes to its codes and terminologies.

Consider a radically different approach to achieving the goal of interoperable health information. First, define interoperable data as data that can be assembled and interpreted in the light of current knowledge, and re-interpreted as knowledge evolves. Re-interpretation requires access to an archive of "raw signal" (voice, image, text, biometrics, etc). Second, require data liquidity – the separability of data from applications so that other applications can use them. Third, limit the use of standard data, by which I mean data that can have only one interpretation, to situations where meaning is explicit and stable over time, e.g. drug ingredients, etc.

In this approach, data about the patient are captured from whatever sources, in whatever form they are available in ways that minimize interruptions but clarify context. Computer algorithms and knowledge-bases work together to analyze this multi-source multi-mode set of "signals". As clinically significant patterns emerge, the computer presents possible interpretations to the clinician and/or the patient for confirmation or correction. This computer-human interpretation and annotation may take the form of the standard codes and terminologies that make up today's electronic health record. However, now the annotations are additional "tags". All of the "signals" and all of the contexts leading up to the interpretation are archived along with the tags. People move freely among levels of detail as they shift from exploring how a patient's problems fit together to drilling down into the basis of one interpretation. As new signals become available, or as biological knowledge advances, the interpretations and annotations may be refreshed.

In this approach, computational techniques are matched to the scale of the problem as depicted in Fig. 2.

For example, connectivity and data mining techniques work together to support information access, such as to a multi-source, multi-mode electronic health record. Data mining and decision support techniques combine to support pattern recognition such as for bio-surveillance. Decision support and automation come together to support informed action such as through evidence-based order sets.

In short, the paradigm shifts from thinking of the electronic health record as a by-product of automating practice – to thinking of it as a visualization of signals accumulated across scales of biology, time and geography. Table 1 summarizes this shift.

This shift breaks up the electronic health record into component parts. Instead of attempting to have one record and practice management system that can be used for many purposes, the set of purposes is met through a set of frameworks for combining components. The scope of individual components are limited and matched to the breadth of coverage and to the depth of function supported by the component. As the breadth of coverage (number of circumstances supported) increases, the depth of functionality (number of features) is reduced so that the combination remains tractable. Limiting scope also achieves a degree of homogeneity among data handled by a component – providing implicit context for data fusion/mining algorithms. Within a framework, components are swapped out as requirements and technology change.

This shift in the paradigm for electronic health records makes possible the flexibility to continually adapt people's roles, process and the technology. It breaks the cycle of ripping out and replacing software to achieve data integration. It cuts the cost and time to implement electronic health records by an order of magnitude.

5.1. A spectrum of electronic health record frameworks

The purpose of an electronic health record, its component parts, and the best framework for putting components together, vary according to the scale it covers. Examples of different scales include: records

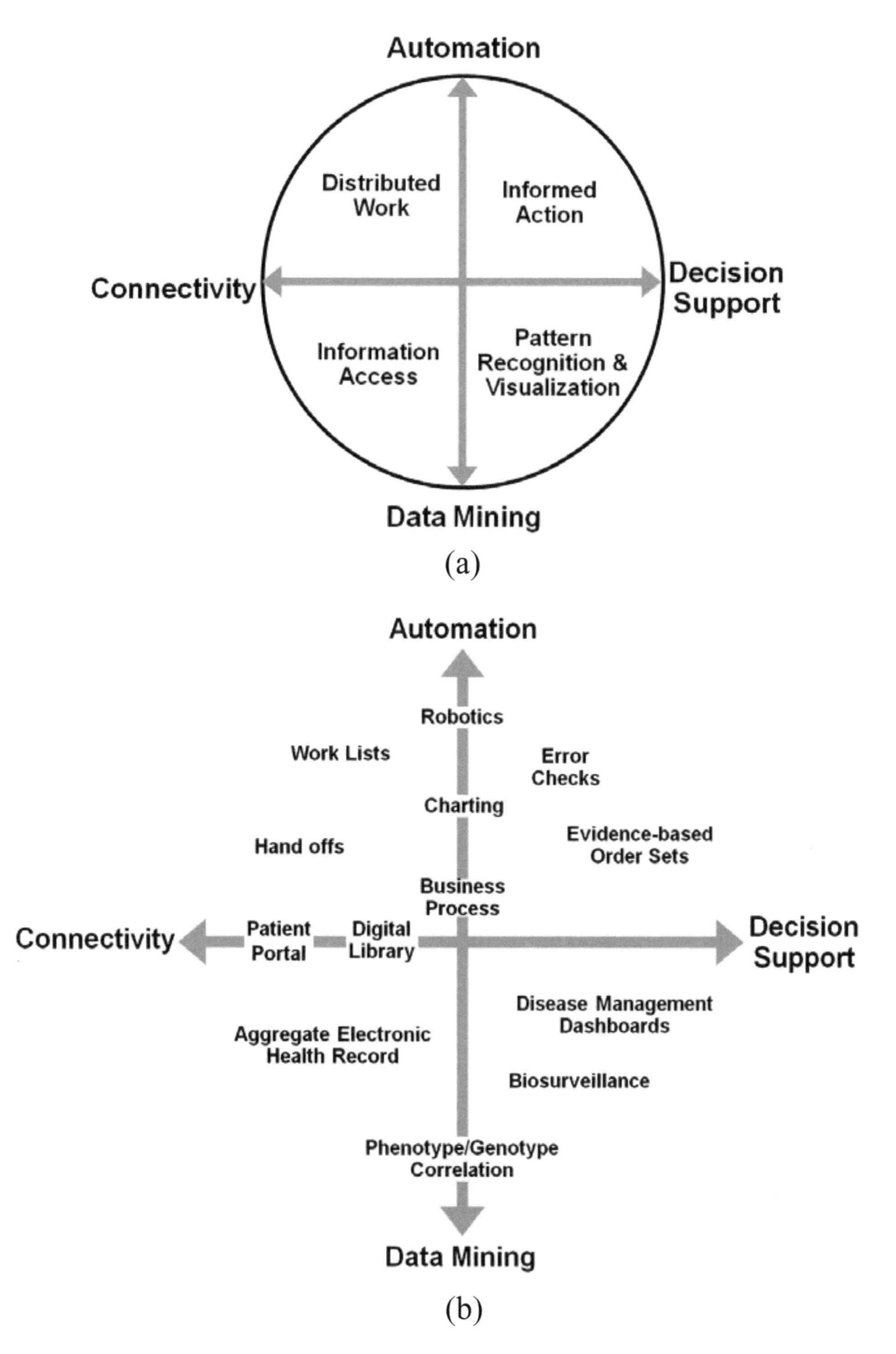

Fig. 2. Match of computational technique to the scale of various electronic health records capabilities. (a) depicts the category of work supported by the two adjacent axes; (b) shows the relative contribution of each to individual capabilities. For example, the aggregate electronic health record is 2 parts connectivity to 1 part data mining.

Table 1

Old	New
One integrated set of data	Sets of data from multiple sources
Capture data in standardized terminology	Capture raw signal and annotate with standard terminology
Single source of truth	Current interpretation of multiple related signals
Seamless transfer among systems	Visualization of the collective output of relevant systems
Clinician uses the computer to update the record during the patient visit.	Clinician & patient work together with shared records and information
The system provides transaction-level data	The system provides cognitive support
Work processes are programmed and adapt through non-systematic work around	People, process and technology work together as a system

of healthcare entities such as integrated care delivery systems; regional data exchanges, such as regional health information organization; personal health records, and population databases.

5.1.1. Healthcare entities

The Vanderbilt University Medical Center (VUMC) enterprise information architecture [16] is an example of data liquidity. It is a framework that separates the management of the healthcare entity's information content from the commercial applications or locally developed informatics tools that provide functionality for the entity's users. Figure 3 is a logical view of the architecture. It represents meaningful

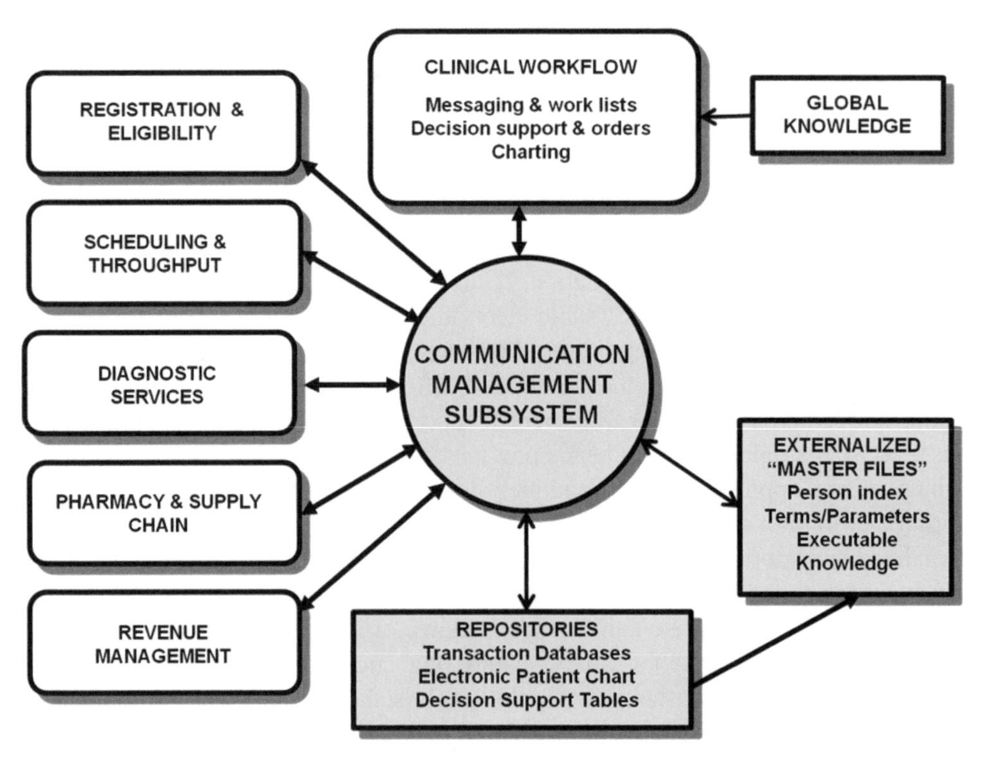

Fig. 3. Logical view of VUMC enterprise information architecture. The shaded components represent information resources managed separately from any application or workflow tool.

content outside of the various application systems, and aligns the applications by importing and using this externally defined content in a standard manner throughout. Information, such as metadata (data about other data) and organizational knowledge that might otherwise be entered into application-specific master files, is externalized in generalized tables. This information is structured to make its meaning explicit and accessible; for example: external tables store the identity of medical center personnel and a mapping to their roles; clinically meaningful orderables are stored externally, with mapping to the administrative equivalents in individual ancillary systems; and, the set of clinical concepts that can be measured in the laboratory is stored externally, with mappings to the various billing codes associated with each concept in ancillary systems. Where possible, applications use these externalized tables directly. It is often necessary to manually copy the information into the profiles of legacy systems. In either case, each new application reuses prior definitional work. Only newly required information needs to be added to the generalized tables, and the relation of such new information to existing information can be made explicit as it is added. This approach cuts implementation time while pre-aligning meaning across otherwise disparate applications.

Similarly, data that are captured or managed by an application, but which are used by more than one application, are externalized into generalized repositories. A set of disparate repositories exploits the strengths of their respective technologies. Collectively they represent VUMC's electronic patient chart. Highly structured, coded clinical data is represented in relational tables, and in contrast, an indexed text repository, organized according to a document paradigm, provides a single logical source for all clinical reports about a patient, be they binary data, images, or text. Some reports are stored in this repository as symbolic links (e.g., links from textual radiology reports to their corresponding images in the Picture Archiving and Communication Systems), while others are copied directly from primary sources and stored directly in the repository, as in the case of EKGs.

The indexed text repository is a non-relational, hyper-indexed database implemented in Perl (a high level interpreted dynamic programming language) on a distributed processing cluster. The lowest tier implements distributed processing, queue-based transaction processing, process control and monitoring, and inter-process communication. The database layer implements permanent data storage; automatic replication across servers in different geographical locations; and conversion of clinical data from all sources into a common internal representation. Common views such as the assembly of documents and data related to a patient into a browsable electronic chart are cached to reduce search demands. The application layer implements transaction and business logic, such as the handling of corrections and updates in stored documents, and the handling of different evolving stages of individual data items (from pending to preliminary to final to corrected report, for example). This layer is shared by all applications that use the repository, and hence provides the single place where transaction and business logic is maintained and applied. It provides request broker functionality to support application interface services, report distribution services, and a number of Web-based interfaces.

The externalized repositories leverage database techniques to solve a class of problems that are difficult to handle through data processing strategies characteristic of transaction processing systems. One of the VUMC repositories is the Enterprise Patient Index, a table of identifying numbers (e.g. medical record number, social security number, etc.), a table of names (e.g. current, maiden, married, etc.) and linkages of those numbers and names to instantiate people. As mistakes are made and corrected, linkages are updated. A query is all that is needed to assemble all record "fragments" for a patient. This approach avoids the complicated processes related to reconciling and merging records characteristic of classic enterprise master patient index systems.

Other aspects of the architecture allow the variety of commercial systems and locally developed informatics tools in use throughout the facilities in the integrated delivery system to interact with the electronic patient chart. For example, the externalized application-independent repositories serve two types of middleware function. First, when an application combines two concepts into one variable, the meaning can be decomposed into a set of granular data on the way into the repository, or assembled from multiple data on the way back into the application. In this fashion, required translation is limited to a "plug-in" between the application and the repository without burdening other applications. For example, an application may represent the combination of the physician's identity and their service as one provider number. If a physician participates in two services, such as trauma and orthopedics, she would have two provider numbers. The external metadata would include a table of physicians, a table of services, valid links among the two and the provider number associated with the link. As applications converge around the external metadata, the plug-ins are removed. Second, when two different processes provide different views of a related datum, those views can be represented "side by side" instead of picking one or the other. For example, the admitting office may be responsible for updating the attending physician field that is used for billing purposes, while the clinical care team on the patient's ward may represent the most reliable source of this information. However the care team does not possess the admitting office's understanding of the correct timing of recording changes to comply with billing requirements. The solution is to record both views of the data (administrative and clinical versions of "attending physician", and to have a process for reconciling differences just before midnight, the deadline for billing corrections).

Commercial "best of class" transaction processing systems operate as components within Vanderbilt's information architecture. Application components connect to the collective externalized tables and repositories through a single logical point, serviced by communication management engines. The Generic Interface Engine (GIE) provides a transaction-processing environment among applications and the repositories including: transaction logging; protocol conversion; one-to-many routing; and request broker functionality. It uses queuing mechanisms to loosely couple inter-application communication. At the same time, it manages acknowledgements so as to insure serialization and logical unit of work across components. Since the proactive end-to-end management of interface transactions provided by the GIE requires application-specific development, a commercial interface engine provides an alternative path for less demanding situations. In addition, efficient query services exist to provide applications with access to some commonly used repositories for transactions that do not result in updates.

Workflow-support and decision-support tools are separate from the transaction processing systems. They draw on information from multiple sources through the repository to construct displays specific to the role and situation. For example, one-patient-at-a-time displays, such as Fig. 4, provide access to the clinical picture for one patient.

Panel management or practice-oriented displays, such as Fig. 5, allow sets of patients to be accessed and reviewed in a single logical operation, including notification, signature, escalation, functionality etc. Patient portal displays allow direct access to portions of their electronic record, together with provider-patient messaging. Since these tools are separate from the application components that automate the various facilities within the enterprise, they can be used as needed across the continuum of care – inpatient, outpatient or home. As decisions are captured through these displays, they are handed off to the application component for processing.

Freedom from having to automate all clinical processes as the means of assembling electronic patient records allows flexibility in sequencing the introduction of information technology. Figure 6 is a schematic showing use of this flexibility to ease adoption by the clinical team. The idea is to introduce change in stages that provide more benefit in clinical workflow than disruption. Information technology is most helpful when easing access to data and most disruptive when data entry is required, just as it is easy to take money out of the bank and hard to put it in. This rule of thumb suggests that Stage 1 is using information aggregation and data mining techniques to assemble the patient record from images, scanned paper, word processing files from transcription, and text reports from data processing systems.

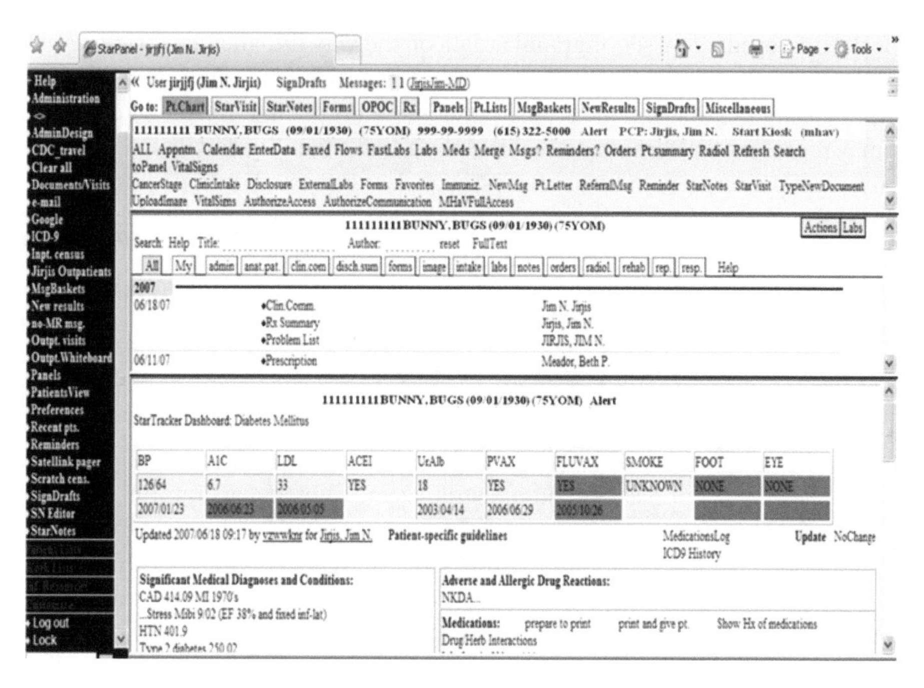

Fig. 4. *Patient* View for Primary Care – Tabs across the top drill down into categories of data such as laboratory. The center section provides a reverse chronological list of new information about the patient & a disease management dashboard specific to the patient's problems. The bottom summarizes problems, medications and allergies. Data are included from multiple systems within and outside of VUMC.

Bed	Patient name	Age	LOS	Orders			Vent	SBT Scrn	SBT Trial	DVT	SUP	RASS Ord.	RASS Pt.	HoB	swab	teeth	hySx
3002B	T, V W	72y	6 d		flowsheet	MAR	v	F		v	v	-4	-4	30			
3003X	N, D	60y	17 d		flowsheet	MAR	v	F		v	v	0	-2	45			
3004B	T, P L	64y	34 d		flowsheet	MAR	v			v	v	-1	-1	30			
3005A	C, D E	61y	7 d		flowsheet	MAR				v	v	0	-1	30	v	v	
3005B	B, J	66y	7 d		flowsheet	MAR	v	F		v	v	-1	-3	30			
3006X	W, A A	20y	66 d		flowsheet	MAR	v			v	v	-1	-2	30			
3007X	W, L E	49y	9:14		flowsheet	MAR				v		0	-1	30			
3008X	P, J L	69y	50 d		flowsheet	MAR	v	F		v	v	0	0	30			
3009X	R, C	72y	15 d		flowsheet	MAR	v	F		v	v	-1	-2	30			
3011A	P, J E	88y	9 d		flowsheet	MAR				v	v	0	0	45	v	v	
3011C	J, W D	69y	2 d		flowsheet	MAR				v	v	0	-1	30			
3011D	P, P J	55y	10 d		flowsheet	MAR	v	P	P	v	v	0	-3	30			
3011E	R, R E	74y	9 d		flowsheet	MAR				v	v	0	0		v	v	
3011F	N, E Y	55y	3 d		flowsheet	MAR				v	v	-1	0	30	v	v	
3012A	S, J D	56y	14 d		flowsheet	MAR	v	F		v	v		0	30			
3012B	R, M	63y	10 d		flowsheet	MAR	v	F		v	v	-2	-2	30			
3013A	N, B D	60y	8 d		flowsheet	MAR	v	F		v	v	-3	-2	30			
3013B	H, S M	66y	16 d		flowsheet	MAR				v	v	0	-1	30	v	v	

Fig. 5. Process Control Dashboard for Ventilator Management – The status of each patient is compared to their plan as a set of flags where green (medium gray) means an aspect of the plan is within control limits, yellow (light gray) indicates a need for action, and red (drak gray) indicates that aspect is out of control. The flag is calculated in *real time based upon inputs from several systems. Reproduced with permission from Stead 2008.*

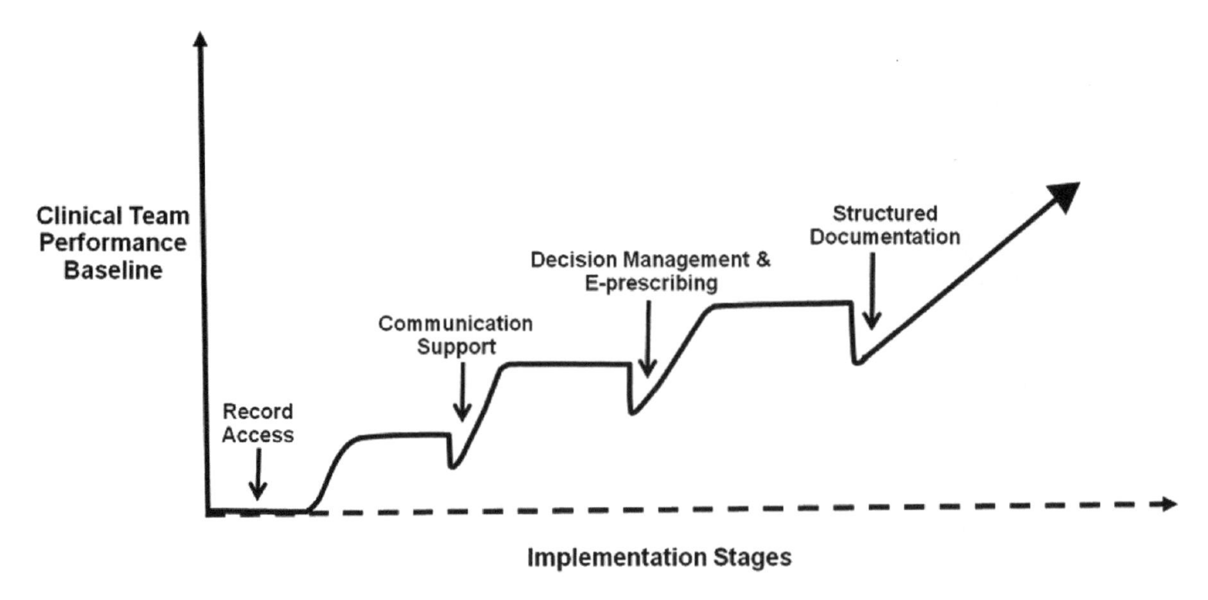

Fig. 6. Impact of staged introduction of electronic health record and associated workflow tools. Dips indicate the cost of learning to practice differently, subsequent up ticks indicate improvement from the change [18].

This Stage is fast and inexpensive. When VUMC adopted this approach in 1996, it took only four months at a cost of less than $500,000 to implement and populate the aggregate electronic health record. The clinical team's first experience is access to the aggregate record via a web browser when and where needed without the downside of change in the rest of their workflow. Roll-out of such a data retrieval capability requires little user support. The 1996 VUMC roll-out was accomplished by giving users an index card with short instructions.

Subsequent stages are more difficult since each involves change in clinical work itself. Figure 6 depicts a drop in performance during the learning curve followed by first gradual and then steeper improvement until a new plateau is reached. The objective is to limit the scope of each stage so team performance never falls below baseline and to time the next stage to start after a period of plateau. In practice this objective is elusive because each new plateau resets the clinical team's expectations. This moving baseline of expectations is offset to a degree because their willingness to tolerate deeper learning curves grows each time they experience such a dip leading to ultimate improvement.

The best sequence for stages of role-process-technology change will vary by healthcare entity reflecting clinical priorities, pain points that present opportunities for early workflow wins, and prerequisite resources. In VUMC outpatient practices, Stage 2 supported communication among the clinical team including notification of new information on their patients as it appears in the aggregate patient record, together with means to note action and manage handoffs. After a short learning curve, Stage 2 saved as much as 20% of the clinical team's time because of the large multi-specialty practice. Stage 3 moved into decision support, adding disease management panel displays and alerts. Stage 3 tools took back some of the time savings from the earlier stages but provided a measurable improvement in quality. Automation such as E-prescribing, capture of ancillary orders and structured data entry were delayed until the earlier stages resulted in the digitally enabled practice ecology to pull these functions in.

5.1.2. Regional data exchanges

Figure 7 depicts a high level framework for setting federal and regional patient data sharing capabilities along side the systems of participating healthcare entities. It shows the relationship of the desired

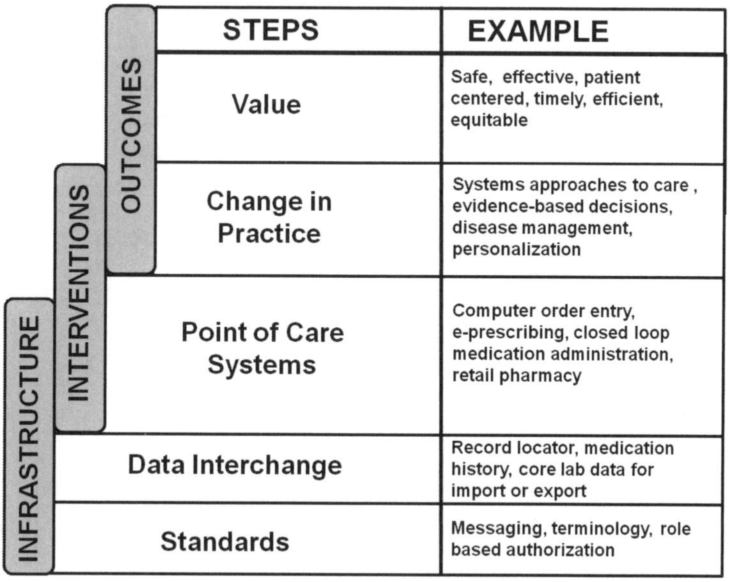

OUTCOMES
INTERVENTIONS
INFRASTRUCTURE

STEPS	EXAMPLE
Value	Safe, effective, patient centered, timely, efficient, equitable
Change in Practice	Systems approaches to care, evidence-based decisions, disease management, personalization
Point of Care Systems	Computer order entry, e-prescribing, closed loop medication administration, retail pharmacy
Data Interchange	Record locator, medication history, core lab data for import or export
Standards	Messaging, terminology, role based authorization

Fig. 7. Layered framework for assembling the information foundation for an engineered system of healthcare.

outcomes to the interventions needed to achieve those outcomes. It then shows the relationship of those interventions to the infrastructure required to enable them. The lower levels provide services or data that decrease the difficulty of implementing the upper levels or increase the value they can provide. In the process, they make the data being made available to them by the upper layers more useful. For example, a regional data interchange based upon data mining techniques may begin by aggregating data across entities and organizing it to support access through a secure web interface. At the same time, standards reduce the effort of implementing the point of care systems while clarifying the meaning of the data they capture. In time, subsets of the data will be captured in, or tagged with, a standard terminology. Those subsets can then be passed directly through to participating point of care systems from the data interchange.

By decomposing the problem into layers, the framework accommodates differences due to breadth and depth of aspects such as form of governance, the nature of the supporting technology, etc. Figure 8 depicts how the appropriate form of governance varies. At the lowest level are efforts of international or national breadth which are best governed through representative processes. Next come layers targeted at one population across business entities which require an alliance or voluntary network approach. The higher levels of point of care systems and change in practice will remain the province of the various entities that make up the healthcare system. At the top are the outcomes managed by consumers and payers.

The MidSouth eHealth Alliance (MSeHA) architecture [5] is an example of a framework to loosely couple the point of care systems of participating entities to the data interchange layer. Figure 9 is a logical view of the architecture. Participating entities publish copies of the transactions that are occurring within their local information systems over a secure network to a "vault" within a common regional databank. Each participating entity has a separate vault. Incoming data are maintained in their original form and remain under the control of the participating entity. The vault includes a database that contains the participating entity's patient identifier plus the additional identifying data supported by their master patient index or equivalent structure. As the participating entity adds or updates data within their local

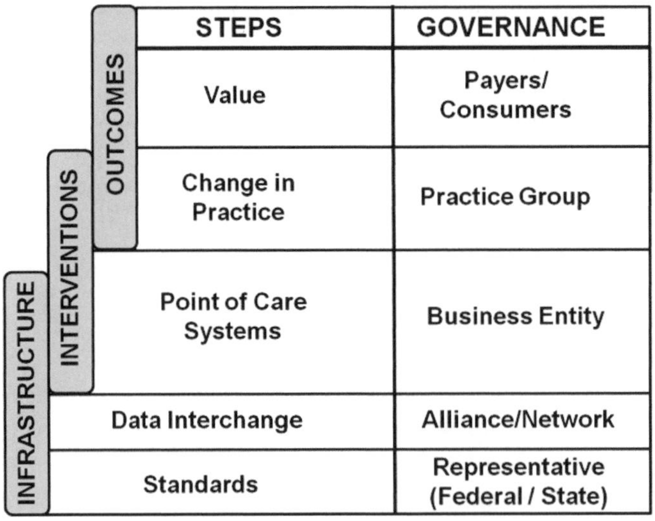

STEPS
GOVERNANCE
OUTCOMES
INTERVENTIONS
INFRASTRUCTURE
Value
Payers/ Consumers
Change in Practice
Practice Group
Point of Care Systems
Business Entity
Data Interchange
Alliance/Network
Standards
Representative (Federal / State)

Fig. 8. Match between governance and layer of the information framework.

Regional Databank
Healthcare Entity Internal Systems
Vaults
Regional Index
Hospital A
Hospital B
Group Practice
Clinic
Nursing Home
Retail Pharmacy
Payer
Entity Patient ID Info
Structured Documents
Person 1 Composite ID Info
Link 1
Link 2
...
Person 2

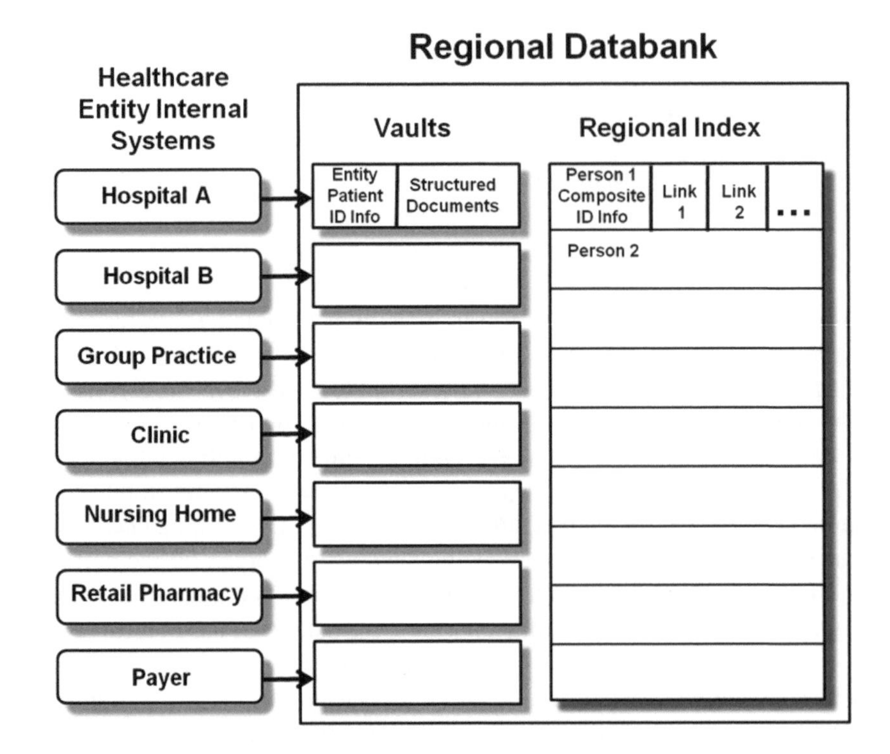

Fig. 9. Logical view of the MSeHA architecture at Stage 1 interoperability. Data is aggregated in the regional databank, but remains in vaults under the control of participating entities.

systems, these changes are passed through to their vault in the regional databank. The vault in the regional databank does not add data management burden for the participating entity. In a sense, the vault is simply a replication of the content of their systems.

Each submission is treated as a record. Upon submission, a link is created in the regional index to other records with matching identifiers within or across vaults. The link is created by heuristic matching algorithms. Matching elements are first name, last name, date of birth, gender and social security number if available. Matching algorithms include the longest common substring method, character transposition checks, SOUNDEX on the last name and the New York State Identification and Intelligence System Phonetic Code on the first name. Each submission is treated as a record and given a unique record ID and added to the set of record IDs with a matching set of identifiers. As new records are submitted the index is updated in real time. However, it is also possible to rebuild the index completely to reflect improvement in the matching algorithms.

The system does not create a unique identifier for each person in the index avoiding the hardware, software and administrative management costs of a master patient index. A record locator service based upon the Markle Connecting for Health Framework instead relates any query to similar records based upon the sets of identifiers in the regional index. The record locator service can be adjusted query by query to the desired balance between false positives and false negatives. Each record is parsed on submission to a vault. Concept matching algorithms tag clinical data by source and type so that related data can be tracked across disparate sources.

Since the participating entities retain control of their vault, the architecture provides the flexibility of a decentralized data interchange with the efficiencies and opportunities for cross entity data mining of a centralized model. Entities can make the decision to submit data in advance of coming to agreement on regional policies regarding use of data across entities. They can clear their vault at any time to accommodate trial and error during initial implementation. As the regional board finalizes data use agreements, access can be granted to all or part of a linked record set for one or more stated purposes. Since data has been accumulating in the various vaults, access can extend to data submitted prior to the agreements. If an entity subsequently has to pull out of the regional databank, they can do so and clear their vault. However, once data are used by another site, records of use and the values resident at that time are retained in audit logs for medical legal purposes.

The regional databank architecture is extensible to achieve interoperability in stages. As described above, Stage 1 makes an individual's data from all participating entities available for viewing through a secure web browser. A cross-entity chronological list of patient encounters allows drill down to individual encounter records in one of the vaults. The viewer can focus in on one type of data for a patient such as radiology reports or a particular type of study. Stage 2 extends the architecture as depicted in Fig. 10 to support a regional integrated patient record. The integrated record is limited to the data that can be tagged with standard terminology or codes. The tagging occurs within the parsers of the regional databank providing consistency while keeping the burden off the participating facilities. At Stage 2 the viewer can present disease management dashboards and graphs of laboratory tests across facilities. Such graphs show both the result itself and the variation in the normal range across entities and time.

MSeHA has achieved Stage 2. Clinical data are currently aggregated on over 1 million people from five competing hospital-based systems, two networks of community clinics, and an academic center medical group. The data are accessible throughout the emergency rooms and clinics, and by the hospitalists, across the three county region in southwest Tennessee. Stage 1 took less than 2 years and Stage 2 costs about two dollars per patient per year.

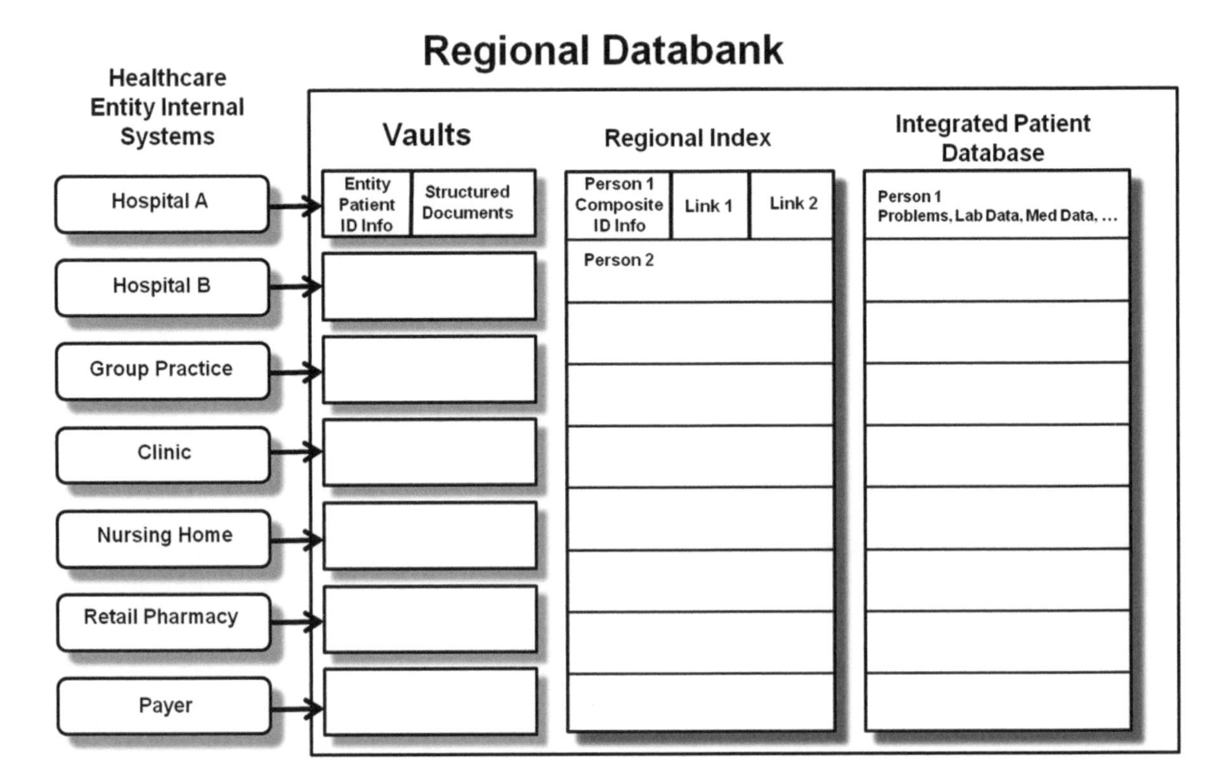

Fig. 10. MSeHA architecture extended to support stage 2 interoperabiltiy. Subsets of data are tagged to a standard terminology and assembled as integrated patient records.

Stage 3 will include export of data from the integrated regional patient record back to the point of care systems. Stage 3 will become possible as the participating entities incorporate standards within their point of care systems.

The architecture allows each participating entity to move toward interoperability at their own pace. The stages co-exist indefinitely. New information sources flow quickly and inexpensively into Stage 1. A subset is then moved to Stage 2 and then an even smaller subset to Stage 3.

5.1.3. Personal health records

The personal health record is an individual's collection of information about their health, health related activities and healthcare. Personal health records have the potential to allow the individual to aggregate a complete picture of their health related activities and control who can access that view of them. Figure 11 depicts the framework VUMC is piloting to relate an individual's personal health record to their electronic health records of the various healthcare entities that care for them, while keeping the records separate.

In this framework, the individual creates and maintains their personal health record using an application service provider (ASP) such as Google Health. She controls the account and its password. The record is governed by the privacy policies of the ASP. She enters information directly, and uploads information from applications on her personal computers, digital sensors, digital cameras, etc.

Separately, she establishes an account with the patient or consumer portal of each of her healthcare entities (providers, payers, retail, etc). She creates each account through the processes of the entity and the account is governed by the privacy policies of the entity. Services range from access to portions

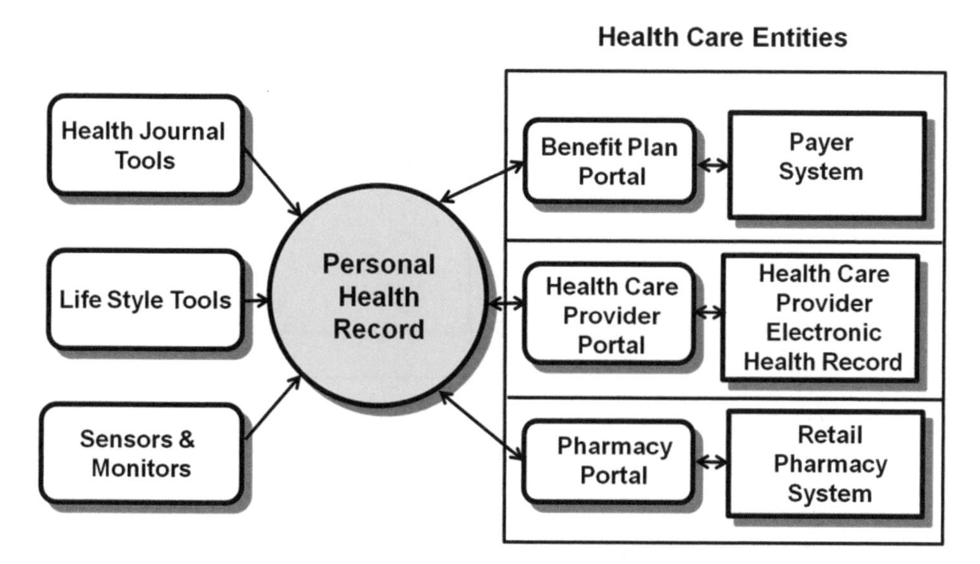

Fig. 11. Logical view of VUMC personal health record framework. The personal health record aggregates information under the patient's control, separate from yet related to the information systems of their healthcare entities.

of her record within the entity to messaging with the team serving her within the entity. The portal interacts with the information and services of the entity's internal systems, but the portal is separate from those systems. In this way, if she elects to submit information to her care provider through their portal's messaging capability, her provider team may review or respond on the information separately from deciding to make it a part of their record.

Next, she creates a link between her personal health record and her portals. This link allows her to open her personal health record, select one of the portals she has subscribed to, and then sign onto that portal as a window within her personal health record. She can then import or export information that she could have otherwise viewed from one to the other. In this way, each party maintains control of their system and record, while allowing information to be passed easily.

5.1.4. Population databases

The preceding frameworks aggregate and present information about an individual to guide decisions about, and manage her care. For individual health care, the information must be sufficiently specific to the individual, complete, and accurate. Management of the information must balance availability as needed with privacy. Population databases aggregate information to support population-scale pattern detection and recognition. Applications include epidemiology, phenotype-genotype correlations, bio-surveillance, post-market drug and device monitoring, etc. For these purposes, the number of records from the population must be large enough to overcome the variations in terminology, completeness, accuracy, etc. In other words, because of the very large number of records, the noise can be greater without preventing detection of the signal.

Figure 12 depicts the framework VUMC uses to exploit this difference in assembling population datasets to support research hypothesis generation and testing [11]. Each patient's aggregate electronic health record is extracted to create a synthetic derivative of the record for research purposes. A one way hash algorithm creates the identifier for the synthetic record from the medical record number. As a result, it is impossible to back track from a synthetic record to the health record it derived from, but it remains possible to pass additional information to the synthetic record as it is added to the health

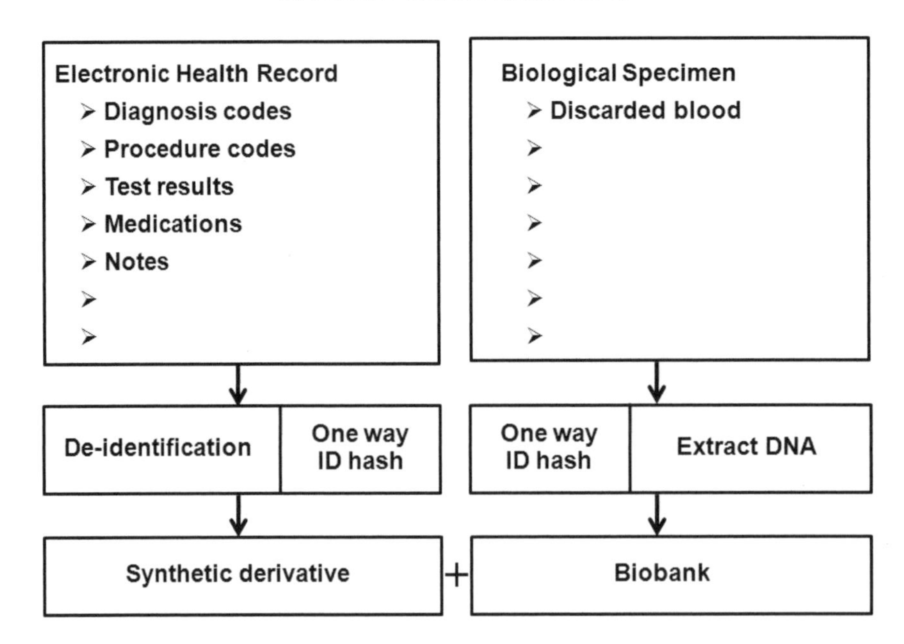

Fig. 12. Logical view of VUMC population dataset framework. Data is extracted from identified records through processes that prevent re-identification.

record. Algorithms remove personal identifiers specified by the HIPAA Privacy Rule in the process of creating the synthetic derivative. In addition, disinformation is introduced to further decrease the chance of re-identification. For example, all dates in the synthetic derivative are shifted within each record so that temporal relationships are preserved, but the dates do not correspond to actual events or dates of healthcare services. The final step in de-identification occurs at query time. The set of synthetic records returned is checked for attributes that are rare enough to provide an unacceptable risk of re-identification. If present, such attributes are removed from the returned set.

If a patient does not opt out as part of her consent to treat, DNA is extracted and banked when blood is left over from clinically indicated testing. This extract is tagged with an ID calculated with the same one way hash algorithm used to create the corresponding synthetic record. It is therefore possible to match the de-identified biological specimen up with the de-identified synthetic record for analysis. Again, disinformation is introduced by randomly excluding a percentage of samples from persons who do not opt out so that no one knows who is and who is not included in the bio-bank. This approach is extensible to other biological specimens.

Because of the attention to de-identification, the synthetic derivative and the bio-bank are not considered to contain individually identifiable data. By federal regulation, their assembly does not require informed consent, although the institution provides extensive education about the program and enables patients to opt-out by simply checking a box on the standard consent to treat form. These data and samples can be used where population-scale data is needed to discover causal relationships and other associations. As associations are discovered they must be confirmed through targeted consented trials using identified data. Similarly, if a discovery results in a change in clinical practice, it is impossible to use the de-identified record to identify and notify the affected patients. Instead, the identified records in the operational electronic health record are searched to identify individuals at risk so that they can be asked to come in for clinical testing.

5.2. A systems engineering approach to standards

Standards are agreements about how to do something where coordinated action is needed. For many people, the word brings to mind the prescriptive standards that grew out of the physical world where something fits or does not. The gauge of train track or an electrical plug, for example, specifies exactly what must be done in a designated situation to the level needed to achieve a fit. Prescriptive standards are appropriate where the need for compatibility is greater than the need for flexibility and they can lay the foundation for explosive growth in the productive use of a technology. Prescriptive standards, however, are good only if they can, in fact, be implemented. Prescriptive standards can have unintended consequences and inhibit progress if they cover too much.

One clear example of the success of prescriptive standards is the World Wide Web. The Internet was used primarily by government and academia from the early 1970s to 1993 when Tim Berners-Lee invented three simple standards – URL, HTTP, and HTML. These standards are prescriptive. The URL defines the address on the network. HTTP defines how to transport the information on the network. HTML specifies how to display material. Although these standards are prescriptive, they specify as little as possible. They say absolutely nothing about the material to be displayed, only how it is displayed. From this combination of limited prescriptive standards with freedom of content arose the World Wide Web, browsers, and the explosive growth and use of the Internet for personal and business use throughout the world, transforming global communications and commerce in a few short years.

The right balance between standardization and adaptability will be key to development of electronic health records suitable as an information foundation for a systems approach to care. Systems engineering principles suggest an approach that combines standards of practice, extensible reference standards, limited prescriptive standards, and performance metrics. The idea would be to couple development of standards with development of metrics to assess if technology built to, or using, the standard achieves the desired result when combined with people and process in real world health setting.

5.2.1. Standards of practice

A standard of practice is agreement on the minimum required process steps or the minimum required outcome of a process step. The barriers to adoption of standards of practices are reduced because of the freedom to innovate around these minimums. They provide a touch stone to test alternative approaches. Practice standards are particularly applicable to the interface between the electronic health record and roles and work process.

Standards of practices are needed to provide a floor under record access management. Examples include minimum criteria to authenticate a person to their record; minimum rules for role-based authorization for access to a record; delegation rules; and minimum elements of data sharing agreements. Standards of practice are also needed to guide design of the person-machine interface to address human factor issues and insure the required minimum level of cognitive support. Finally, standards of practice are needed to force a shift toward data liquidity by requiring a separation of data from applications.

5.2.2. Reference standards

Reference standards are a new concept made possible by computers [17, pp. 116–117]. They allow computers to speak a common language, thus facilitating information exchange. A single, framework of information is created allowing multiple levels of specificity. "Tagging," data to that framework provides a common language and also specifies the format in which the data will be expressed: a text document, an Excel spreadsheet, an image. Each tag, then, describes a "category of interest", which in the example below, is body part, interspersed with the actual name of the data element, which in the example is the word limb.

<body-part>limb</body-part>

A properly constructed framework of information can evolve over time as knowledge advances. Continuing the example, the framework could expand to include categories of interest for limb type and body side. (see below).

<body-part>limb</body-part>
<limb-type>arm</limb-type>
<body-side>left</body-side>

A reference standard can be put to use as soon as the major categories at the top of the framework are understood. No meaning is lost because the raw data is retained in addition to the tag. Precision increases over time as the framework is fleshed out.

5.2.3. Terminology frameworks

A terminology framework manages the relationships among concepts as a knowledge-base. The National Library of Medicine's Unified Medical Language System (UMLS) [8] is the best example of this approach. UMLS includes a number of terminology knowledge sources. The UMLS Metathesaurus is a vocabulary database containing information about health-related and biomedical concepts, their various names, and the relationships among them. It has been assembled from the electronic versions of many different thesauri, classifications, code sets, and lists of controlled terms used in patient care, health services billing, public health statistics, research, and indexing the biomedical literature. The 2008 version contains 1.88 million concepts and 7.56 million distinct concept names in 17 different languages. The UMLS Semantic Network consists of Semantic Types that provide a consistent categorization of concepts and Semantic Network Relations that provide a consistent representation of relations among Semantic Types. The UMLS SPECIALIST Lexicon contains syntactic, morphological and orthographic information for biomedical terms and commonly occurring English words. The UMLS Metathesaurus establishes synonomy among terms from its many source vocabularies. In other words, the links among the source vocabularies contain information not in any of the sources.

Natural language processing algorithms, working in conjunction with the UMLS knowledge sources, can compute concept matches to interpret text or other vocabularies [2]. Figure 13 depicts the terminology management framework VUMC is evolving toward. It uses concept matching along side human curation. The concept matching algorithms scan available sources of text, such as external terminology knowledge-bases, standard terminologies, internal terminology databases, documentation templates and text notes. The idea is to accept a term or phrase and to display all uses of the term and all concepts that relate to it as a broad scan to guide the human curation process. With this aid, the human terminology editor populates the internal terminology database with the external standard where applicable. If a more specific internal term is required, she can visualize the appropriate links to internal and external concepts and represent them in the internal terminology database. This curation process increases the terminology knowledge available to the concept matching algorithms, improving performance with time.

5.2.4. Standard product identifiers and vocabulary

Other industries have achieved interoperability by attaching computer readable information at the point of product manufacture. For example, manufacturers of retail products include a bar code with all the information needed to manage the distribution, sale and replenishment of the product. In healthcare, it is not yet practical to attach a physical tag to every drug or test result to contain the needed information.

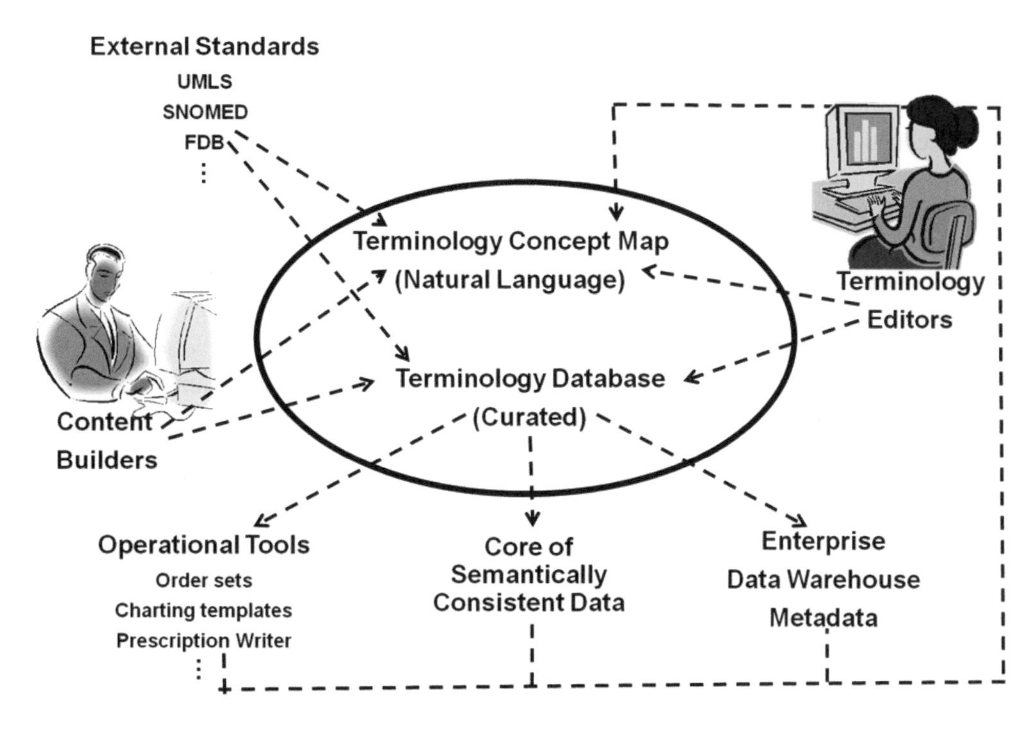

Fig. 13. Logical view of VUMC terminology management infrastructure. Content builders use the terminology database to build templates for operational tools. Terminology editors curate the terminology database. Both are informed by the aggregate terminology concept map.

It is practical to identify the product with a standard identifier, to include that identifier in a national database, and to link it to all relevant information according to the appropriate terminology framework [1, p. 6]. Manufacturers of drugs, devices and test kits could then include standardized identifiers in labels, packaging, and data outputs of devices and test kits. Downstream, participants in the information "supply chain" could then use this information within their local system much as the retail industry leverages product bar codes. The idea is to apply the standard at the point of manufacture instead of applying it at the inter-connections among systems.

6. Summary

An engineered system of healthcare delivery requires electronic health records that aggregate multi-source, multi-modal data about highly variable individuals across time, geography and change in biomedical knowledge and that can be linked into rapidly evolving patterns of work and support diverse perspectives. The scale of this challenge requires a radically different approach to achieving the goal of interoperable health information.

This chapter describes such an approach. The approach redefines interoperable data as data that can be assembled and interpreted as knowledge evolves. The approach breaks the electronic health record up into component parts, starting by insuring separation of data about an individual from applications that support her care. It matches computational technique used to implement a component – automation, decision support, connectivity and data mining – to the scale of the problem handled by the component. It permits staging of change in workflow and supports iterative refinement in practice. It allows governance and control to be managed at the level of the component. It achieves the balance between standardization and adaptability to support an engineered system of healthcare. It cuts the cost and time to implement electronic health records by an order of magnitude.

Acknowledgments

The thoughts in this chapter reflect concepts I learned working with Dr. C. Frank Starmer on the Duke Cardiovascular Disease Databank, Dr. W. Edward Hammond on TMR, Dr. Randolph A. Miller on terminology and knowledge-bases, Dr. Dario Giuse on aggregation of an electronic chart, Dr. Mark E. Frisse on regional data exchange, Dr. Jim N. Jirjis on patient portals, Dr. Joshua C. Denny on concept mapping, and Dr. Dan R. Masys on extracting research datasets.

References

[1] Commission on Systemic Interoperability. Ending the document game: connecting and transforming your healthcare through information technology. Washington, D.C.: US GPO. http://endingthedocumentgame.gov/medicationRecord.html, 2005,
[2] J.C. Denny, J.D. Smithers, R.A. Miller and A. Spickard, III, "Understanding" medical school curriculum content using KnowledgeMap, *J Amer Inform Assoc* **10**(4) (2003), 351–362.
[3] C.M. DesRoches, E.G. Campbell et al., Electronic health records in ambulatory care – a national survey of physicians, *N Engl J Med* **359** (2008), 50–60.
[4] R.S. Dick and E.B. Steen, The computer-based patient record. Institute of Medicine Report, Washington, D.C.: National Academies Press, 1991.
[5] M.E. Frisse, J.K. King, W.B. Rice, L. Tang, J.P. Porter, T. Coffman et al., A regional health information exchange: architecture and implementation, *AMIA Annual Symposium Proceedings* (2008), 212–216.
[6] Y.Y. Han, J.A. Carcillo, S.T. Venkataraman et al., Unexpected increased mortality after implementation of a commercially sold computerized physician order entry system, *Pediatrics* **116** (2006), 1506–1512.
[7] R. Hilllestad, J. Bigelow et al., Can electronic medical record systems transform health care? Potential health benefits, savings, and costs, *Health Affairs* **24**(5) (2005), 1103–1117.
[8] B.L. Humphreys, D.A.B. Lindberg et al., The Unified Medical Language System: an informatics research collaboration, *J Am Med Inform Assoc* **5** (1988), 1–11.
[9] Institute of Medicine (US) Committee on Quality of Health Care in America. Crossing the quality chasm: a new health system for the 21st century. Washington, D.C.: National Academies Press, 2001.
[10] A.K. Jha, C.M. DesRoches et al., Use of electronic health records in U.S. hospitals, *Special Article N Engl J Med* **360**. Published at www.nejm.org on March 25, 2009 (10.1056/NEJMsa0900592).
[11] D.M. Roden, J.M. Pulley, M.A. Basford, G.R. Bernard, E.W. Clayton, J.R. Balser and D.R. Masys, Development of a large-scale de-identified DNA biobank to enable personalized medicine. *Clin Pharmacol Ther* **84**(3) (2008), 362–369. Epub 2008 May 21.
[12] S.T. Rosenbloom, F.E. Harrel, C.U. Lehmann et al., Perceived increase in mortality after process and policy changes implemented with computerized physician order entry, *Pediatrics* **117** (2006), 1452–1455.
[13] W.W. Stead and W.E. Hammond, Computer-based medical records: the centerpiece of TMR, *MD Comput* **5**(5) (1988), 48–62.
[14] W.W. Stead, A quarter-century of computer-based medical records, *MD Comput* **6**(2) (1989), 75–81.
[15] W.W. Stead, R.A. Miller, M.A. Musen and W.R. Hersh, Integration and beyond: linking information from disparate sources and into workflow, *J Am Med Inform Assoc* **7** (2000), 135–145.
[16] W.W. Stead, R.A. Bates et al., Case study: the Vanderbilt University Medical Center, clinical information system, in: *Clinical information systems: a component-based approach*, R. Van de Velde and P. Degoulet, eds, New York: Springer-Verlag, 2003, pp. 253–264.
[17] W.W. Stead, B.J. Kelly and R.M. Kolodner, Achievable steps toward building a national health information infrastructure in the United States, *J Am Med Inform Assoc* **12** (2005), 113–120.
[18] W.W. Stead, Rethinking electronic health records to better achieve quality and safety goals, *Annu Rev Med* **58** (2007), 14.1–14.13.

[19] W.W. Stead and J.M. Starmer, Beyond expert-based practice, in: *Evidence-based medicine and the changing nature of health care*, M.B. McClellan, J.M. McGinnis, E.G. Nabel and L.M. Olsen, eds, IOM Annual Meeting Summary. Washington, D.C.: National Academies Press, 2008, pp. 94–105.

[20] W.W. Stead and H.S. Lin, eds, Computational technology for effective health care: immediate steps and strategic directions. Committee on Engaging the Computer Science Research Community in Health Care Informatics. Computer Science and Telecommunications Board, National Research Council. Washington, D.C.: National Academies Press, 2009.

William W. Stead, M.D. is Associate Vice Chancellor for Health Affairs, Chief Strategy and Information Officer, and McKesson Foundation Professor of Biomedical Informatics and Medicine, Vanderbilt University Medical Center. The Informatics Center blends units that manage the Medical Center's information technology infrastructure, the academic Department of Biomedical Informatics (research and education), the Eskind Biomedical Library (knowledge management), and the Center for Better Health (accelerating change). Dr. Stead received his B.A., M.D, Internal Medicine, and Nephrology training at Duke University. His interest in computer-based patient records dates to 1968. At Vanderbilt, his team has translated informatics research into approaches to information infrastructure to reduce cost to implement and barriers to adoption. The resulting enterprise-wide electronic patient chart and communication/decision support tools support his current focus on system-supported, evidence-based practice and research leading toward personalized medicine. He is a Founding Fellow of both the American College of Medical Informatics and the American Institute for Engineering in Biology and Medicine. He is an elected member of the Institute of Medicine of the National Academies and the American Clinical and Climatological Association. He served as Chairman of the Board of Regents of the National Library of Medicine, and as Chairman of the Board of Regents Working Group on Health Data Standards. He was a Presidential appointee to the Commission on Systemic Interoperability, and is co-editor of the NRC report *Computational Technology for Effective Healthcare: immediate steps and strategic directions.* Dr. Stead was recipient of the American Medical Informatics Association President's Award, 1997; the Donald AB Lindberg Award for Innovation in Informatics, 2005; and the American College of Medical Informatics Morris F. Collen Award of Excellence, 2007. In addition to his academic and advisory responsibilities, he is a director of Healthstream. Dr. Stead is co-inventor of two patient medical record products – one licensed to McKesson HBOC, Inc., and one licensed to Informatics Corporation of America – from which he receives royalties through Vanderbilt University.

Information Knowledge Systems Management 8 (2009) 145–157
DOI 10.3233/IKS-2009-0156
IOS Press

Chapter 9

Evidence-based medicine

Engineering the Learning Healthcare System

J. Michael McGinnis
E-mail: mcginnis@nas.edu

Abstract: Whether for the generation or application of evidence to guide healthcare decisions, the success of evidence-based medicine is grounded in principles common to engineering. In the Learning Healthcare System envisioned by the Institute of Medicine's (IOM) Roundtable on Evidence-Based Medicine, evidence emerges as a natural by-product of care delivery, which is thoroughly documented, pooled for continuous monitoring and analysis, integrated with insights from related studies, and fed back seamlessly to improve the consistency and appropriateness of care decisions by clinicians and their patients. Drawing from lessons shared at the IOM/NAE symposium, *Engineering a Learning Healthcare System,* this paper provides an overview of the state-of-play in health care today, some of its key challenges, the vision and features of a learning healthcare system, applicable commonalties and principles from engineering, and potential collaborative opportunities moving forward to the benefit of both fields.

1. Introduction

Engineering principles set the standard to which medical care aspires. As the science most devoted to the design, organization, and improvement of systems that marshal knowledge to maximize performance – effectiveness, efficiency, and reliability – against a targeted goal, engineering's aim is, in effect, at the heart of what the Institute of Medicine's (IOM) Roundtable on Evidence-Based Medicine seeks in its work to foster the evolution of a *learning healthcare system* that delivers the best care every time and improves with each element of the care experience [10].

Today, the performance of the healthcare system falls far short of this goal, and far short of the results that many Americans expect and believe they are getting. Americans have high expectations as they look to cutting-edge biomedical research and innovation to protect and improve their health and health care, and as they see striking innovations in the diagnosis, treatment, and long-term management of disease. Breakthroughs in just the past decade in human genomics, stem cell biology, proteomics, and immunology offer glimpses of new approaches that could heretofore only be imagined. Yet, with respect to improving the effectiveness and efficiency of health care for Americans, the promise of health progress from these discoveries in biology will be little more than illusory imaginings without fundamental attention to improving the structure and processes of the healthcare system charged with their application.

2. Health status and health care for Americans

Ultimately, the effectiveness of health care must be judged on its performance in improving health status – of matching available evidence with societal need. At some level, there have been striking advances on that count. Infant mortality has reached an all-time low for American babies, in part because of improved prenatal care, but also in part due to dramatic improvements in the capacity to care for babies of high risk and low birth weight. Among children, treatment of several childhood cancers – such as soft tissue sarcoma, leukemia, and Hodgkin's lymphoma – has advanced dramatically. For adults, advances in the treatment of high blood pressure, elevated serum cholesterol levels, coronary artery disease, HIV, and certain types of cancer – paired with lifestyle improvements such as reduced tobacco use, shifts away from saturated fat consumption, greater focus on physical activity levels, and use of seat belts – have ushered in unprecedented reductions in adult death rates and in disability rates among older people.

Still, if we take the experience of other countries as an indication of what should be readily attainable for a nation so richly invested in health care, the deficiencies leave us far short of what should be expected. Our infant mortality rate ranks 29th in the world, and at 6.3 deaths per 1000 live births is far higher than that of Singapore (2.3) or Sweden (2.8) [18]. Obesity increasing at alarming rates among adults and children alike is offsetting progress against other risk factors for heart disease and cancer. Diabetes and Alzheimer's disease are leading killers whose toll is actually increasing among Americans. Similarly, disparities in health among socioeconomic groups, both in access to health care and in progress against risk factors, have led to actual reductions in life expectancy in certain clusters of people with low income. At 75 years for men and 80 years for women, we rank 27th and 30th, respectively, in life expectancy at birth [4]. In a World Health Organization rating of overall health care system performance, the U.S. ranks 37th in the world [26].

Numerous studies have documented a persistent variation in the adoption of proven health care interventions. U.S. adults reportedly receive only about half of recommended care for conditions assessed, with quality varying significantly by medical condition. For example, only about 45% of established care is delivered for diabetes, 23% for hip fractures, 65% for hypertension, and 54% for asthma [16]. This problem has been shown to be ubiquitous, affecting even the most prestigious academic medical centers. Such quality deficiencies result in increased mortality and morbidity, as well as decreased quality of life and a less productive workforce.

Several factors contribute to these shortfalls, ranging from the disparities noted in access to needed health care, perverse economic incentives that emphasize payment for volume of services rather than outcomes, a fragmented delivery system that predisposes to discontinuities in the care process, and an inability for the production of evidence to keep up with the pace at which new interventions are proposed. Some very public examples exist for the too rapid adoption of unproven interventions, including hormone replacement therapy, COX-2 inhibitors for pain relief, autologous bone marrow transplants for advanced breast cancer, and fluoride treatment for osteoporosis. It is clear that, from an engineering perspective, the individual elements of our health care system, as sophisticated and impressive as they may be in appearance, do not engage in the synchronous fashion necessary for effective system performance.

3. Health costs

Even less impressive than the effectiveness of the U.S. health care system, is its efficiency. U.S. healthcare expenditures in 2009 amount to nearly 17% of GDP – approximately $2.5 trillion – close to about twice the per capita average of other developed nations, and 50% more than the second highest spending nation. In the recession year from mid-2008 to mid-2009, overall prices for goods and services in the U.S. economy declined by about 1.5%, while health prices increased about 6%. These costs will continue to rise and are predicted to reach 20% of the GDP by 2015 [2].

While medical progress has improved health care for many, rising costs are a growing burden for households, businesses, and governments. More individuals than ever are reporting that out-of-pocket health expenses present a problem for their household budgets, and the availability of health insurance benefits is one of the strongest determining factors of job choice. At the same time, rising health care costs are also increasingly associated with reductions in the depth and breadth of employer-based health insurance coverage for U.S. workers, and are often cited as a factor reducing the ability of companies to remain competitive. Up until the recession of 2008–2009, chief executive officers of U.S. companies consistently cited health care costs as their number one economic concern – a concern compounded by questions about the quality of the return on that investment.

The efficiency of health care delivered in the United States is therefore at least as significant a concern as its quality. With spending double that of other nations, population health status results ought not to be so inferior. Many studies of the appropriateness of health care services, including the variability of service intensity for a given condition, suggest that far too high a proportion of our health investment – perhaps 30% – goes toward? activities that do not improve patient outcomes, and in some cases, may even be detrimental [25]. Again, from an engineering perspective, the inability to take advantage of such substantial resources to produce concomitant health gain is testament to the existence of a very inefficient enterprise – one clearly in need of change.

4. Evidence-based medicine

As awareness has grown of the substantial shortfalls in health care among Americans, a number of recent initiatives, some by patient groups and some by medical and scientific groups, have emphasized the need for health care to focus more on the delivery of effective and efficient, evidence-based care. Among the most notable in this regard was the 2001 report of the Institute of Medicine, *Crossing the Quality Chasm*. In this report, the IOM Committee explicitly cast aside what they termed as the approach of "decision making based on training and experience", in favor of what they called the new rule of "decision making (that) is evidence-based [9]."

Although the language of "evidence-based medicine" is relatively new – tracing to Eddy's use of the term "evidence based" in a 1990 *JAMA* article [6] and Guyatt *et al's* 1992 article, also in *JAMA*, on "evidence-based medicine [7]." – the notion of testing of different medical interventions for their efficacy has been recorded in writings dating back to healers in the ancient Chinese, Greek, and Roman civilizations. Its development as a systematic contemporary science was given voice in the 1970's by Professor Archie Cochrane, a Scottish epidemiologist, and taken up in the formal methodologies espoused by a number of clinical groups and investigators, including, perhaps most prominently, Guyatt and Sackett of McMaster University.

Over the past quarter century, a number of activities have been undertaken aimed at applying structured evaluative approaches to the medical literature in the development of recommendations for practice grounded in the strength of the studies that constitute the scientific support base. These include the work of the Canadian Task Force on the Periodic Health Examination, the U.S. Preventive Services Task Force, the Oxford Centre for Evidence-based Medicine, the Grade Working Group, and the largest, the international Cochrane Collaboration which has about 50 groups involved in the ongoing review of the medical literature. Most such efforts employ decision rules that give greatest weight to studies of treatments offered to well-defined populations that have been subjected to randomized, double-blind, placebo controlled trials. They place very little stock in professional or patient opinions based on experience rather than formal study.

The field of evidence-based medicine is one rich with perspectives and opinions as to the most appropriate approaches and methods, the strengths of some and the weaknesses of others. Are rigorously structured trials in narrowly selected populations so far removed from the prevailing circumstances of populations that they may sometimes negate the ability to draw conclusions that might be practically applied? If so, under what circumstances? Is the "noise" that inevitably is part of observational data so distorting with respect to the influence on outcomes of one factor or another that reliable insights are virtually impossible? What is the appropriate use and phasing for different research approaches and how does it vary by clinical circumstance?

All these, and many more, are important issues for ongoing exploration. But the core common element underlying the notion of evidence-based medicine is that of a dynamic learning process in which structured insights are systematically captured and fed back to improve the knowledge base for decisions and practice. In principle, this is the fundamental notion of any "well engineered" activity. Accordingly, noted below is the applicability of sound engineering philosophy to the IOM's notion of a Learning Healthcare System. But also noted is the dependence of the system's effectiveness on key elements such as the components of the feedback processes in the system and the incentives to ensure synchrony in the functions of the system elements.

5. Evidence-based medicine and the learning healthcare system

At a basic conceptual level, seamless application of engineering principles underlies the essence of the *learning healthcare system* which is the dominant focus of the IOM Roundtable on Evidence-Based Medicine ("the Roundtable"). This is evident in the Roundtable's Charter (see Fig. 1), which defines "evidence-based medicine broadly to mean that, *to the greatest extent possible, the decisions that shape the health and health care of Americans – by patients, providers, payers and policymakers alike – will be grounded on a reliable evidence base, will account appropriately for individual variation in patient needs, and will support the generation of new insights on clinical effectiveness.*"

The Roundtable Charter also describes the *learning healthcare system* as one "designed to generate and apply the best evidence for the collaborative health care choices of each patient and provider; to drive the process of discovery as a natural outgrowth of patient care; and to ensure innovation, quality, safety, and value in health care." Much of the work of the IOM Roundtable has been devoted to characterizing in greater detail how this learning healthcare philosophy translates operationally in terms of its 10 core features [12].

1. *Learning-driven care.* Continuous improvement is the fundamental focus of the learning healthcare system. Trusted validation of new insights leads naturally to their systematic introduction and assessment for ongoing and routine improvement of the care process.
2. *Care-driven learning.* The point of care is the knowledge engine. Given the rate at which new interventions are developed, along with new insights about individual variation in response to interventions, the care delivery process must become the central focus for the continuous learning process.
3. *Best practice every time.* Established best practice, and consistency and reliability in its delivery – every time – is the expectation and the starting point of the care process for every patient. Departures, as appropriate to circumstance, are monitored and reported with the care warranted for new contributions to the evidence base.

The Institute of Medicine's Roundtable on Evidence-Based Medicine has been convened to help transform the way evidence on clinical effectiveness is generated and used to improve health and health care. We seek the development of a ***learning health care system*** that is designed to generate and apply the best evidence for the collaborative health care choices of each patient and provider; to drive the process of discovery as a natural outgrowth of patient care; and to ensure innovation, quality, safety, and value in health care.

Vision: Our vision is for a health care system that draws on the best evidence to provide the care most appropriate to each patient, emphasizes prevention and health promotion, delivers the most value, adds to learning throughout the delivery of care, and leads to improvements in the nation's health.

Goal: By the year 2020, ninety percent of clinical decisions will be supported by accurate, timely, and up-to-date clinical information, and will reflect the best available evidence. We feel that this presents a tangible focus for progress toward our vision, that Americans ought to expect at least this level of performance, that it should be feasible with existing resources and emerging tools, and that measures can be developed to track and stimulate progress.

Context: As unprecedented developments in the diagnosis, treatment, and long-term management of disease bring Americans closer than ever to the promise of personalized health care, we are faced with similarly unprecedented challenges to identify and deliver the care most appropriate for individual needs and conditions. Care that is important is often not delivered. Care that is delivered is often not important. In part, this is due to our failure to apply the evidence we have about the medical care that is most effective—a failure related to shortfalls in provider knowledge and accountability, inadequate care coordination and support, lack of insurance, poorly aligned payment incentives, and misplaced patient expectations. Increasingly, it is also a result of our limited capacity for timely generation of evidence on the relative effectiveness, efficiency, and safety of available and emerging interventions. Improving the value of the return on our health care investment is a vital imperative that will require much greater capacity to evaluate high priority clinical interventions, stronger links between clinical research and practice, and reorientation of the incentives to apply new insights. We must quicken our efforts to position evidence development and application as natural outgrowths of clinical care—to foster health care that learns.

Approach: The IOM Roundtable on Evidence-Based Medicine serves as a forum to facilitate the collaborative assessment and action around issues central to achieving the vision and goal stated. The challenges are myriad and include issues that must be addressed to improve evidence development, evidence application, and the capacity to advance progress on both dimensions. To address these challenges, as leaders in their fields, Roundtable members will work with their colleagues to identify the issues not being adequately addressed, the nature of the barriers and possible solutions, and the priorities for action, and will marshal the resources of the sectors represented on the Roundtable to work for sustained public-private cooperation for change. Activities include collaborative exploration of new and expedited approaches to assessing the effectiveness of diagnostic and treatment interventions, better use of the patient care experience to generate evidence on effectiveness, identification of assessment priorities, and communication strategies to enhance provider and patient understanding and support for interventions proven to work best and deliver value in health care.

Core concepts and principles: For the purpose of the Roundtable activities, we define evidence-based medicine broadly to mean that, *to the greatest extent possible, the decisions that shape the health and health care of Americans—by patients, providers, payers and policymakers alike—will be grounded on a reliable evidence base, will account appropriately for individual variation in patient needs, and will support the generation of new insights on clinical effectiveness.* Evidence is generally considered to be information from clinical experience that has met some established test of validity, and the appropriate standard is determined according to the requirements of the intervention and clinical circumstance. Processes that involve the development and use of evidence should be accessible and transparent to all stakeholders.

A common commitment to certain principles and priorities guides the activities of the Roundtable and its members, including the commitment to: the right health care for each person; putting the best evidence into practice; establishing the effectiveness, efficiency and safety of medical care delivered; building constant measurement into our health care investments; the establishment of health care data as a public good; shared responsibility distributed equitably across stakeholders, both public and private; collaborative stakeholder involvement in priority setting; transparency in the execution of activities and reporting of results; and subjugation of individual political or stakeholder perspectives in favor of the common good.

Fig. 1. Elements of a Learning Healthcare System.

4. *Clinician as steward.* The clinician in the learning healthcare system is a partner in the decision processes, the informed navigator for the introduction and application of the best evidence for the circumstance, the vigilant monitor of the results, and the facilitator of broader learning from each experience.
5. *Patient at the center.* The patient's lens provides the optical perspective in shaping and assessing the care process. Care decisions and shared decisions, performance evaluation is aimed at learning how the care experience is affecting its outcome, satisfaction, convenience and affordability for patients and their families.
6. *Seamless cycle feedback.* In a learning healthcare system, evidence development follows a new clinical research paradigm – one that draws clinical research more closely to the experience of clinical practice, advances new study methodologies adapted to the practice environment, and engages cultural incentives to foster more rapid learning.
7. *IT-based knowledge engine.* The rate of learning – both the application and development of evidence – depends on the full and essential application of electronic health records as a prerequisite for long-term change. Large electronically-based data sets offer important new sources for new evidence development and quality improvement.
8. *Clinical data as a public trust.* Meeting the potential for using new data sets as central sources of evidence on the effectiveness and efficiency of medical care requires recognition of their qualities as a public good, including assessing issues related to ownership, availability, and use for real-time clinical insights.
9. *A trusted scientific intermediary.* Greater synchrony, consistency, and coordination in the determination of what constitutes best practices, and how priority setting, development, interpretation, and application of new clinical evidence, requires a trusted, neutral scientific intermediary to broker the perspectives of different parties.
10. *Networked leadership.* Strong, visible, and multifaceted leadership from all involved sectors is essential to marshal the vision, nurture the strategy, and motivate the actions essential to create the learning healthcare system needed.

The aim, then, of the learning healthcare system is continuous improvement of all aspects of system performance, leading to the most effective, efficient and reliable delivery of value and outcomes possible real-time in the care delivery process. This is where the practical application of lessons from the engineering sciences is directly in play.

6. Engaging complex systems through engineering concepts

Health care is a complex adaptive system, but one that currently is not adapting well to apply the best evidence, to generate needed evidence, to produce value for dollar, or to improve health. Myriad continuously changing inputs, throughputs, and outputs, often disconnected from each other and from the central production function – better health – represent central feature of the enterprise. It is this complexity, and the utility of engineering concepts in engaging it, that prompted the sponsorship of an IOM/NAE symposium dedicated to exploring the issue. One co-editor of this volume, William Rouse, was the chair of the planning committee for the symposium, and the other, Denis Cortese, is the chair of the IOM Roundtable on Evidence-Based Medicine that was its principal sponsor. Noted below are some of the points emphasized in that meeting that offer relevant considerations in contemplating the prospects for evidence-based medicine to take better advantage of the conceptual synergy with the engineering field.

Systems engineering perspectives on health challenges. Rouse, in describing some of the potential utility of systems engineering approaches to addressing the complexity in health care, has noted not only the common elements of focus on control loci, predictive modeling, and feedback elements, but also the importance of tending to a clearer understanding between the healthcare and engineering vocabularies. He has cautioned on the need not to take for granted the common interpretation of seemingly straight forward engineering terms, including *controls* (the ability to measure a system's state); *feedback* (comparing expected and actual outcomes and correcting for the differences); *design* (structured relationships between inputs and outputs); *analysis* (understanding input – output relationships, including uncertainties); *synthesis* (designing input – output relationships to achieve objectives); *production* (creating systems that embody desired relationships); and *sustainment* (creating mechanisms to ensure realization of future objectives) [22].

Engineering systems analysis tools. As a science devoted to the systematic assessment of the relationship between people and the technologies they use to improve the effectiveness and efficiency of system performance, operations research (OR) is a natural tool for health care. In the IOM symposium, Richard Larson illustrated ways in which OR has been used to enhance the application of evidence with an example from cancer chemotherapy employing optimization modeling and computational techniques to offer safer and more reliable treatment. The approach Larson described eliminate simulation-required imaging before and after surgery, helped save an estimated $459 million per year, and dramatically reduced complications associated with the older treatment model [15]. Many other potential applications exist, although the payment incentives are not often aligned to encourage their use.

Engineering systems design tools. Creating an evidence-driven learning healthcare system conforms directly to the system design activities described by James Tien in his discussion of the tools that engineering can bring to design and decision making in managing the people, processes, and products of service systems. The key to decision making in the informatics age is that data production and engineering modeling, can generate new and quicker perspectives to inform conclusions and decisions. This is certainly the situation in health, in which there is increasing need for real-time, adaptive decision making within systems, especially systems characterized by such complex, customized, and personalized products and services (see mass customization below) [24].

7. Engineering principles and learning healthcare systems

The advantages of drawing on lessons from engineering have been a central interest in most key recent assessments of the need to improve effectiveness and efficiency in healthcare. Many of the insights and recommendations in the IOM's *Crossing the Quality Chasm* report, for example, were drawn from engineering. The Study Committee drew particular attention to five such principles in underscoring the potential to improve the extent to which healthcare delivery is based on evidence available about care that works, about the nature of the population served, and the impact of the care delivered. The Committee was, in effect, not only highlighting to the utility of engineering concepts to health care, but the dependence on reliable, validated evidence for those concepts to be successfully implemented (Ibid).

System design using the 80/20 principle. The 80/20 principle is also referred to as the Pareto Principle, and plays to the notion that process design should be focused on the usual case, and the remainder addressed with tailored efforts. In health, this means that an initial challenge is gathering information on the profile of the patient population on the key dimensions of interest, and based on that evidence, instead of building care systems to accommodate all possible occurrences, develop standardized, low cost processes to ensure that reliability and efficiency are natural feature of most care, with contingency triage rules for matching the small number of patients who need it with higher-skilled, technology-intensive capacities.

Design for safety. In 2000, the IOM report *To Err is Human* pointed out that health care in America can be dangerous, accounting for 44,000 to 98,000 otherwise preventable deaths per year [8]. This underscores how easy it can be to violate the most fundamental medical principle of "first do no harm", without designing systems around the prevention of errors by simplifying and standardizing key processes, rather than relying on memory and vigilance to ensure safety. Two other dimensions of this watchword reside in efforts to make errors visible when they occur and in designing procedures to mitigate harm from errors.

Mass customization. The concept of mass customization helps organizations address the unique interests and needs of their customers with the efficiencies of mass production, by developing the evidence and insights on their nature and distinctions, clustering or grouping them into sub-categories. In hotels, this is accomplished, for example, by identifying and registering returning customers according to their preferences. In health care, there are several dimensions on which this sort of stratification may occur, such as disease risk, stage, or severity.

Continuous flow. Continuous flow has also been called a "batch size of one" and refers to the development of system queuing capacity so that it matches demand. It is the theoretically optimal situation in which there is no clumping, aggregation or back-up of units or people in the production or service system. Many healthcare organizations manage demand by using barriers, such as waiting, to discourage utilization. It is essentially designed to accommodate some stated notion of system capacity or function. With continuous flow, the assumption is that, on average, patient flow is reasonably steady and predictable, and, rather than introduce the uncertainty of canceled appointments that often occur if, for example, a two-week wait is required, the need is met immediately. The most advanced example is open access in which a wait is never required.

Production planning. Production planning is the means of allocating staff, resources, and equipment to best match the flow of the needs of customers. It requires a detailed understanding of the details of the necessary work processes, including those that may be particularly repetitive. Knowing the natural ebb and flow of the processes allows for much more efficient and effective dedication of resources to match the demand, and is critical to preparing a busy clinical care enterprise for delivery of the care that the evidence suggests is most appropriate for the patient population of concern.

Reinforcement of the applicability to health care delivery of engineering principles, such as these, were offered by several presenters in the IOM/NAE symposium. Brent James, of Intermountain Healthcare in Utah, for example, underscored the importance of these principles to addressing five areas in which he felt health care's current failures could be substantially reversed: 1) the well-documented, unjustified, and wasteful variation in practice intensity; 2) high rates of inappropriate care; 3) unacceptable rates of preventable care associated with patient injury and death; 4) a striking inability to "do what we know works;" and 5) delivery inefficiencies leading to substantial waste and spiraling prices.

James observed that, in the face of growing complexity of care and the current reliance on inherently limited subjective judgment, "re-engineering" approaches is essential. He proposed four specific areas for attention by engineering professionals to help in the development of approaches to alleviate these shortfalls: 1) addressing clinical complexity; 2) developing a more robust capacity of knowledge management in a learning system; 3) improving systems for care delivery via team versus independent experts; and 4) designing health care as a coordinated system of production [13].

In that same session, Donald M. Berwick, of the Institute for Healthcare Improvement, underscored the potential of benefits for health care that could stem from a deeper understanding of system dynamics.

He identified seven issues as of particular importance: 1) the need to emphasize interdependence in the healthcare system; 2) the need to make the redesign of processes more visible; 3) the need to recognize the importance and value of dynamic learning and local adaptation as scientific learning processes; 4) the question of waste, which health care must confront with systematically gathered knowledge and targeted action; 5) the need for a sufficient platform for robust multidisciplinary research and development at the intersection of health care and engineering; 6) the need to enrich professional education and development in health care – for example, with more attention to teamwork and systems thinking; and 7) the reform of health care in a way that would result in a radically different, integrated systems design of the fundamental healthcare infrastructure.

Berwick illustrated the importance of genuinely understanding and mapping systems of care by noting how minor differences in merely the perspectives of different caregivers can yield vast variation in the care process. Referencing the observation that the human mind can typically only consider between 5 and 9 factors at any one time for a clinical decision, he pointed out that the actual number needing to be addressed is typically many more – 40, for example, in the case of ventilator settings in ICU patients with acute respiratory distress syndrome. If every time a physician or nurse is subconsciously, and perhaps at random selecting only six or seven factors to optimize, the widely observed variation should not only not be surprising, it should be expected.

In such circumstances, merely relying on incentives or other approaches to encourage effort – the dominant notion in popular theories of healthcare change today – would not likely be successful. Berwick notes that the management guru, Dr. W. Edwards Deming, pointed out that when the fundamental problem is one of system design, trying harder is the worst plan. Despite the public policy currency aimed at "try harder plans," the straightest path to healthcare designed to ensure application of the best evidence is by re-engineering the processes.

In another observation important to the acceptance of evidence-based medicine – the recognition that it is not an approach that slavishly treats all patients in the same manner – Berwick draws on the words of Taichi Ohno, who was responsible for the development of the Toyota Production System, who said, "When waste is at a minimum, every customer can be seen as an individual." The lesson here is that, a system tuned to precision in process, if done properly trying to meet the needs of the individual, drives costs down, not up [1].

8. Large scale engineering challenges for evidence-driven health care

Healthcare culture. William W. Stead has pointed out that opportunities for individualized patient care will continue to be missed unless the healthcare culture fundamentally changes in areas such as decision-making processes, payment mechanisms, and care planning. All of the incentives, practice patterns, and stakeholder silos are now structured to accentuate independent, non-team, unassisted, and sometimes untrusting activities and decision-making. The challenges of this situation are heightened by increasing needs for knowledge about new interventions that exceeds individual ability to keep apace. In moving from episodic and segmented care to patient- and population-based care, a simultaneous shift away from expert-based, mediated use of evidence to the systematic delivery and use of clinical evidence is necessary. Attention to re-engineering the practice environment to facilitate teamwork, mutual support and decision assistance is possible, and can counter these influences in the interest of delivering best practices to the patient. Taking advantage of these prospects will require reorienting recruiting and education practices to emphasize individual recognition of clinicians' own limits and comfort with trusting the system – including teammates – to foster the right performance [23].

Diagnostic and treatment technologies. Evidence-driven introduction of new diagnostic and treatment technologies is another area in which the use of engineering principles can be naturally applied – assuming the availability of the tools and incentives – to assure that performance feedback loops guide the most efficient, effective and appropriate use of the technologies. Despite the potential of new technology to improve quality of care and outcomes, the technologies – including information technology, laboratory/radiology/imaging systems, and monitoring equipment – remain often disconnected and therefore, ultimately contribute to overuse. Rita F. Redberg has described these issues in the cardiovascular arena, underscoring that inefficiencies stemming from technology overuse often far exceed patient benefit. She notes that, by engineering into care the systematic collection of data and establishment of registries, patients and clinicians would make better informed care decisions, as well as promote a culture oriented to review of evidence on clinical benefits of new technologies as a matter of routine [21].

Clinical data systems and clinical decision support. As long as clinical data systems remain in a disorganized state, the nation's ability to maximize the role of evidence in health care, or to take advantage of engineering approaches to system improvement, will be fundamentally impaired. An effective clinical data system is at the heart of the notion of the learning healthcare system and the ability to both generate and aid the delivery of evidence in clinical care. Michael Chase notes that, at least in terms of the deployment and use of electronic health records, it may also be the most underleveraged resource available today for the systematic improvement of healthcare in the United States. Data are often located in a variety of applications, cul-de-sac databases, and paper forms, inherently limiting their use. Chase's description of progress in the Kaiser system offers important insights into the potential for progress as well as some of the processes and barriers to be engaged in reorganizing this basic resource for consistent, reliable, and smoothly functioning clinical care [3].

Care coordination and linkage. Another fundamental and systemic flaw prevalent in today's U.S. healthcare system, is found in its fragmented, disorganized, and disconnected nature. Amy Deutschendorf has observed the increasing presence of factors that add complexity with a propensity to dysfunction, including an aging and chronically ill population, decreased lengths of stay, acute care capacity issues, convoluted payer structures and incentives, and higher consumer expectations. Deutschendorf notes that the evidence we have on the right care for the right person can simply not be effectively applied until these issues are addressed. She emphasizes the importance of systems of care that are truly designed around the patient, fully engaging all members of the healthcare team; with care planning much more aggressive, emphasizing prevention; and with the provider infrastructure fully integrated. Health care must go from "silo" to "systems" thinking, with stronger communication among all stakeholders. New structures must be created, including new models of care based on evidence, expedited care delivery and increased monitoring and surveillance [5].

Information knowledge and development. Continuous generation of new knowledge through constant feedback on performance provides the engine of progress for the learning healthcare system. This must be "hardwired" into the design of the care process. Eugene C. Nelson describes the ways basic, translational, and outcomes research can be facilitated by a system that focuses on "feed-forward" and "feedback" data systems to both improve patient care and generate and manage new information. Nelson illustrates the principles and methods of feed-forward data systems with a case from the Dartmouth-Hitchcock Spine Center's work, which focuses on the centrality of patient-reported data embedded into the process of healthcare at multiple levels. Particularly challenging are some of the complexities associated with developing patient-centered, feed-forward data systems, which require embedding dynamic decision support evidence into the natural care delivery process – but essential to engage if care is ultimately to be evidence-driven in a seamless fashion [19].

9. Systems engineering and complex adaptive health systems: Two cases

Numerous examples exist, in health care and elsewhere, of systems engineering's successful application in revolutionizing performance and results. One prominent example is that of airline safety, in which engineering solutions have transformed the safety outcomes for air travel. The fundamental approach in this case was two-fold: installation of feedback systems associated with detecting and managing mechanical problems; and assurance of "exquisite redundancy." The basic working assumption is that humans are imperfect and systems can be structured to correct – and even anticipate – human errors through training programs, procedure standardization, and variable minimization [17]. Two examples of the application of this approach in health care, are the reform experiences in the VA health system, and in Ascension Healthcare.

Veterans Health Affairs. The Veterans Health Administration in the U.S. Department of Veterans Affairs (VA) was founded in 1946, and is the largest integrated healthcare system in the United States. It was lauded for its specialized services during its early years, but by the 1990s, it was widely criticized for providing fragmented and disjointed care that was expensive, difficult to access, and insensitive to individual needs. Kenneth W. Kizer describes the radical re-engineering of VA health care that was launched in 1995, in a program aimed at a fundamental re-engineering of the system to: (1) create an accountable management structure and management control system; (2) integrate and coordinate services across the continuum of care; (3) improve and standardize the quality of care; (4) modernize information management; and (5) align the system's finances with desired outcomes. Kizer describes a result that was transformational, creating a continuum of consistent, predictable, high-quality, low-cost, patient-centered care. He points out that attention to often small elements at the system interfaces, can have a considerable impact on overall performance [14]."

Ascension Health. Ascension Health is the largest not-for-profit delivery system in the United States, the largest Catholic healthcare system, and the third largest system overall (after the VA and the Hospital Corporation of America). David Pryor describes the results of their system reform efforts in Ascension Health's "Call to Action." The work focused on three goals: health care that works, health care that is safe, and health care that leaves no one behind. In addressing safety in the system environment, simultaneous efforts were directed to the challenges in culture, the infrastructure, the business case, standardization, and how staff worked together. By engaging leadership throughout the staff, strategies were developed for each challenge, and targets were set for progress in key priorities such as hospital mortality, adverse drug events, Joint Commission National Patient Safety Goals, nosocomial infections, falls and fall injuries, pressure ulcers, perinatal safety, and surgical complications. The result was striking improvements in each area, attributable to the focus on broad scale process engineering that also created changes in culture, orientation, teamwork, and focus on patient needs [20].

10. Various insights engineering has produced for health care

Described above, and emphasized in the joint IOM/NAE work are a number of insights important to the development of evidence-based medicine that delivers effective and efficient care to the patient. These include [11]:

- *Center the system's processes on the right target – the patient experience.* Health care is by its nature highly complex, involving multiple parallel activities that sometimes take on a character of their own, independent of patient needs. To ensure that processes support patients – and patients are not forced into processes – patient needs and perspectives must be the central focus pointing process design.

- *System excellence is created by the reliable delivery of established best practice.* Identifying and embedding practices that work best, and developing the system processes to assure their delivery, every time, defines excellence in system performance. In health care, this means establishing practices from the best available evidence and building them as routines into practice patterns, as well as developing systems to document results and update best practices as the evidence evolves.
- *Complexity compels reasoned allowance for tailored adjustments.* Established routines may need adjusting in certain circumstances, either because of differences among individuals in the appropriateness for them of the established healthcare regimens, variation in caregiver skill, the evolving nature of the science base – or all three. Mass customization and other engineering practices can help assure the consistency that can accelerate the recognition of need for tailoring.
- *Learning is a non-linear process.* Our focus on an established hierarchy of scientific evidence as a basis for evaluation and decision making cannot accommodate the fact that most sound learning in complex systems is occurring in local and individual settings. To avoid a cost to knowledge growth, a means must be found to bridge the gap between formal trials and local improvement.
- *Emphasize interdependence and tend to the process interfaces.* A system is most vulnerable at links between its processes. In health care, attention to the nature of relationships and hand-offs between elements of the patient care processes is therefore vital.
- *Teamwork and cross-checks trump command and control.* Especially in systems designed to guarantee safety, system performance that is effective and efficient requires careful coordination and teamwork throughout, as well as a culture that encourages parity among all with established responsibilities.
- *Performance transparency and feedback serves as the engine for improvement.* Continuous learning and improvement in patient care requires transparency in process and outcome, as well as capacity to capture feedback and make adjustments.
- *Expect errors in the performance of individuals, perfection in the performance of systems.* Human error is inevitable in any system and should be assumed. On the other hand, safeguards and designed redundancies can deliver perfection in system performance. Mapping processes, embedding prompts, cross-checks, and information loops can assure best outcomes, and allow human capacity to focus on what cannot be programmed – compassion and individual patient needs.
- *Align rewards on key elements of continuous improvement.* Incentives, standards, and measurement requirements can serve as powerful change agents. It is vital then that they be carefully considered and directed to the targets most important to improving the patient and provider experience.
- *Develop education and research to facilitate understanding and partnerships between engineering and the health professions.* The relevance of certain basic systems engineering principles to health care, as well as the impressive transformation brought to other industries, speaks to the merits of developing common vocabularies, concepts, and ongoing joint education and research activities that will help generate stronger questions and solutions.
- *Foster a leadership culture, language, and style that reinforces teamwork and results.* Positive leadership cultures foster and celebrate consensus goals, teamwork, multidisciplinarity, transparency and continuous monitoring and improvement.

References

[1] D. Berwick, (2008). Presentation, in IOM, *Engineering the Learning Healthcare System,* 2010, *in preparation.*

[2] Bureau of Labor Statistics. (2009). *Consumer Price Index-August 2009* http://www.bls.gov/news.release/pdf/cpi.pdf (accessed October 2, 2009). Centers for Medicare and Medicaid (CMS). 2009. *National Health expenditure Data Overview*. http://www.cms.hhs.gov/nationalhealthexpenddata/01_overview.asp (accessed June 1, 2009).
[3] M. Chase, (2008). Presentation, in IOM, *Engineering the Learning Healthcare System,* 2010, *in preparation.*
[4] CIA World Factbook, Accessed October 9, 2009, https://www.cia.gov/library/publications/the-world-factbook/index.html.
[5] A. Deutschendorf, (2008). Presentation, in IOM, *Engineering the Learning Healthcare System,* 2010, *in preparation.*
[6] D.M. Eddy, Practice Policies: Where Do They Come From? *Journal of the AmericanMedical Association* **263**(9) (1990), 1265, 1269, 1272, 1275.
[7] G. Guyatt, J. Cairns, D. Churchill et al., Evidence-based medicine. A new approach to teaching the practice of medicine, *JAMA* **268** (1992), 2420–2425.
[8] IOM (Institute of Medicine). (2000). *To Err is Human.* P. 31 Washington, D.C.: National Academy Press.
[9] IOM (Institute of Medicine), *Crossing the quality chasm: A new health system for the twenty-first century*. Washington, DC: National Academy Press, 2001, p. 76, pp. 120–127.
[10] IOM (Institute of Medicine). (2007). *The Learning Healthcare System,* Washington, D.C.: National Academy Press.
[11] IOM, (2010). *Engineering the Learning Healthcare System, in preparation.*
[12] IOM (Institute of Medicine), (2008). Roundtable on Evidence-Based Medicine, *Learning Healthcare System Concepts,* NAP: Washington DC.
[13] B. James, (2008). Presentation, in IOM, *Engineering the Learning Healthcare System,* 2010, *in preparation.*
[14] K. Kizer, (2008). Presentation, in IOM, *Engineering the Learning Healthcare System,* 2010, *in preparation.*
[15] R. Larson, (2008). Presentation, in IOM, *Engineering the Learning Healthcare System,* 2010, *in preparation.*
[16] E.A. McGlynn, S.M. Asch, J. Adams, J. Keesey, J. Hicks, A. DeCristofaro and E.A. Kerr, The Quality of Health Care Delivered to Adults in the United States, *New England Journal of Medicine* **348**(26) (2003), 2643.
[17] J. Nance, (2008). Presentation, in IOM, *Engineering the Learning Healthcare System,* 2010, *in preparation.*
[18] National Center for Health Statistics. (2008). "Recent Trends in Infant Mortality in the United States", Centers for Disease Control and Prevention. p. 2.
[19] E. Nelson, (2008). Presentation, in IOM, *Engineering the Learning Healthcare System,* 2010, *in preparation.*
[20] D. Pryor, (2008). Presentation, in IOM, *Engineering the Learning Healthcare System,* 2010, *in preparation.*
[21] R. Redberg, (2008). Presentation, in IOM, *Engineering the Learning Healthcare System,* 2010, *in preparation.*
[22] W. Rouse, (2008). Presentation, in IOM, *Engineering the Learning Healthcare System,* 2010, *in preparation.*
[23] W. Stead, (2008). Presentation, in IOM, *Engineering the Learning Healthcare System,* 2010, *in preparation.*
[24] J. Tien, (2008). Presentation, in IOM, *Engineering the Learning Healthcare System,* 2010, *in preparation.*
[25] J.E. Wennberg, E.S. Fisher and J.S. Skinner, Geography and the debate over Medicare reform, *Health Aff* (*Millwood*) Supp Web Exclusives: W96–114, 2002.
[26] World Health Organization. (2000). "The World Health Report 2000 – Health Systems: Improving Performance". p. 200.

Michael McGinnis is Senior Scholar and Director of the Institute of Medicine's Roundtable on Evidence-based Medicine, as well as an elected IOM Member. Much of his policy leadership stems from his continuous four-Administration tenure, perhaps unique among federal appointees, through the Carter, Reagan, Bush, and Clinton Administrations as point person for disease prevention and health promotion policy. Several still prominent initiatives were launched under his guidance, including the *Healthy People* national goals and objectives process, the *Dietary Guidelines for Americans* and the U.S. Preventive Services Task Force. He has also served as Chair of the Secretary's Task Force on Smoking and Health, Chair of the HHS Task Force on Health Risk Assessment, Chair of the IOM Committee on Food Marketing to Children and Youth, and Chair of the NIH State-of-Science Review of the Role of Multi-Vitamin Supplements in Chronic Disease Prevention. Internationally, he served in India, in 1974-5, as epidemiologist and State Director for the successful WHO smallpox eradication program, and in Bosnia, in 1995-6, as Chair of the World Bank/European Commission post-war task force for reconstruction of the health system.

Information Knowledge Systems Management 8 (2009) 159–175
DOI 10.3233/IKS-2009-0158
IOS Press

Chapter 10

Transforming healthcare through patient empowerment

Leslie Lenert
E-mail: leslie.lenert@gmail.com

I will prescribe regimens for the good of my patients according to my ability and my judgment and never do harm to anyone. Hippocrates

Abstract: The United States faces tremendous challenges with its healthcare system. By any standard, it is expensive and performs poorly in most measures of health and thus, is in great need of reform. But how do we reform things without making the situation worse? Some of the more fundamental problems arise from the combination of a fee-for-service payment system for physicians with insurance-based financing care. This combination results in conflicts among the interests of patients, physicians and payers. This paper examines this issue from a decision analytic perspective, starting with a definition of the patient-centered view, and an assessment of the practicality of controlling costs by making healthcare more patient-centric. It then illustrates how fee-for-service models corrupt decision-making and other solutions designed to reign in the abuses of the fee-for-service model and also negatively impacts the quality of decision making for individual patients. Whatever the strategies for health reform, the degree of patient-centeredness of care is a benchmark that allows policy makers to understand how far they have had to deviate from optimal to achieve the desired ends of cost control.

1. Introduction

While the United States is the world's largest economy, it is not the most prosperous. On a per capita basis, the United States ranks 9th on most measures of per capita income. But we spend by far and away, the most on healthcare in terms of the percentage of Gross National Product devoted to healthcare. Further, one might expect the most prosperous economy to have the highest average physician salary, but the United States is number #1 in physician salaries world-wide. So, not only do we have a system that performs poorly, we reward the leaders of that system (physicians) more highly than countries more prosperous than us. Clearly we value health in this country, but why is what we buy such a poor value? One of the reasons is the type of system that has evolved in the United States – a largely fee-for-service system where two-thirds of the physicians are specialists, with wide discrepancies (300% or more and hundreds of thousands of dollars) in income between the generalists who care for people, and the specialists who treat diseases. Physician salary costs are only about 10% of total health expenditures. But, as the gatekeepers and frequently the promulgators of new, expensive technologies, it is not the amount that physicians earn that is the problem. As Arthur Relman, former editor of the New England Journal of Medicine has suggested, the problem may be the way that they earn it. Physicians as a by product of insuring fee-for-service activities frequently consume other scarce resources (diagnostic tests, hospital days, pharmaceuticals, etc.) The power of the checkbook, based on their contributions to both tactical and strategic medical decision making, rests with the medic, limited only by the procedures of the payer for authorization of reimbursement and their ability to convince patients that what is recommended is in their interest.

The upshot of this chapter is that there are fundamental conflicts of interest between patient and physician and between patient and payer. Resolution requires that abstraction to the patient perspective and an explicit focus on actions in patients' best interests. How do we devise structures for care processes that are patient-centered and maximize the focus on patients' interests? Is there a role or a need for policies to limit patient centered decision making to prevent excessive use of resources? Or, would putting patients in charge of resource utilization through patient empowerment, cure what ails health care?

2. More is not better

In systems that produce and sell other types of goods or services, a capitalist perspective is good. More goods and services produces benefits. In health, this is not true – more services sometimes leads to worse health outcomes. One famous example from the Veterans Affairs Health System looked at enhanced access to primary care services in diabetes, congestive heart failure, and obstructive lung disease after discharge from hospital [1]. The intervention, which clinically makes sense – more supervision by doctors and nurses of patients post discharge of sicker patients – actually raised readmission rates without impact on other physiological parameters. Paradoxically, patients were more satisfied with care that was more likely to lead to readmission, probably because their perceptions of quality of care were based on the amount of services they received.

The effect is also illustrated by studies of the process of dying in the United States. There is always a question in medicine of how much to try to extend life near the end, and wide variability in preferences between patients and families on how they want end of life care managed. But, there seems to also be wide variability in how aggressively physicians marshal resources in the fight against an inevitability of death. Does this added intensity buy what is hoped – a chance for restoration of health and quality of life? In a study I led on decision-making in managed care and fee-for-service environments, we examined this issue. The approach used an outcome called Potentially Ineffective Care (PIC) [2]. PIC was based on how a common business model divides care into four quadrants based on relative performance (high cost high benefit care, low cost high benefit care, low cost low benefit care, and high cost low benefit care). To find the proportion of care in the intensive care units that was PIC, we mapped both costs and outcomes to a graph. Costs were defined based on charges adjusted for hospital cost structures using Medicare data. Benefit was defined as the duration of survival after discharge from the hospital. Potentially Ineffective Care was defined as costs in the upper 90% of resource utilization and post discharge survival of 100 days or less. One of the first things we learned in our study was that it was easier to predict PIC than in hospital mortality. Death in the hospital is often an unexpected outcome. But death after a long hard fight that utilized many resources, was something that could be foreseen, in many patients, by their response over the first five days of treatment.

We then went on to study differences in the rates of PIC across fee-for-service and managed care environments [3]. While 100-day mortality HMO and fee-for-service patients is similar, patients in a managed care environment had far less risk of falling in the PIC. Why was this? One potential explanation is the fee-for-service environments provide few incentives for physicians to use clinical judgment to limit services in end-of-life situations, and as a result, they don't. Whereas, if a physician is a part of a culture that aims to use care most efficiently, there are incentives to limit ineffective care near the end of life. The data from this study shows that it is possible to do so without harming patients' long term survival using medical judgment. But physicians have to be motivated to apply their knowledge.

There is a fundamental inequality of knowledge between physician and patient. Further, in that context, the knowledge imbalance is linked to how a physician earns her income in a fee-for-service environment [4]. Cardiologists advocate for the use of angioplasty and stenting. Thoracic surgeons advocate for bypass surgery. Moreover, when a patient asks the physician performing a service for their opinion, how can that opinion not be tied to both the physician's beliefs about the efficacy of their the physician own skills and, in the background, the economics how the physician generates their income. To be fair to my colleagues in procedural specialties, one certainly chooses to employ a procedure or a technology because one has come to believe in its efficacy. Further, the more one knows about the details of a procedure, the cognitive theory argues the more one believes that they understand what goes wrong and why, and how to control the risks [5]. But in the end, there are only the statistics on the outcomes and the costs (both material and personal).

What is wrong with the healthcare system is not the system of insurance or the costs of technology, but the locus of control of decision making and the context for flow of information. In fee-for-service medicine linked to high cost, high technology services, there is a strong driver toward delivery of care at the margins of effectiveness (or past those) not necessarily based on evidence but rather on some optimistic view of the physician on his or her impact on health [6]. A further paradox is that a physician can believe herself to be ethical in offering the service, because she has the belief it offers some benefit to the individual, but the return for the individual may ultimately be less than the financial benefit to the physician (i.e., it is ethical to offer services where, on the whole, the physician benefits more than the patient.) Similarly, the structure of information flow is focused on the healthcare system itself, directed at financial reimbursement and provider business process management, rather than the patient care management. Yes, it is important to move information to insure that business partners in the medical enterprise are paid. But, what if the same efforts were put into moving information to insure that patients receive the care they need in a coordinated fashion?

What is the route out of the present difficulty? One option is a patient centric approach to both decision making and to movement of information for care management. If patients were empowered to make decisions, patients acting in their own self interest would make better decisions that more completely balance risk and benefit. As a result, patients would avoid minimally beneficial, high cost care. Similarly, if patients were able to tailor follow up and management of their disease to their own unique circumstances, through patient centered information flow management, patients and family members could begin to experience continuity of care and accrue the health benefits and cost reductions associated with such.

3. A simple model

Helping patients make a better decision through technology and other means, presumes that such help is a good thing, and that people make rational decisions. But what is a rational decision and how do we know when we are helping people make a better decision? The foundation of any approach based on helping patients make better decisions is that decision making is rationale or normative, that is to say, decision making is based on the careful weighing of costs and benefits.

To describe decision models, we will use a notation developed by Matheson and Howard called Influence Diagrams [7,8]. Influence diagrams excel at capturing the conditional dependencies between factors in a model and are computable. While we will not offer calculations in this paper, the models could be readily enhanced with appropriate data to yield predictions.

In its ideal form, medical decisions should be simple. Nodes in the model are shown in *italics*. As shown in Fig. 1, there are two relevant factors influencing the choice (circles): the *patient's physiology and pathology* and the *physician's knowledge about treatments*. These factors may or may not be known completely and are variables under the control of nature with ranges of outcomes determined by chance. *Choice of treatment* is a decision, represented by a square. The optimal choice is based on maximizing the expected value of the decision relative to what treatment to undertake, under uncertainty. No one can know which treatment will prove best for an individual until after it is implemented. Random chance will always play a role. Influence diagrams do not attempt to show every possible choice or alterative (this is perhaps better represented using a Decision Tree). Rather, they attempt to show what factors depend on other factors and areas of dependence between those factors and areas of independence.

The approach does allow for generation of models that are computable. Given a full specification, a normative (e.g. rational) individual should make the best choice given his or her knowledge of his or her own physiology and the types of treatments available (again, knowledge of what a treatment does in an individual is imperfect at best, and the degree to which a patient or a physician may study the options is variable, as is the conclusions they may reach about the effects of treatment). A normative patient, however, will chose the treatment option that maximizes his or her utility, the overall *outcome* (the sum of the probability of different potential outcomes multiplied by value each outcome has to the decision maker). Underlying all theories of intervention in medical decision-making is an assumption that individuals will do what they believe will maximize their utility. However, as we will discuss later, this assumption is not borne out in real world decision-making in some circumstances. Sometimes people make decisions based on goals of minimizing risk or maximizing the chance of one particularly desired outcome, even if this is not in the overall best interests.

4. A more realistic model

To understand how complexity impacts decision making, we need to expand the model shown in Fig. 1. Figure 2 introduces additional complexity related to the patient. The state of *patients' physiology pathology* and the degree of damage from disease (pathology) is only incompletely known. Some of the triggers for disease or the risk factors are known. The *demography* of the patient (age, gender), the *genetic profile* and family history, exposures in the *environment*, and the *symptoms* that the patient experiences, all inform (but do not define) the state of physiology and pathology in the patient. Diagnostic testing, sometimes at risk or cost, better defines what the *physiology and pathology* of the patient is. Diagnostic testing sometimes poses risks that can adversely affect a *patient's post treatment state*. Concurrently with this, and frequently as important, patients value health outcomes differently. They have different beliefs about what quality of life is, about how long they hope to live, and about the level of physical and mental functioning to which they aspire or demand. The optimal choice of treatment for an individual often depends on their values, and the trade-offs between risk, length of life and quality of life that they are willing to accept, as much as their physiology. Of course, a good choice of treatment does not guarantee a good outcome for a patient. The post treatment state of the patient depends on the underlying physiology, physician's skill and the patient's fortune. Whatever this state is determines the ultimate value of the treatment to the patient. Out-of-pocket costs for care might also influence the ultimate value of the outcome to the patient. The model shown in Fig. 2, as complex as it is, is still a highly simplified model of decision making. However, it is a patient centric model. If we model a decision for allocation

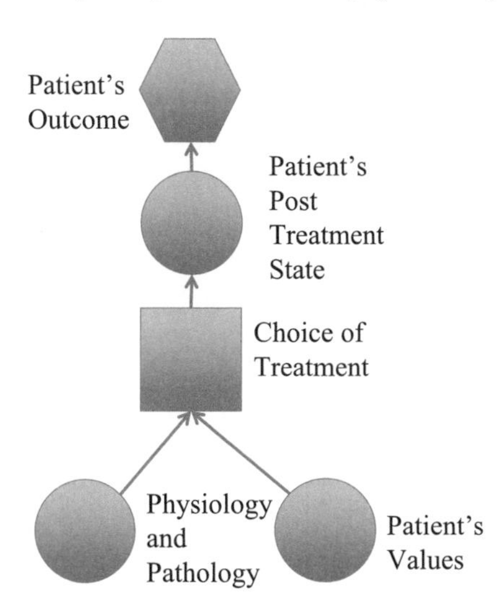

Fig. 1. Simplified model of a medical decision. Circles are things that can be known about a patient's decision but not precisely. The square indicates a choice between one or more treatments. The hexagon represents the utility (value) of the outcome to the patient. This is determined probabilistically by what happens during treatment (the types of complications, successes, etc.) and how the individual values each outcome.

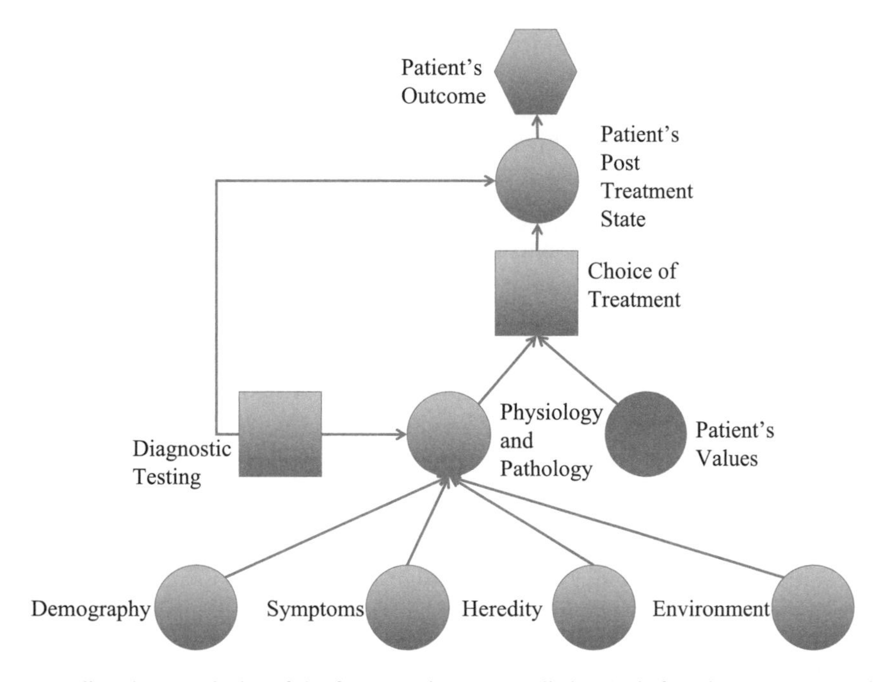

Fig. 2. Diagram expanding the complexity of the factors to be more realistic. As before, hexagons are "value nodes" or the utility to each party, the square is the choice to be made, and the circles represent things that happen but which cannot be known in advance.

of resources using this framework, decisions are optimized based on their outcome for the patient. This is the essence of the patient-centric approach – medical care that does what is best for the individual without compromise [9].

5. Methods for implementing patient-centered decision making

The limitations of a model where a doctor acts as a proxy for the patient in decision making have long been recognized. Early efforts looked at how models could improve physician decision making by better computation and closer tailoring of decisions to individuals. Tailoring diagnostic tests and treatments to individual patients using mathematical models and computers is a 50 year-old idea. Initial efforts focused on individualization of diagnostic strategies using Bayes theorem, and descriptions of this were published in Science in 1959 [10,11]. Even in the early 1960's, efforts to apply these strategies focused on the use of computers as an aid to calculations necessary to tailor care to individuals [12].

Starting in the mid 1970's, physicians in academic institutions began to experiment with the use of formal decision models to understand complex medical choices [13] and eventually to begin to help guide decisions for individual patients [14], using what was then the new technology of microcomputers to perform calculations [15]. Efforts to use formal models to guide medical decision making for individuals probably reached their zenith in the late 1980's with the creation of consultative services that used decision analysis to advise patients and physicians on difficult cases [16]. These services were not designed for profit, but to train physicians in formal decision methods. The work involved in creating a custom model often precluded completion of the modeling task in a relevant time frame. As researchers worked to make it easier to tailor models to individuals [17] they began to understand the complexities of tailoring predictions to the multiple causative factors in individual physiology. Further, problems arose with the procedures measurement of patient values for inclusion in decision models. Researchers discovered that the results of measurements for modeling purposes were sensitive to the frame used (chance of survival versus risk of death) the model for capture of trade-offs, methods for search for indifference points in trade-offs, how health outcomes were described and a myriad of other factors [18] that seemed to make it impossible to represent values with a single number. These factors led to a split in the field in the late 1980's and 1990's, with the majority of researchers focusing on using models to develop educational materials to help patients make medical decisions.

The group of researchers who used models as a guide for more qualitative efforts developed *decision aids* – systematic tools that would describe alternative treatments, present numeric descriptions of the probabilities of outcomes, and help patients clarify their values for trade-offs. Some of these aids were implemented in computer programs [19]. Others were brochures and still others a combination of brochures and audiotapes and other presentation methods [20–22]. Decision aids were developed for a wide variety of clinical conditions, but as they moved away from formal modeling efforts, decision aids became progressively difficult to distinguish from "patient educational" materials [23]. Ultimately, the researchers had to develop a survey instrument to assess the degree to which instruments conformed to their paradigm! There is strong evidence supporting the concept that decision aids improve patients' knowledge and reduce the sense of internal conflict they feel about the trade-offs in a decision [24]. However, some have questioned the importance of patients being "conflict free" when facing a difficult trade-off or a risky choice [25].

The limitation of the decision aid approach is that the patient is the calculating engine, subject to the same cognitive biases and lapses, if not more severe ones due to the emotional stress of illness, that prompted physicians to want to use models to support decision making in the first place [26]. Further, patients may be excessively optimistic about the likely outcome of their illness or feel the need to take action against it, even it if causes harm [27,28]. The effect of decision aids on the quality of decisions is not known [25].

Researchers who continued on the path of applying models to individual patients have developed progressively more automated approaches to applying models to individuals to ascertain the best choice [29–31]. Researchers at the University of Bristol [32–34] have shown it is practical to do this in clinical settings, albeit in randomized trials. The results are often surprising, particularly with regard to patients' willingness to accept risk or inconvenience for long term benefit, as discussed below. The question that prevents widespread use of this approach is what to do about the inconsistencies in patient responses [18]. Outcomes frequently have different rank orders when preference is measured by different procedures, calling into question the validity of direct measurement. While such errors can be repaired by prompting patients about the inconsistencies [35], the meaningfulness of the results is debated.

Both decision aids and decision models are difficult to maintain. Medicine evolves rapidly and the evidence that a treatment is efficacious comes long before we know how effective it is individuals. An accurate prediction of the quantitative benefits to an individual from a procedure requires much more data than knowing a treatment shifts the average response in a group. As a result, procedures may evolve faster than the ability to make statistically valid individualized predictions from data on their performance. Further, as we identify genetic linkages and environmental effects, prediction becomes a more and more difficult task. As much as analysts work toward an objective probability of outcomes, the evolving nature of medicine suggests a continuing role for expert judgment on probabilities of outcomes for individuals.

With the dissemination of the Internet across American society starting in the mid-1990's, patients have gained much more access to educational materials on diagnosis and treatment choices [36]. While there are widespread problems with the quality of information, it is possible for patients to gain access to information, highly independent of their physician, through web search and use of web-based tools. Patient organizations have sponsored web sites to help patients better understand the risk that they face and that even have calculators that predict outcomes [37], based on their disease profiles. Other sites collect patients' experiences on and off treatment and share these experiences, so that the patient considering a treatment can better understand impacts of a disease [38]. However, the complexities can seem overwhelming to some and there has been a renewed call for health professionals whose job is to assist patients with decision-making [39]. These might be doctors, nurses, or even lay persons with training in the domain of the decision under consideration. Despite our progress, models, educational tools, and decision aids remain guides to decision making which may be (still) best performed by linking the patient to well informed unbiased professionals who uses his or her experience to help integrate treatment options for the individual and to make a recommendation.

Of course in a world of limited resources, payers – whether they be private parties such as insurance companies or the government – fear increasing marginal use of resources. In the patient centered model, the only factors that might limit the use of medical resources for a person are risks. Diagnostic tests carry risks that might limit their use. Treatments have risks of complications, pain, inconvenience and adverse effects. Under patient centric models of decision making, we might predict that patients would be very judicious in use of treatments that carry risks for them. This is in fact what is seen in the literature. For treatments with up front risks, when a patient centric approach is implemented to decision making, through *decision aids* and other technologies to support decision making, in settings where treatments carry risks, patients tend to be conservative, and in practice, fewer medical resources are used. As shown in Exhibit 1 [40], in risky situations, such as decision making for surgery or decision making for prevention of stroke with drugs that pose risks of bleeding, patient-centered approaches appear to reduce costs. These studies use a qualitative approach, based on creation of decision aids that allow patients to participate more fully in medical decisions. There are a limited number of studies where researchers have employed models such as shown in Fig. 2, and tailored those models to a patient's physiology and values through measurements. These studies confirm that in selected situations, using a model driven by patient preferences would result in less aggressive use of therapies and may, when shared with patients, change the rate of use of invasive procedures such as elective caesarian section for birth.

However, there are a growing number of situations with expensive therapies that pose few risks, offer small marginal benefits to patients, and have high costs. Examples of this type of treatment include use of certain novel anti-cancer drugs to attempt to extend life in advanced cancer and use of biological therapies for autoimmune disorders. Because the risks of treatments are low, rates of adverse effects are low, even if benefits are small, there is no reason for a patient not to want the treatment, if there are no financial costs.

In some situations, patient centered decision making may be suboptimal because of cognitive biases. For example, in situations where patients feel an acute sense of loss due to their injury, Prospect Theory [26,41] may become operative. In this setting, because of perceived losses, patients might be willing to take more extensive risks, and accept greater risk benefit trade-offs than they would under circumstances where they were not experiencing such loss. They might "clutch at straws." In such settings, the patient centric approach might lead to inappropriately risky interventions and higher costs.

6. Multiple participants in medical decisions

The patient centered approach is a simplification. At the minimum, at least two parties are involved: the patient and his or her physician. Many would consider this the ideal state – the patient and his or her caring physician share decision making with regard to costs or other constraints. But the nature of decision-making is fundamentally changed by adding a second party, who experiences different outcomes and has different values to the decision process.

What goes on in the consultation suite or the examination room, between physician and patient, when deciding about a treatment, has been the subject of numerous studies and surveys. Much of the work has focused on who leads and who follows. In studies of patient preferences for decision making for medical care, typically explored with a question similar to, "In decision making on treatments, who should make the decision on what therapy to use?" and with categorical responses of, "mostly my doctor", "mostly myself", "shared with doctor and myself" [42]. While data vary, the largest group prefers "shared decision making" in most studies. The locus of control is associated with age (older patients more frequently preferring "doctors" to make decisions for them) and with education (more educated patients more frequently prefer to make decisions themselves [43,44]).

In the context of applying this to our problem, limiting the use of higher cost, limited efficacy therapies, theories of decision control illustrate two problems. What if a patient wants everything that could be done, to be done, even if it is not wise? In this setting, a prescriptive model is required where the health provider has to confront values that he or she believes to be harmful to the patients' best interest. These values may be associated with religious beliefs or social norms for cultures, and may not be amenable to change. The opposite context is also an issue. In settings where the patient defers decision authority to the physician, limiting resource use based on patient preferences works only in the context of interventions that the patient will want to choose. Again, culture or religious values may need to be addressed in any intervention that attempts to help patients take more control of medical decision-making.

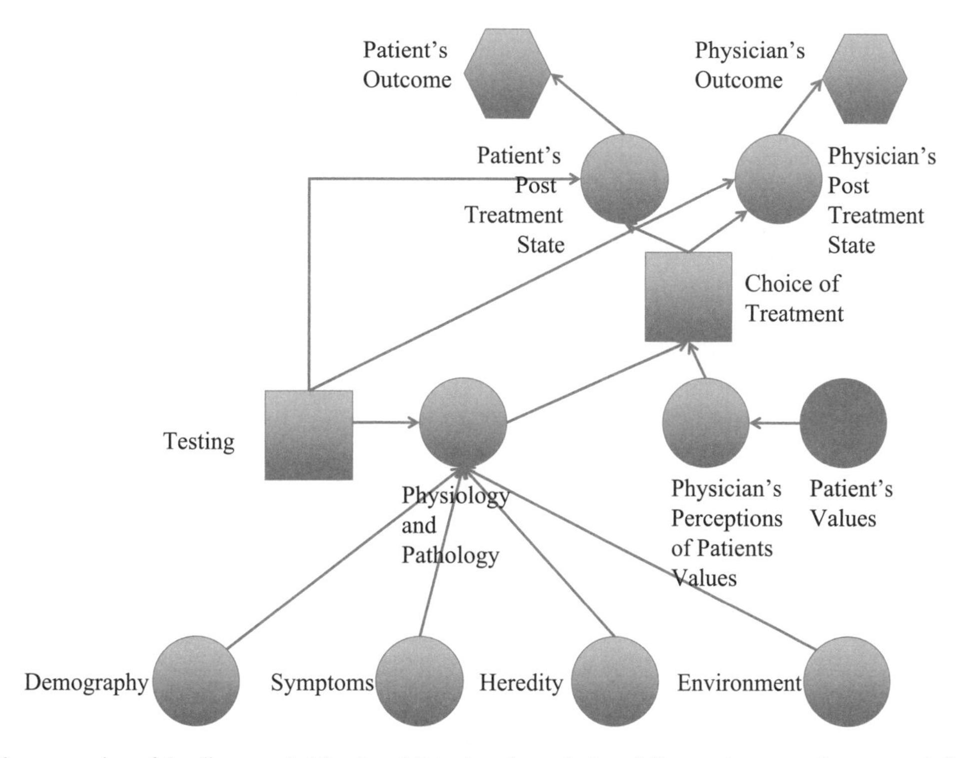

Fig. 3. Further expansion of the diagrams in Figs 1 and 2 to show how choice of diagnostic tests and treatment influences both patient and physician outcomes and values.

7. Physician interests influence decision making

Figure 3 is a model that explicitly identifies the physician as one of two parties in a medical decision. In previous diagrams we've explored the figures from the bottom up. In this section we will explore it from the top down. As shown in Fig. 3, the assumption that the interests of the patient and the physician are not identical results in their being two "value" nodes in the diagram (hexagons): a physician's outcome and a patient's outcome. If the reader questions whether this split is possible, he or she might remember the adage about the "operation was successful, but the patient died." No patient could take this perspective.

In addition to outcomes physicians experience other outcomes separately from patients. Sometimes this may be financial, other times in satisfaction (fighting a good fight may still be satisfying, even if the patient dies). Outcomes of each party in this decision are experienced separately. They may influence each other, but each is distinct. Patients' values are influenced by their post treatment state. Let us assume that the physician outcome is influence by both the post treatment state (good physicians care for their patients) and the physician's benefits from the process, both financial and psychological. This could be influenced by the choice of treatment (a cardiologist choosing angioplasty) and the diagnostic testing performed (the same choosing to perform a catheterization or other study from which he reaps financial benefit). In this setting the process used to chose the treatment becomes critical. Or a physician might minimize the risk of an outcome that they experience differently. For example, in a study we did of resident physicians [45], they placed more weight on death due to adverse effects of treatment than on death due to progression of disease (obviously, the outcome for the patient is the same).

While we can expect physicians to chose treatments that they believe are not causing harm to patients, this belief may more reflect the incomplete knowledge of the physician than the truth. The choice, when in the physicians' hands, should be influenced by patients' values, but in this setting, it is the physician's perception of the patient's values that largely matters, rather than the values themselves. Physicians will be more or less skilled at eliciting what those values are and then integrating them into decisions. What the patient knows about his or her medical problems, about treatment options, and how they feel about different outcomes, may all be influenced by the descriptions of his or her physician. Other factors in the model are still operative. The right choice for each patient is influenced by his or her physiology and pathology. What is known of that is determined by diagnostic testing strategies (some of which provide additional benefit to the physician), and by demography, symptoms, genetics and environment influenced factors.

The structure of this model does give cause for concern in a fee-for-service environment. There are powerful incentives for physicians to maximize service delivery level to patients, in order to increase their own benefits. The only factor limiting delivery of services for either diagnosis or treatment is perceived benefit. The temptations under this model are extreme. A recent article in the *New Yorker* [46] detailed the excesses in McAllen Texas – a poor community with the highest per capita healthcare costs in the United States. In McAllen, more and more invasive and expensive diagnostic tests come into play as culture surrounding care makes it permissible for physicians to reasonably conclude that actions are in the interests of patients.

Perceptions of benefit are based on physicians medical reasoning, much of which is model dependent. Models can be highly persuasive to physicians (and to patients). Unfortunately, conceptual models do not always predict what happens when patients are treated with medications or therapies. For example, in the 80's there were widespread beliefs that dangerous cardiac arrhythmias could be controlled by empiric therapy with arrhythmia suppressing drugs such as procainamide. While these drugs did suppress the arrhythmias detected with the diagnostic procedures of the day, they did not save lives – in fact they placed patients at greater risk for sudden death. Similarly, orthopedists of recent have used injections of platelet rich plasma in deep connective tissue sites to reduce inflammation and speed healing of damaged tendons. While plausible and costly, a recent study showed this treatment to be no more effective than placebo injections of saline [47].

Physician interests in decision making has huge potential to impact costs. Every patient becomes a candidate for the procedure that benefits the physician. New technologies disseminate beyond the realm of proven effectiveness at great cost because of physician incentives. A world where physician led decision-making goes unchecked is not practical.

8. Influence of third party financing on decision making

The majority of medical services in this country are paid for by either government or private insurance. In this setting, decision making becomes even more complex. Figure 4 illustrates how the model changes. There is a third "value" node based on the outcome the payer experiences. This is largely determined by the *payer's cost* for the episode of care being modeled. The factors influencing this, including the patients' post treatment state (how much more resources might they need afterward for further recovery or because of complications, and for some employers who are payers, how their outcome influences patients' productivity), by the choice of treatment and the costs entrained by that, and by the costs of diagnostic testing. Payers learned long ago that physician decision making would often not optimize the outcome the payer experienced. Therefore, payers set up policies and controls that limit diagnostic testing choices and treatment choices in certain contexts. These policies are shown in the figure, represented as a square node, indicating that the payer has made decisions about policies that influence how diagnostic

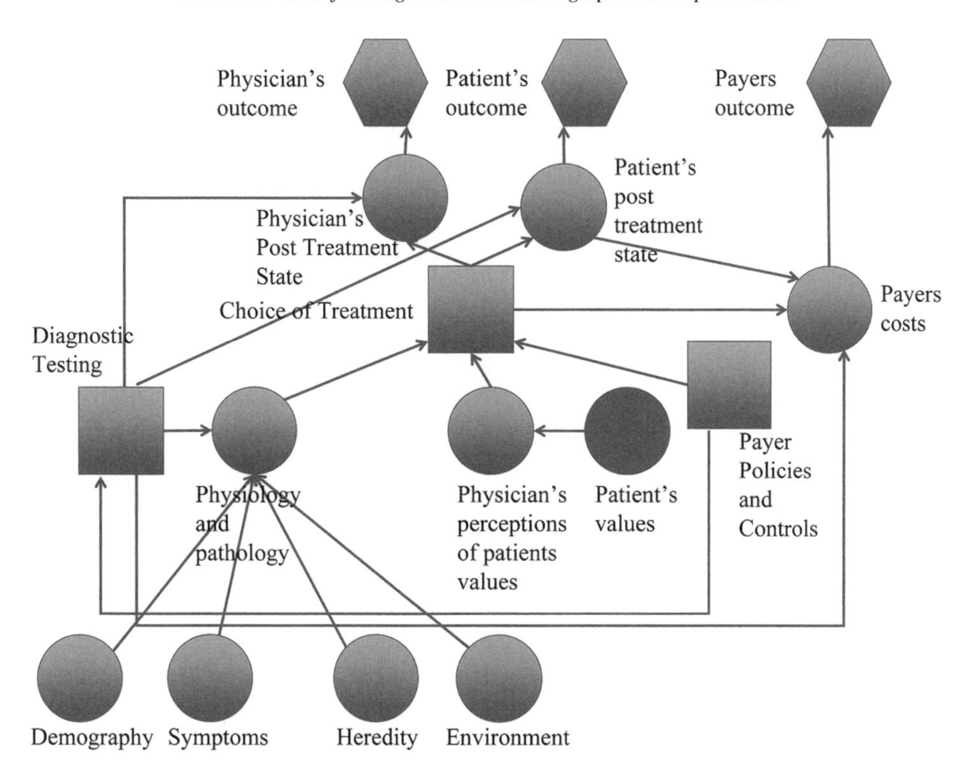

Fig. 4. Diagram of how the additional complexity added by considering a third party payer's values, such as an insurance company, influences choice of diagnostic tests and treatment.

tests and medical treatments can be used. These policies take the form of guidelines, pre-approval for testing or treatment, documentation policies and other forms. The intent is to decrease the potential for physicians to drive the system to maximize their gains, through choice of treatment and diagnostic testing. Optimistically, this might also improve outcomes for patients but, as shown in the diagram, patients outcomes are independent of payers, except in how the outcome influences future costs for the payer. Therefore, as the model shows explicitly, patient outcomes and payer outcomes are not closely aligned and it is possible for payers to create policies that are detrimental to patients.

Overall, though, the complexity of this system does little to guarantee that the choices made optimize the outcome for the patient. This model is the simplest representation of current decision making for healthcare under a fee-for-service model. Other interested parties could be introduced with different values and outcomes. For example, separating hospitals from physicians would create another set of issues and more potential opportunities for decision making to be corrupted and depart from the optimal decision under the patient centered perspective. The more value nodes that are introduced into the model, the more likely that decisions will become arbitrary, reflecting a balance of the interested parties rather than what is optimal for the patient. Therefore, it is critical that policies attempt to create conditions that enhance the patient-centeredness of medical decision making, even while attempting to control costs.

9. Multiple payers and a single payer system

While Fig. 4 shows the complexity of decision making for an individual patient, physicians rarely have the luxury of a single set of policies to constrain their diagnostic and therapeutic decision making behavior. In a system with multiple payers, decisions made for patients with different payers are made under different constraints. The professional must try to balance each payer and patient combination of restrictions against the patient's interests and his or her own. This complexity probably reduces the quality of the decisions made under such a system.

10. Solutions that try to contain costs: Single payer systems and salaried physicians

As discussed above, while single payer approaches reduce administrative costs and prevent physicians and patients from having to deal with multiple types of constraining policies, just converting to a single payer system does nothing to simplify Fig. 4. As long as physicians and other providers have a financial interest in healthcare, decision making suffers by having multiple parties pursuing different objectives. From a modeling perspective, if the financial aspects of physician interests could be taken from the equation, this would simplify the model and at least make the distinctions between patient interest and payer interest more clear. Removing the financial tie between the decision and the physician's financial interest might also help control costs. With less incentive to undertake procedures and treatments to enhance their own outcomes, care might be more patient centric and cost effective.

Not surprisingly, this idea has been implemented and tested. In 1970's and 1980's, one solution proposed to the problem of increasing costs was the development of the Health Maintenance Organization. Health maintenance organizations removed direct financial incentives from providers and hospitals, these entities being part of the payer organization. These organizations of salaried physicians, were hoped to align decision making to patients long term benefit and to control costs.

Figure 5 is a representation of decision-making between patient, physician and an HMO payer. As we can see, in the diagram the direct link between the decision and the physician's outcome and value is broken. However, a new link is created. The decision, is still subject to constraints by policies of the payer. Without the physician as an advocate for the patient (and himself or herself), the outcome may be less favorable for the patient. Some policies may highly constrain healthcare to the detriment of the patient. A practical example of this is when, in the late 1990's, Northern California Kaiser Permanente (KP) set up its own renal transplantation program and attempted to convert all transplant care in its patient population to its own program as a cost containment measure. Outcomes of the program were much worse than competing universities and other centers and still the payer persisted in requirements for use of their system. Only after there was an outcry from patients (and the *Los Angeles Times*), did the policy change [48]. The issues with the link between payer interests and physician interests in decision making are represented in the figure by the link between the payer's outcome and the physician's outcome. This might be through partnership with the provider (as in the case of KP) or through financial incentives to the salaried physician to actions that control costs.

HMO organizations have had limited penetration in the US market, largely due to concerns about poor quality of care due to excessive alignment between physician interests and payer interests. Recently, Relman has proposed a model based on this notion of separating physician interests from patient interests by putting delivery of healthcare by salaried physicians [4]. The approach requires healthcare delivery institutions such as hospitals to be not-for-profit and focuses on delivery of medical services through community-based multi-specialty not-for-profit clinics with salaried staff. Relman's approach would require a massive shift in the way healthcare is delivered in this county. Currently, more than 50% of physicians practice in groups of 5 or less. This approach would essentially convert all outpatient medical practice to large groups. As a result, it may not be culturally acceptable to physicians or to patients.

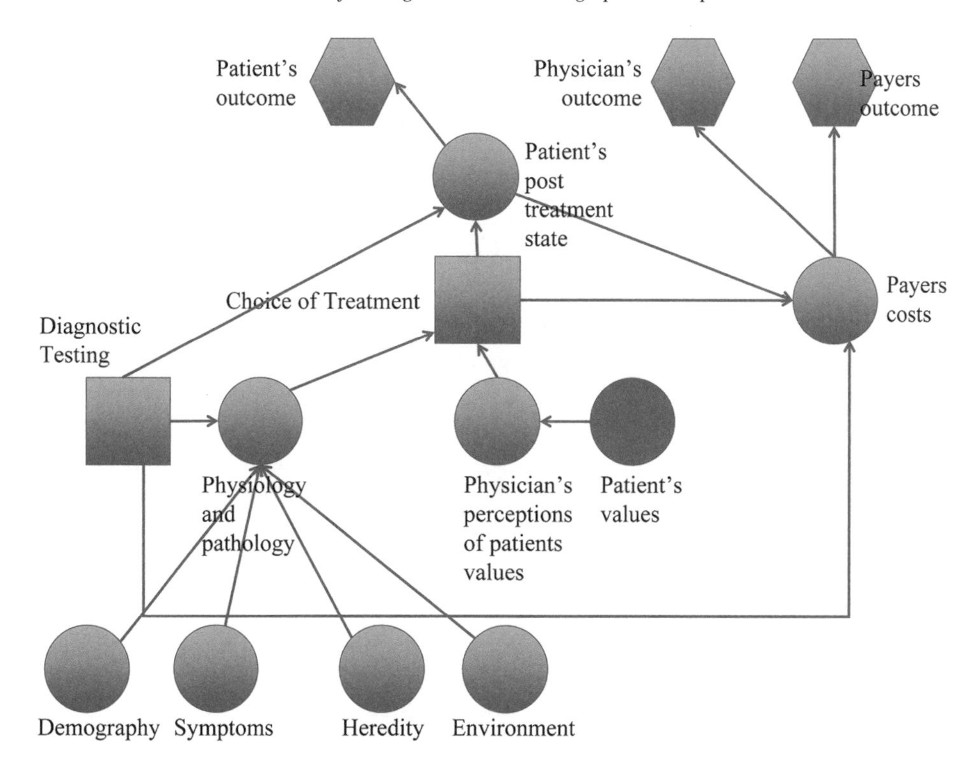

Fig. 5. Representation of decision making for a staff model Health Maintenance Organization. Physician and Payer interests are aligned.

11. Consumer directed healthcare

One approach to limit costs of care that has risen in popularity of the past years is consumer directed healthcare. This model of care combines a high deductible insurance plan (which is often low cost), with a (non-taxable) healthcare savings account [49]. Decision making on the use of this savings account for healthcare (funds are limited to use for health-related services and products) is driven by the patient, informed by the physician and by education from other sources. Amounts above the deductible are covered by the insurance program. The result is a model that is a hybrid of Figs 2 and 4. For the deductible monies, decision making resembles Fig. 2. Patients' interests alone drive the model. But, because the model now includes other competing uses for the money, the patient is forced to decide which health benefits are of greatest value to him or her. The result, as shown in experiments of consumer directed health plans, is similar to the case when there a deductibles for prescriptions, medications are refilled somewhat less frequently, causing patients to miss treatments [49,50]. Preventative services may be neglected by patients (having little direct immediate return), and as a result, some consumer directed plans exempt preventative services from the deductible. The situation becomes more complicated, as shown in Fig. 6 when we take into consideration two other practical issues. First, health plans cover both individuals and families and when they do this, the healthcare savings account must provide for care for all the individuals in a family, setting up some degree of competition between individuals for resources. Second, the education of the patient and/or his or her family to participate in the decision may be incomplete or there may be erroneous sources of data used in decision making (for example, fears of a parent about vaccines causing autism). The incompleteness of transfer of information for an informed decision and the multiple parties involved within a family, who all share resources, creates further

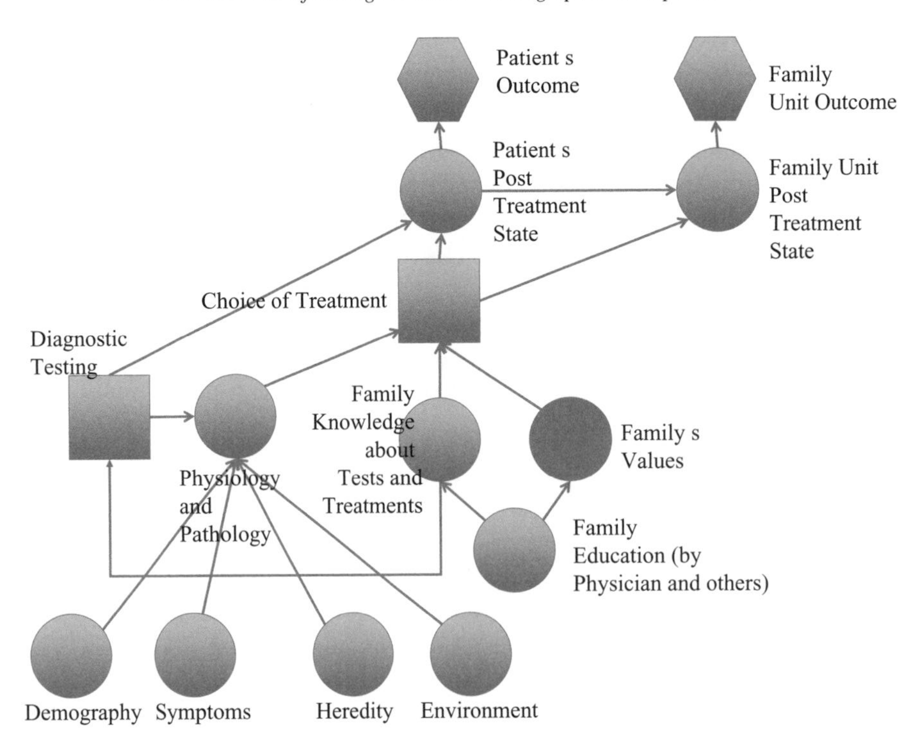

Fig. 6. Consumer Driven Healthcare Systems. These high deductible plans place patients and their families in charge of medical decision making below the deductible. Complications of the approach include variable quality of education, family vs. patient values, and competition for health resources among family members.

complexity. Recent data suggest that financial responsibility does not necessarily increase information seeking [50].

Above the deductible, the model reverts to Fig. 4. Savings in the model are driven by consumers' more careful use of resources and by co-funding of the health savings account by the consumer. Because the model for decision making on amounts above the deductible is the same, this approach may not have great impacts on costs. Regina Herzlinger, a Harvard economist, has proposed further extensions to the Consumer Directed Healthcare Model that would allow patients to direct healthcare choices above the deductible for healthcare savings accounts [51]. She proposes that patients with identified diseases be given annual allowances determined by arbitrage, to pay for care for their illnesses. Unused funds would be carried over to a consumer healthcare savings account and could be used for other purposes or after a period, converted to retirement funds. Advised by health counselors, patients would chose from among providers who would offer all health services needed for the year for a fixed fee. A new class of health entrepreneurs, would develop "health factories" that could efficiently provide all the needed services for a particular disease, at a reduced price through mass production techniques and specialization. The result of Herzlinger's model is intended to be the idealized Fig. 2. Guided by fee for service advisors, patients make rational choices that optimize their health at a reasonable cost. The reality (this idea has not been tested) may be a bewildering model that is a combination of Figs 4 and 5, where family member needs compete with patient needs, where physician financial interests determine the types of options available (with few alternatives to the patient tracked to one hospital) and there are still substantial constraints imposed by insurance companies and other payers on decision making. The complexities of the ecology proposed by Herzlinger may make for an efficient system. But will it make for a patient centric one?

12. Conclusions

In this essay, we have discussed a number of the factors that can influence the quality of a medical decision. A medical decision is patient centric when the diagnostic test performed and the treatment option ultimately chosen, capture a patient's physiology and his or her values, and maximize his or her expected utility. While this does not guarantee a good outcome or a cost-effective care strategy, it does represent the best choice for the individual. Introduction of objectives for other individuals, corporations, or for society, impact the choice of treatment and reduce the patient-centeredness of decision making, and necessarily, reduce the quality of medical decisions. Strategies to control costs through policies that restrict services, remove financial incentives for physicians, ask patients to balance medical needs among family members or that create of complex financial ecologies (e.g., Herzlinger), should be assessed based on the gold standard of their impact on the patient centeredness of the decision. Strategies to control costs should do the minimal harm to the patient centeredness. Mathematically, this would be the difference between the expected utility under a patient centric model and the policy implemented. Practically, this means policy decision makers should design health systems that result in as few corruptions to the idealized patient centric model in Fig. 2 as possible.

References

[1] W. Weinberger, E.Z. Oddone and W.G. Henderson, Does increased access to primary care reduce hospital readmissions? Veterans Affairs Cooperative Study Group on Primary Care and Hospital Readmission, *N Engl J Med* **334**(22) (1996), 1441–1447.
[2] L. Esserman, J. Belkora and L. Lenert, Potentially ineffective care. A new outcome to assess the limits of critical care, *JAMA* **274**(19) (1995), 1544–1551.
[3] D.J. Cher and L.A. Lenert, Method of Medicare reimbursement and the rate of potentially ineffective care of critically ill patients, *JAMA* **278**(12) (1997), 1001–1007.
[4] A.S. Relman, *A Second Opinion: Rescuing America's Healthcare: A Plan for Universal Coverage Serving Patients Over Profit*, (1st ed.), 2007, New York: PublicAffairs. xvii, 205 p.
[5] A. Tversky and D. Kahneman, Judgment under Uncertainty: Heuristics and Biases, *Science* **185**(4157) (1974), 1124–1131.
[6] B. Sirovich et al., Discretionary decision making by primary care physicians and the cost of U.S. Health care, *Health Aff (Millwood)* **27**(3) (2008), 813–823.
[7] Stanford Research Institute. Decision Analysis Group et al., *Readings in Decision Analysis*, (2d ed.), 1976, Menlo Park, Calif.: Decision Analysis Group, Stanford Research Institute. vi, 609 p.
[8] R.A. Howard and J.E. Matheson, Influence Diagrams, *Decision Analysis* **2** (2004), 127–143.
[9] D.M. Berwick, What 'patient-centered' should mean: confessions of an extremist, *Health Aff (Millwood)* **28**(4) (2009), w555–w565.
[10] R.S. Ledley and L.B. Lusted, Probability, Logic and Medical Diagnosis, *Science* **130**(3380) (1959), 892–930.
[11] R.S. Ledley and L.B. Lusted, Reasoning foundations of medical diagnosis; symbolic logic, probability, and value theory aid our understanding of how physicians reason, *Science* **130**(3366) (1959), 9–21.
[12] R.S. Ledley and L.B. Lusted, Biomedical electronics: potentialities and problems, *Science* **135** (1962), 198–201.
[13] S.G. Pauker and J.P. Kassirer, Therapeutic decision making: a cost-benefit analysis, *N Engl J Med* **293**(5) (1975), 229–234.
[14] S.G. Pauker and J.P. Kassirer, Decision analysis, *N Engl J Med* **316**(5) (1987), 250–258.
[15] S.G. Pauker and J.P. Kassirer, Clinical decision analysis by personal computer, *Arch Intern Med* **141**(13) (1981), 1831–1837.
[16] D.A. Plante et al., Clinical decision consultation service, *Am J Med* **80**(6) (1986), 1169–1176.
[17] S. Holtzman, *Intelligent Decision Systems*. Teknowledge series in knowledge engineering. 1988, Reading, Mass.: Addison-Wesley. xv, 304 p.
[18] L. Lenert and R.M. Kaplan, Validity and interpretation of preference-based measures of health-related quality of life, *Med Care* **38**(9 Suppl) (2000), II138–II150.
[19] M.J. Barry et al., Patient reactions to a program designed to facilitate patient participation in treatment decisions for benign prostatic hyperplasia, *Med Care* **33**(8) (1995), 771–782.

[20] A.M. O'Connor et al., The Ottawa patient decision aids, *Eff Clin Pract* **2**(4) (1999), 163–170.
[21] A.M. O'Connor, H.A. Llewellyn-Thomas and A.B. Flood, Modifying unwarranted variations in health care: shared decision making using patient decision aids, *Health Aff (Millwood)* Suppl Web Exclusives, p. VAR63-72, 2004.
[22] A.M. O'Connor et al., Decision aids for patients facing health treatment or screening decisions: systematic review, *BMJ* **319**(7212) (1999), 731–734.
[23] M. Holmes-Rovner, International Patient Decision Aid Standards (IPDAS): beyond decision aids to usual design of patient education materials, *Health Expect* **10**(2) (2007), 103–107.
[24] A.M. O'Connor et al., Decision aids for people facing health treatment or screening decisions, *Cochrane Database Syst Rev* (3) (2009), CD001431.
[25] W.L. Nelson et al., Rethinking the objectives of decision aids: a call for conceptual clarity, *Med Decis Making* **27**(5) (2007), 609–618.
[26] D.A. Redelmeier, P. Rozin and D. Kahneman, Understanding patients' decisions. Cognitive and emotional perspectives, *JAMA* **270**(1) (1993), 72–76.
[27] A. Fagerlin, B.J. Zikmund-Fisher and P.A. Ubel, Cure me even if it kills me: preferences for invasive cancer treatment, *Med Decis Making* **25**(6) (2005), 614–619.
[28] L.A. Allen et al., Discordance between patient-predicted and model-predicted life expectancy among ambulatory patients with heart failure, *JAMA* **299**(21) (2008), 2533–2542.
[29] D.J. Cher and L.A. Lenert, Rapid approximation of confidence intervals for Markov process decision models: applications in decision support systems, *J Am Med Inform Assoc* **4**(4) (1997), 301–312.
[30] L.A. Lenert and R.M. Soetikno, Automated computer interviews to elicit utilities: potential applications in the treatment of deep venous thrombosis, *J Am Med Inform Assoc* **4**(1) (1997), 49–56.
[31] G.C. Scott and L.A. Lenert, What is the next step in patient decision support? *Proc AMIA Symp* (2000), 784–788.
[32] A.A. Montgomery et al., Two decision aids for mode of delivery among women with previous caesarean section: randomised controlled trial, *BMJ* **334**(7607) (2007), 1305.
[33] A.A. Montgomery et al., Evaluation of computer based clinical decision support system and risk chart for management of hypertension in primary care: randomised controlled trial, *BMJ* **320**(7236) (2000), 686–690.
[34] A.A. Montgomery, J. Harding and T. Fahey, Shared decision making in hypertension: the impact of patient preferences on treatment choice, *Fam Pract* **18**(3) (2001), 309–313.
[35] L.A. Lenert, A. Sturley and M. Rupnow, Toward improved methods for measurement of utility: automated repair of errors in elicitations, *Med Decis Making* **23**(1) (2003), 67–75.
[36] Pew Internet and American Life Project, *Pew Internet and American Life project*, Pew Internet and American Life Project: Washington, DC.
[37] M. Markman, J. Petersen and R. Montgomery, An examination of characteristics of lung and colon cancer patients participating in a web-based decision support program. Internet-based decision support programs, *Oncology* **69**(4) (2005), 311–316.
[38] Patients_Like_Me. *Web site*. 2010; Available from: www.patientslikeme.com.
[39] A.M. O'Connor, D. Stacey and F. Legare, Coaching to support patients in making decisions, *BMJ* **336**(7638) (2008), 228–229.
[40] J.E. Wennberg et al., Extending the P4P agenda, part 1: how Medicare can improve patient decision making and reduce unnecessary care, *Health Aff (Millwood)* **26**(6) (2007), 1564–1574.
[41] A. Tversky and D. Kahneman, The framing of decisions and the psychology of choice, *Science* **211**(4481) (1981), 453–458.
[42] R.B. Deber, N. Kraetschmer and J. Irvine, What role do patients wish to play in treatment decision making? *Arch Intern Med* **156**(13) (1996), 1414–1420.
[43] R.B. Deber et al., Do people want to be autonomous patients? Preferred roles in treatment decision-making in several patient populations, *Health Expect* **10**(3) (2007), 248–258.
[44] R. Say, M. Murtagh and R. Thomson, Patients' preference for involvement in medical decision making: a narrative review, *Patient Educ Couns* **60**(2) (2006), 102–114.
[45] L.A. Lenert, D.R. Markowitz and T.F. Blaschke, Primum non nocere? Valuing of the risk of drug toxicity in therapeutic decision making, *Clin Pharmacol Ther* **53**(3) (1993), 285–291.
[46] A. Gawande, The Cost Conundrum. What a Texas Town Can Teach Us About Healthcare, in The New Yorker, New York City, 2009.
[47] R.J. de Vos et al., Platelet-rich plasma injection for chronic Achilles tendinopathy: a randomized controlled trial, *JAMA* **303**(2) (2010), 144–149.
[48] R. Lin, Kaiser Permanente to settle renal transplant claims for $1 million, in Los Angeles Times, Lost Angeles, 2009.
[49] K. Davis, Consumer-directed health care: will it improve health system performance? *Health Serv Res* **39**(4 Pt 2) (2004), 1219–1234.

[50] A. Dixon, J. Greene and J. Hibbard, Do consumer-directed health plans drive change in enrollees' health care behavior? *Health Aff (Millwood)* **27**(4) (2008), 1120–1131.
[51] R.E. Herzlinger, Who killed health care? America's, 2007, New York: Mc-Graw Hill. vii, 304 p.

Leslie Lenert, MD, MS, FACMI is a graduate of the University of California, Riverside and the University of California, Los Angeles, School of Medicine. Trained in Internal Medicine at the University of Texas Southwestern School of Medicine and in Clinical Pharmacology and in Medical Informatics at Stanford University School of Medicine, Dr. Lenert has held faculty posts at the Department of Medicine at Stanford and the University of California San Diego (UCSD). At UCSD, he was promoted Professor of Medicine, was the Director of the Health Services Research Unit at the San Diego VA Healthcare System, and was Associate Director (Medical Informatics) at the California Institute for Telecommunications and Information Technology (Calit2), an interdisciplinary institute with more than 200 faculty, focused on translational research in computing and wireless technologies. In 2007, Dr. Lenert became the first permanent Director of the National Center for Public Health Informatics (NCPHI) at the Centers for Disease Control and Prevention (CDC). At NCPHI, Dr. Lenert led the agency's efforts to meet public health information needs through improved linkages with the clinical care system based on "cloud computing" technologies, including linkage of public health providers to the National Health Information Network (NHIN). He also help to found a new Global Public Health Informatics program at CDC and championed the migration of public health systems to Open Source development methods. Currently a consultant in population health informatics, Dr. Lenert has published over 100 original articles and book chapters, is a Fellow of the American College of Medical Informatics and was a past member of the Board of Directors of the American Medical Informatics Association and serves on the editorial boards of the Journal of the American Medical Informatics Association, the Journal of Biomedical Informatics, and the International Journal of Medical Informatics. His current research interests focus upon the application of information technology to enhance continuity of care in community settings.

Section 3: Incentives

Information Knowledge Systems Management 8 (2009) 179–193
DOI 10.3233/IKS-2009-0155
IOS Press

Chapter 11

Health economics

Gail R. Wilensky
E-mail: gwilensky@projecthope.org

Abstract: Health care spending and more importantly, health care spending growth rates, are unsustainable. Past strategies of price controls, reliance on administered pricing for Medicare and the dominance of a la carte fee for service reimbursement have been part of the problem and do not represent promising strategies for the future. Too much time has been spent debating whether Medicare has done better or worse than the private sector since neither represents an acceptable path going forward. Understanding the effects of innovative payment strategies – including those that affect the patient – will be an important part in learning how to "bend the curve". Making sure that there are strategies to implement the results of successful pilots and demonstrations will also be important.

1. Introduction

The study of rising health care expenditures in the United States has been the focus of numerous articles and books over the last 50 years. During that period, the country has seen health care spending increase from about $143 per person in 1960 to $7421 person in 2007 and total health care spending growing from around 5 percent of the GDP to more than 16% of GDP [6]. Current expectations from the actuaries of the Centers for Medicare and Medicaid Services, the official arbiters of national health spending projections, are that the average annual growth in national health spending for the next decade will be 6.2% per year – which is 2.1 percentage points faster that the average growth in the economy as measured by the GDP that is expected over the same period of time. If this in fact materializes, health care is expected to account for more than 20% of the economy, with about half of the spending coming from public sources of payment [6]. None of these numbers builds in the potential effects of health care reform, which has as one of its objectives, slowing down spending on health care, although initially health care reform is likely to substantially increase health care spending as all or most of the 15% of the population without insurance coverage becomes insured.

This chapter reviews the implications of continued health care spending that substantially exceeds the growth in the economy, the drivers of that growth as well as some of the strategies that have been proposed to slow the growth in health care spending. Particular attention is paid to the use of price controls and administered pricing–the traditional tools of other countries (along with global budgets) and of Medicare (without global budgets) and to the use of changed incentives to impact how health care is organized and delivered and thus affecting health care spending. Various strategies that have been proposed to increase the value of health care spending – including different payment mechanisms – such as paying for value or performance, better information and combining better information with changed incentives are also reviewed. More detailed discussions of changing reimbursement systems and how they can impact spending and value are discussed more fully in the next two chapters.

2. Implications of continued health care spending growth

For at least the last two decades, health policy analysts and budget experts, among others, have commented on the pressures which the continued growth in health care spending places both on the Federal budget and also on the ability of employers to provide increasing cash wages to their employees. The President has repeatedly claimed that economy recovery cannot be separated from health care reform and finding strategies that restrain the growth in health care spending [17]. The Congressional Budget Office, in its most recent Outlook, has once again indicated that the Federal budget is on an unsustainable path – that is, that the federal debt will continue to grow faster than the economy, and that rising costs for health care along with the growth of the US population will continue to cause federal spending to rise rapidly under current law [12].

If current law does not change, federal spending on Medicare and Medicaid as a share of GDP will double in about 15 years, growing from 5% of GDP today to 10% in 2035. If this were to continue over the long term – 2080 – federal spending for these two programs would be about 17% of the GDP which is close to historical averages of federal spending on all government programs and services [12, p. 26]. This is not to suggest that anyone expects that current law will prevail for the next several decades but rather to indicate the level of pressure for change that exists.

Similarly, rising health care costs have not only contributed to the decline in employer-sponsored coverage over the past decade but have also been associated with rising health insurance premiums that have consistently outpaced the rate of increase in cash wages. Even in years when premium increases have been relatively modest, as they were in 2008 when they increased by 5%, the increase was faster than wage growth. Over the past decade, premiums have doubled while wages have increased by only 34% and general inflation increased by 29% [20].

The experiences during the current decade shouldn't be surprising. Only the 1990's has deviated from this trend when health care spend grew unusually slowly – largely driven by aggressive actions by managed care – while the economy grew at a robust rate. The inability to moderate health care spending has meant that employers are allocating more of their employee's compensation to health care even while they are increasing deductibles and copayments and using other benefit design changes to limit the cost of the health coverage that they provide.

In short, finding ways to slow the rate of growth in health care spending is critical if the country is to get its fiscal house in order and if we are to see cash wages begin to grow in a more robust way than has been possible during the current decade.

3. Key drivers in health care spending

People often speak about the high cost of health care in this country. Indeed spending in the United States, at almost $7500 per person is far greater than spending in any other country, whether measured in dollars per person or share of the economy devoted to health care. For example, when the U.S. was spending more than 15% of its GDP on health care in 2006, OECD countries were spending just under 9% [4]. What is of even greater concern than the absolute level of spending, however, has been the increased rate of spending – the 2 to 2.5% percentage points faster growth in health care spending relative to the growth in the rest of the economy. In terms of growth rate, the U.S. is closer to the average of OECD countries than it is in terms of absolute spending levels although the growth rates have been greater for the U.S. than most other countries [2].

This distinction between absolute levels and growth rates is an important distinction to keep in mind because some potential savings may be "one-off savings" that once they occur, will not provide going-forward savings while other changes may indeed affect the growth rate in spending.

For example, many of the industrial engineering efficiencies that would make physician offices function more efficiently or reduce the costs associated with hospital operating rooms or admissions processes are likely to be "one-off" savings. Once they are implemented, they reduce the base costs of providing services but not the growth rate of spending. Other changes, such as learning to adopt and disseminate new technologies in a more prudent fashion, could reduce the growth rate in spending as well. To be clear, if the country can find a series of strategies that reduces the level of spending on a one-time basis, this would give us some breathing room to introduce changes that might lower the growth rate in spending but require a number of years to implement. It would also mean experiencing a slower growth rate that starts from a lower base line of spending

There have been many attempts to parse out the drivers of health care spending growth. Partly it depends on how the question is approached. Chronic disease is associated with most health care spending in the United States – as much as 75% by some estimates. Conditions such as obesity that are associated with the increased prevalence of certain types of chronic disease such as diabetes and hypertension can be viewed as significant drivers of health care costs. Indeed, some estimates have attributed more than 25% of the increase in health care spending between 1997 and 2005 to rising rates of obesity [13].

For some years, HCFA – the name formerly used for the agency that is responsible for administering Medicare, now called, CMS – estimated the growth in Medicare spending attributable to population change, general inflation, medical inflation, utilization and a residual that was generally attributed to technology. A number of authors have attempted similar designations. Medical inflation has generally been associated with no more than 20% of the total increase, aging about 2% and the largest impact, the effects of technology, responsible for as much as 60% of the increase in spending by some estimates [16]. Most of the studies that show technology as being the dominant factor continue to define technology as a residual but even those that use just proxies for technological change have come up with technology being a major factor in the growth of health care spending [16]. However, as noted in a recently released article, technology does not expand in a vacuum but rather is fueled by rising incomes and expanding insurance coverage. When the interactive effects of income and insurance are taken into account, the role attributed to technology diminishes some, although may still be as high explaining 48% of the health care spending since 1960 [26].

While the studies have been quite consistent with regard to the smaller weight attributable to aging and medical specific inflation compared to technology in explaining spending growth trends, those that have attempted to explain cross-national difference in health care spending attribute a greater role to prices [3]. This is important in understanding why the US spends so much more than other countries at a point in time but differential levels of pricing do not have a similar relevance in explaining the growth in health care spending – the most serious aspect of the problem confronting the sustainability of health care in the U.S. A recent study that projected health spending through 2018, projected a larger importance to the growth in medical prices compared to utilization changes but did not attempt to allocate any role to new technology which, as indicated, other studies have found in the single biggest factor associated with spending growth [25].

4. The impact of price controls

The use of price controls as a strategy to control spending has a long history. Some trace their use all the way back to the Old Testament and proscriptions regarding the use of interest charges. In the United States we have occasionally attempted to control prices with wage and price controls, although generally the U.S. has not had sustained periods with price controls. Most frequently price controls have been used to prevent inflation in certain areas of shortage or for prices during periods of war. The U.S. used them during both World War I and World War II and also the Korean War. The most recent attempt was when President Nixon used wage and price controls in the early 1970's to combat what had been regarded as intolerable rates of inflation by historical standards, 4%–6%. These were mostly dismantled by 1974 even though later in the decade, inflation was much worse than it had been during the early 1970's [32].

The wage and price controls used during WWII have had a major impact on health care because they were the genesis of the differential tax treatment between employer contributions to employer-sponsored health insurance and the treatment of employee wages. Employers began offering health insurance to their employees as a way to increase employee compensation without violating the wage controls that were in place during WWII, claiming that the employer contributions were not wages and should not be treated as employee wages for purposes of calculating an employee's income. The distinction was not an issue for the employers since any type of employee compensation is deductible for purposes of calculating employer income. Not treating employer contributions to employer sponsored insurance as part of the employee's wage in calculating taxable income was reaffirmed by the Internal Revenue Service in 1954 and thus became a permanent part of employee compensation for most of the employed population.

Most economists believe that the differential tax treatment between employer contributions to insurance and wages is the single, most important reason that employer-sponsored insurance is the dominant source of insurance for the under 65 population [23]. The current tax treatment has also been regarded as introducing a significant distortion in the choice of taking compensation as taxable wages or as a non-taxed fringe benefit, and has lead to increased purchases of insurance which has in turn, has been a contributing factor to the rate of increase in spending on health care. In addition, the current tax exclusion is regarded as inequitable and unfair because the value of the exclusion increases as the individual's income increases. Various efforts to date to change the tax laws, including the proposal by John McCain during the 2008 Presidential campaign to substitute a refundable credit in place of the tax exclusion, have met with resistance from a variety of sources, including some large employer groups and several labor unions.

It remains an issue of discussion because it also represents a very large loss of tax revenue to the Treasury, currently estimated to be approximately $240 billion per year [11].

5. Administered pricing under medicare

The most pervasive form of price controls in the U.S. has been the use of administered pricing in Medicare. While Medicare over time has changed the type of reimbursement it uses for most providers of services to Medicare beneficiaries – moving towards more bundled payments – the reimbursement for the bundled payments continues to be set by administered pricing strategies. Prior to 1983, for example, hospitals had been paid on a per diem basis using a rate set by Medicare. Since the introduction of DRG's (Diagnostic Related Groups) in 1983 as the basis of payment to hospitals, hospitals have received a single payment for all services provided during a hospital stay (other than for physician services who continue to be paid separately from the hospital). The reimbursement they receive continues to be set through an administrative pricing process although the DRG payments were originally constructed based on historical costs associated with treating the diagnosis. The relative weights associated with labor and other costs that were part of the historical cost base are periodically adjusted to reflect more current factors. Over the last decade, the reimbursements used for outpatient hospital services, home care and nursing home services have moved toward bundled payments and away from reimbursements for individual services. The bundled payments for each of these services are set through an administered pricing process that is established by law as had the more disaggregated forms of reimbursement that had previously been in use.

Reforms to the way physicians are reimbursed under Medicare are the exception to the move to more bundled payments. The major reform in physician payment, introduced in 1992 with the implementation of the Resource Based Relative Value System (RBRVS), continued the use of a disaggregated fee schedule, unlike the changes made to other parts of Medicare. The relative value scale was designed to reflect the work effort associated with more than 7000 services coded under the CPT (Current Procedure Terminology) system which is combined with an estimate reflecting practice costs and also a geographic adjuster. Prior to the adoption of the relative value scale, Medicare payments to physicians had in large part reflected historical prices set by private insurers. In its earliest days, Medicare payments to physicians was based on "usual, customary and reasonable" fees used by private insurance but the use of UCR-like reimbursements was eliminated because of the belief that it was not only inherently inflationary because of its reliance on fee-for-service reimbursement but that it also perpetuated the distortion towards excessive payments for specialty care versus primary care and towards care provided in urban settings versus care provided in rural settings.

Although the RBRVS was designed to rebalance payments in favor of services mostly provided by primary care physicians, there is continuing evidence that this has not occurred and CMS has recently proposed reducing payments for cardiologists and oncologists so that it can increase payments for primary care services on a budget neutral basis [6].

Unlike other parts of Medicare, reimbursements used for physicians are also subject to a spending limit. This limit is now called the "Sustainable Growth Rate" (when the limit that was first introduced in 1992, it was called a Volume Performance Standard) and is based on the growth in the economy. The rationale for using a relative value scale combined with a spending limit is based on the experiences from the 1980's. During that time, spending under Part B Medicare with its disaggregated fee schedule increased even faster than spending for the rest of Medicare. As a result of this experience, the RBRVS, which continued the use of a disaggregated fee schedule – although one that was based on relative values rather than historical charges – was passed with a spending limit to "guarantee" that spending would not exceed legislatively-determined amounts. Reimbursements under Medicare that have moved toward more bundled payments have not used spending limits [1]. There are some concerns about volume increases, even with bundled payments from time to time, as is evident from the proposal by the Obama administration to not pay for certain types of hospital readmissions that occur with the first 30 days of discharge from a hospital [5]. In general, however, concerns about inappropriate increases in service volume are primarily associated with disaggregated reimbursement rather than with more bundled forms of payment. While the spending limit will limit the effects on spending of inappropriate service volume increases – assuming they are actually used – there are some concerns that inappropriate distortions may be introduced by having spending limits in place in only one area of Medicare.

Provider reimbursements under Medicare are also updated by an administered process. Here, again, there is a distinction between the process that is used for providers other than physicians and the one used for physicians. For most non-physician providers, payments are increased annually based primarily on an estimate of inflation, assumed productivity enhancements and changes introduced by legislation. Physician reimbursements are updated based on the rate of increase in spending that actually occurred relative to the amount that was legislated to have occurred. From 1992 to 1997, the amount of the allowable increase in spending was specified each year by the Congress and adjustments were made to fees that reflected the difference between the allowable change and the actual change that occurred two years in the past. Since 1997, the update has been based on the growth in the economy although in most years since 2002, the Congress has ignored the reductions in fees that would have resulted from a direct application of the law and either held fees flat or increased them by a small amount. Because the Congress only provided the financing needed to fix physician fees temporarily, under current law fees are scheduled to be reduced 20% as of January of 2010. No one believes that will actually occur and the Administration has a "place holder" in its budget indicating that the physician fees will be kept "whole" although it has not indicated how it will pay for the fix.

The use of administered pricing has been Medicare's strategy to moderate spending because by providing an essentially unlimited choice of providers, it has left a minimal role for price competition. Getting administered pricing "right" is always a challenge as so many countries, including our own, have found during their brief ventures with price controls. Administered pricing is particularly challenging in industries such as health care which are characterized with rapid technological change. Unfortunately, not only has administered pricing not been a very successful tool for limiting expenditures in Medicare but its structure has had powerful and frequently unintended and undesirable effects on the services that are provided [27].

For example, the introduction of DRG's produced shorter inpatient hospital stays but also led to an increased use of hospital outpatient visits, and increased use of nursing homes and home care. These changes led to the changed reimbursements strategies for outpatient hospital stays, home care and nursing homes, which have also struggled with some of their own unintended consequences [27].

Neither the relative value based reimbursement for physicians nor the various bundled payments used for other providers under Medicare reflect the value of services provided to the people receiving them nor do they vary by clinical appropriateness or quality as judged either objectively or by the seniors receiving the services. Movements in this direction have been the subject of many reform proposals – specifically made for Medicare and also those discussed for non-Medicare reimbursement. This is an issue that is discussed more fully in the next chapter.

6. Incentives: Medicare versus the rest of health care

Most of the incentives in Medicare to moderate behavior or change spending rates have been placed on the providers. Beneficiaries pay substantial amounts of money out of pocket on health care but most of the payments relate to services not covered by Medicare or to pay for insurance that supplements Medicare. Because the supplemental insurance generally covers the deductibles, co-payments and at least some of the catastrophic protection that Medicare does not provide, beneficiaries tend to face little or no cost at the point of use for services covered under Medicare.

While most beneficiaries face few financial constraints to accessing care under Medicare, they may face other types of constraints. In some areas of the country, for example, new Medicare patients have been reporting difficulties getting appointments with primary care physicians. This is in addition to places with limited health care capacity where beneficiaries have historically reported difficulty accessing care [29]. In general, however, Medicare beneficiaries report good access to health care providers and the vast majority of providers accept. Medicare patients and accept Medicare as payment in-full. That is not really surprising given the amount of health care used by the Medicare population and the limited ability to charge more than Medicare reimburses that exists under the law.

Over the years, economists and others have considered the implications of the widespread use of supplemental coverage for Medicare and the increased spending its presence has meant for Medicare. There have been proposals to tax supplemental coverage to pay for the increased costs to Medicare, and occasionally even to ban supplemental coverage. The more promising proposals, however, have been to redesign Medicare's benefits to make the use of supplemental coverage unnecessary and also to allow for the more judicious use of cost sharing to accomplish various policy goals such as encouraging the use of high value services and discouraging the use of low value services and reinforcing other types of payment system reforms. MedPAC is once again raising a Medicare benefit redesign as a strategy to be explored not only to improve incentives for beneficiaries but also as a strategy to help improve Medicare's sustainability [21].

Medicare's incentives for providers vary according to the reimbursement strategy for the various services provided under Medicare. For those services that receive payment as a bundled payment – which includes hospital inpatient care, hospital outpatient care, home care and nursing home care, the incentive is to provide fewer and less costly services for the services covered by the payment. Also, if possible, there is an incentive to select healthier than average patients. There is also an incentive to increase the number of bundled payments, to the extent that is possible, such as by readmitting patients to hospitals or by providing multiple episodes of home care. The discrete nature of the bundled payment makes it more difficult to increase the volume for these types of payments but as the current interest in hospital readmissions indicates, not impossible. In addition, the reimbursement is also affected by the treatment that is selected for what may be similar disease states-such as bypass surgery versus angioplasty.

For services that are provided under a fee schedule, which most notably includes physician services, the incentive is to increase the volume, especially for those services that are well compensated relative to their costs or, at the least, to code them accordingly. The sustainable growth rate compensates in the aggregate for the incentive to provide more services by reducing the payment for all physician services whenever total spending on physician services exceeds the level suggested by the growth in the economy but the incentive that the individual physician faces remains that of providing more services. Some have even argued that since no one physician or physician practice is large enough to affect total spending on physician services, the sustainable growth rate may in fact encourage volume growth by individual physicians since physician fees will be reduced if other physicians provide more services irrespective of what any individual physician does [31].

The incentives in the private sector are more diverse because not all insurance plans use the same reimbursement strategies although many use some variation of the ones that are used by Medicare. Also unlike Medicare, private plans have made much greater use of strategies that combine incentives for patients or plan enrollees to moderate spending rather than placing all of the pressure on providers. Privately insured enrollees are much more likely to face financial pressures in the form of deductibles or coinsurance at the point of use than are Medicare beneficiaries. Increasing numbers (although still a relatively small part of the privately insured population) have high deductible plans, usually with some type of tax-favored account to use for care received under the deductible. Many enrollees are part of network plans where the amount of the coinsurance or protections for out of pocket costs varies according to whether or not the provider is part of the network. Some insurance plans are beginning to experiment with differential co-payments for enrollees who chose providers that are deemed to be more efficient and who provide higher quality services.

7. Medicare versus the private sector: Who has moderated spending or improved value more effectively?

There is an ongoing debate over whether Medicare with its administered pricing has done a better job than the private sector in terms of moderating spending and improving the value of the health care provided. The answer depends in part on what time period is considered, how spending is adjusted for differences in coverage and how value or clinical appropriateness are defined. What seems most readily apparent is that neither Medicare not the private sector have done very well in terms of delivery health care that is sustainable or that provides good value (i.e. outcome relative to cost).

With regard to spending rates, the differences between the private sector and Medicare are greatest when short, discrete periods of time are considered. For example, private sector spending growth was very slow during the early 1990's until the time around the passage of the Balanced Budget Act in 1997. Since then, at least in part because of the manage care backlash that occurred later in the 1990's, Medicare has been growing slower than the private sector [29].

MedPAC has reported that Medicare has grown about 1 percentage point slower than private insurance over the 32 years from 1970 to 2002 – excluding spending on outpatient prescription drugs to make the spending streams more comparable. However, during that period private sector benefits have expanded and in particular, cost-sharing arrangements have declined while Medicare benefits have stayed relatively unchanged. Attempting to adjust the spending streams for these differences is very challenging but not making an adjustment makes it difficult to compare appropriate spending streams that reflect comparable benefits [21].

During the current period and in the next 10 years, Medicare is expected to grow at a faster rate than private insurance. The most recent estimates suggest that Medicare spending increased at a rate of 7.2% in 2007 and 8.1% in 2008 while private insurance increased at a rate of 6.5% in 2007 and 6.3% in 2008 Over the period 2007–2018, Medicare is expected to grow at an average rate of 7.3% and private insurance at 5.4% [25]. These are annual average rates of spending and not real spending rates per capita.

The likelihood that Medicare can or could sustain different, that is lower, spending rates compared to spending in the private sector over any extended period seems very low. To do so would lay the program open to charges that seniors were being provided differential access to new technology or to high priced providers like academic health centers. Unless there was convincing evidence that the care being provided to seniors was superior in objective and measurable ways, any sustained differential is politically untenable. It is even less credible to imagine a sustainable differential occurring once the baby boomers start to retire in significant numbers. By the time all of the baby boomers will have retired, the numbers on Medicare will have doubled and the share of the population over the age of 65 will have approximately doubled as well. Given the higher voting rates of seniors compared to younger populations, Medicare beneficiaries will represent a very formidable power bloc.

This does not mean that Medicare and the private sector cannot or should not learn from each other. There are a variety of important and interesting innovations that are currently underway in the public and private sectors and it is important that each learn from the successes that the other is experiencing.

8. Innovative payment strategies

There is increasing recognition that the current strategies for reimbursing physicians and institutions used either by Medicare or by the private sector are not consistent with the need to produce sustainable spending growth rates or improved clinical outcomes. There are many different experiments that are underway in both the public sector – primarily Medicare – and the private sector to identify strategies that both encourage efficiency and reward quality.

Medicare has mounted several major pilot projects during this decade that attempt to reward improved quality and efficiency. The first two of these is a hospital pilot project involving Premier and a group practice demonstration. The hospital pilot primarily focused on rewarding quality but found that participating hospitals not only had larger increases in quality improvements but for at least some medical conditions, had lower costs as well [6]. The group practice demonstration rewards group practices whose patients show spending growth that is slower than the growth in spending for other beneficiaries in the area, as long as the group practice also passes a quality screen. This has proven more difficult than the ten well-established large group practices had expected. Only two had sufficient savings to qualify for any reward the first year although more qualified the following year [6]. Interestingly, even those that did not qualify reported that they believed that participation in the demonstration resulted in better care being provided, just not always with enough savings to qualify for a bonus.

Congress has directed CMS to engage in a variety of other payment or care coordination demonstrations over the past few years. A care management demonstration that was geared towards high-cost beneficiaries with complex needs was started in 2006. Although it was believed that a chronic care improvement program for patients in fee-for-service Medicare with congestive heart failure and diabetes would be able to save money and the fees to the organizations providing the services was contingent on demonstrating pre-specified levels of savings, the demonstrations has since been stopped when it appeared that the demonstration was costing money rather than producing savings [22].

Several other demonstrations have begun in the past two years. These included a demonstration to permit "gain-sharing" between physicians and hospitals that are not part of integrated delivery systems or financially at-risk in a joint enterprise. Others involved small and medium-sized physician practices, some in rural areas that focus on fee-for-service, which is important since this is representative of most physicians practices. Attempts to promote primary care which is regarded as a way both to indirectly slow spending and improve care coordination are also underway. The medical home pilot, which is one such example, provides monthly payments for each beneficiary covered so that the medical practice can conduct care management and care coordination. There are a variety of criteria that must be met by any group seeking medical home funds including the use of health information technology for clinical decision support, have a formal quality improvement program, keep up-to-date advance directives, and have a written understanding with the patient that designates the provider as a medical home.

Although Medicare's history is that even successful demonstrations have been difficult to translate into new legislation and thus implementation at the national level, it is possible that these newer demonstrations will have a different fate. Clearly the need to find strategies that can slow spending and/or improve quality and clinical outcomes is well-understood.

A variety of strategies and experiments have been tried in the private sector as well. Early in the decade a variety of pay for performance strategies were initiated, frequently by private payers – either insurance companies or employers. California has put in place one of the largest on-going attempts that involves seven of the large payers in the state, 225 physician organizations and 35,000 physicians. It started in 2002 and has gradually moved from rewards and recognition that primarily reflected process measures to increasing inclusion of outcome measures [18]. A variety of other broad payment reform models are also in progress. This include a primary care capitation with performance incentive model in Massachusetts, the on-going work associated with the Prometheus project that is developing global case rates for specified conditions, including risk stratification and performance incentives based on a comprehensive score card, and the episode-based payment that Geisinger is developing first for elective coronary artery by-pass grafting and also for other types of acute episodes [24].

9. Value-based insurance design: incenting consumers

Most of the examples of innovative designs being developed and piloted by public and private payers such as the ones described above focus their efforts on changing provider behavior – primarily changing physician behavior. A different and potentially important adjunct to these provider-focused initiatives is the concept of a valued-based insurance design (VBID) [14]. Under VBID, cost-sharing is varied so as to encourage the use of high value services and discourage the use of low value services. It can be considered an extension of the logic of the tiered co-payment structure that has been used by PBM's (Pharmacy Benefit Managers) to encourage the use of generic and preferred branded drugs relative to other branded drugs but in the case of VBID, the differentiation is based on the clinical value and/or appropriateness of the service or therapy rather than the purchasing power of the PBM.

Generally VBID is used in two different ways. One way is to vary the co-payment (or co-insurance – the variation can either be targeted to the dollar value of the cost-sharing or the percentage value) according to the value of the service on average, without differentiating how it might affect different patient of subgroups. The other (and preferred) strategy, assuming enough information is available, is to differentiate cost-sharing so as to target patients with specific clinical diagnoses and to lower the cost-sharing for the groups of patients that would benefit. As more and more information becomes available in what is now being labeled the move to "precision medicine", the use of VBID would suggest cost sharing should be lowest for those groups of patients with biomarkers indicating a high likelihood of clinical benefit with certain types of interventions and cost sharing higher for others. The development of a biomarker for the use of Herceptin for women with advanced breast cancer and estrogen positive receptors is the type of scientific advancement that could lend itself to use with VBID.

The potential to use VBID, in this case reduced cost sharing as a way of improving compliance for treating seniors with chronic disease, has been included in proposed legislation as a strategy for Medicare to test [15]. Although it is still relatively early in its development and use, the potential for VBID to impact spending in ways that could both slow growth rates and improve clinical outcomes should be enhanced with the increased attention being given to the development of comparative effectiveness research (CER). CER will be an important adjunct to identifying high value services and the subgroups of the population most likely to benefit from these services. The expansion of health IT will further increase the potential of VBID as it becomes easier, faster and cheaper to generate information about differential clinical outcomes associated with ongoing variation in the use of different therapeutic interventions.

10. Comparative effectiveness research

The focus on comparative effectiveness research – that is, understanding what works best, for whom, and under what circumstances–is not new but has received renewed interest in the United States as part of a set of strategies that could help slow spending in health care without adversely affecting health care and in fact, maybe improve health care outcomes. This belief has been reinforced by the research by John Wennberg, Elliot Fisher and others that indicates that areas of the country where there are high rates of health care spending have no better health care outcomes and are not more responsive to patients preferences than areas with lower rates of spending [28].

Many countries have used information on comparative effectiveness to support coverage or reimbursement decisions for drugs and devices as part of their national health insurance decision-making. These countries typically also have strict controls in place in terms of how many and what types of medical specialists are trained and licensed to bill their national health systems, how many new imaging or other high tech centers will be allowed and where they will be located, and the numbers, bed size and location of any new hospitals. Thus focusing CER primarily on drugs and devices may make some policy sense since there are already tight controls in place for other aspects of health care that are likely to increase spending. In the U.S., which does not have national controls in any of these areas and state controls vary in their focus and reach, CER needs to be regarded as an important source of information both for existing drugs and devices and also for medical procedures – maybe even more so for medical procedures since spending is so much greater for procedures than it is for drugs and devices [30].

Several attempts were made to pass legislation that would have provided very modest funding for comparative effectiveness in 2007 and 2008 including HR 3162, the so-called "CHAMP" bill that passed the House of Representatives in 2007 but was not passed in the Senate and the Baucus/Conrad bill that was introduced in 2008. In what was somewhat of a surprise, the stimulus bill signed into law early in 2009 included $1.1 billion for comparative effectiveness research which was allocated in approximately equal shares to the AHRQ (Agency for Health Research and Quality), the NIH and the office of the HHS Secretary. There was disagreement between the House and the Senate about whether the research should be limited to include only research on comparative clinical effectiveness as the Senate desired or be silent on whether work could also be supported on cost-effectiveness as the House preferred. The House language survived the conference process although conference language indicated that the funds should only be used to support research and dissemination of information and not be used to mandate coverage or reimbursement [30].

The issue of whether and how to bring in information on cost-effectiveness to augment the work on clinical effectiveness and how to make use of such information is a debate that is yet to be played out in this country. Most observers believe that as important as better information is, by itself it will not change physician or patients' behavior. However used in conjunction with changed incentives for clinicians and patients, including but not limited to such strategies as VBID and with a better alignment of incentives between clinicians and institutional providers, CER could become an important driver in the effort to slow health care spending and improve clinical outcomes.

11. "Bending the curve"

Strategies to realign incentives to improve value and particularly to slow down spending have been given the term "bending the curve". What that means is slowing down the trajectory of spending growth – focusing on slowing the growth rate as opposed to changes only in the absolute level of spending.

Actually, the last two sections of this chapter have already addressed this issue. Two of the important sets of strategies that can be used to slow spending in health care involve changing how we reimburse clinicians and institutions for the services they provide and making better information available so that clinicians, institutional providers, patients and payers can make better-informed decisions.

There is growing acknowledgement that the current fee-for service system drives and rewards much of the behavior that needs to be changed. Instead of rewarding the provision of more and more complex services, which is inherent in fee-for-service reimbursement, we need to develop reimbursement strategies that reward providers for taking care of the health needs of their enrolled populations, in ways that satisfy their enrollees and produce good health outcomes. It is within this context that many of the innovative payment strategies are being piloted. These strategies include developing more episode-based payments, such as is now used for home-care in Medicare, bundling payments for chronic care delivery, using pay for performance that blends patient outcome and satisfaction measures into the reimbursement, piloting accountable care organizations that allow physicians and hospitals to share savings produced by achieving spending and satisfaction targets, and developing new strategies that encourage both providers and patients to seek out new ways to integrate the delivery of services that work in communities that have thus far been resistant to such efforts.

One of the important changes that will need to occur is to facilitate the more rapid adoption of demonstrations and pilots that "work" into Medicare practice. The history in this area is not encouraging and indicates the need for more rapid learning and adoption strategies. Even demonstrations that have produced promising results have rarely become law or taken years for the statute to change. The Medicaid program started in Arizona in 1983 introduced strategies to coordinate care for its urban and rural populations to provide them with access to ambulatory care and keep them out of emergency rooms. This was done as part of an R&D waiver since it violated current Medicaid requirements and remained as an R&D waiver for about 15 years until the Medicaid law was sufficiently changed as to allow for it. If CMS is to help guide payment changes, it will need the authority and flexibility not only to engage in rapid testing and evaluation strategies but will also need the authority to implement the changes that produce desirable outcomes. Otherwise the likelihood of being able to make effective use of strategies that slow spending and/or improve outcomes – or hopefully to do both – will remain low.

The flip-side of a willingness to allow for a faster adoption of strategies that "work" is the understanding that downward payment pressure will need to be placed on providers and institutions that attempt to stay in the traditional a la carte fee-for-service environment. The ability to solve the spending challenges the country faces will be very limited if only rewards and inducements are considered for promising new strategies as opposed to a "push and pull" system.

In addition to adopting payment strategies that reward the types of behavior that we want to encourage in a reformed delivery system, it is also important to provide better information on comparative clinical effectiveness and to adopt appropriate incentives consistent with its use. That means a willingness to fund investments in new research and the synthesis and dissemination of existing research which unfortunately does not seem to be happening. After the initial bolus of money for CER in the stimulus bill of $1.1 billion, the various health care reform bills introduced in mid/late 2009 have allotted far smaller amounts to CER on a going-forward basis [19]. What is needed are annual investments in the billions of dollars rather than the $100 to $150 million per year being proposed. As discussed earlier, it is also important to put in place reimbursement strategies that encourage the use of information developed as part of CER such as the value based insurance design or VBID.

Although not really the subject matter of this chapter, two other issues need to be at least mentioned in a chapter on the health economics of a re-engineered health car system. The first is the need for a strategy that protects clinicians and institutions that practice in a conservative style from concerns of medical liability. Instead of focusing on caps for punitive damages, clinicians and institutions that follow a standard set of patient safety measures and where care is provided using the clinical guidelines developed by the respective medical specialty societies should be protected against liability suits unless there are provable claims of criminal negligence. It is unreasonable to expect individuals to put themselves at financial and reputational risk without such protection. An appropriate mechanism to help pay for the care of individuals who have adverse outcomes should be developed separately. The second issue is the need for a work force that is consistent with the reshaped health care system that is being considered and a payment system that recognizes the various participants that will be needed to provide services in a reorganized delivery system.

12. Conclusions

Health care spending in the United States is notoriously high – whether measured in terms of spending per person or as a percentage of the GDP. But curbing the growth rates in spending is even more critical than reducing the absolute level of spending. As the President has made clear, reducing these growth rates are critical to getting our fiscal house in order. It is also critical to maintaining any ability to keep the promises made to generations to come of seniors.

Although many factors contribute to the high and unsustainable spending growth, the use and dissemination of new technology is particularly important – much more so than inflation in medical prices or the aging of the population although both of these are also contribution factors. The country's fleeting use of price controls in health care – primarily during periods of war–has not been particularly effective although indirectly had a lasting impact since it produced the current tax treatment of employer sponsored insurance which has had a significant effect on spending.

A review of Medicare, with its reliance on the use of administered pricing, has indicated that administered pricing has not resolved the problem of unsustainable spending – not surprising in a sector that is dominated by technological change. This is not to suggest that Medicare has done worse than the private sector but it has not done particularly better either, especially if adjustments are attempted that reflect the changing benefits in Medicare versus the private sector. Projections for the next ten years, suggest Medicare is likely to grow at rates that will exceed the growth rate in spending in the private sector.

This suggests that that if we are to slow spending, the country will need to find new, more innovative payment strategies that are more consistent with producing sustainable growth rates and improved clinical outcomes than the administered pricing of Medicare or the reliance on fee-for service payments, particularly for physicians, that has dominated both Medicare and private insurance. CMS has been sponsoring a variety of interesting pilots to improve efficiency and quality. Some started relatively early in the decade and others are just coming on board. Whatever their results, it will be important for CMS to find ways that allow for the more rapid introduction of new reimbursement systems that "work". Provisions in various versions of health care reform that give the Secretary of HHS authority to implement promising changes in reimbursement will help resolve what has been an important impediment to change – promising demonstrations that are never translated into statutory change.

Most of the innovations in both the public and private sectors – care management, pay for performance or pay for results, gain-sharing, etc. are focused on changing provider behavior. At least one important innovation – value-based insurance design – attempts to use cost-sharing to encourage the use of high value services and discourage the use of low value services – brings in the patient as well in terms of changed behavior. To the extent that progress is made in research on comparative clinical effectiveness, it is possible to imagine a world where variable cost-sharing links to what is know about which services are likely to benefit various subgroups of the population and incentives are provided to encourage this type of behavior. As with health information technology, comparative effectiveness research could become an important enable of learning how to treat patients more effectively as well as learning how to spend at more sustainable rates.

Comparative effectiveness research, value-based insurance, moves to pay for results or accountable care organizations are all examples of what has now been dubbed "bending the curve" – that is slowing the growth rate in spending. Understanding better how specifically to bend the cost curve is our challenge.

References

[1] American Medical Association, The Resource Based Relative Value Scale. Available at http://www.ama-assn.org/ama/pub/physicians-resources/solutions-managing-you r-practice/coding-billing-insurance/medicare, 2009.

[2] G. Anderson and B. Frogner, Health Spending in OECD Countries: Obtaining Value Per Dollar, *Health Affairs* **27**(6) (November/December 2008).

[3] G.F. Anderson, U.E. Reinhardt, P.S. Hussey and V. Petrosyan, It's the prices, stupid: why the United States is so different from other countries, *Health Affairs* **22**(3) (May/June 2003).

[4] A. Caitlin, C. Cowan, M. Hartman and S. Heffler, National Health Spending in 2006: A Year of Change for Prescription Drugs, *Health Affairs* **27**(1) (January/February 2008).

[5] Centers for Medicare and Medicaid Services. CMS Proposes to Expand Quality Program for Hospital Inpatient Services in FY 2009. Available at: http://www.cms.hhs.gov/apps/media/press/release.asp?Counter=3041, 2008.

[6] Center for Medicare and Medicaid Services. CMS Proposes Payment, Policy Changes for Physician Services to Medicare Beneficiaries in 2010. Available at http://www.cms.hhs.gov/apps/media/press/release.asp?Counter=3469, 2009.

[7] Center for Medicare and Medicaid Services. National Health Expenditures, Historical Data, Table 1, at http://www.cms.hhs.gov/NationalHealthExpendData/downloads/tables.pdf, 2009.

[8] Center for Medicare and Medicaid Services. NHE Fact Sheet at http://www.cms.hhs.gov/NationalHealthExpendData/25_NHE_Fact_Sheet.asp, 2009.

[9] Centers for Medicare and Medicaid Services. Premier Hospital Quality Incentive Demonstration. Available at: http://www.cms.hhs.gov/HospitalQualityInits/35_hospitalpremier.asp, 2009.

[10] Centers for Medicare and Medicaid Services. Medicare Physician Group Practice Demonstration. Available at: http://www.cms.hhs.gov/DemoProjectsEvalRpts./dowloads/PGP_Fact_Sheet.pdf, 2009.

[11] L. Clemans-Cope, S. Zuckerman and R. Williams, Changes to the Tax Exclusion of Employer-Sponsored Health Insurance Premiums: A Potential Source of Financing for Health Reform. Urban Institute. Available at http://www.taxpolicycenter.org/uploadedpdf/411916_tax_exclusion_in surance.pdf, 2009.

[12] Congressional Budget Office. The Budget and Economic Outlook: An Update, summary available at http://www.cbo.gov/doc.cfm?indix=10521, August 2009.

[13] R. DeVol and A. Bedroussian, "An Unhealthy America: The Economic Burden of Chronic Disease". Milken Institute. October 2007. Available at http://www.milkeninstitute.org/publications/publications.taf?function=detail&ID=38801018&cat=resrep, 2007.

[14] A. Fendrick and M. Chernew, Value-Based Insurance Design: Aligning Incentives to Bridge the Divide Between Quality Improvement and Cost Containment, *American Journal of Managed Care* **12**(Special Issue) (2006), SP5-SP10.

[15] M. Fendrick and M. Chernew, Value Based Insurance Design: Maintaining a Focus on Health in an Era of Cost Containment. Expert voices. NICHM Foundation. June 2009. Available at: http://www.nihcm.org/pdf/EV_Fendrick_Chernew_FINAL.pdf, 2009.

[16] P. Ginsburg, High and rising health care cost: Demystifying U.S. health care spending.(Research Synthesis Report No. 16) Princeton, NJ: Robert Wood Johnson Foundation. Table 1, 2008.

[17] http://www.whitehouse.gov/issues/health_care/.

[18] Integrated Health Care Association. Advancing Quality Through Collaboration: The California Pay for Performance Program. Available at http://www.iha.org/wp020606.pdf, 2006.

[19] Kaiser Family Foundation (2009). Focus on Health Reform: Health Care Reform Proposals. Available at: http://www.kff.org/healthreform/upload/healthreform_tri_full.pdf.

[20] Kaiser Family Foundation and Health Research and Education Trust. Yearly Premiums for Family Health Coverage" News Release. Available at http://www.kff.org/newsroom/ehbs092408.cfm, Sept. 2008.

[21] Medicare Payment Advisory Commission. Improving Incentives in the Medicare Program, Report to the Congress. Washington: Medpac. Available at: http://www.medpac.gov/documents/Jun09_entirereport.pdf, June 2009, pp. xi–xvii.

[22] Medicare Payment Advisory Commission. Medicare Payment Policy, Report to the Congress. Washington: Medpac. Available at: http://www.medpac.gov/documents/Mar09_entirereport.pdf, March 2009, pp. 3–32.

[23] M.V. Pauly, *Health Benefits at Work*, Ann Arbor: University of Michigan press, 1997.

[24] M. Rosenthal, Beyond Pay for Performance, *New England Journal of Medicine* **359**(12) (2008), 1197–1200.

[25] A. Sisko, C. Truffer, S. Smith, S. Keehan, J. cylus, J. Poisal, M. Clmens and J. Lizonitz, Health Spending Projections through 2018: Recession Effects Add Uncertainty to the Outlook. Health Affairs. DOI 10.1377/hlthaff.28.2.w346, 24 February 2009.

[26] S. Smith, J.P. Newhouse and M.S. Freeland, I ncome, Insurance, and Technology: Why Does Health Spending Outpace Economic Growth? *Health Affairs* **28**(5) (September/October 2009).

[27] G.R. Wilensky and J.P. Newhouse, "Medicare: What's Right? What's Wrong? What's Next?" *Health Affairs* **18**(1) (January/February 1999).

[28] G. Wilensky, Developing a Center for Comparative Effectiveness Information, *Health Affairs* **25** (7 November 2006): w572-w585. (published on-line 7 November 2006; 10.1377/hlthaff.25.w572.)

[29] G.R. Wilensky, The Challenge of Medicare, in: *Restoring Fiscal Sanity*, A.M. Rivlin and J.R. Antos, eds, Washington: Brookings Institution Press, 2007, pp. 81–104.

[30] G. Wilensky, The Policies and Politics of Creating A Comparative Clinical Effectiveness Research Center, *Health Affairs* **28**(4) (25 June 2009), w.719–w.729.

[31] G.R. Wilensky, Reforming Medicare's Physician Payment System, *New England Journal of Medicine* **360**(7) (Feb. 12 2009).
[32] D. Yergin and J. Stanislaw, Nixon Tries Price Controls. Commanding Heights, http://www.pbs.org/wgbh/commandingheights/shared/minitextlo/ess_nixongold.html, 1997.

Gail Wilensky, Ph.D., is an economist and a Senior Fellow at Project HOPE, an international health education foundation. She serves as a trustee of the Combined Benefits Fund of the United Mine Workers of America and the National Opinion Research Center, is on the Board of Regents of the Uniformed Services University of the Health Sciences and the visiting committee of the Harvard Medical School. She recently served as president of the Defense Health Board, a federal advisory board to the Secretary of Defense and chaired their health care subcommittee, was a commissioner on the World Health Organization's Commission on the Social Determinants of Health and co-chaired the Dep't of Defense Task Force on the Future of Military Health Care. From 1990 to 1992, she was Administrator of the Health Care Financing Administration (now called CMS). She also served as Deputy Assistant to President (GHW) Bush for Policy Development. From 1997–2001, she chaired the Medicare Payment Advisory Commission and previously chaired a predecessor commission, the Physician Payment Review Commission. From 2001 to 2003, she co-chaired the President's Task Force to Improve Health Care Delivery for Our Nation's Veterans. In 2007, she served as a commissioner on the President's Commission on Care for America's Returning Wounded Warriors (also known as the Dole/Shalala Commission). Dr. Wilensky's work focuses on the policies and politics of health care reform, and on strategies to produce sustainable health care spending as well as establishing a comparative clinical effectiveness strategy. Dr. Wilensky testifies frequently before Congressional committees and speaks before professional, business and consumer groups. She is an elected member of the IOM and served two terms on its governing council. She earned her Ph.D. in economics at the University of Michigan.

Information Knowledge Systems Management 8 (2009) 195–207
DOI 10.3233/IKS-2009-0141
IOS Press

Chapter 12

Pay for value

Robert Smoldt
E-mail: smoldt.robert@mayo.edu

Prologue: Texas Bix Bender is not a known health economist. In fact, he's not an economist at all. He is the author of "Don't Squat with Yer Spurs On! The Cowboy's Guide to Life", and in that book he provides some insight into the issues that affect improving healthcare effectiveness and efficiency. One of his guides to life is as follows: "If you find yourself in a hole, the first thing to do is stop digging" [3].

1. Introduction

In healthcare we find ourselves in a hole. For many years, we have been expounding that our healthcare system does not provide the quality we desire and that it is too expensive. Indeed, back in the 1970's, President Richard Nixon declared that healthcare in the United States was in a crisis. Since that time, similar pronouncements have been made by many people. But what have we done? Basically, we have continued to dig, even though we were finding ourselves in a hole. It is time for a different approach.

In my opinion, the editors of this book have correctly stated the goal we should be pursuing: "We do not think that people want the lowest cost, universally available healthcare system. We think the central issue should really be the creation of a healthcare system that provides the highest value." It is similar to what Warren Buffet has said – price is what we pay, value is what we get.

The editors also identify a constructive approach for defining value when they say that it "includes the quality of health outcomes, the safety of the process of delivery, and the service associated with the delivery process." These factors would basically be the numerator of the value equation. The denominator would be cost. But cost can viewed from several different perspectives in the healthcare field. It could be the cost per line item. For instance, what is the cost of a chest x-ray? An MRI scan? A blood glucose lab test? Alternatively, costs could be viewed from the standpoint of the cost per visit with the healthcare delivery system. Under this approach, cost would include the encounter with the physician or allied health professionals plus testing, imaging, etc. A third approach could be cost for an episode of care – for instance, built around a hospitalization, thus including more line items and visits in the total. Or alternatively, we could think of it as cost per certain types of patients over a longer period of time, perhaps a year or longer. For example, cost per transplant patient per year (thus picking up readmissions, etc.)

It is interesting that when viewed within the perspectives outlined above, most people would agree that the best way to analyze cost from a value standpoint would be to take costs over a period of time. However, the actions taken to date to try and stem costs have been predominantly aimed at holding down the price per line item. Indeed, the Medicare program since the mid 1980's has imposed price controls as a prime method of trying to control costs. It has not worked. A pertinent quote from George Will comes

Table 1
The Medicare Price Control Cycle

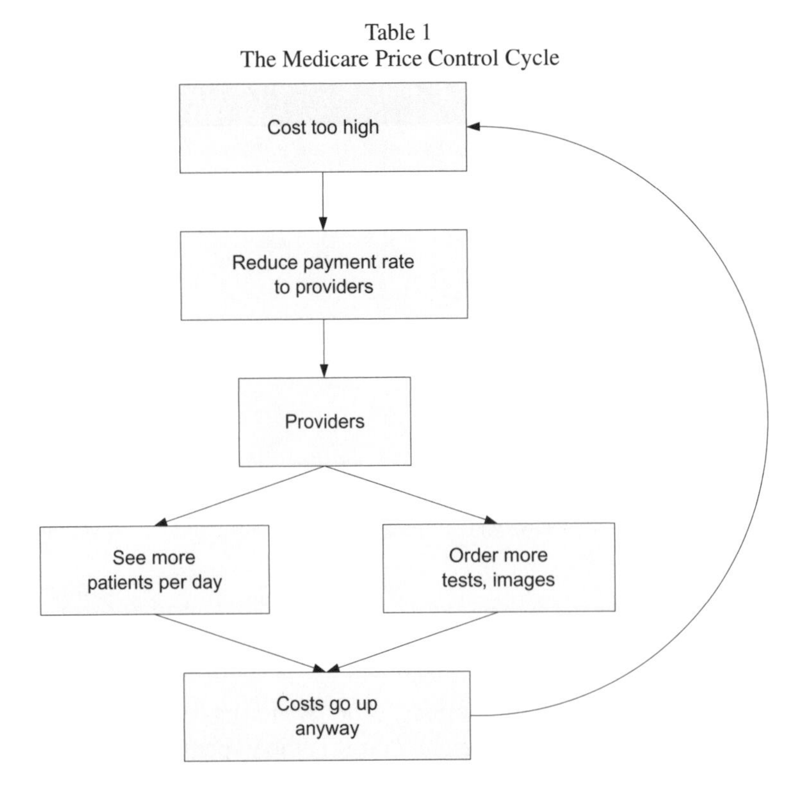

to mind: "...a policy that has a record, running from Roman times to the present, that is unblemished by success. It is the policy of price controls." [22].

The fact that Medicare price controls have not led to better effectiveness nor efficiency of care is heightened when one looks at recent studies that show that Medicare payment rates have now on average gone below the cost of providing care. Therefore, there is a significant cost shift that is included in private insurance premiums that are subsidizing care provided to patients on government programs [9, 12].

And what are the results of this healthcare delivery "experiment" of the line-item price control approach trying to controlling cost? 1) Patient time with physicians is down. As their payments have been reduced, physicians have increased the number of patients they see per day and spend less time per patient visit – thus, making the patient encounter less satisfying [7]. 2) Utilization of ancillary services is up. Partly because less time is devoted to the patient visit, more tests and images are ordered to discover the underlying nature of the problem and cover for possible legal issues if a medical problem is missed. Therefore, even though line item prices are constrained, total costs go up anyway. And as total costs go up, the government then restricts the payment levels even more, and the cycle continues. See Table 1. 3) Medical decision making not based on evidence or knowledge continues. The result is that more things are done to people, more medications are prescribed, and more devices are used. The approach provides no incentive to define what is most appropriate for specific individual medical cases nor to distribute the knowledge that is available for medical decision making.

The Commonwealth Fund has reported data that has shown this result for Medicare overall by looking at two time periods – one four-year period where Medicare physician fees increased and one four-year period where Medicare physician fees decreased. Interestingly, the overall physician service cost per beneficiary went up the same in each four year time period.

Table 2

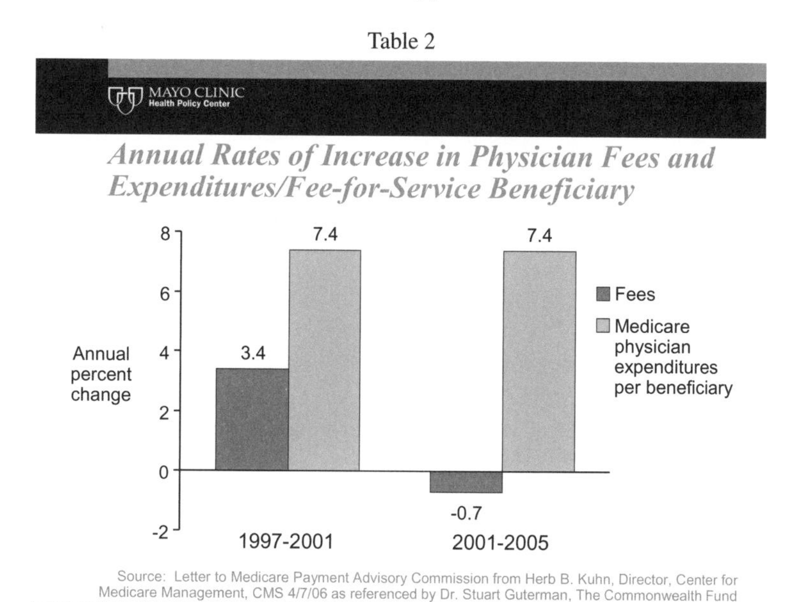

And to make matters worse, the price control payment levels are now reaching points where more and more physicians are and will be refusing to see new Medicare patients or Medicare patients at all [2]. This scenario is basically playing out in the manner economists indicate is the typical pattern for price controls – reduced access, compromised quality and costs increasing anyway. We need a better approach.

The fortunate thing is that a better approach is available. There are large variations in spending on healthcare within regions of the United States, and between healthcare institutions in this country. This has been studied for decades by the Center for Evaluative Clinical Sciences at Dartmouth. When comparing high cost areas with low cost areas, the Dartmouth team has observed that total health cost is derived from a simple formula: Total cost = cost per item of service x use rate of services. They go on to conclude that "utilization contributes substantially more than price per unit of care (line items) to variations in per enrollee spending." [6] In other words, high spending regions and institutions cost more primarily because they use more physician visits, more hospitalizations, more intensive care unit days, and more surgeries than those that cost less. Yet the increased use of resources comes without a demonstrated improvement in the outcomes, safety, or service.

Indeed, Dr. Jack Wennberg, the person who has conducted the most studies on the variations in cost of care between regions in the United States, has concluded that, contrary to what most people believe, price is not the key factor.

So if we want to stop digging our hole deeper, what should we do? If the premise of this book is correct, we desire a) good patient outcomes, b) a safe environment, c) satisfied patients, and d) efficient healthcare delivery with reasonable costs per patient over time. If physicians and medical institutions are paid for this package of desired endpoints (value), they will be much more likely to deliver it. In short, we need to move towards pay for value.

2. Pay for performance vs. pay for value

In recent years pay for performance has become a common phrase in the healthcare field. Indeed, there are numerous projects under way where changes in payment rates are made under a pay for

Table 3
Financial impact on two academic medical centers under present direction of pay for performance

	Academic medical center A	Academic medical center B
Hospital days†	11.2	24.4
Physician visits†	31.2	79.3
Financial results	$25,800	$44,000
Total CMS payments per Medicare Patient†		
Hypothetical		
Percentage "incentive" for completing processes	5%	5%
Pay for performance "incentive"	$1,290	$2,200

†Calculated on the basis of services provided during the last 6 months of life from Dartmouth Atlas of Health Care.

performance scheme. Most of these incentives target a mix of process and structural measures, with less emphasis on patient satisfaction and overall patient outcomes [18]. As stated in the Mayo Clinic Proceedings [20], these programs have varying payment approaches, but quality bonuses are common. Typically, payers give physicians and medical institutions an annual "bonus" or percentage for meeting a goal (such as prescribing angiotensin-converting enzyme inhibitors at hospital discharge for acute myocardial infarction) or withhold a small percentage of payment until the requirements are met.

The theory is that the process steps being measured represent good quality. Therefore providers following these processes should get a bonus. However, if the payment is given as a percentage of total spending per patient at the facility, it will also inadvertently give the greatest payment bonus to the most inefficient medical centers, as shown below.

In Table 3, provider A and provider B are actual academic medical centers from the same state. Assume that both complete the desired quality processes and are paid an additional 5% of the total CMS payment for meeting CMS standards. Both have a similar mix of patients and similar outcomes. However, utilization patterns (e.g., intensive care unit days/patient, physician visits/patient, etc.) vary greatly between the providers. Given the circumstances of this comparison – similar patients, similar outcomes – and the country's desire to improve healthcare cost efficiency, the efficient provider should be the one with the greatest payment incentive. However, under the present pay for performance direction, the opposite will happen. As Table 3 shows, the inefficient provider will receive the largest reward.

Years ago, Walter McNerney, who oversaw the integration of Blue Cross and Blue Shield and helped shape the debate leading to Medicare and Medicaid stated, "Although quality assessment is gathering institutional momentum, its value still hangs in the balance... poorly conceived or mismanaged, it can heighten cost and quality problems and, through narrow focus, keep the public's attention off the larger picture" [11]. McNerney cautioned about a burgeoning quality assessment movement that was permeating health care at that time. His concern was that overly simplified assessments of quality may not be relevant to the complexities of medical care and may subsequently compromise both quality and cost [11].

Payers creating pay for performance programs face the same issues. They have the challenge of selecting what to measure, designing a fair incentive plan, and marshalling sufficient numbers of patients so that physicians and medical institutions will take notice. Epstein [8] in the January 22, 2004, issue of *The New England Journal of Medicine* noted that

"incentives based on a handful of measures of quality may encourage physicians to focus their efforts on improving quality in the areas targeted by the programs, neglecting other important aspects of care. In contrast, incentives based on too many measures may overwhelm physician practices."

In their book *Redefining Health Care: Creating Value-Based Competition on Results,* Michael Porter and Elizabeth Teisberg [17] argue that many pay for performance efforts are not about quality results but are about completing processes, which may or may not lead to better results. "These current (P4P) efforts... carry some risks. Most... are not actually about quality results, but processes. Most "pay for performance" is really pay for compliance. Compliance to too many process standards... runs the risk of inhibiting innovation by the best providers." They go on to write; "The only truly effective way to address value in health care is to reward ends, or results, rather than means, such as process steps."

Results from a *Journal of the American Medical Association* report entitled "Hospital Quality for Acute Myocardial Infarction: Correlation among Process Measures and Relationship with Short-Term Mortality" [4] lends credence to this observation. In that study, the authors analyzed hospital performance on the CMS/Joint Commission on Accreditation of Healthcare Organizations process measures for acute myocardial infarction (i.e., use of angiotensin-converting enzyme inhibitors at hospital discharge, smoking cessation counseling, etc.) They found that hospital performance on these measures explained only 6% of the hospital-level variation in short-term, risk-standardized mortality rates for patients who had a heart attack. As a result, the researchers suggested that reporting short-term, risk-standardized mortality rates – outcomes – is a better approach to characterize hospitals' overall quality of care.

A more recent study by Landrum et al. analyzed care provided to colorectal cancer patients in varying regions. They separated the regions into low spending regions and high spending regions. Interestingly, they found that high spending regions had a higher percentage of recommended processes being accomplished on their patients. However, the higher spending regions also had a higher use of processes that were not recommended, a higher use of processes with uncertain benefits (such as using treatments when co-morbidities indicate no expected benefit), and most interestingly, the patient outcomes in terms of three-year mortality were no different between the low spending regions and the high spending regions [10].

On the basis of studies such as those discussed above, as well as their own detailed analyses, researchers at Dartmouth recently concluded the following: "Efforts to improve the quality and cost of US health care have focused largely on fostering adherence to evidence-based guidelines, ignoring the role of clinical judgment in more discretionary settings... Clinical judgment, not clinical guidelines should be the focus of policy efforts to improve the quality of care and address disparities in spending" [19].

In short, if we want to improve health care cost efficiency as well as effectiveness, we must move away from pay for performance approaches that reward process achievement, and move toward paying for value. Dr. Robert Nesse, a panelist at the Mayo Clinic National Symposium on Health Care Reform in 2006, used the following analogy:

> "What would the cost of a hamburger be if, instead of paying for the outcome of good food delivered in a congenial location by friendly service, we actually just paid for the number of cooks... and how many wait staff went by... The economics of health care are not dramatically different. We are paid for the process. We are not paid for the outcomes."

3. Moving towards pay for value

The models for how we might pay providers for medical services range from fee for service to full capitation. There is no perfect method. Both ends of the spectrum have strengths and weaknesses. As

Table 4

Growth in National Health Spending (NHS) versus Gross Domestic Product (GDP) 1990-2005

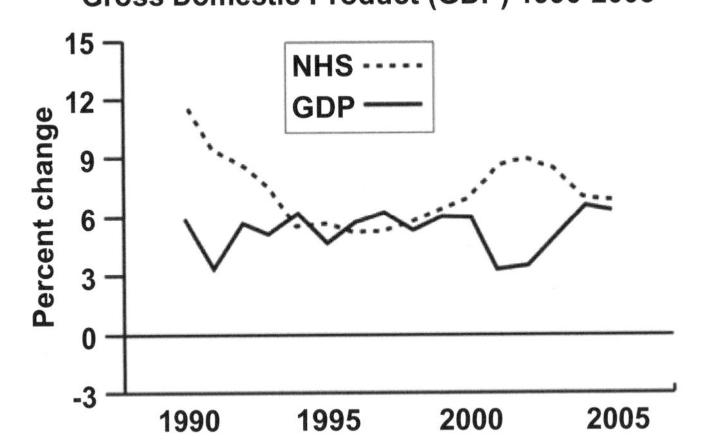

Sources: Centers for Medicare and Medicaid Services, Office of the Actuary, National Health Statistics Group, U.S. Department of Commerce, Bureau of Economic Analysis; and National Bureau of Economic Research.

stated by Margaret O'Kane and a diverse group of leaders in the May/June, 2008 issue of *Health Affairs:* "Fee for service theoretically aligns providers and patients interests by removing any incentive to deny or refuse potentially beneficial care, as long as the patient can pay what providers want to charge. Fee for service also protects clinicians from substantial financial risk for the contingent and unpredictable health needs of patients. The downside is that fee for service creates incentives to provide ever more narrowly defined, specialized, and higher priced services, even when the expected clinical value added is doubtful or non-existent. Providers gain from delivering more care, but are not rewarded, and will often lose revenue from evidence-based parsimony. On its own, fee for service payment does little to align patients and providers interests in improving outcomes while minimizing costs. Capitation is intended to give providers strong incentives favoring efficiency, but it also carries the potential to be abused. Needed care may be withheld, especially if capitation is not combined with transparency about outcomes and patients experiences. In the 1990s, questions about inappropriate restrictions on access to care led to a tremendous public backlash" [14].

In the zeal to change payment schemes, it is important to remember this public backlash in the mid 90's. Society is saying we need to reduce health cost increases. Yet in the managed care era of the mid 90's, health cost increases were actually relatively the same or lower than GDP growth. (Table 4) But as the O'Kane article appropriately reported, society rebelled. People felt that health resources were being inappropriately withheld. Thus as changes in payment approaches are made, the need for transparency of outcomes and patient satisfaction cannot be emphasized too much. The transparency is needed so that patients who experience lower resource use can see whether the outcomes from the provider are good.

This chapter argues for a move from a fee for service payment system to pay for value approaches. However, there is a category of patients for whom fee for service may be the most appropriate payment scheme – the complex, difficult to diagnose patient. Christianson and his colleagues [5] discuss this group in their recent book "The Innovator's Prescription" They argue that "solution shops" are needed for the complex patients. Solutions shops are defined as "institutions structured to diagnose and recommend solutions for unstructured problems." They go on to explain that solution shops exist outside of healthcare as well. They conclude that, "almost always, solution shops charge their clients on a fee-for-service basis... there are simply too many variables in addition to the consultants' diagnosis and recommendations that affect the outcome... and because diagnosing the cause of complex problems and devising workable solutions have such high subsequent leverage." Thus, even in an environment of changed approaches to pay for medical care, there is still a place for fee-for-service.

Fortunately, there are a number of models for changing how health services are paid that lie between these extremes. Also important is the fact that the payment models described below are not all mutually exclusive. Thus, some of them could be implemented in series or at the same time. In addition, they could be applied selectively to certain medical conditions. What follows are some payments schemes that would begin to reward value:

4. Shared savings

Under the shared savings concept, groups of high cost patients (such as patients hospitalized for diabetic-related complications) would be identified. A payer would determine the annual cost per patient for each separate provider system. The payer would share this information with each provider system, and offer to share savings in total cost per patient with each provider system that can deliver such savings while maintaining or improving patient outcomes. Employers (as payers) have an added advantage in that they can measure potential lower absenteeism and the resulting increased productivity from the workforce. This method of calculating both savings from reduced medical expenses as well as increased productivity of workers has been used in the Seattle area by large employers working collaboratively with Virginia Mason Medical Center. Interestingly, in those applications, the benefits of increased productivity and lower absenteeism were more substantial than were the actual reductions in medical costs.

While the shared savings approach has many positive features, it will be easier for medical centers in high cost areas and medical centers that are presently high cost themselves to achieve these savings. Thus, it provides less incentive to providers who have already been functioning efficiently. In addition, if there is no corresponding penalty for high cost providers, those who elect not to participate in the program would likely continue their high-spending ways. In other words, there is no across the board incentive to move to a more efficient care delivery approach. And there are huge variations in cost per patient – even between medical centers in the same state and in the same multi-hospital organization. As an example of these variations in spending per medical center, Dr. Wennberg et al., in an article in the November/December 2007 issue of *Health Affairs,* comment on the differences in Medicare spending per decedent during the last two years of life. For instance, they cite that Catholic Health Care West hospitals in the Los Angeles area spent $79,002 per decedent, whereas those in Sacramento spent $46,866 [21]. In this real world example, utilization again is the differentiator. The Los Angeles hospital used 87.6 hospital bed inputs per 1,000 decedents, compared to 47.9 in Sacramento. ICU bed use (the most expensive setting in health care) was even more dramatically different, with the Los Angeles hospital using 35.8 ICU bed inputs per 1,000 decedents compared to 16.9 in Sacramento. Now let's assume the Los Angeles hospitals reduce their costs halfway toward the Sacramento rates and that there is a 50–50 shared savings for the cost reduction between the payer and provider. In this hypothetical situation, that would still put the Los Angeles hospital cost per patient at $62,934 compared to Sacramento's $48,866. Yet the Los Angeles hospital would receive a bonus of $8,034 per patient while Sacramento's "bonus" for providing care that is still 25% less expensive would be nothing. In the long run, payment systems that actually reward all efficient delivery of care are needed – not just those to deal with the most inefficient.

Table 5

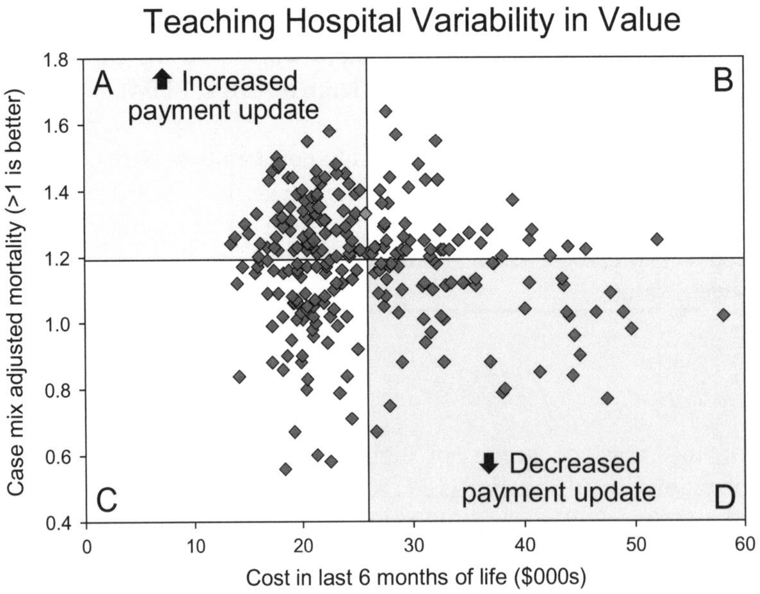

Teaching Hospital Variability in Value

A ⬆ Increased payment update
B
C
⬇ Decreased payment update D
Case mix adjusted mortality (>1 is better)
Cost in last 6 months of life ($000s)

[6]

5. Variable provider payment updates

Under this payment approach, a payer would risk adjust patient outcome measures (mortality, safety, patient satisfaction) on a provider specific basis as well as cost over a span over time – such as the Dartmouth Atlas costs in the last six months of life, or cost per cardiac surgery patient, etc. One might use hospital-based episodes of care since hospitalized patients account for the majority of health care expense. These data would be used to determine which care systems are delivering the best value (outcomes over cost). Providers delivering the best value would receive larger payment updates when the usual annual payment change is determined. Providers who are not delivering high value care would receive lower updates or perhaps no updates at all.

To give an indication of how this might play out for a subcategory of hospitals, consider Table 5. It shows every teaching hospital in the United States on an outcome measure (case mix adjusted mortality where 1.0 is average for the United States, and anything higher than 1.0 is better than the US average). It also looks at costs in the last six months of life from the Dartmouth Atlas. Each dot reflects a hospital in the United States. The graph has been divided into four quadrants; those in the lower right have poor mortality rates and high costs, those in the upper left have good mortality rates and lower costs. Under the scheme being suggested, when a payment update was scheduled, those medical centers in the upper left quadrant would receive a higher than normal payment update. Those in the lower right quadrant would receive a lower than normal payment update, and those in the upper right and lower left quadrants might receive a normal payment update. Clearly, such a scheme could be made to be "budget neutral" by having the percentage of increased payment update for the high value providers be the same as the percentage lower payment update for the low value providers.

In addition, this scheme does provide an incentive for every medical center to be an efficient provider. Thus, it overcomes one of the weaknesses of the shared saving approach described above. This payment approach could be phased in as well. For instance, rather than basing the update for all services, one

Table 6

Quality and Costs of Care for Medicare Patients Hospitalized for Heart Attacks, Hip Fractures, or Colon Cancer, by Hopsital Referral Regions, 2004

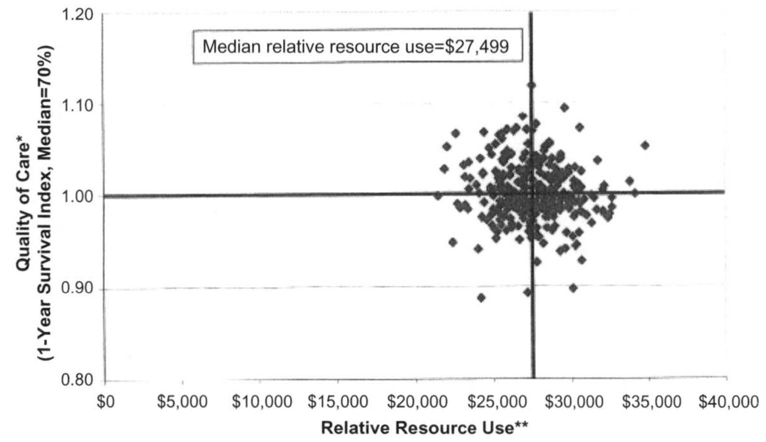

* Indexed to risk-adjusted 1-year survival rate (median=0.70).
** Risk-adjusted spending on hospital and physician services using standardized national prices.
Data: E. Fisher, J. Sutherland, and D. Radley, Dartmouth Medical School analysis of data from a 20% national sample of Medicare beneficiaries.
Source: Commonwealth Fund National Scorecard on U.S. Health System Performance, 2008

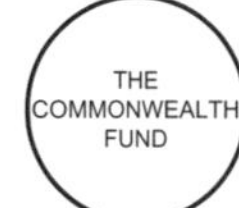

could start with variable updates just for the (Diagnosis Related Groups (DRGs) that cost a payer the most. For a few of these DRGs, teams could decide on appropriate outcome measures as well as how the cost per episode would be calculated. Then one would start the variable update just for those DRGs and gradually expand the number of DRGs covered. For instance, Dartmouth and Commonwealth have produced a similar chart for a more targeted group of patient conditions.

6. Chronic condition coordination payments

Under this approach, patients with one or more chronic conditions would choose a "medical home" (an organization with resources and infrastructure to coordinate chronic disease patient care over time) for their care management, preventive and minor care associated with those chronic conditions. The medical home would receive a periodic, prospectively-defined "care management payment" to cover those services. Acute patient care episodes would be paid separately under regular insurance coverage rules.

As the US population ages, an increasing percentage of our population is living with one or more chronic diseases. Especially when there are multiple chronic diseases, coordination of the care and assuring that patients are following treatment regimens becomes more important. Otherwise, over time, increased acute episodes cause costs to increase.

However, if immediate health cost savings are desired in the first year or two after implementation of these medical home programs, it would be wise to start them for patients who have been hospitalized for a condition related to one or more of the chronic diseases [15]. From the experience at Geisinger Health System, there were benefits from having a care coordinator for all chronic disease patients. However, those who had been hospitalized were the patients where such care coordination showed short term cost savings through reductions in readmissions to the hospital. It is understandable that the other patients will not show immediate cost savings because their chronic disease is not yet to the point where it is causing complications. In fact, for those patients, costs in the short term may actually increase. For example, an uncomplicated diabetic patient who is not taking her/his medications, is not coming in for eye exams, or regularly checking their glycosylated hemoglobin levels will likely be low cost in the upcoming year. A medical home would probably increase the costs for these patients, because of the additional health services that would be consumed. However, the potential payoff from avoiding complications in the future (perhaps avoiding heart surgery, amputations, etc.) could very well be happening many years into the future.

A Medicare demonstration project following chronic disease patients in 15 locations from 2002 to 2005 found a similar result. "... care models (that) enroll patients while they are in the hospital... have shown large reductions in readmissions... making this... (hospitalized chronic disease patient) a potentially rewarding one [16].

Thus, if a Medical Home program will be evaluated on cost savings in the short run, it is highly recommended that it be targeted to those chronic disease patients who have already sustained an acute hospital episode.

7. Shared decision making

Under this payment approach, all patient candidates for selected, elective treatment options or surgery, (for example, spinal fusion or bed rest, coronary artery bypass graft or prescription drugs etc.) would be offered an approved educational decision aid related to their specific disease/condition. This decision aid would provide education about the disease or condition. It would also explain the advantages and disadvantaged of each treatment option. A number of such Internet-based educational systems exist and they are gradually expanding the medical conditions and procedures that are being covered.

Under this scheme, medical centers would be separately compensated for offering an independent educational program to the patient. In addition, it would likely be beneficial for payers to create incentives for patients to complete the educational sessions. These incentives could include the payer reducing or eliminating co-pays for patients who take the education.

Some may ask whether there would be enough difference in the rate that procedures would be done with this type of education to warrant the efforts. However, the potential is larger than one might initially assume. It has been previously noted that Dartmouth has shown wide variability in the use rates for procedures in the United States. Henry Aaron [1] of the Brookings Institution in his book entitled "Can We Say No?" commented on the rate that coronary artery bypass grafts and coronary angioplasty combined is done per million population in the United States. He noted that the U.S. rate of 5,967 was almost four times higher than the United Kingdom. However, does the United States do too much, does the United Kingdom do too little, or are both rates questionable? Dartmouth has indicated that integrated delivery systems tend to do fewer procedures. Thus, using internal data from Mayo Clinic as an example of an integrated delivery system, the rates for doing coronary artery bypass grafts and coronary angioplasty on an age and sex adjusted basis for the same year was 3,179 per million population, or about 40% less than the United States as a whole. So what do U.S. patients choose after taking an independent shared decision making educational program? With regard to coronary revascularization for angina, the rate of patients selecting surgery was reduced by 30% – close to the integrated delivery system difference with the US rate [13]. Thus, the potential for substantial savings appears to be significant.

Table 7
Applicability of potential pay for value schemes

Payment approach	Acute conditions		Chronic conditions		Prevention
	Procedures	Complex, difficult to diagnose problems	High cost	Low cost	
Shared Savings (FFS)	√	√	√		
Variable Payment Upgrades (FFS)	√	√	√		
Chronic Care Coordination Payment			√	√	√
Shared Decision Making	√				
Accountable Care Organizations	√		√	√	√
Episode Based Payments	√		√		
Full Capitation	√		√	√	√

8. Accountable care organizations

Under this approach, a group of physicians and a hospital would be responsible for quality and overall annual spending for their patients. Physicians could be paid at normal fee for services and DRG rates, and then receive added payments for meeting resource use and quality targets over the course of a year. Since added payments would depend on meeting use rate and quality targets, it would likely lead to forming virtual accountable care organizations based on physician hospital referring relationships.

Such an approach is designed to create incentives for physicians and hospitals to work together to provide better value care. At the same time, in order for the virtual accountable care organizations to develop, it may be necessary to change some of the legal rules prohibiting collaborative efforts between independent physicians and hospitals. Since achieving cost savings is a prime objective, once again it would make sense to evolve into this payment approach by starting with those hospital DRGs accounting for the highest cost.

9. Episode based payments for hospitalized patients – 0r mini-capitation

This approach would provide a single bundled payment to hospitals and physicians managing the care for patients with major acute episodes. One lump sum payment for both hospital and physician services is different from the present Medicare DRG payment that only covers the hospital service. The new approach is intended to encourage the two groups (hospitals and treating physicians) to effectively integrate patient care.

Focusing episode based payments on hospitalized patients concentrates efforts where the large costs are. An advantage of this approach is that one does not get bogged down trying to change payment schemes for all medical services. This is especially pertinent, since 10–15% of patients will account for 80% of total costs. As Len Nichols, director of the health policy program at the New American Foundation said before the Committee on the Budget of the United States Senate on June 26, 2007: "The secret is not, however, to re-jigger 10,000 prices in 3,000 counties so that we get them right once and for all (or until medical knowledge or technology or input prices change again). The secret is to pay for what we want... while bundling ever-larger sets of services into one payment, which frees clinicians and providers to find more efficient ways to deliver health."

This approach would basically expand what currently happens with most transplants in the United States. Mayo Clinic has the largest total transplant program in the country. Almost all of our transplant patients are covered by mini-capitation packages. These can even cover periods of time that are greater than the hospitalization itself.

10. Conclusion

The need to improve efficiency of health care in the United States is evident. The theme of this book about systems thinking and engineering clearly needs to be embedded in our healthcare systems. We need much better application of process flow analysis, LEAN thinking, and various quality improvement techniques. In doing so, however, we should remember that the use rate of service is the real key to efficiency. It is important to do a heart surgery procedure or an MRI scan as efficiently as possible. However, it is even more important to have integrated systems in place that do no more heart surgeries or MRI scans than are needed.

How we pay for health services can not by itself correct the problems that we face of inefficient healthcare delivery. But they can help and there are a number of alternatives available. Table 7 shows that alternative payment approaches discussed and where they might be most applicable. It is time to get started.

References

[1] H. Aaron, "Can We Say No?" *Brookings Institution*, 2005.
[2] AMA, "Focused on Change", *AMA Voice* (July 2007), 4–5.
[3] T.B. Bender, *Don't Squat With Yer Spurs On! A Cowboy's Guide to Life*, Layton, UT: Gibb Smith Publishers, 1992.
[4] E. Bradley, J. Herrin, B. Elbel et al., Hospital quality for acute myocardial infarction: correlation among process measures and relationship with short-term mortality, *Journal of the American Medical Association* **296** (2006), 72–78.
[5] C.M. Christensen, J.H. Grossman and J. Hwang, *The Innovator's Prescription,* New York: McGraw Hill, 2009.
[6] Dartmouth, "The Care of Patients with Severe Chronic Illness; Ch. 5: The Problem of Overuse of Acute Care Hospitals in Managing Chronic Illness: A Regional Analysis." *Dartmouth Atlas Project*, May 2006.
[7] R. Eiselberg, Op-Ed, *Seattle Post-Intelligencer*, 15 January 2008).
[8] A.M. Epstein, T.H. Lee and M.B. Hamel, Paying physicians for high-quality care, *New England Journal of Medicine* **350** (2004), 406–410.
[9] D.P. Kessler, "Cost Shifting in California Hospitals: What is the Effect on Private Payers", *Stanford University Graduate School of Business*, 6 June 2007.
[10] M.B. Landrum, E.R. Meara, A. Chandra, E. Guadagnola and N.L. Keating, "Is Spending Always Wasteful? The Appropriateness of Care and Outcomes among Colorectal Cancer Patients", *Health Affairs* **27** (1 January/February 2008).
[11] W.J. McNerney, The quandary of quality assessment, *New England Journal of Medicine* **295** (1976), 1505–1511.
[12] Milliman Consulting, Inc, "Hospitals and Physician Cost Shift Payment Level Comparison of Medicare, Medicaid, and Commercials Payers." December, 2008.
[13] A.M. O'Connor, H.A. Llewellyn-Thomas and A.B. Flood, "Modifying Unwarranted Variations in Health Care: Shared Decision Making Using Patients Decision Aids." *Health Affairs Web Exclusive* (7 October 2004).
[14] M. O'Kane, J. Corrigan, S.M. Foote, S.R. Turris, G.J. Isham, L.M. Nichols, E.S. Fisher, J.C. Ebeler, J.A. Block, B.E. Bradley, C.K. Cassel, D.L. Ness and J. Tooker, "Crossroads in Quality", *Health Affairs* **27** (2008), 3.
[15] R.A. Paulus, K. Davis and G.D. Steel, "Continuous Innovation in Health Care: Implications of the Geisinger Experience", *Health Affairs* **27**(5) (2008), 1235–1245.
[16] D. Peikes, A. Chen, J. Schore and P. Brown, "Effects of Care Coordination on Hospitalization, Quality of Care, and Health Care Expenditures among Medicare Beneficiaries", *JAMA* **301**(6) (2009), 603–618.
[17] M.E. Porter and E.O. Teisberg, *Redefining Health Care: Creating Value-Based Competition on Results*, Boston, MA: Harvard Business School Press, 2006.
[18] M.B. Rosenthal, R. Fernandopulle, H.R. Song and B. Landon, Paying for quality: providers' incentives for quality improvement, *Health Affairs* **23** (2004), 127–141.
[19] B. Sirovich, P.M. Gallagher, D.E. Wennberg and E.S. Fisher, "Discretionary Decision Making by Primary Care Physician and the Cost of US Health Care", *Health Affairs* **27**(3) (May/June 2008).
[20] R.K. Smoldt and D.A. Cortese, "Pay for Performance or Pay for Value?" *Mayo Clinic Proceedings* (February 2007).
[21] J.E. Wennberg, E.S. Fisher, J. Skinner and K.K. Bronaer, "Extending the P4P Agenda: Part II: How Medicare can Reduce Waste and Improve the Care of the Chronically Ill, *Health Affairs* (Nov/Dec 2007).
[22] G. Will, "McCain's Housing Restraint," *Washington Post* (6 April 2008).

Robert K. Smoldt is Chief Administrative Officer Emeritus of Mayo Clinic. He served as a member of Mayo Clinic Board of Trustees and Mayo Clinic Executive Committee from 1990 through 2007; and is presently pursuing U.S. health reform in close partnership with Mayo Clinic's president and chief executive officer. Mr. Smoldt earned the B.S. degree from Iowa State University and the M.B.A. degree from the University of Southern California. He has given numerous presentations and is a recognized speaker on the health care environment. Mr. Smoldt has provided leadership at Mayo Clinic facilities in Rochester and Scottsdale. He has completed two terms as secretary of Mayo Clinic Rochester Board of Governors and served on the Mayo Clinic Scottsdale Board of Governors as a senior advisor from 1998 to 2000. He has been involved in health care administration for over 30 years – both with the U.S. Air Force and Mayo Clinic. Mr. Smoldt joined Mayo in 1972, and he has worked in a variety of administrative positions in both medical and surgical departments. Prior to his CAO role, he served as chair of the Department of Planning and Public Affairs. Mr. Smoldt also has been active in Medical Group Management Association, along with other members who manage and lead medical facilities across the nation – and work together to improve their knowledge, skills and the effectiveness of medical group practices. He has chaired the organization's research and marketing committees and has acted as moderator of its international conference in London, England. Most recently, he was a member of the Medical Group Management Association National Awards Committee, which honors those who make significant leadership contributions to health care administration, delivery or education in medical group practice and presents the following awards: Harry J. Harwick Award for Lifetime Achievement Award, Physician Executive Award, Fred Graham Award and Medical Practice Executive of the Year Award.

Information Knowledge Systems Management 8 (2009) 209–227
DOI 10.3233/IKS-2009-0142
IOS Press

Chapter 13

Reform incentives to create a demand for health system reengineering

Alain Enthoven
E-mail: enthoven@stanford.edu

Abstract: America needs a far more efficient health care financing and delivery system than the one we have. Our present system is a serious threat to public finances and is pricing itself out of reach. At the root of the problem are incentives and organization. The present fragmented fee-for-service small practice model is filled with cost-increasing incentives. There are some relatively efficient organized delivery systems, mostly based on large multi-specialty group practices. Unfortunately, most consumers are not offered the opportunity to save money and get better care by choosing such a system. This situation presents great opportunities for improvement in performance by re-engineering the system. However, for this to happen, incentives must be fundamentally changed so that everyone is cost conscious and care is organized in accountable care systems seeking improvement.

1. Introduction

The performance of America's health services industry is unsatisfactory in terms of its cost, quality and accessibility. (I do not say "health care system" because with a few distinguished exceptions, we do not have a *system*.)[1] What we have is made up of loosely connected independent actors each with their own objectives and purposes.

Physicians. Most doctors practice independently, alone or in small single-specialty groups. They have undergone many hard years of training, work hard now, probably left medical school in debt, and reasonably expect a good livelihood for their efforts. Doctors went to medical school because they want to care for patients. If they just wanted to make money, they would have gone to business school which takes much less time. Most doctors are paid fees for individual services ("fee-for-service"), a method of payment historically demanded by the organized medical profession. As increasing numbers of Americans are coming to understand, fee-for-service rewards volume of services, but not quality. It rewards pleasing patients who, once insured, may want more and more services, whether or not evidence supports their efficacy. And fee-for-service rewards doctors for resolving uncertainties in favor of more services, more tests, and more complex and costly procedures. And medicine is filled with uncertainties. Doing more, such as ordering more tests may also be a defense against malpractice claims.

Doctors want to be paid promptly and sue insurance companies that do not do so. Doctors often chose their profession because they value autonomy, that is, ability to exercise their own independent judgment

[1]The exceptions include real systems like the Mayo Clinic, Kaiser Permanente, Intermountain Health Care, the Geisinger, Ochsner, Billings, Palo Alto, Fallon, Dean, Marshfield, Park Nicollet Clinics and perhaps several dozen others.

in each case, not constrained by collective norms. This value of professional autonomy leads many doctors to be reluctant to share medical records with other doctors, which contributes to the general lack of coordination of care in the traditional fee-for-service small practice sector.

Hospitals. Most American hospitals are non-profit community service organizations. There are some very profitable non-profits.[2] Their goals are to serve their communities with high quality hospital care, and to do this, they want to keep their beds filled and to deploy the most advanced technology (sometimes referred to as "the medical arms race"). Hospitals compete to attract doctors with amenities and advanced technologies the doctors can use in treating their patients.

The Payers: Employers, Workers, Government, Insurance Companies. Who pays? These services are paid for, ostensibly, by a very large number of different entities, each with their own histories and objectives.

Insurance Companies. For example, non-profit Blue Cross and Blue Shield plans were created, respectively by hospital associations and medical societies to assure these providers that they would not only be paid for services, but would be paid in a manner satisfactory to them. Among the best known payers are insurance companies, now mostly investor-owned, that either bear risk by actually insuring individuals or members of employment groups, or that merely process claims on behalf of employers who are the real payers. Either way, insurance companies compete for business, both for free standing individuals and for employment groups. In the case of individuals, it is important to them to avoid insuring people likely to have high medical costs, and they employ many strategies that give insurance companies a bad reputation.[3] In the case of employers, they emphasize low administrative costs, because that is valued by employers. Most employers know or understand little about health care. They want to provide an attractive employee benefit, they would like it to be done simply and cheaply, and they do not want to antagonize employees by visibly trying to cut costs, other than raising coinsurance rates or deductibles. Each insurance company wants to be the sole supplier of health insurance or administrative services to their employer customers and they offer better prices if they can have that role. Seeing traditional fee-for-service solo practice as the norm, employers see little point in offering their employees a choice of insurer. Most do not.

Government: Medicare and Medicaid. The largest payer is the Federal Government through the Medicare program, which is the Federal program for the aged and disabled. Medicare is an open-ended entitlement. As long as a Medicare beneficiary obtains care from a licensed physician, and the doctor submits a bill, the bill will be paid up to the allowable amount in the Medicare fee schedule. Practically the only way that Medicare can save money is by reducing the prices it will pay doctors and hospitals. The value of this method is limited by the fact that expenditures are determined by volumes as well as prices, and doctors can and do make up for fee cuts with higher volume. As to hospitals, employers

---

[2]John Carreyrou, "Nonprofit Hospitals Flex Pricing Power," *The Wall Street Journal,* August 28, 2008, page A1.

[3]Reflecting the views and expectations of their constituents, politicians criticize insurance companies for their actions to avoid covering sick people. Part of the problem is a fundamental difference in understanding of the appropriate role of insurance companies. The companies see themselves as businesses, responsible to maximize shareholder wealth. On the other hand, many people think that insurance companies are or should be part of a social insurance scheme that should cover everybody, especially the sick. The Dutch have developed a model that reconciles these perspectives. In Holland, where they have mandatory universal health insurance, private insurance companies compete to serve individual cost conscious consumers, in a model in which they have to accept all who would enroll with them, but the Dutch government has created a system called risk equalization whereby the insurance companies are compensated for enrolling predictably sick patients, so they have no incentive to avoid enrolling sick people. The Committee for Economic Development has proposed a similar system for the United States. See www.ced.org/.

complain that hospitals shift to private payers, ultimately employers and employees, the costs they could not cover from Medicare payments.

Medicare is predominantly a fee-for-service small practice program – it had to be at its inception in order to gain the acquiescence of the medical profession. Medicare is caught at the intersection of powerful political forces that lobby and make campaign contributions: the medical profession including many specialty organizations, the hospitals, the drug and device manufacturers, and many other service providers who make their livelihood serving Medicare patients. Like the private insurers, Medicare suffers from considerable amounts of fraudulent claims. Congress will not let Medicare consider costs in coverage decisions, and will not let Medicare make suppliers of durable equipment compete with each other on price. Medicare/Congress sets the prices.

Other important payers include the various state Medicaid programs. Medicaid is a joint federal-state program to pay for medical care for "the deserving poor", that is mainly women with dependent children, disabled and poor elderly. This constituency is less powerful than the Medicare constituencies, and states are more motivated to save money on Medicaid. One main way they do this is by low pay for doctors, which leads many doctors to choose not to participate in Medicaid programs.

Ultimate payers. *But the ultimate payers are workers as employees or as taxpayers or self-employed and other individual premium payers. So called "employer contributions" really come out of the total compensation that would otherwise be paid in wages.*

Not a System. In short, the health services industry, for the most part, is not a system or a collection of systems each motivated to improve quality and efficiency. Delivery systems process redesign and re-engineering is the exception, not the rule.

Economic Consequences. The economic consequences include the fact that American health care expenditures are soaring, in 2009, likely to reach 17.6% of GDP.[4] National Health Expenditures (NHE) have been growing about 2.5 percentage points per year faster than total GDP for many years. Many public and private attempts to moderate this trend – Comprehensive Health Planning and Professional Standards Review Organizations by Medicare, Federal price controls by President Nixon, have failed to make a dent. "Managed care" introduced by employers in the 1990s did temporarily slow the growth in expenditure, relative to GDP growth. But the anti-managed care backlash led to some weakening of its controls, and expenditure growth faster than GDP resumed. Because about 60% of NHE is a drain on public sector budgets (including the exclusions from employee taxable income of employer contributions to health care, and health insurance for public employees, as well as Medicare and Medicaid) health expenditures now burden public finances at the rate of about 10% of GDP. That can be compared to the 28% of GDP the public sector takes in total tax revenues. So the burden is very large.

In 2008, health care's drain on the Federal Budget exceeded one trillion dollars (again including the tax exclusion and public employees' health care). Its continued growth faster than the GDP, and therefore faster than the incomes on which tax revenues are based, poses a serious threat to public finances and the ability of the Federal Government to borrow indefinitely at reasonable rates.

The rising cost of health insurance, in turn, has been driving up the number of people without health insurance as the health services industry prices itself out of reach for families of moderate means, or their employers, or taxpayers who might want to help them if the price were affordable. In 2007, the number of Americans without health insurance reached 45 million. With millions of people losing their jobs in 2008-09, it seems certain that the number of uninsured will soar. Many of these people will get their

[4]See Sisko, A, Truffer C., Smith s., et al. "Health Spending Projections Through 2018: Recession Effects Add Uncertainty to the Outlook," *Health Affairs* Web Exclusive, 24 February 2009. w. 346–357.

urgent care in emergency rooms where hospitals are obliged by law to treat them regardless of ability to pay. This is a very expensive way to provide care.

At the same time, indicators of poor quality abound: hospital-acquired infections, errors in drug dosing, equipment failures, errors of omission often raise costs and worsen outcomes.[5] These are symptoms of an almost complete lack of care management systems and processes to measure, control and improve quality. (Again, there are a few distinguished exceptions.)

Candidate Obama's Proposals. When he was a candidate, President Obama proposed some ideas for cutting health care costs, but adoption of his proposals will not come near to creating the savings we will need. He suggested, for example, that electronic medical records could save Americans nearly $80 billion per year. But information technology cannot bring meaningful savings if it is used in a health care non-system that regularly rewards waste and punishes efficiency, as ours does. Health information technology is more a matter of physician culture than it is of computers and software. For it to produce meaningful savings, doctors have to want to use it to improve quality and reduce health expenditures and be willing to organize appropriately to do so. Otherwise, just throwing money at information technology will be a waste, and may even make matters worse by giving a good idea a bad name.

Similarly, Mr. Obama proposed to save more than $80 billion per year by better management of chronic conditions like high blood pressure, heart disease, diabetes and asthma, and by preventing more diseases in the first place. It is true that most American doctors are weak on prevention and chronic disease management. But they will not improve until they have economic incentives to organize for these tasks, to buy the equipment and hire the personnel needed actually to deliver these services.

The Only Solution. The only truly promising way to save substantial amounts of money is to change fundamentally the way health care is organized and delivered. Instead of the predominant uncoordinated small practice fee-for-service model, we need to make the transition to large multi specialty group practices and similar organized delivery systems in which doctors work together to improve quality and keep costs low. Payment systems need to reward keeping people healthy while conserving resources, not just paying for volume of services. The most promising example is per capita prepayment, characteristic of prepaid group practices like Kaiser Permanente, Group Health Cooperative and others.[6] Their doctors share values and cultures of teamwork. They keep comprehensive electronic medical records, they share information with each other, and they emphasize disease prevention and chronic disease management as a matter of course. These doctors are usually paid salaries, not fees for services. Research and experience suggests that these practices and systems can reduce costs by 30 percent compared to the traditional sector.[7]

And the way to begin to get there from here is to convert our present health insurance system based on open ended commitments to employees and retirees to pay for traditional fee for service coverage to a system of choice of health plan (including those affiliated with efficient organized systems of care) and defined contributions toward consumer choices of health plan, which would make people cost conscious in their choices. Some employers do offer choices and fixed dollar contributions. For example, the

[5]The Institute of Medicine of the National Academy of Sciences, *To Err Is Human,* Washington 2000.

[6]See Enthoven, AC and Tollen, LA, *Towards a 21stCentury Health System: The Contributions and Promise of Prepaid Group Practice,* Jossey Bass, San Francisco, 2004.

[7]J.P. Newhouse, *Free for All:Lessons From the RAND Health Insurance Experiment,* Harvard, Cambridge 1993. Also the Dartmouth Institute for Health Policy and Clinical Practice, *An Agenda for Change, Improving Quality and Curbing Health Care Spending: Opportunities for Congress and the Obama Administration, December 2008.* The authors report that if everyone practiced like the Mayo Clinic, Medicare would cost 30% less. If Intermountain Healthcare, another large integrated healthcare delivery system, were the benchmark, costs would be 40% lower.

University of California and Stanford University offer employees choices and fixed dollar contributions, and 81% choose HMOs. In the State of Wisconsin, state employees are in a similar model, and over 90% choose HMOs. Hewlett Packard and Wells Fargo also offer fixed dollar contributions and choices of plan, and also have high market penetration by organized delivery systems. So market forces, that is, informed cost conscious consumer choice, could drive the transition to efficient organized health care delivery systems. In short, the whole situation calls out for a model of competing organized delivery systems which, in turn, would have to engage in large scale system redesign and re-engineering to reduce errors and reduce costs.

2. A thought experiment

To deepen our insight into this problem, consider a thought experiment in which each principle is taken to its extreme. Imagine three countries: one is the USA as it is today with its mixed and complex health care financing arrangements; another is Country A, just like the USA today except that all insured people get coverage from employers and government programs that offer open-ended commitments to traditional uncoordinated fee-for-service; and Country B with a universal health insurance model based on defined contributions for everyone combined with informed, cost-conscious, individual, choice among Accountable Care Systems, and managed competition.[8]

Country A is "the land of the free (health care) and the home of the broke." Country B is "the land of responsible choice and the home of sustainable finances."

In **Country A,** practically all employers offer employees a single insurance plan, traditional "free choice" fee-for-service[9] in which each patient has complete freedom of choice of provider at all times and an insurance arrangement that does not discriminate among providers. Or employees might have coverage through so-called Preferred Provider Organizations (PPOs) which are no more than discount fee-for-service.[10,11]

A few large employers offer employees a few choices of insurance plan and possibly carrier, including some with narrower networks, but in all cases they pay 80–100% of the premium of the plan of the

---

[8]Accountable Care systems are organizations that have in place processes for monitoring and improving quality of care and cost, and that are capable of accepting responsibility for managing them for an enrolled population. See Shortell SM and Casalino LP, "Health Care Reform Requires Accountable Care Systems," *JAMA* 2008; 300 (1) 95–97. Managed competition is a framework in which insurers, teamed up with provider organizations, compete to provide better care at a lower cost. This is explained later in this chapter. See Enthoven AC, "The History and Principles of Managed Competition," *Health Affairs* Supplement 1993; 12: 24–48.

[9]"Free choice" of doctor is in quotes because it refers to a particular historic demand of the medical profession that each insurance plan must offer complete "free choice" of doctor at all times, and may not discriminate against some providers because they charge more. See Weller, Charles, "Free choice" as a restraint of Trade in American Health Care Delivery and Insurance, Iowa Law Review, 69/5, July 1984. This freedom does not include the freedom of a consumer to limit his choices to one medical group for a year at a time in exchange for what he perceives to be better benefits at a lower cost.

[10]The name PPO was chosen to rhyme with the better known "HMO". The trouble with that name is that there is no care delivery *organization* there. It would be more accurate to call them "preferred provider insurance plans," because they are traditional fee-for-service insurance plans with the exception that they negotiate with doctors for fee discounts under threat that if they do not agree to discount prices, the insured patients will have to pay more out of pocket to access them. However, out of fear of antagonizing some employees, employers resist very selective networks and high payment differentials for using providers outside the network.

[11]The bargaining power of preferred provider insurance carriers is further degraded by so called "any willing provider laws" in some states, under which any contract made with some doctors must be offered to all similar doctors. This blocks the ability of the insurance plan to trade patient volume for price by directing patients to some, but not all doctors.

employee's choice, the most costly of which is invariably fee-for-service. In this scheme, employees have little or no financial incentive to choose plans with narrower networks because they can't save for themselves much or any of the premium savings. So, insurance companies have little incentive to offer such plans.

The employers who do not offer choices have to offer a single plan that satisfies everyone because they don't want employees to be angry because their favorite doctors are not included, or only included at a large extra out of pocket cost. That means, in effect, that if the insurance plan is of the preferred provider sort, it still has minimal bargaining power. Most doctors know that they have to be included. So the threat of exclusion from the preferred provider network is not a powerful bargaining tool. Also, in Country A, employer contributions to employee health insurance are all in the form of open-ended commitments to pay for all or most of the cost of traditional uncoordinated fee-for-service insurance.

Consequences For Health Care in Country A. Everyone in Country A is locked into fee-for-service. What are the consequences?

First, Country A. has a 19th century health system because they are unable or unwilling to subject their health systems to competition.

Second, the health care system can be said to be in "economic gravity free space" in which no provider is held responsible for the total health care costs per person or, except in extreme cases, the quality of the care. As I pointed out earlier, fee-for-service pays for volume, not for quality or for finding less costly ways to solve the patient's problem. Fee-for-service pays providers more for doing more things, whether or not more is necessary or beneficial to the patient's health. In fact, fee-for-service rewards poor quality care. If the patient acquires an infection in the care process, the doctors and hospitals collect more money, sometimes substantially more, for caring for the complications. Or if the joint implant comes loose, the doctors and hospitals are paid in full for doing the revision surgery. In fact, by reducing the revenues of cost-reducing innovators, fee-for-service punishes those who innovate in ways that reduce patients' need for medical care.

A few years ago, the famous Virginia Mason Hospital and Clinic in Seattle, a large multi specialty group practice, were under pressure from local employers to do something to reduce their costs. They did not have an engineered process for managing patients who presented with lower back pain, but they routinely gave most such patients MRI scans. Under employer pressure, the doctors reconsidered their care processes and wrote a new protocol which began the process with a visit to a physical therapist. (Physical therapists are the most appropriate providers in most of such cases.) The change reduced their revenue per case from a profitable $2100–2200 to an unprofitable $900–1000, from a financial winner to a loser. I doubt Virginia Mason will be motivated to search out many more such opportunities.[12]

Third, fee-for-service is based on treatment for episodes, not for the kind of continuous contact and support needed for the management of chronic conditions. For example, fee-for-service often does not pay for the nurses and other allied professionals whose services cannot be captured in a "doctor office visit." (To correct this problem, some specialized "disease management companies" were created that contracted with insurance companies to provide the nurse and other provider staff to contact patients and support them in management of their conditions. It would be more effective if this were simply

[12]See Vanessa Fuhrmans, "A Novel Plan Helps Hospital Wean Itself Off Pricey Tests, 1, *Wall Street Journal,* January 12, 2007. Also Hogangmai Pham, Paul Ginsburg, Kelly McKenzie, and Arnold Milstein, "Redesigning Care Delivery in Response to a High Performance Network: The Virginia Mason Medical Center, *Health Affairs* web exclusive July 10, 2007. The *Wall Street Journal* story goes on to report that the employers and the insurance company agreed to increase payments for physical therapists by 16% to mitigate the loss in profits. But the insurance company, Aetna, only accounted for 10% of the medical center's business and the other insurers, at least at the time of the publication of the story, had not agreed to such a change.

integrated into the process of medical care to begin with.) But some 75–83% of the costs of care are for people with one or more chronic conditions. Fee-for-service payment doubtless has much to do with the inadequate treatment of chronic disease patients in the traditional sector – inadequate treatment for prevention and management, but generous payment when the patients need to be hospitalized with an acute episode.

The New York Times reported that "Insurers, for example, will often refuse to pay $150 for a diabetic to see a podiatrist, who can help prevent foot ailments associated with the disease. Nearly all of them, though, cover amputations, which typically cost more than $30,000." [13]

Fourth, in Country A, uncoordinated fee-for-service small practice is not threatened with any competitor that can offer better value for money to attract patients, because typical fee-for-service insurance offers patients little or no financial saving for choosing more economical providers. There might be savings for limited episodes whose costs are below the patients' deductibles (that is, less than the $1500 or so per year that patients must pay out of pocket before insurance starts to pay), but most health expenditures are on costly patients who have exceeded their deductibles and out-of-pocket spending limits and are therefore in the "cost unconscious zone".

In Country A, there are no "Hondas or Toyotas of health care" that can threaten to drive out costly small practice uncoordinated fee-for-service. Some doctors did attempt to create efficient care systems in which they could offer superior quality at a lower total cost, but they were brutally suppressed by the medical profession that accused them of inferior quality. An anti-trust action against the conspiracy against such an organization went to the Supreme Court that ruled the actions of Organized Medicine to be an illegal conspiracy in restraint of trade, but that came too late to save the victim. [14]

Fifth, new technologies are seized upon and diffuse rapidly without proper benefit-cost evaluation. In fact, there is no cost-benefit analysis of medical technology in Country A because nobody is interested in it. Payers are firmly instructed not to take costs into consideration in making coverage decisions, as is the case in Medicare in the USA. There were proposals to create a new institute for comparative evaluation of new technologies, but the institute was not allowed to factor comparative costs into their analyses. And even these proposals were not enacted.

Sixth, occasional pressures on unit prices from some payers could be offset, often easily, by increasing volume. Doctors tell sick patients to come back in two days, instead of weekly, and appear to the cost unconscious patients to be giving particularly good care. Or they might order a few more diagnostic tests performed in their offices. Doctors might visit hospitalized patients daily, or even twice a day, even if they don't do anything for the patients on those visits. When President Nixon imposed price controls on doctors, the doctors were able to protect their real (inflation adjusted) incomes by just increasing volume of visits.[15] And the Medicare Program in the USA has an Office of Volume Response to estimate how much each proposal for cost reduction by lowering fees will be offset by increasing volume of services. [16]

Seventh, in responding to rising costs, some health plans and employers wanted to experiment with "Tiered High Performance Networks" in which serious cost sharing is used to motivate patients to choose doctors who rank highly in quality and economy of resource use. But consumers resisted because they didn't want their choices to be limited. And physicians resisted because they resist any form of economic

[13]Ian Urbina, "In the treatment of Diabetes, Success Often Does Not Pay," *The New York Times,* January 11, 2006

[14]Paul Starr, The Social Transformation of American Medicine, Basic Books, Harper, New York 1982. See also Charles Weller, *op.cit.*

[15]See Enthoven AC, *Health Plan: The Practical Solution to The Soaring Costs of Medical Care,* Beard Books, Washington 2000.

[16]See http://www.cms.hhs.gov/ActuarialStudies/downloads/PhysicianResponse.pdf.

competition among doctors. The medical societies brought suit against an insurance company that tried it and political and legal action forced the company to back down. There is no shortage of sophisticated arguments against any method of cost and quality comparison in Country A.

Physician culture in Country A emphasizes physician autonomy, not teamwork. The physician is 'Superman' who flies in and fixes the patient's problem and then flies away. Complex processes tend to be executed better by team players, but in Country A, this is a foreign thought. Patients too want to regard their doctors as Supermen. They derive comfort and prestige from saying "My doctor is the best" even in the complete absence of any scientific information to support that belief. Doctors in Country A do not systematically track patient outcomes. (Systematically here refers to having a full or large unbiased sample of patients tracked over the time period relevant for observing the outcome of interest.) Why don't they do so? The problem is partly the episodic fee for service culture. To be able to track all patients over time would require a costly cooperative effort which has not been a compelling interest of doctors in Country A. This lack of information makes it very difficult or impossible to compare the effects of different doctors or treatments on outcomes, which doubtless contributes to physician lack of interest in reporting such information.

Moreover, the culture of all health care providers is biased toward greater and greater cost. "Come back and see the doctor more often" not less often. Take the extra precaution, do the extra test. While some might ascribe this to income maximization, it can be explained as just a natural outcome of wanting to protect the patient in a cost unconscious situation. This culture is reflected in state laws limiting the scope of practice for non-MDs, as well as in the implicit norms of community standards of care used in malpractice suits.

Cost reducing innovations, such as "Minute Clinics" staffed by nurse practitioners working under physician-directed protocols are seen as suspect, a danger to health, not as a response to the needs of rational adults who have to pay for the services and may otherwise have to wait a long time to get them.

In short, costs rise inexorably in Country A because there is no incentive for health care providers to innovate in ways that reduce health expenditures, which innovations would reduce their incomes.

There is another large problem in health care in Country A. Government sets prices for physician services, an extremely difficult task considering the variety of specialties, services, and locations. Traditionally, fees are set when services are newly introduced and then very costly. As costs come down with experience, these fees tend not to be adjusted downward. Government inevitably makes errors in pricing, if an error means failing to set a price that elicits the desired volume of services at the lowest cost. Some fees are set too high in complex specialties such as diagnostic radiology and cardiology, which are therefore very profitable.[17] And some prices are set too low, as in the case of primary care, leading to unwillingness on the part of medical school graduates to choose primary care residencies. Unlike a normally functioning market, in this case the errors are not self-correcting. The winners recycle their windfall profits back into the political process in the form of campaign contributions. The losers have no surplus to use in this way.

Where is process engineering in Country A? There may be some directed to efforts to maximize throughput and revenue from existing facilities or personnel. What doesn't exist is engineering and re-engineering to find less costly ways of meeting patients' needs because that would lead to a loss in revenue.

[17]Ginsburg PB , Grossman JM. "When The Price Isn't Right: How Inadvertent Payment Incentives Drive Medical Care," *Health Affairs* Web Exclusive, August 9, 2005.

Country B "the land of responsible choices and the home of sustainable finances" is completely different, almost a polar opposite from Country A from the point of view of economic incentives. *Everyone* has significant financial incentives to consider the cost implications of their choices. In Country B, each consumer receives a "premium support payment" from government (or possibly an employer) a fixed dollar amount, usable only as a contribution toward the purchase of a qualified health insurance plan, meeting standards of quality and coverage, and participating in the regulated market. The contribution amount is set to approximate the premium of the low-priced health plan in their region, so that everyone can save money personally by choosing a less rather than more costly plan and everyone can have a standard plan at little or no cost. Everyone sees the premium of the health plan of their choice, which encodes total per capita cost, and everyone is responsible for premium differences. Consumers make an informed cost conscious choice at the time of annual enrollment, when they are likely to be able to make a considered choice, and not at the point of service when they may be suffering pain, anxiety, and uncertainty.

Medicare as we know it has been replaced by a model of consumer choice and regulated competition, along the lines of the concept recommended by the National Bi Partisan Commission on the Future of Medicare chaired by Senator John Breaux and Congressman Bill Thomas, in the late 1990s.[18]

Country B has a 21st Century health system because competition forced the health sector to innovate and modernize.

In Country B, the great majority of providers of health care services work for or in affiliation with a health plan that must compete with others for the business of cost conscious consumers. By organizational culture or contracts, each health plan must control costs so that it can give value for money and survive in business, and it must motivate its providers to be conscious of value for money. A large and increasing number of the participating health plans are sponsored by multi-specialty group practices.

Everyone is offered a wide choice of health care financing and delivery plan, including some "free choice" fee-for-service, as long as there is a demand for it, some preferred provider insurance plans, some with wide networks, some with narrow networks, also Prepaid Group Practices and other multi-specialty group practices with their affiliated insurance plan, individual practice associations, plus some selective Tiered High Performance Networks, etc. People are interested in these alternatives to "free choice" fee-for-service because by choosing them, they can save money and receive better coordinated care. The competitive market is managed, i.e. exchanges operated, by an independent Federal Agency patterned after the Federal Reserve with its long and staggered terms, independence, and expertise.

Managed Competition. The rules of the market include "guaranteed issue" (i.e. anybody who chooses a plan during the enrollment process is guaranteed coverage by that plan); community rating (i.e. the same price is paid for the same coverage regardless of the health status of the insured); risk equalization (i.e. a statistical process whereby the predicted health costs of each enrollee are estimated, based on electronic medical records, and each health plan is paid an amount that compensates it for enrolling predictably sick people); and standardized coverage contracts to make it easy for people to understand their choices and compare plans. The exchanges make serious efforts to simplify choices and to make shopping and switching easy. (The exchanges might be web sites. All this is the way competition is managed in Holland.)[19]

---

[18]National Bi Partisan Commission on the Future of Medicare, Chaired by Senator John Breaux and Congressman Bill Thomas, March 16, 1999. see http://thomas.loc.gov/Medicare/bbmtt31599.html (accessed February 9, 2009.)

[19]This paragraph summarizes the rules of "managed competition." See Enthoven, "History and Principles of Managed Competition," *op.cit.*

Standardization of Coverage Contracts. There were arguments in Country B against standardizing coverage contracts on the grounds that some people don't need and want some services (e.g. infertility treatment), and that standardization limits their freedom of choice. But the wanting or not wanting some insured services was seen as a way for some people to escape the risk pool, and contrary to the social-insurance goals of the program which include spreading risks widely. In Country B, people understood and accepted that taxpayer subsidized health insurance is social insurance.[20] People who don't want the standardized coverage are always free to forfeit their government premium support contribution and to go out onto the open market and find insurance. (This would be analogous to the situation in the USA regarding public and private schools.) That is the same freedom enjoyed by e.g. Federal employees, Stanford employees and others in such employer sponsored arrangements.

Standardization was seen as necessary because health insurance contracts are extremely complex, filled with technical language, read by practically nobody, understood by fewer and necessary to make people willing to make comparisons and to switch to save money, in confidence that the lower priced plan was not achieving its lower costs by not covering something important. The purpose of this, in the terminology of economists, was to make demand "price elastic", that is, that health plans could gain revenue by cutting prices. Also standardization can lead to much cost reduction and simplification for exchanges, consumers, health plans and providers. Doctors' offices would not be confronted with a bewildering array of different insurance contracts with different coverages and cost sharing provisions. (Maybe standard with a few variations or add-ons would accomplish this.) Good publicly-reported measures of quality and customer satisfaction were developed in Country B, and people relied on them as well as on the experiences of their friends.

Country B was considering "individual mandates", that is laws giving people strong incentives to sign up for insurance, but it was not clear that would be needed because people could always enroll in the low priced plan at little or no cost. Country B had a default insurance plan for people who had not enrolled.

Country B will look very familiar to people who belong to those few employer groups that have choices and fixed dollar employer contributions in the USA today – most notably, the Federal Employees Health Benefits Program (FEHBP), State of Wisconsin Employee Trust Funds, State of California (CalPERS), State of Washington, a few Universities (Stanford, Harvard, California), a few large private sector employers (Wells Fargo in California, Hewlett Packard) and some others. It will be less familiar to people working for large employers that do offer choices and pay 80–100% of the premium of the plan of the employee's choice, because these people will have a chance, under Country B's plan, to keep 100% of the savings from choosing a less costly plan.

Accountable Care Systems. Experience with these "fixed dollar" groups tells us that a high and growing percentage of people will migrate to what they see as value for money, usually among the lower cost plans. Gradually and voluntarily, Country B's health care financing and delivery system will become dominated by what Shortell and Casalino call *"Accountable Care Systems."* An Accountable Care System (ACS) is an entity that can implement organized processes for improving quality and controlling the costs of care and be held accountable for the results."[21] They mention five different kinds of entity in the USA today that could be candidates for the ACS role: multi specialty group practices,

[20] Wikipedia defines social insurance as any government-sponsored program with the following four characteristics: 1. the benefits, eligibility requirements and other aspects of the program are defined by statute; 2. explicit provision is made to account for the income and expenses; 3. it is funded by taxes or premiums paid by (or on behalf of) participants (although additional sources of funding may be provided as well); and 4. The program serves a defined population, and participation is either compulsory or the program is heavily enough subsidized that most eligible individuals choose to participate.

[21] Shortell and Casalino, *op.cit.*

some of which are prepaid and therefore ACS today; hospital-medical staff organizations; Physician-Hospital Organizations (PHO); interdependent physician associations (IPA) and Health-Plan provider organizations. In Country B, most of the above moved rapidly to ACS status because the competitors in Country B's marketplace have to bear risk for total per capita costs, and compete on value for money.

Providers have a choice: don't join or form an ACS, maintain their freedom of practice and autonomy, and have their insured services marketed through the wide-access PPOs or "free choice" fee-for-service plans, or practice independently outside the insurance system. Some prosper offering "concierge medical practices". In fact, some offer concierge practices to people insured with the various ACS and serve as convenient primary care physicians as well as guides to their patients' ACS providers. But most ACS's compete by offering excellent primary care so that the extra expense of a concierge doctor is not needed.

Comparative Cost-Benefit Evaluation. Country B has created a well-funded independent Institute for Comparative Cost-Benefit Evaluation to study new and established medical technologies and to publish findings as to whether they are "proven"" and not "experimental", and on their effectiveness, safety and cost compared to alternatives. The Institute needs to be well funded because its role includes organizing and conducting clinical trials, where needed or likely to have a large impact on outcomes or costs or both. And it needs to be independently funded, in a manner analogous to the Federal Reserve, so that its funding will not be vulnerable to annual Congressional appropriations. In Country B, they learned that some technologies that are found to be wanting are made in the home district of some member of Congress, or are made by some generous campaign contributor, and it is very important that the Institute can do its deliberations without fear of retaliation in case their findings displease someone. Their product is unbiased evaluative information, and not decisions about what is covered. The independent ACS's are responsible for that.

Expectations for Health Care in Country B. What might one reasonably expect of the health care financing and delivery system in Country B? First, it would become a vital economic necessity for most providers to form and join an ACS, to improve quality and reduce risk-adjusted total per person cost. (As noted above, some could choose to work independently outside the system.) Because of the risk equalization system, care systems would not need to be afraid of developing a reputation for excellence in the care of some chronic condition. On the contrary, if paid for, e.g. the average costs of a diabetic, they might judge that with their superior treatment processes, their diabetic patients would cost substantially less than the average, and they would be able to make a good profit while delivering excellent care. (There is a basis in actual fact for this example in the Dutch health care system.)

At first, every ACS would grab the low-hanging fruit, eliminating unnecessary tests and procedures, and improving outpatient management of chronic conditions to prevent patients from needing hospital.

Then they would begin to change the personnel mix. Every ACS would understand that excellence in primary care is a necessary foundation for an effective economical care system. Primary care physicians advise patients how to stay or become healthy, monitor for chronic conditions, then, in consultation with appropriate specialists, organize and carry out the management of their conditions. The primary care physician coordinates all of the patient's care.

Then ACS's would pursue higher-hanging fruit, such as reviewing all care processes against evidence and redesigning them appropriately. The evidence would include analysis of their own experience as described in their comprehensive electronic records systems. They would re-engineer processes, seeking to improve effectiveness and safety, and to reduce costs. When the ACS is responsible for and paid by total per capita costs, the savings from such process improvement fall right to the bottom line.

Examples of Process Redesign in the USA. One example of process redesign occurred in a large clinic in Minnesota in the 1980s. The previous practice was that when a patient called the nurse and asked for an appointment with the doctor, the nurse arranged the appointment, the patient came in, often a day or two later, the doctor examined and prescribed, the patient took the prescription to the drugstore, filled the prescription and began the treatment. Then the patient came back again to see the doctor a few days later just to make sure things were all right. Some of these patients were women with urinary tract infections. Under the new process, the nurse asked the patient about her problem. If the answers suggested urinary tract infection, the nurse asked a prescribed set of questions. If the answers indicated urinary tract infection, the nurse would say to the patient "please tell me the most convenient drug store for you, and I will telephone your prescription on behalf of the doctor. Follow the directions. Then if you aren't better in several days, we will arrange for you to see the doctor." In most cases, the prescription cured the patient. This process redesign cut out two doctor visits and initiated treatment much sooner than if the patient had had to wait a few days to see the doctor. One visit to the convenient drug store led to the solution of her problem. The transition to the new process was facilitated by a parallel transition from fee-for-service payment to doctors, to salaries. That change meant the doctors could adopt the new protocol without fear of loss of income.

Electronic Patient-Provider Interface. A large class of process improvement now being done in the USA involves improvements in the customer/patient interaction with the provider system by deployment of Information Technology. Banks are improving customer service with ATM's and electronic access to account information and bill paying. Airlines are reducing their service costs by allowing (or rewarding) passengers to make reservations on the internet. Leading multi-specialty group medical practices, like Kaiser Permanente and the Palo Alto Medical Foundation are using the Internet to allow patients to access their doctors on secure email; to make appointments; to receive test results; to have prescriptions sent to the pharmacy electronically; to request prescription refills, and now to request a complete Electronic Medical Record on a memory device. The Electronic Medical Records facilitate the work of primary care physicians in reviewing the status of their chronic disease patients to be sure the recommended actions have been taken, and they permit multiple doctors caring for the same patient to share complete information on the patient conveniently.

Two more examples were provided by my former student, Martha Gilmore, MBA, now Medical Group Administrator for Kaiser Permanente Medical Center, South San Francisco. In the first example, a woman with a suspicious breast lump enters a complex world of physician consultations and imaging tests. This is a very stressful time for the patient and dealing with a complex system can increase anxiety. While clinical care has improved over time with changes in technology and physician expertise, in many healthcare systems, the individual patient must schedule her own appointments and track the process between the physicians in primary care, radiology and surgery.

In early 2000, the physicians and staff at Kaiser Permanente San Diego set a goal to reduce the amount of time from suspicion to diagnosis.

Dr. Steven Feitelberg, Physician Director for Quality and Assistant Medical Director and his administrative partner pulled together a team representing all the clinicians, technical staff and clerical staff who touch the patient – the primary care physician, the mammography service, the radiologist, the surgeon, the nurse case manager and the appointment scheduler.

The group found multiple departments owning parts of the workup, also found several opportunities to improve the coordination between the departments. The team mapped out the current process starting with all the ways a suspicious lump is first detected – by the primary care physician, as a result of a screening mammogram or by the woman. Each subsequent step was carefully documented and discussed, concluding with the communication of final diagnosis to the woman. The process picture was highly complex and fraught with variation. The team found opportunities to eliminate steps and decrease the variation in performance. The end result was markedly fewer sleepless nights for the patients and most patients getting an answer within 1–2 days.

The key system changes are noted below:

- The Radiologists agreed to assume responsibility for the care of a type of breast lump that was previously referred to a surgeon. New stereo-tactic technology allowed radiologists to perform a mammogram, followed with an ultrasound if needed, and finally, if indicated, conduct a radiologically-directed biopsy. This process change saved a number of appointments and decreased the wait time for the diagnosis.
- The Radiology department structured a case-manager-appointment scheduler role so one person could work with the patient in timely scheduling of follow-up appointments.
- Measurement tools were developed and tracked regularly on each step in the system, including from the initial call to booking an exam, from screening mammogram to ultrasound, from ultrasound to stereo tactic breast biopsy and ultimately to definitive therapy – reassurance or surgery.
- Surgical access improved dramatically as the surgeons only received appropriate candidates for surgical intervention.
- Role of the breast care coordinator was enhanced to include specific accountabilities for coordinating the care and ensuring timely follow-up of patients.

The lean process simplified the workup creating capacity all along the care delivery system. The changes greatly improved both patient and physician satisfaction.

A second example, one of Continuous Quality Improvement in action,[22] was the recognition that in the case of acute heart attacks, time is heart muscle. Ten years ago, it commonly took one or more hours for the patient to receive drug therapy to dissolve the blood clot and save heart muscle. The physicians at Kaiser Permanente South San Francisco decided to redesign the process through careful study and collaboration. The community standard at the time involved three different physicians – the Emergency Room physician, the hospital-based Internist and the Cardiologist to determine the patient's treatment course. The clock ticked by as each of these physicians came to assess the patient. Kaiser Permanente physicians, nurses, pharmacists, management and tech staff were convinced they could improve the process of delivering this care, and significantly improve the outcomes.

Representatives from each of these groups of professionals sat down with the goal of improving the efficiency and effectiveness of the care. This multidisciplinary team did a process map to document the many steps and handoffs, set targets based on national standards and developed measurement and data collection tools. The hospital and physician leadership empowered the team to make changes and supported examination of data for continued improvement to the process. Dr. William Plautz, Physician Director for Quality and an Emergency Room physician, is proud of the outcome of the team. Today, every patient receives appropriate drug treatment in less than 30 minutes.

The global measurement was "Door to Drug". The team made significant changes in each of the three major process steps: Door to Data, Data to Decision and Decision to Drug.

Door to Data:

- All Emergency Room RNs were trained to quickly evaluate chest pain and prioritize obtaining an EKG. This required the RNs to abandon old practice patterns and move patients directly into a bed prior to obtaining a complete history. The RN staff also needed reassurance that the physicians would support their assessment.

[22]For a description of Continuous Quality Improvement, see Berwick DM, *Curing Health Care,* Jossey Bass, San Francisco, 1990.

- The RNs, Techs and physicians reached agreement on a system to assign patients to an available bed.
- All staff – nurses and techs – became competent in acquiring an EKG.

Data to Decision:

- The RNs and MDs reached agreement on which MD would be assigned to these patients to avoid confusion and delays. The completed EKG is physically handed to the appropriate MD.
- The Internists, Cardiologists and Emergency Room physicians agreed that the Emergency Room physician would read the EKG and make the decision about thrombolytic treatment. The Cardiologists agreed to be available to receive faxes of EKGs (now available electronically) if the Emergency Room physician needed decision making support. Initially all cases were retrospectively reviewed for education and quality improvement purposes.

Decision to Drug:

- The thrombolytic drug was removed from the pharmacy and placed in a unique locked box in the Emergency Department along with preprinted thrombolytic orders, a tool for assessing and recording indications and contraindications and other necessary supplies.

The team of front line staff and physicians eliminated steps, streamlined care based on the physical constraints of the department and achieved large savings in heart muscle. [23]

Country B would be a very good place for people like industrial engineers who specialize in care process engineering. Initially, a great deal of the work would be making sure that the delivery system took full advantage of the opportunities for process improvement offered by the deployment of information technology. However, most of this work does not require people with degrees in Industrial Engineering. Much of it takes training in Continuous Quality Improvement and similar techniques. "Quantitative common sense" and the ability and willingness to gather and analyze data using basic statistical methods plus a good understanding of the care processes are good qualifications. [24]

ACS would be strongly motivated to use personnel efficiently, as in the case of the number of surgeons retained to meet the needs of their enrolled populations. Compared to the oversupply of specialists in Country A, country B's systems would retain just the right number of specialists so that they would be fully occupied seeing the patients that need to be seen by them, making a good living at a low cost per case because they would have full schedules. They would be proficient and, in the case of surgeons, not tempted to recommend inappropriate operations because they would be fully occupied with patients that need them.

Disruptive Innovation. Christensen, Grossman and Hwang write of *disruptive innovation.* "The products and services offered in nearly every industry, at their outset, are so complicated and expensive that only people with a lot of money can afford them, and only people with a lot of expertise can provide them or use them.... At some point, however, a force transformed other industries, making their products and services so much more affordable and accessible that a much larger population of people

[23]In 2002, the California Office of Statewide Health Planning and Development published a report comparing risk adjusted 30 day mortality for heart attacks in different hospitals in California. The average for Kaiser Permanente hospitals was 8% whereas the average for non-Kaiser hospitals was 13%. See California Hospital Outcomes Project: Heart Attack Outcomes 1996–1998, Volume 1, Office of Statewide Health Planning and Development, 2002.

[24]As a business school professor, I cannot resist suggesting that the training our MBAs receive is very well suited to quality improvement work.

could purchase them, and people with less training could competently provide them and use them."[25] *Disruptive innovation* consists of "a sophisticated technology whose purpose is to simplify. It routinizes the solution to problems that previously had required unstructured processes of intuitive experiment to resolve;" a 'business model innovation [that] can profitably deliver these simplified solutions to customers in ways that make them affordable. . . " and a value network, a commercial infrastructure that facilitates the innovation." One can imagine care systems seeking technologies that routinize specialist tasks so that primary care physicians can perform them, or even nurse practitioners. A key part of cost reduction will be reduction in need for extremely highly trained and therefore expensive people through task simplification and process redesign. In Country B, many industrial engineers would be at work on just such efforts.

As one example, years ago I read a journal article describing a clinical trial in which specially trained nurse practitioners and gastroenterologists did colonoscopies. The nurses did just as well as the gastroenterologists. I mentioned this to a visiting group from an Academic Health Center, and one of their doctors said "we did a similar trial comparing heart catheterizations done by cardiologists and by technicians, and the technicians did just as well. After all, it is mainly hand-eye coordination."

Engineers could work with the high priced specialists to see at each step "doctor, how can this process be made simpler and easier for you so that you can be more productive?"

Knowledge Management. An important part of the processes of the ACS is knowledge management and guidelines development. Chassin reported that it takes 17 years for a new scientific discovery to make its way into ordinary medical practice.[26] Practicing doctors are often too busy to keep up with the scientific literature. One sees evidence for this in the piles of medical journals in their offices, still in their wrappers. What organized systems need to do is to form committees in each specialty, assisted by health services researchers, to review the literature and translate it into appropriate and up to date practice guidelines, transmitted to the front-line doctors through their electronic information systems, in a process similar to Minnesota's Institute for Clinical Systems Improvement or Kaiser Permanente's Care Management Institute. The guidelines recommendations need to come from doctors who are conscious of the need for efficient use of resources. Guidelines produced by specialty society doctors in Country A in fee-for-service small practice risk being produced by a single specialty bias and a cost unconscious perspective.

Another important part of the process needs to be similar careful evaluation of alternative drugs, followed by effective procurement practices to secure good prices when there are competing alternative drugs. Another is the similar evaluation and cost-effective procurement of devices.

Guidelines development and well-informed choices of drugs and devices are large and costly activities, so the costs might best be shared among several care systems to obtain economies of scale.

An important adjunct to procurement of drugs and devices is to develop and maintain registries so that the experience of patients using the different products can be tracked over time, with the results analyzed and conclusions fed back into medical practice quite promptly.

A major negative consequence of Country A's model is that doctors generally do not have any *systematic* data on what happens to their patients after they leave the hospital, data that can be analyzed and fed back in to practice. Paul Ellwood has called for "Outcomes Management: A technology of patient experience," in which patients would be followed continuously, including asking them about their medical results,

[25]Christensen, CM, Grossman J.H., and Hwang, J. *The Innovator's Prescription: A Disruptive Solution to the Health Care Crisis,* McGraw-Hill, 2009, p.xx.

[26]Chassin, M. Milbank Quarterly.

and the data analyzed and conclusions fed back into practice improvement.[27] To do this, it is necessary to have a reasonably stable and continuous patient base where people are in regular contact over time with the care system of their choice. If care systems do a good job and satisfy their patients, they are likely to experience such patient loyalty as to make this possible.

Accountable Care Systems in Country B offer two types of insurance products: "Exclusive Provider Organizations" ("EPO's") or "lock in" where patients agree to get *all* their covered services from or through the ACS, in a manner similar to HMOs in the USA, and "Point of Service Products" ("POS") for people who want the advantages of well organized care systems, but who would be willing to pay extra for a coverage that allowed them to go outside of the system for care, partially covered by insurance, after paying a substantial deductible.

Incentives Aligned. So in brief, incentives are aligned in Country B. Consumers have strong incentives to seek and choose high quality affordable care, and they are likely to migrate to it. That puts pressure on providers to "follow the money" and create and join and operate high quality, affordable care systems, and to pursue continuous quality improvement. The fact that individual consumers have a choice gives care systems' providers incentives to make care "consumer centered." In Country B, there will be a large and ongoing demand for process redesign and engineering.

Other institutions in society would find themselves under pressure to align themselves with cost reduction. . For example, state and federal regulation that grew up in an era of provider protectionism, cost unconsciousness and lack of consumer choice, and has been a cost-increasing force would gradually change under the pressures of cost conscious consumers and providers who would favor increasing latitude for cost reducing innovation. And legislators who had to vote the taxes to pay for the government's contributions to support of the system would be more interested in creating space for cost reduction. For example, scope of practices for nurses could be widened, under protocols approved by doctors in the ACS's. The tort system would realign under the same pressures. The fact that providers would be more regularly working to generally agreed practice guidelines, and also increased use of quality improvement systems would likely reduce the incidence of tort claims. Public confidence in the health care system would improve. The important element of consumer choice would also improve the tort atmosphere as people would feel empowered and able to choose the system they prefer.[28]

Whether or not Country B will have brought the growth of its health expenditures into line with growth in the GDP is uncertain. Country B is creating a path in uncharted territory. But the incentives to contain or reduce costs are strong. The incentives to develop cost reducing technologies would also be strong. At a minimum, Country B will have a much more efficient effective health care system than Country A. All we know about economics and our experience should tell us that. While the trajectory of costs are uncertain, a reasonable educated guess is that over two decades, Country B's health expenditures could be half what they will be if we in the USA stay pretty much on the same track as we are on now.

Countries A and B are compared in Table 1.

3. Back to the real world of the USA

Today, the USA is more than 90% like Country A and less than 10% like Country B, measured by the number of people who, in their employment or public programs, are offered multiple choices, including

---

[27]Ellwood ,P M. "Shattuck Lecture: Outcomes management, a technology of patient experience," *New England Journal of Medicine,* 19__.

[28]Riemer, DR. "Follow the Money: The Impact of Consumer Choice and Economic Incentives on Conflict Resolution in Health Care," 29 Hamline Journal of Public Law and Policy 423, Spring 2008.

Table 1
Countries a and b compared

Aspect	Country A	Country B
Medical Organization	uncoordinated FFS Small practice	Large multi-specialty group practice
Main Provider Incentive	Do More whether Needed or not	Innovate to provide value for money
Information Technology	Few doctors use it To coordinate care	Electronic Records plus full IT functionality
Main Insurance Model	Independent companies Or Self-insured employers	Insurers Affiliated with Provider Systems
Process Engineering	Practically Non-existent	Ubiquitous
NHE as a % of GDP	20% and growing	12–14% and stable
% of Population Insured	80% and falling	100%
Consumer Choice Of Insurer	Almost None	Wide Cost-Conscious Consumer choice
Consumer Choice of Provider	"free choice" of individual providers	Wide choice of Systems of Care
Consumer Economic Incentive	Cost-Unconscious demand	Cost-conscious choice of system
Technology Assessment	Little, Cost not Considered	Cost-benefit Analysis for all Technologies

ACS, and fixed dollar employer contributions. So in the mixed USA, we see some promising examples of Country B phenomena, mainly among the prepaid group practices and other large multi specialty group practices, and in the successful operation of competitive cost conscious multiple choices of health plan models offered to employees. It is attractive to think in terms of gradually moving from A to B.

But effective Accountable Care Systems need economies of scale, and less than 10% of the population of a metropolitan area on cost conscious consumer choice, especially if spread randomly across the population, is usually not enough scope for one or two, not to mention the several ACS needed for competition. Also, the 90+% of health care that is cost unconscious in the USA produces wastefulness that spills over into the community standards of care and regulatory environment, as well as prices provider systems have to pay for supplies and personnel. Cost unconscious consumers lobby their legislators for regulations that increase costs. So, in my view, for the transformation to competing ACS to happen before growth in National Health Expenditures has done great and irreparable damage to the rest of our economy, we need to move much faster than we have in the past. How could this be done?

CED's Proposal for a Smooth Transformation to Value Conscious Choice. In 2007, the Committee for Economic Development (CED), a business and university-sponsored, non partisan, non profit virtual public policy research organization based in Washington DC published a proposal that contains a road map.[29]

A "Health Fed" to Create and Oversee Exchanges. CED begins with creation of a national system of exchanges, organized and run by a new independent Federal Agency, the "Health Fed". Exchanges would cover every part of the country. (An exchange is an institution to which buyers and sellers, of health insurance in this case, come together to do transactions according to rules.) Their role would be to sponsor competitive health plan offerings as much as possible in every area, and to set the rules

[29]See *Quality, Affordable Health Care for All: Moving Beyond the Employer-Based Health-Insurance System,* A Statement by the Research and Policy Committee of the Committee for Economic Development, available at www.ced.org/. Washington, 2007.

under which they would compete. Initially, all employers of 100 employees or less would be required to buy their coverage through the regional exchange. At the same time, the Congress should cap the tax exclusion at the estimated price of an efficient health plan in each region. Employers would have to buy through the exchanges in order to keep the tax exclusion for employer contributions – an incentive strong enough to give even relatively healthy groups an incentive to join. (Experience teaches that purely voluntary exchanges, without such an incentive, are vulnerable to adverse selection. If the exchange is only for employers having trouble obtaining health insurance, the participating population is almost certainly biased in favor of sicker people, in which case premiums would be high and the employers would be unhappy, and healthy groups would not join voluntarily.) But if a representative population of employers participates in the exchanges, there will be many advantages for them. Today, small employers are less likely to offer their employees *any* insurance. Through the exchange they can offer a choice and a defined contribution. Small employers are far too small for the spreading of risks, especially in an era in which exotic biotech drugs can cost as much as $300,000 per year for an afflicted patient. Through the exchange, risks can be spread very widely. Small employers lack expertise in health care and health insurance, and they lack economies of scale. The experience of CalPERS, a large exchange in California for public employees, that brokers health insurance for 1.3 million people in over 1000 employment groups, is that its administrative costs are less than one half of one percent of premium. So through the exchange, employers will be able to obtain more competitive insurance and more stable premium rates. The cap on the tax exclusion will help to make employees more cost conscious, and the rules might require participating employers to make whatever contributions they choose to make in the form of fixed dollar amounts. Capping the tax exclusion would also save the Federal and State budgets tens of billions of dollars that could be used to enhance subsidies for poor people.[30] So the problem of inadequate access could be addressed both by making insurance more affordable, more available to small employers, and by generating savings that could be used to help the uninsured.

This move would open up a very large market of cost conscious multiple choices in which ACS's could enroll people and compete for members. Roughly one third of the labor force would be available. Moreover, processes might be developed to allow single self-employed people to participate. (There must be care that individual self employed are not too free to choose to be insured or not lest adverse selection be created in the exchange. I think it likely that solutions could be found, one of which would be an "individual mandate", a requirement that people buy health insurance, as in Massachusetts.

As the exchanges proved themselves to be efficient and effective, the threshold for joining could be progressively increased to 200, 500, and more employees until every employed insured person was covered through the exchange. (Very large employers might be exempted if they wanted to be as a class.) Then public programs for poor people could support their purchases through the exchange, at least to the extent practical. (Not all Medicaid patients would fit well in a model for employed insured people.) With the tax exclusion capped, many people in larger groups will want access to the exchange.

The "Health Fed" would be patterned after the Federal Reserve with long terms, expertise, and a significant degree of political independence. The Health Fed would operate under broad guidelines and goals set by Congress, and it would report regularly to Congress. The goals would include making coverage universal and affordable with improving quality motivated by extensive public reporting of quality and consumer satisfaction.

---

[30]The Staff of the Joint Committee on Taxation of the Congress of the United States estimated that in 2007, the Federal Budget lost $145.3 billion from exclusion of employer contributions from the income tax liability of employees, and $100.7 billion from the exclusion from FICA taxes. See *Tax Expenditures for Health Care,* July 30, 2008, JCX-66-08, Washington 2008.

Recall, nobody would be forced to accept a delivery system they dislike. Fee-for-service is likely to be available for a long time. But employer and public contributions could be keyed to the low priced plan, not to the most costly fee-for-service plans.

Regulation of Health Insurance. The CED also recommended that the Health Fed take over regulation of health insurance from states, with uniform federal rules for participation in any exchange to lower costs and simplify processes. This would open the market to participation by many insurers around the country, not limited to the particular state in which they are now regulated. This could simplify the process for insurers in some states to enter more states.

Accountable organized delivery systems with more and more of the attributes of the modern firm would eventually come to dominate the scene as the qualitative advantages of having a well organized "medical home" with primary care and electronic records would be too great for most people to prefer uncoordinated fee-for-service. (But some would prefer the traditional model and should be free to choose it in a responsible manner.)

The same principles could and must be applied to Medicare along the lines recommended by the majority (but not super majority) of the Bi Partisan Commission headed by Breaux and Thomas. In fact the case for applying coordinated care to Medicare is even stronger than for younger people because many more Medicare beneficiaries have multiple chronic conditions and greatly need primary care in a coordinated care system.

All this would create the powerful incentives in which everyone would have to engineer evidence-based care processes, track patient experience and feed back the results into process improvement.

Alain C. Enthoven is the Marriner S. Eccles Professor of Public and Private Management (Emeritus) in the Graduate School of Business at Stanford University. He holds degrees in Economics from Stanford, Oxford and MIT. He has been an Economist with the RAND Corporation, Assistant Secretary of Defense, and President of Litton Medical Products. In 1963, he received the President's Award for Distinguished Federal Civilian Service from John F. Kennedy. In 1977, while serving as a consultant to the Carter Administration, he designed and proposed Consumer Choice Health Plan, a plan for universal health insurance based on managed competition in the private sector. He is a member of the Institute of Medicine of the National Academy of Sciences and a fellow of the American Academy of Arts and Sciences. He is Chairman of Stanford University's Committee on Faculty/Staff Human Resources and a consultant to Kaiser Permanente, the former Chairman of the Health Benefits Advisory Council for CalPERS, the California State employees' medical and hospital care plans. He has been a director of the Jackson Hole Group, PCS, Caresoft Inc., and eBenX, Inc. He was the 1994 winner of the Baxter Prize for Health Services Research and also the 1995 Board of Directors Award, Healthcare Financial Management Association. In 1997, Governor Wilson appointed him Chairman of the California Managed Health Care Improvement Task Force. Commissioned by the State legislature, the Task Force addressed healthcare issues raised by managed care. In 1988, he gave the De Vries Lectures in Rotterdam, called *Theory and Practice of Managed Competition in Health Care Finance,* which provided the theoretical foundation for the Dutch model of universal health insurance based on managed competition. In 1998-99, he was the Rock Carling Fellow of the Nuffield Trust of London and also Visiting Professor at the London School of Hygiene and Tropical Medicine. He wrote the Rock Carling Lecture *In Pursuit of an Improving National Health Service* recommending further Introduction of market forces in the National Health Service. He and Laura Tollen recently edited a book called *Toward a 21*st *Century Health System: The Contributions and Promise of Prepaid Group Practice* (Jossey Bass, San Francisco, 2004). He is a member of the Research Advisory Board of the Committee for Economic Development (CED) and since 2006 served as project director for a recently published CED report *Quality, Affordable Health Care for All: Moving Beyond the Employer-Based Health-Insurance System.* November 2007. In 2008, he was awarded the honorary degree of Doctor of Public Policy by the RAND Graduate School.

Section 4: Engineering Approaches

Information Knowledge Systems Management 8 (2009) 231–240
DOI 10.3233/IKS-2009-0139
IOS Press

Chapter 14

Systems engineering and management

William B. Rouse and W. Dale Compton
E-mail: bill.rouse@ti.gatech.edu

Abstract: This chapter offers a systems view of healthcare delivery and outlines a wide range of concepts, principles, models, methods and tools from systems engineering and management that can enable the transformation of the dysfunctional "as is" healthcare system to an agreed-upon "to be" system that will provide quality, affordable care for everyone. Topics discussed include systems definition, design, analysis, and control, as well as the data and information needed to support these functions. Barriers to implementation are also considered.

1. Introduction

The healthcare system in the United States was not designed; it just emerged as a federation of a very large number of entrepreneurs with no one in charge. The result is a highly fragmented system rife with seams across which information does not flow and care processes cannot be coordinated. Further, we have created, over time, a business model that focuses on reimbursing the costs of procedures and other activities rather than the value of outcomes. Put simply, healthcare is at the craft stage of development much as the automobile industry was almost 100 years ago.

This chapter argues that systems engineering can provide the means to transform healthcare to be a high value and integrated provider of health services. This integration requires a process-oriented approach to understanding, supporting, and enhancing the ways in which value is understood, provided, and rewarded. This integration requires that the system be redesigned – be engineered – to provide quality, affordable healthcare for everyone.

This conclusion is far from new. The National Academy of Engineering and Institute of Medicine have pursued this line of reasoning in great detail [23]. This effort resulted in the following nine findings:

1. The health care delivery system does not function as a system – at least not in the sense of a traditional system [26]
2. A systems view of health care cannot be achieved until organizational barriers to change are overcome
3. Systems-engineering tools have been used in many industries to improve quality, efficiency, safety, and/or customer-centeredness
4. Health care has been very slow to embrace systems-engineering tools
5. Systems-engineering tools for the design, analysis, and control of complex systems and processes could potentially transform the quality and productivity of health care
6. Neither the engineering community nor the health care research community has addressed the delivery aspects of health care adequately

7. Information/communication systems will be critical to taking advantage of the potential of existing and emerging systems design, analysis, and control tools to transform health care delivery
8. The current organization, management, and regulation of health care delivery provide few incentives for the use or development of systems engineering tools that could lead to improvements.
9. The widespread use of systems engineering tools will require determined efforts on the part of health care providers, the engineering community, federal and state governments, private insurers, large employers, and other stakeholders.

Based on these findings, the Academies provided the following recommendations:

1. Private insurers, large employers, and public payers, including the Federal Center for Medicare and Medicaid Services and state Medicare programs, should provide more incentives for health care providers to use systems tools to improve the quality of care and the efficiency of care delivery
2. Outreach and dissemination efforts by public and private sector organizations that have used systems engineering tools in health care delivery should be expanded, integrated into existing regulatory and accreditation frameworks, and reviewed to determine whether, and if so how, better coordination might make their collective impact stronger.
3. The use and diffusion of systems engineering tools in health care delivery should be promoted by a National Institutes of Health Library of Medicine website that provides patients and clinicians with information about, and access to, systems engineering tools for health care. In addition, federal agencies and private funders should support the development of new curricula, textbooks, instructional software, and other tools to train individual patients and care providers in the use of systems engineering tools.
4. The use of any single systems tool or approach should not be put "on hold" until other tools become available
5. Federal research and mission agencies should significantly increase their support for research to advance the application and utility of systems engineering in health care delivery, including research on new systems tools and the adaptation, implementation, and improvement of existing tools for all levels of health care delivery. This should include support for multi-disciplinary research, development, demonstration and teaching centers.

This chapter is concerned with how systems engineering can support pursuit of the above recommendations. It, in conjunction with Chapters 15–19, provides the engineering concepts, principles, models, methods, and tools for enhancing healthcare delivery in the ways sought by the NAE/IOM initiatives. The other appropriate chapters will be identified as the broad discussions in this chapter are developed.

Systems engineering is the management technology that plans and orchestrates the total life-cycle process of a system, which involves and results in the definition, development, deployment, and sustainment of a system that is of high quality, trustworthy, and cost-effective in meeting stakeholders' needs. The breadth of this definition has caused this endeavor to be more broadly termed systems engineering and management [33]. The management involves planning and orchestrating the processes of definition, development, deployment, and sustainment. Thus, the concern is not just with creating and manufacturing artifacts and distributing them. Systems engineering and management is also concerned with ongoing system operations, maintenance, and support and, increasingly, with the end of life, retirement, and disposal (e.g., recycling) of the system.

There are many other definitions of systems engineering. For example, the International Council on Systems Engineering defines systems engineering to be an interdisciplinary approach and means to enable the realization of successful systems [14]. In general, the range of available definitions are compatible, although there are differences in the extent to which systems engineering is viewed as responsible for a system once it is deployed. For instance, there are differing opinions about whether a well engineered automobile that fails in the marketplace represents a systems engineering failure. We are inclined to think it is.

In this chapter, we will discuss systems engineering and management in the context of large, disaggregated systems. Such systems are quite different from self-contained systems such as airplanes and automobiles, although even these systems are not so self contained when seen as elements of transportation systems. In pursuit of understanding large, disaggregated systems, we need to understand the "architectures" of these systems, both in terms of how current architectures enable and constrain performance, and in terms of how new architectures could enhance performance.

Not surprisingly, there are many tradeoffs in moving from the "as is" architecture of healthcare delivery to the "to be" architecture. Put simply, to what extent, and over what time horizon, can we morph the system while it continues to operate under stress? Further, how is the answer to this question affected by the quite divergent stakeholder positions on what should change and how? Clearly, there will be a large number of interactions and trade-offs involved in addressing these questions.

As we pursue these questions, this chapter will provide descriptions of several families of systems engineering models, methods, and tools. For many of these, descriptions will be brief and reference later chapters in this book. The primary goal in this chapter is to catalog the possibilities and show where they fit into systems engineering and management processes.

2. The need for good data

Both science and engineering tell us that data should drive our conclusions about the nature of phenomena of interest. Data collection should, to the extent possible, be theory or hypothesis driven. Somewhat simplistically, one hypothesis might be that the healthcare system provides the highest quality care possible. The data complied by the IOM [15,16] leads us to reject this hypothesis. Our healthcare system over-utilizes procedures, under-delivers value, and results in far too many avoidable accidents and deaths. We have a major problem.

There are many ways that are advocated for fixing the system. Evaluation of these possibilities poses a problem, however. The "gold standard" in medical science is the randomized clinical trial. This time-consuming and expensive approach has proven to be effective for evaluation of clinical interventions. In contrast, organizational interventions cannot be evaluated in this manner. Quite simply, we cannot operate the healthcare system under multiple different reimbursement schemes and find the true "best" scheme. There are too many contextual factors to allow such a pristine approach to be useful.

Instead, we can take advantage of the millions of pieces of data generated by the healthcare system every day. Every patient in every hospital for every procedure generates an invaluable data point that can contribute to understanding what works, for who, and where. There is no lack of data; there is, however, an extreme fragmentation of information systems. What is learned about "who" when they entered the system cannot be aligned with "what" happens to them throughout their care, and with "where" and "when" this care happens. Were Wal-Mart to operate like the healthcare system, "everyday low prices" would become "everyday high prices, increasing every day."

Other chapters in this book address solution of these information fragmentation problems – see Chapters 7–10. In this chapter, we will assume that information can be made available to support analysis, modeling, and evaluation of alternative means to improve the value delivered by the healthcare system. Indeed, we feel that the ultimate benefit of information integration concerns what you can then do with this information. This chapter outlines a wide range of ways to use this information.

3. System definition methods and tools

System definition is concerned with formulation of the requirements that the system of interest should satisfy [2]. It further involves considering alternative concepts for satisfying these requirements, particularly in terms of how alternative concepts align with the concerns, values, and perceptions of key stakeholders [25]. Beyond conceptual design, there are alternative system architectures within which these concepts can be realized [19]. Requirements, concepts, and architectures are key elements of defining a system.

These notions are particularly important for healthcare. The current system addresses requirements that are dysfunctional. Do we really want the lowest-cost healthcare system that can assure a minimum of care to everyone? Or, do we seek a healthy, educated, and productive workforce that can compete successfully in the global marketplace? Low cost is easy if we do not seek a healthy, educated, and productive workforce.

Our current concept involves millions of nearly independent entrepreneurs running their family practice, specialty practice, or laboratory service trying to deliver enough procedures to pay their nurse, receptionist, and office manager, pay their malpractice insurance, and earn a decent living. For example, of the nearly 700,000 clinicians in the US, 80% practice in groups of 10 or less. Is this the right concept for providing quality, affordable healthcare for everyone? If this were the right concept, we would still have separate retail stores for each of the almost 50,000 products that are on the shelves of major retailers. One store for salad greens, another for salad dressing, and another for salad condiments.

The current system of healthcare delivery was not architected; it just emerged over decades [26, 34]. The highly-fragmented system concept with which we are very familiar involves each participant generating, capturing, storing, and retrieving information on patient transactions. The result can be, in our personal experience, an individual patient completing patient history records several times in one day for each provider involved in the care process of interest, perhaps all on the same floor of the same building. Of course, they do not really think of it as a process. They are simply selling MRIs or colonoscopies, not actually providing care.

System architecting, as an element of system definition, is concerned with defining information elements and how they flow through the organization to enable provision of the value that the organization strives to deliver. The current system is viewed as an artifact of old assumptions, old practices, and a lack of impetus on integration to provide value. Architecting focuses on how the whole system will operate rather than just one practice or one process.

System architecture can be viewed, most simply, as involving three levels:

- Operational level at which people, or perhaps robots, interact with the system to perform work and receive services
- Systems level at which various functions are performed ranging from information processing to physical control functions
- Technical level at which the system interacts with the broader environment to sense and access information either physically or through information networks

Ideally, the definition of the operational level should drive the lower levels. Thus, the desired nature of work and workflow [30] would define the required interactions with the system. This, in turn, would determine what functions are required, which would then determine what is needed at the technical level.

Even if we were engineering a system of healthcare delivery from scratch, this system definition task would be quite complicated, but not as difficult as the real task at hand. We have to somehow dovetail the desired "to be" architecture with the legacy "as is architecture" to enable significant change – overcoming the inertia of the status quo – while also providing continuity of current system operations.

This pursuit is complicated by the fact that our system of healthcare delivery is a complex adaptive system [24,26]. The characteristics of such systems include:

- They are *nonlinear, dynamic* and do not inherently reach fixed equilibrium points. The resulting system behaviors may appear to be random or chaotic.
- They are composed of *independent agents* whose behavior can be described as based on physical, psychological, or social rules, rather than being completely dictated by the dynamics of the system.
- Agents' needs or desires, reflected in their rules, are not homogeneous and, therefore, their *goals and behaviors are likely to conflict* – these conflicts or competitions tend to lead agents to adapt to each other's behaviors.
- Agents are *intelligent, learn* as they experiment and gain experience, and change behaviors accordingly. Thus, overall systems behavior inherently changes over time.
- Adaptation and learning tends to result in *self-organizing* and patterns of behavior that emerge rather than being designed into the system. The nature of such emergent behaviors may range from valuable innovations to unfortunate accidents.
- There is *no single point(s) of control* – systems behaviors are often unpredictable and uncontrollable, and no one is "in charge." Consequently, the behaviors of complex adaptive systems usually can be influenced more than they can be controlled.

For systems with these characteristics, one cannot, using any conventional means, command or force these systems to comply with behavioral and performance dictates. The agents in such systems are sufficiently intelligent to game the system, find workarounds, and creatively identify ways to serve their own interests. Consequently, it will be necessary to identify the right mix of incentives and inhibitions (e.g., regulations) that will enable and motivate the agents in the system to morph in ways that will, over time, create the desired "to be" system.

4. Systems design methods and tools

Once one or more system concepts and architectures are defined, attention shifts to system design. There are a range of methods and tools available to support design. A particularly useful approach is concurrent engineering [18]. Concurrent engineering is the practice of considering the entire system life cycle, from design to disposal, in an integrated design process.

While this may seem like the intuitively right approach, it is not common. For example, it is indeed rare to pursue the design of healthcare delivery infrastructure, e.g., information systems, in ways that can be easily upgraded and not plagued, in the future, by legacy systems. Of course, there are many tradeoffs and there are often limits on how much one can invest in possible future upgrades and changes.

Quality function deployment [1] and design structure matrices [4] can provide strong support for addressing these tradeoffs, as well as a plethora of tradeoffs that emerge throughout system design. These two methods, referred to as QFD and DSM, provide matrix-based representations for portraying relationships among system attributes at several levels [6]. For example, there is usually some mapping between stakeholders' desires, the functions within a system, and the realization processes (e.g., manufacturing) for creating the system. The tools associated with QFD and DSM enable depicting and managing these relationships in ways that make tradeoff analyses more understandable and manageable.

Both of these procedures accept that the "wants and needs" of the stakeholders must be first identified and then consistently incorporated into any plans for the end processes and products.

It is also important to consider how systems are likely to fail, abilities to maintain them, and the implications for system availability [22]. Tools such as failure mode and effects analysis (FMEA), fault tree analysis (FTA), and root cause analysis RCA) can help to pursue these issues. Note that FMEA, FTA, and RCA are also useful for diagnosing why a system has failed or why it has availability problems.

Human systems integration (HSI) is also central to system design [3]. Healthcare delivery is labor intensive. Consequently, the manpower, personnel, and training implications of the design of this system are critical. Central questions include how many people will be needed, what aptitudes they will need, and how they will be trained. Further, the design of efficient and effective human-machine interfaces is central to assuring the desired system behaviors and performance. HSI provides a set of methods and tools for addressing these questions. This toolset also includes approaches to designing system interfaces and job aiding, including decision support systems.

5. Systems analysis methods and tools

There is a range of methods and tools for analyzing systems, both existing systems and alternative system designs emerging from the processes discussed above. Some of these methods and tools support analytic representation of system attributes and their relationships – QFD and DSM are good examples. For static deterministic attributes and relationships, these approaches may be sufficient.

However, there are many situations where we are interested in system performance over time, including how performance is affected by variability. (Chapter 15 discusses the nature and sources of variability in healthcare.) In these situations, modeling and simulation are the typical approaches adopted [29, 35]. Various methods and tools are available for modeling and simulating representations based on queuing theory, system dynamics, and behavioral and social science theories. These are referred to as discrete-event simulation, system dynamics simulation, and agent-based simulation.

Many methods and tools are available for optimizing the performance of systems [13]. These approaches may involve use of similar models and simulations. However, many mathematical programming approaches (e.g., linear, integer, and dynamic programming) employ deterministic representations to compute the best allocations of resources – within the assumed structure of the problem. Chapter 15 discusses several applications of these approaches within healthcare.

There are also methods and tools available for considering the whole enterprise as a system [27]. There is an emerging body of data, theories, and models for addressing fundamental change of complex organizational systems. Table 1 summarizes how systems engineering can enable enterprise transformation.

The enablers listed in Table 1 are supported by methods and tools for economic valuation of investments [35], service system management (see Chapter 16), process reengineering (see Chapter 17 [32];) supply chain management (see Chapter 19), and risk management [12].

Another class of methods and tools for system analysis concerns access and management of information and knowledge [31]. This class includes approaches to data mining and modeling for purposes such as measuring and monitoring productivity, identifying best practices, and predictive health. Integrated information systems are central to healthcare delivery organizations being able to take advantage of these methods and tools.

Of particular importance, information and knowledge management are concerned with the diffusion of learning, not just the capturing, archiving and retrieval of data and information. As data is generated in multiple locations, one would like to fuse the evolving data sets to enable a breadth of learning that

Table 1
Executives' concerns & systems engineering enablers

Executives' concerns (Given forces and intent to change)	Systems engineering enablers (For addressing executives' concerns)
Identifying Ends, Means & Scope and Candidate Changes	System Complexity Analysis to Compare "As Is" and "To Be" Enterprises
Evaluating Changes in Terms of Process Behaviors & Performance	Organizational Simulation of Process Flows and Relationships
Assessing Economics in Terms of Investments, Operating Costs & Returns	Economic Modeling in Terms of Cash Flows, Volatility, and Options
Defining the New Enterprise In Terms of Processes and Their Integration	Enterprise Architecting in Terms of Workflow, Processes, Levels & Maturity
Designing a Strategy to Change the Culture for Selected Changes	Organizational & Cultural Change Via Leadership, Vision, Strategy & Incentives
Developing Transformation Action Plans in Terms of What, When & Who	Implementation Planning in Terms of Tasks, Schedule, People & Information

could be disseminated broadly across the system. There are collaborative tool suites that enable this in other domains such as marketing, sales, and product management. These capabilities would greatly facilitate system-wide learning in healthcare delivery.

6. System control methods and tools

System control involves comparing actual system outputs (or outcomes) to desired system outputs and using any differences to adjust controls such as performance expectations, service standards, and allocations of resources. Classically, control has been based on estimates of system state. Feedback control involves use of current and past state information while feedforward control involves using current and projected state information.

In the context of healthcare delivery, knowledge of the state of the system is critical to controlling the system [28]. Medical science has focused quite effectively on defining, measuring, and controlling the states of patients. However, the state of the overall system includes variables that medical science seldom addresses. Examples of such broader state variables include:

- The health state of each and every patient in the hospital at the moment, rather than on average
- The distribution of labor hours per patient versus types of procedures and interventions today, rather than on average
- The levels and locations of inventory for all consumables at the moment, rather than on average

These types of variables are, quite rightly, not within the purview of clinicians providing patients with state of the art benefits of medical science. Yet, these types of variables have enormous impact on the costs of healthcare. Consequently, many have argued of late that we need a "science of healthcare delivery" that draws upon best practices in systems engineering, in companion with medical best practices gleaned from medical science [5,23]. Indeed, a recent report by the Institute of Medicine [17] presents priorities for comparative effectiveness research with substantial emphasis on how to make service delivery more effective.

System control can also involve the use of methods and tools such as statistical process control, control charts, and forecasting methods. Of particular relevance in this arena are Six Sigma, the Toyota Production System, and the Baldrige National Quality Program [21]. It is important to note that these approaches squeeze the greatest productivity and quality from the "as is" system architecture. They do not inherently morph the architecture, although they may inform the process of rethinking the architecture.

Chapter 15 on operations research addresses a range of operations management issues including demand forecasting, patient scheduling, outpatient scheduling, inpatient scheduling, and workforce planning and scheduling. This chapter also addresses management decision making in terms of clinical decision making, decision analysis and dynamic influence diagrams, performance improvement (i.e., diagnostic accuracy, testing strategies, and treatment of disease), cost effectiveness and cost benefit analyses, disease management, epidemic control of contagious and other population-wide diseases (see also Chapter 18), screening and control of non-contagious diseases for an individual, and computational biology and biomedicine. Chapter 15 is quite rich in terms of providing many examples of healthcare applications.

7. Conclusions

This chapter has discussed a wide range of concepts, principles, models, methods, and tools for addressing the issues raised by the NAE and IOM, as well as pursuing the recommendations provided by NAE and IOM. There are a range of reasons why this has not yet happened to any great extent.

First and foremost, the system of healthcare delivery in the United States in highly fragmented with hundreds of thousands of mostly small and highly specialized enterprises and no one in charge. Consequently, no one has the responsibility, purview, and resources to undertake systemic change. There are enormous policy and market barriers to reducing this fragmentation. As emphasized by *The Economist* five years ago, any efficiencies and cost savings entertained directly affect various stakeholders' incomes [7]. The forces for preservation of the current business models in healthcare are very strong.

Despite very well articulated illustrations of the shortcomings of the current system [9,10], organizational and managerial obstacles are ubiquitous. Providers' organizations have been designed and tuned to prosper based on fee-for-service reimbursement by third parties. The more services provided, the greater the revenue, regardless of whether health outcomes are enhanced. Indeed, as many of the chapters in this book compellingly report, there is ample evidence that health outcomes are not enhanced by these increased expenditures. Further, there is increasing evidence of disparate expenditures across the country that are not related to local income levels or health outcomes [11].

Beyond these economic, social, and political barriers, there is the straightforward fact that the highly fragmented system of healthcare delivery does not have the integrated information systems needed to take full advantage of the approaches outlined in this chapter. Lots of data are captured on paper, but little information is created from this enormous store of data. It is difficult to adopt best practices when these practices are premised on knowing the state of the system – as illustrated earlier – and controlling the system based on this information. Integrated health information systems are essential to moving beyond the current crisis.

Finally, there are educational barriers. For the most part, physicians are in control of the system – at least to the extent that anyone has any control. Physicians are not trained to take a systemic view of the overall care processes within which they are involved [20]. Physicians are not trained to work as members of teams associated with these processes. Indeed, most physicians are independent private practitioners and inherently must focus on keeping their small businesses solvent [8].

Of course, we should keep in mind that physicians are compensated for the procedures they perform, not the value produced by the overall process in which they participate. Thus, they are behaving quite rationally by focusing on just their activities in this process. We might reasonably expect that outcome-based compensation will lead physicians to pay much more attention to the overall process that produces outcomes. As found in many other domains, this will inherently lead to greater attention being paid to teamwork.

There is progress in training physician teamwork (see Chapters 20–22). However, there is not yet widespread recognition that engineering the system of healthcare delivery is not a problem of medical science, and that it is a problem of systems engineering and management. Broadly based recognition of this reality, combined with incentives to surmount the other barriers outlined above, is central to agreeing on and creating the "to be" system that will provide quality, affordable care for everyone.

References*

[1] J.A. Armstrong, Jr., Issue formulation, in: *Handbook of Systems Engineering and Management*, A.P. Sage and W.B. Rouse, eds, 2nd Edition. New York: Wiley, 2009.
[2] T. Bahill and F.F. Dean, Discovering system requirements, in: *Handbook of Systems Engineering and Management*, (2nd Edition), A.P. Sage and W.B. Rouse, eds, New York: Wiley, 2009.
[3] H.R. Booher, R.J. Beaton and F. Greene, Human systems integration, in: *Handbook of Systems Engineering and Management*, (2nd Edition), A.P. Sage and W.B. Rouse, eds, New York: Wiley, 2009.
[4] T.R. Browning, Using the Design Structure Matrix to design program organizations, in: *Handbook of Systems Engineering and Management*, A.P. Sage and W.B. Rouse, eds, 2nd Edition. New York: Wiley, 2009.
[5] C.M. Christenson, J.H. Grossman and J. Hwang, The innovator's prescription: A disruptive solution for health care. New York: McGraw-Hill, 2008.
[6] W.D. Compton, Engineering Management: Creating and Managing World Class Operations. New York" Prentice Hall, 1997.
[7] Economist, Survey of Healthcare Finance, *The Economist* (15 July 2004).
[8] V. Fuhrmans, Replicating Cleveland Clinic's Success Poses Major Challenges, *Wall Street Journal* (23 July 2009), A4.
[9] A. Gawande, Complications. A Surgeon's Notes on an Imperfect Science. New York: Picador, 2003.
[10] A. Gawande, Better: A Surgeon's Notes on Performance. New York: Metropolitan Books, 2007.
[11] A. Gawande, The cost conundrum: What a Texas town can teach us about health care, *New Yorker* (1 June 2009).
[12] Y.Y. Haimes, Risk management, in: *Handbook of Systems Engineering and Management*, (2nd Edition), A.P. Sage and W.B. Rouse, eds, New York: Wiley, 2009.
[13] K.W. Hipel, D.M. Kilgour, S. Rajabi and Y. Chen, Operations research and refinement of courses of action, in: *Handbook of Systems Engineering and Management*, A.P. Sage and W.B. Rouse, eds, 2nd Edition. New York: Wiley, 2009.
[14] INCOSE, Systems Engineering Handbook: A Guide For System Life Cycle Processes And Activities (Ver. 3.1). Seattle, WA: International Council on Systems Engineering, 2007.
[15] IOM, To err is human: Building a safer health system. Washington, DC: National Academies Press, 2000.
[16] IOM, Crossing the quality chasm: A new health systems for the 21st *century*, Washington, DC: National Academies Press, 2001.
[17] IOM, Initial National Priorities for Comparative Effectiveness Research. Washington, DC: Institute of Medicine, 2009.
[18] A. Kusiak and N. Larson, Concurrent engineering, in: *Handbook of Systems Engineering and Management*, (2nd Edition), A.P. Sage and W.B. Rouse, eds, New York: Wiley, 2009.
[19] A.H. Levis, Systems architectures, in: *Handbook of Systems Engineering and Management*, A.P. Sage and W.B. Rouse, eds, 2nd Edition. New York: Wiley, 2009.
[20] S. Long and R. Alpern, Science for future physicians, *Science* **324** (5 June 2009), 1241.
[21] J. Melsa, Total quality management, in: *Handbook of Systems Engineering and Management*, (2nd Edition), A.P. Sage and W.B. Rouse, eds, New York: Wiley, 2009.
[22] M. Pecht, Reliability, maintainability, and availability, in: *Handbook of Systems Engineering and Management*, (2nd Edition), A.P. Sage and W.B. Rouse, eds, New York: Wiley, 2009.

*Note that many of the references refer to chapters in the recently published 2nd Edition of the *Handbook of Systems Engineering and Management*. These chapters, in turn, provide a wealth of references for key sources on the many topics discussed in this chapter.

[23] P.P. Reid, W.D. Compton, J.H. Grossman and G. Fanjiang, Building a better delivery system: A new engineering/health care partnership. Washington, DC: National Academies Press, 2005.
[24] W.B. Rouse, Managing complexity: Disease control as a complex adaptive system, *Information · Knowledge · Systems Management* **2**(2) (2000), 143–165.
[25] W.B. Rouse, People and Organizations: Explorations of Human-Centered Design. New York: Wiley, 2007.
[26] W.B. Rouse, Healthcare as a complex adaptive system, *The Bridge* **38**(1) (2008), 17–25.
[27] W.B. Rouse, Engineering the enterprise as a system, in: *Handbook of Systems Engineering and Management*, (2nd Edition), A.P. Sage and W.B. Rouse, eds, New York: Wiley, 2009.
[28] W.B. Rouse, Engineering perspectives on healthcare delivery: Can we afford technological innovation in healthcare? *System Research and Behavioral Science* **26**(1) (2009), 1–10.
[29] W.B. Rouse and D.A. Bodner, (2009). Organizational simulation, in: *Handbook of Systems Engineering and Management*, A.P. Sage and W.B. Rouse, eds, 2nd Edition. New York: Wiley, 2009.
[30] W.B. Rouse and A.P. Sage, eds, Work, Workflow and Information Systems. Amsterdam: IOS Press, 2007.
[31] W.B. Rouse and A.P. Sage, Information technology and knowledge management, in: *Handbook of Systems Engineering and Management*, A.P. Sage and W.B. Rouse, eds, 2nd Edition. New York: Wiley, 2009.
[32] A.P. Sage, Systems reengineering, in: *Handbook of Systems Engineering and Management*, A.P. Sage and W.B. Rouse, eds, 2nd Edition. New York: Wiley, 2009.
[33] A.P. Sage and W.B. Rouse, eds, Handbook of Systems Engineering and Management (2nd Edition), New York: Wiley, 2009.
[34] R.A. Stevens, C.E. Rosenberg and L.R. Burns, eds, History & health policy in the United States. New Brunswick, NJ: Rutgers University Press, 2006.
[35] C.E. Van Daalen, W.A.H. Thissen, A. Vergraeck and P.W.G. Bots, Methods for the modeling and analysis of alternatives, in: *Handbook of Systems Engineering and Management*, A.P. Sage and W.B. Rouse, eds, 2nd Edition. New York: Wiley, 2009.

William B. Rouse, is the Executive Director of the Tennenbaum Institute at the Georgia Institute of Technology. He is also a professor in the College of Computing and School of Industrial and Systems Engineering. His research focuses on understanding and managing complex public-private systems such as healthcare and defense, with emphasis on mathematical and computational modeling of these systems for the purpose of policy design and analysis. Rouse has written hundreds of articles and book chapters, and has authored many books, including most recently *People and Organizations: Explorations of Human-Centered Design* (Wiley, 2007), *Essential Challenges of Strategic Management* (Wiley, 2001) and the award-winning *Don't Jump to Solutions* (Jossey-Bass, 1998). He is editor of *Enterprise Transformation: Understanding and Enabling Fundamental Change* (Wiley, 2006), co-editor of *Organizational Simulation: From Modeling & Simulation to Games & Entertainment* (Wiley, 2005), co-editor of the best-selling *Handbook of Systems Engineering and Management* (Wiley, 1999, 2009), and editor of the eight-volume series *Human/Technology Interaction in Complex Systems* (Elsevier). Among many advisory roles, he has served as Chair of the Committee on Human Factors of the National Research Council, a member of the U.S. Air Force Scientific Advisory Board, and a member of the DoD Senior Advisory Group on Modeling and Simulation. Rouse is a member of the National Academy of Engineering, as well as a fellow of four professional societies – Institute of Electrical and Electronics Engineers (IEEE), the International Council on Systems Engineering (INCOSE), the Institute for Operations Research and Management Science (INFORMS), and the Human Factors and Ergonomics Society (HFES).

Dale Compton is the Lillian M. Gilbreth Distinguished Professor (Emeritus) of Industrial Engineering at Purdue University. He joined the Purdue faculty in 1988. From 1961–70 he was at UIUC as a Professor of Physics. From 1965–1970 he was Director of the Coordinated Science Laboratory. From 1970–1986 he was with the Research Laboratories of the Ford Motor Co. – the last 13 years as Vice-President Research. He was the first Senior Fellow of the National Academy of Engineering before joining Purdue. He is currently a member of St. Vincent Hospital (Indianapolis) Quality Committee and a past member of the IHI National Advisory Committee on Pursuing Perfection. Between 2000 and 2008 he served as Home Secretary for the National Academy of Engineering.

Information Knowledge Systems Management 8 (2009) 241–276
DOI 10.3233/IKS-2009-0152
IOS Press

Chapter 15

Operations research

A valuable resource for improving quality, costs, access and satisfaction in health care delivery

William P. Pierskalla
E-mail: william.pierskalla@anderson.ucla.edu

Prologue: In *Evita*, Andrew Lloyd Webber and Tim Rice wrote: *Politics, the Art of the Possible*. To those of us in the operations research community, we postulate: *Operations Research, the Science of Better* – (i.e. better processes, better systems and better decisions). Using our own and other scientific, engineering, mathematical, and social sciences methodologies, operations researchers help decision makers make better decisions; decisions leading to improvements: greater quality, lower costs, greater revenues, better access, better scheduling, lower risks, more satisfaction – *with the goal of always striving for the best or optimal decisions*.

1. Introduction

There is a rich history of applying operations research in health care delivery and medicine. Beginning in the 1950s with the work by N.T.J. Bailey in the UK and Charles Flagle and his colleagues and students at Johns Hopkins University there has been a steady progression of applications now numbering in the thousands. Some surveys of his work have been done [33,34,78]. Furthermore there is an excellent introductory textbook by Ozcan [73], *Quantitative Methods in Health Care Delivery* that is used to teach students pursuing a career applying operations research to health-care management and delivery. For some of the latest research in applying operations research to health-care see the book edited by Brandeau [13], *Operations Research and Healthcare: a Handbook of Methods and Applications* and for the application of operations research in hospitals the book by Gaucher and Coffey [36].

The operations research community has professionals who work in developing the theory and/or methodologies of stochastic processes, mathematical programming, simulation, decision analysis, the sciences of marketing, finance, and service and production supply chain processes and at times the theory and methodologies of other disciplines such as statistics, economics and computer sciences.

However, the majority of operations research professionals work in the area of applying operations research theory and methodologies to practice. These applications range from strategically optimizing capacity and location decisions, optimally running a call-center, locating warehouses or depots, forecasting sales and revenue, planning and mobilizing for terrorist attacks, developing and operating military logistics systems, preventing, ameliorating or curing a disease, evaluating the risks involved in any activities, maintaining and/or preventing equipment malfunctions, designing and implementing marketing plans, optimizing a portfolio of investments, optimally organizing and running supply chains,or scheduling people, machines, and products or services to optimize yields, speed response times and meet demands. The settings for these applications occur in myriad business sectors, military and government sectors, health-care sectors, and virtually every other sector in which strategic or operational decisions must be made to improve planning, performance and outcomes.

Most operations research applications involve analyzing complex situations. The approach taken begins by looking at the complex situation from a systems perspective. Inside the system, processes are diagrammed and analyzed and a model is constructed based on the flows of people, products, services, technologies and information. Using this structure, the approach models the objectives desired to be achieved, the fixed and variable constraints on the system, all available options for decisions, evaluation of all possible outcomes, estimation of risks and bringing to bear the latest tools and techniques leading to improved or optimal decisions on system operation and outcomes. In most applications, it is frequently the case that multiple objectives such as to improve quality, lower costs, improve access and improve satisfaction are simultaneously achieved. In some cases, multiple objectives trade-off against one another and the decision maker has to weigh these objectives and choose among them. In this latter situation, operations research also provides decision analytic methodologies for optimally weighing and choosing among competing objectives.

Because this book is about "Engineering the Health Care System", this chapter will be devoted to operations research applications in health care delivery with mentions of theory and methodologies as appropriate. We have space to cover only some of the applications from the thousands available but hope to do so with enough breadth of topic and depth of description to give a flavor for the capabilities of operations research in developing better or best solutions for many complex health care issues. If one wishes to have a brief introduction to the theory and methodologies mentioned in this chapter see Gass and Harris [35] and the website Wikipedia, http://en.wikipedia.org/wiki/Main_Page.

Operations research has been used in the development of theories and methodologies and in applications in many areas of health services delivery. Some of these areas are strategic in decision making and others are operational. Some examples are:

1. Health care and health care systems strategic planning and design: types and levels of services offered, technologies chosen and used, site locations, capacity levels for health delivery facilities, emergency services deployment, business and enterprise planning, estimates of future resources needs and the deployment of those resources.
2. Healthcare systems design and operation: management of appointment systems and waiting lines for clinical services, ancillary services, and administrative services for both inpatient and outpatient facilities, determining staffing levels and scheduling, determining optimal levels and locations of inventories, material requirements planning, supply chains management, forecasting short and long-term demands, facility layouts, evaluating medical technologies and deploying health-care personnel, equipment and vehicles.
3. Support of clinical activities: modeling of diseases, optimizing diagnostic tools usage, therapy programs and procedures, patient care flows, drug usage for interactions and contraindications, choosing from available therapies and/or technologies and in helping solve complex problems in genetic modeling and bioinformatics.
4. Public health systems design, planning and operations: modeling disease epidemiology, health promotion, incidence, prevalence and mortality of diseases, screening programs and public health services delivery and operation.

An important observation should be stated at the outset. Although many complex problems faced by operations researchers in health care are not analytically different from problems in other industries, many others are *quite unique* due to certain characteristics of health care delivery systems. Some of these

Table 1
Health care delivery objectives with matching operations research capabilities

Health care delivery objectives	OR capabilities
• Low Costs	• Cost Containment
• High Quality	• Quality Improvement
• Rapid Access	• Access Improvement
• Choices of Providers	• Greater “Client” Satisfaction
• Latest Technologies	• Greater Effectiveness
• Broad Coverage	• Increased Efficiency and Productivity
• Income Protection	• Technology Assessment and Risk Management

unique characteristics are the uncertainty of needs, decisions, delivery and outcomes at all levels, largely uninformed/unknowledgeable consumers (asymmetric knowledge), the possibilities of death, pain or low quality of remaining life, the often greater difficulty in measuring quality and value of outcomes, the sharing of many decisions among several decision makers (patients, families, physicians, nurses and administrators), consumers usually not the direct or primary payers, and the concept of health care delivery as a right of citizens in society. This chapter attempts to focus on some areas involving these unique characteristics.

There are other features of the health-care system that are not as unique, but still in many cases significantly different when solving problems in health care delivery. Some of these features are technology is largely cost increasing, there are many choices of treatment modality and treatment regimes, some treatment processes are reasonably inflexible and consumers are of all ages, both sexes and myriad demographic characteristics with thousands of presenting symptoms and thousands of possible diseases. Furthermore, there is a complex set of institutional, societal and individuals’ goals and objectives some of which may be complementary or conflicting. There is heavy governmental involvement in private individuals’ and institutions’ actions, costs and incomes. Actions/inactions by individuals can impose costs or create benefits for others. Finally, there is a lifelong progression of health care from well-being to death involving intermediate care, intensive care, self-care, continuing care, extended care, home care and/or hospice care.

Table 1 above illustrates some of the key health care delivery objectives in the United States. Paralleling those objectives are shown the OR capabilities which have demonstrated proven success in many areas of health care delivery but even more so in many other sectors of the economy.

2. Four big issues facing health care delivery in the US today

Although there are many issues facing health care delivery today and many that have been addressed in one form or another by operations researchers, the models discussed in this chapter will be focused on four of the major issues facing health care delivery today – costs, quality, technologies, and access. Each of these issues will now be briefly discussed. Later, examples will be given on how operations research has addressed these issues in various application areas.

2.1. Costs

In the United States health-care costs have been rising exponentially since 1960. The following two Figs 1 and 2 show the actual costs for health care. From 1960 through 2006, the total costs can be fit extremely well by a quadratic polynomial equation ($R^2 = 0.9957$). Since there are not likely to be

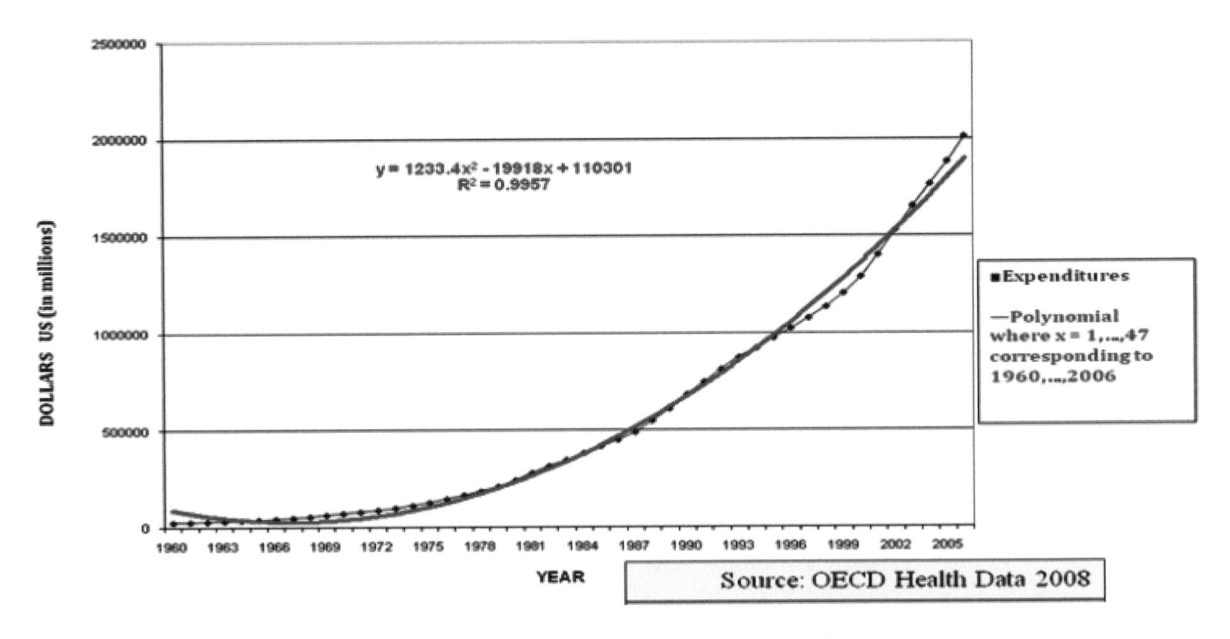

Fig. 1. United states total HC expenditures 1960–2006.

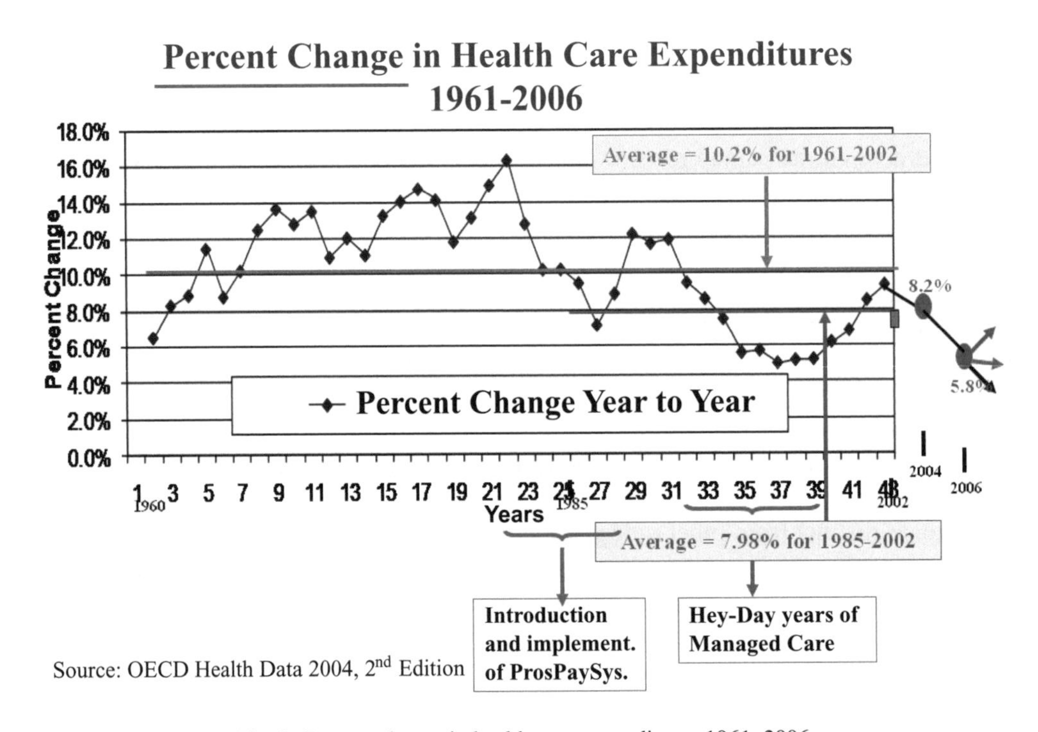

Fig. 2. Percent change in health care expenditures 1961–2006.

significant changes in the way health care is actually delivered by physicians and hospitals in the near future, there is good reason to believe that this trend will continue for some years yet into the future.

The second graph illustrates the *annual increases* in health care costs from 1961 through 2006. The

Table 2
Accounting for the increase in health costs 1940–1990

Factor	Increase Due To		Share of Total	
Static Factors				
Demographics	14		2	
Income	37		5	
Spread of Insurance	100		13	
Relative Price Change	147		19	
Administrative Expense	101		13	
Factor Rents	0		0	
All Static Factors		399%		51%
Residual (**technology/intensity**)		**391%**		**49%**
Total Increase		790%		100%

Source: David M. Cutler, "Technology, Health Costs and NIH," Harvard University and NBER paper presented at the NIH Economics Roundtable on Biomedical Research, October, 1995.

average annual increase for the whole period was just over 10%. Most of this increase occurred in the late 1960s, the 1970s and the early 1980s. This was the time when Medicare and Medicaid were introduced as federal programs, and the delivery of healthcare to the very poor and elderly took off. In the last two decades, 1985 to 2006, the annual rate of increase was approximately 8%. These rates of increase exceeded US annual economic growth, i.e. the annual rate of increase in GDP, by two to three times (meaning that every year more and more of the nation's GDP is going to health care). Again, there's little reason to believe these rates will be brought down significantly in the future.

2.2. *Technologies*

As shown in Table 2 Cutler [20] and other studies, the *primary driving force* behind these annual rates of cost increase, accounting for about 50% of the increase, are the introduction of new technologies and the increasing intensity of use of these and older technologies by more and more patients. Also contributing to some of the annual rate of increase are the aging of the population, the rise in the administrative expenses of regulations and insurance and a general increase in income and insurance coverage in the population.

In health care, as distinct from other industries, most new technologies are cost increasing and indeed significantly cost increasing. It is now possible to replace many parts of the body. In the near future we may be able to replace or assist every part of the body. Furthermore, with the advent of new genetically manufactured therapies for curing disease, preventing disease and replacing organs (specifically designed for each individual), the rate of cost increases in providing health care delivery will most likely accelerate. A role for engineering and operations research in the future will be to aid not only in the development of these technologies but also in their design and manufacture to be more cost efficient and cost effective.

Another quirk of the introduction of new technologies in health care is that: 1. They often do not replace old technologies for a long time and 2. They are often used for many diagnoses and therapies for which they were not designed. Consequently, new therapies for a particular use most often add to the armamentarium of available therapies without reducing costs or often significantly changing behavior.

2.3. Quality, satisfaction and safety

Institute of Medicine [49,50] studies have pointed out the large number of deaths, disabilities and pain and suffering caused annually by medical errors. In many, if not most, cases these adverse events can be traced to poor systems, procedures, communications and conflicting goals and objectives of the service providers.

Furthermore, another factor contributing to a large fraction of the total cost of care delivery is waste and inefficiency, including overuse, underuse, misuse, and duplication of drugs, procedures and technologies and system failures and poor communications, resulting in about 30%–40% of the total health care costs and amounting to more than half a trillion dollars in 2004 [68]. These wastes and inefficiencies can be controlled with better use of operations research methods and procedures.

In fact as shown in other industries, over 85% of most waste and inefficiency is usually caused by poorly designed and operating systems and procedures and can usually be eliminated by improved operations research analysis. Furthermore, these system improvements not only lead to significant cost reduction but at the same time significant improvements in the quality of care delivered.

2.4. Access

The issue of access to health care services has many dimensions. The one most often heard about in the newspapers relates to the fact that approximately 45 million persons in the United States do not have health care insurance at any one point in time. This problem is exacerbated in times of economic stress and unemployment.

However, there are many other types of access issues. There are the problems of waiting lines that, in many countries, inhibit access to care. In United States these waiting lines often occur in emergency rooms, walk in clinics and physicians' offices. But they also occur inside hospitals, nursing homes and other care delivery sites. For example, in hospitals there are frequently waiting lines for operating rooms, ICU beds, ancillary facilities and admissions and discharge. Speed and timeliness of access to health care delivery may also be a problem in emergency cases. The appropriate location and deployment of emergency vehicles and personnel are often critical for life-saving access. It is these types of access barriers and operations researchers have successfully removed for overall health care systems improvement.

As can learned from this brief discussion of these four big issues in health care delivery in the United States, the rate of increase in costs (i.e. the slope of the health care cost curve) is largely being driven by the introduction of new technologies and the intensity of use of all technologies. Consequently, to reduce his rate of increase it is necessary to restrict the introduction of new technologies or use more cost-saving technologies. With the expenditure of over $50 billion each year in US health care research and development by the NIH and private companies, we are not likely to see significant restrictions on the introduction of new technologies. However, there are operations research methods for restricting introduction of new technologies, now being used in other parts of the world that are discussed later in this chapter. The other approach to reducing costs is to pursue cost savings that lower the level of the healthcare cost curve. This can be done by introducing better methods of delivering care so that wastes and inefficiencies are removed, as well as introducing cost-saving procedures and improving processes used throughout the delivery system. The bulk of the operations research work done today and discussed in this chapter is primarily directed toward lowering the cost curve by making continuing cost savings and by improving quality of care at the same time.

The applications in this chapterare presented in three major sections. First is management of operations, which examines uses of operations research methods at the operational and tactical levels of management. Second is medical management and biomedicine, which involves patient disease prevention, detection and/or treatment at the policy, at the patient and at the cellular levels. Third is system design and planning, which deals with strategic decisions, both at the policy level and at the operational level.

3. Management of operations

What has been learned in many industries over the past century is that the quality and safety of production and services can be greatly improved, costs greatly reduced and throughput significantly increased by reducing unnecessary variability in the delivery (production) processes. Perhaps the most famous example is Henry Ford's use of the assembly line where variability of the production process was reduced to a minimum, worker safety improved, automobile quality stabilized and continually increased and costs reduced year on year. Although health care delivery is not a production line such as automobile production, the approach of eliminating unnecessary variability also will work to improve quality, costs and throughput in health care delivery [64,65].

The variability phenomenon that is working in health care delivery involves the random arrival of patients on an emergency basis usually through the emergency room competing for scarce resources in the clinic or hospital with the arrival of scheduled patients. Generally speaking the arrival of emergency patients typically follows a compound Poisson or truncated Poisson distribution that has natural variability. The knowledge of this natural variability with its mean arrival rates and variances can be used for planning the availability and amounts of resources needed for these emergency patients with any required high-level of probability (95% or higher). The problem compounds, however, when the scheduled patients are not properly scheduled into the workload with the randomly arriving emergency patients. This latter happens when there is unnecessary or "artificial" variation in elective scheduled arrivals at the clinic or hospital. The peaks of these combined flows of arrivals are higher and the valleys of low activity are deeper so that many undesirable consequences follow. There are not enough nurses, other personnel, OR rooms, recovery beds, ICU beds, etc. to handle the peaks leading to long overtime hours, errors, adverse events, forgotten tasks, bumped elective patients and lower throughput. And there are often too many nurses, other personnel, empty facilities, etc. which are wasted in the valleys. Furthermore, higher patient congestion than available resources can properly handle will cause more mortality than would occur otherwise [2,50]. It is always a mystery why health care delivery seems to think that their personnel are "superhuman" and can "handle" these excessive peaks and valleys whereas industry, airlines, utilities and others know that their workers, engineers, pilots, etc. are not able to do so without the proper workload balance and rest.

Fortunately for health care delivery, these peaks and valleys can be greatly smoothed, workloads put into better balance and resources used much more effectively and efficiently. The artificial variation is usually an artifact of the surgical block scheduling regimes or specialty bed allocation rules used in the operating rooms and/or other units that create unnecessary bottlenecks and backlogs. Eliminate this artificial variation first to begin to smooth the incoming workload. Once the incoming patient workload is smoothed, then tackle smoothing the other bottleneck flows of patients and resources in the institution including the scheduling of nursing, ancillary and administrative services and patient transfers and discharges. It is essential to tackle the incoming workload *first* because often the downstream congestion, waste and workload problems are the result of the peaks and valleys of the initial input processes that later create artificial downstream bottlenecks and variation. An excellent example of the

Exhibit 1: Staff Bulletin May 2009, Volume 45 Issue 5
For the Medical Staff and Alumni of Cincinnati Children' s Hospital Medical Center
A CFO's Perspective
Improved patient flow and placement boosts capacity

Scott Hamlin, CFO and senior vice president, Finance, has long been touting how improving the quality and safety of care is beneficial to the medical center's bottom line. Now, he's spreading the word about how improved patient flow and placement can have a similar effect.
In a recent presentation to the Finance Committee of the Board, Hamlin noted that in FY2004, Cincinnati Children's had a maximum physical inpatient capacity of 425 beds, or what he calls "theoretical capacity." It was theoretical because we never actually were able to use all those beds, thanks to inherent glitches in the system, such as:

- Uneven scheduling of elective admissions
- Bottlenecks in key flow areas (ED, Post Anesthesia Care Unit, Intensive Care, etc.)
- Inadequate discharge planning
- Inefficient physical layout constraints and patient placement not designed with capacity as part of criteria

These glitches meant that we were really only able to really count on using about 325 beds which Hamlin dubbed our "practical capacity." So in effect when we were at the peak of practical capacity we were only at 76 percent of our theoretical maximum capacity.
But things have changed.
Over the past four years, Cincinnati Children's staff has been focusing on smoothing scheduling, discharge planning, patient flow and physical layout in key bottleneck areas and re-examining patient placement to allow for greater use of resources and space. With renovations at College Hill and with efforts to recapture inpatient bed space by moving office space to 3244 Burnet, today our "theoretical capacity" is at 490 beds, But more importantly because we're improving flow processes, over the past four months we've been able to frequently handle a peak daily census in excess of 450 patients. That translates to expanding our practical capacity to 91 percent of theoretical capacity.

What it means
Most importantly, our ability to accommodate more patients in a safe, timely and efficient manner means better outcomes, experience and value for our families. But the added capacity also boosts the bottom line by giving us the potential to generate $ 375,000 of additional net billing revenue each day ($137 million each year) from our existing assets and staffing.
To date in FY2009, we have been able to capture about 24 percent of the total additional capacity we have created through offering state of the art programs that remain in high demand. This combination of extraordinary program offerings and finding ways to better utilize the existing assets to accommodate that demand have allowed us to avoid the construction of 102 additional beds that would have been required to meet today's volume if we were still operating at 76 percent practical capacity. That adds up to a savings of more than $100 million in construction costs.
Says Hamlin: "This is an amazing achievement given the current economic climate. It shows that while we have always worked hard, it's equally important to work smart. And Cincinnati Children's staff has proven, time and time again, that they're experts at doing both."

great value of workloads smoothing is illustrated in the sidebar Exhibit 1, shown below, giving results from the Cincinnati Children's Hospital Medical Center.

The key operations research methodology used in studying variation in services is queueing theory and methods [32,67]. Every day almost everyone in the world is involved in at least one and usually many queueing processes whether it is waiting in traffic at intersections, for checkout in retail stores, for meals in restaurants, for data bytes whizzing from some other electronic devices to your electronic devices and the like. Queueing processes can be simple or complex but they all involve "customer" arrivals, usually with some natural or artificial randomness, a waiting line where they queue and some servers that provide the service desired by the customer where the time and level of service may also involve some randomness. The output of this process is the throughput of the queueing system. The throughput can have many characteristics such as numbers served, speed of service, waiting time, quality of service, satisfaction, etc. But there are only three ways that this queueing process can be managed for improvement. First, manage the arrivals of customers, second, manage the waiting lines and third, manage the service delivery. Of course the more complex the queueing processes, such as a hospital, the more complex the management but this complexity should not be a deterrent to tackling improvement.

In the previously referenced papers [64,65,67] these authors show these significant improvements in throughput, costs and quality of care delivered by appropriately using queuing methodologies to smooth the emergency and scheduled arrivals of patients for surgical procedures. Indeed Exhibit 1 is an example of the use of these methodologies.

In the province of British Columbia, Canada, it was noted that there were many bottlenecks in the provision of surgical services for the population [84]. examined this problem to look for ways they could increase the throughput of patients through the surgical process. It was necessary to build a model involving the capacities of the operating rooms, surgical beds and other facilities in the hospital, the schedules and availabilities of surgeons and the waiting lists of patients for surgery. They also used a mixed integer programming model for scheduling surgical blocks in the operating rooms by specialty in order to maximize throughput of surgical patients. The results were improved utilization of resources in the hospital and reduction in waiting lines for patients.

An often overlooked management activity is revenue enhancement at the same or lower costs. Texas Children's Hospital [9], optimized the performance of reimbursement contracts with insurers to increase direct revenues by $17 million annually with the use of operations research forecasting, risk measurement and nonlinear optimization models. The hospital used PROS revenue management software to quantify expected future demand via forecasting, risk analysis for measuring contract performance and incorporating these inputs into a cost and revenue model which told the hospital the net cost or profit of each procedure and activity. (This model is an adaptation of revenue enhancement models used in airlines, car rentals and other industries that have inventories whose values cannot be stored such as an empty seat, an empty bed, a car in the lot if is not used that day). The revenue management model then informed the hospital's contract negotiators on which items to renegotiate contracts with insurance providers in order to maximize total revenue with no increase in costs. This analysis also informed hospital management in their analysis of internal operations and processes on where to put more emphasis in cost control and performance improvement. The enhanced revenues enabled the hospital to continue to provide the highest quality patient care, research and teaching services.

Other operations research applications involve direct and indirect cost improvements via improved efficiency and effectiveness in the delivery of clinical, ancillary and administrative services. Many of these improvements can be realized by *process analyses* of how the work is currently being done and how unnecessary steps, waste or errors can be eliminated. It is always surprising to this author how little attention is given to the operations of seemingly mundane tasks in a hospital such as patient location and scheduling, patient transport, patient meals, inventories, etc. and yet how big an impact they often have on the smooth or in many cases dysfunctional operation of the processes of care delivery. Take patient transport, for example. If the patient is not in the correct place at the correct time, there are delays and disruptions in ancillary tests, surgeries, ICUs, wards and other locations leading to personnel and facilities downtimes and excessive patient waiting for service and/or rescheduling [41], studied this problem for large German hospitals and designed a computer-based programming model that supports all phases of transportation flows including booking, dispatching, delivery and monitoring and reporting in real time so that smooth timely flows of patients to required locations are accomplished.

Another mundane example of waste occurred in the food/dietary department of a large urban hospital [79]. Presbyterian Hospital had positioned itself as a premier healthcare provider. Yet the quality of its food delivery system was very poor resulting in excessive costs due to waste of food and labor time and also resulting in patient dissatisfaction and frustration among clinicians and nurses. This problem in Food Services was only one of many cost and quality problems in the hospital. Each day in Food Services on average 800 meals were delivered in the hospital at a cost exceeding six dollars per meal. Also each day 62% of these meals were wasted and discarded. Treating this problem as a systems problem and using process flow analysis along with simple methodologies such as flow diagrams, Pareto analysis, fishbone diagrams and statistical control charts, the root causes of this waste was understood and systems changes were introduced. Thousands of dollars per day were saved in food costs alone as well as significant savings made in better labor utilization of food service personnel, nurses' time and physician interactions.

3.1. Demand forecasting

Work smoothing begins with forecasting and with understanding the structure and flows of the demand processes arriving for services. How can you plan ahead and obtain and deploy needed revenues and resources without having a good idea of what demand will be or of what demand would be after changes to the system? Yet very few institutions do any formal forecasting but prefer to operate on the basis of intuition for the future or on the expectation that the future will be like the recent past. Of course this approach is a form of forecasting but at the most naïve and primitive level. It frequently leads to unpleasant surprises: unplanned shortfalls, quality deterioration and cost overruns.

The operations research literature is replete with good forecasting models and applications at all levels and in all types and manners of industries and sectors of the economy. When they are used, health care tends to employ existing and well-known operations research models developed for use in other industries rather than invent unique approaches. With the more recent exception of forecasting for revenue enhancement [9] the examples of the use of forecasting for better decision making largely appears in the earlier health services research literature.

Forecasting models fall into two categories: qualitative models and quantitative models. The chief differences between qualitative and quantitative models are the degree to which subjective judgment influences the model and the levels of analytic methodologies used. Some models, such as the Delphi technique, attempt to formalize explicit expert judgment. Others, such as econometric modeling, make other implicit assumptions and judgments in the specification of the inputs and structure of the model. This impact of judgment, whether explicit or implicit, on the outputs of the demand forecasting model can be strong as [42,47] describe in their reviews of models used in health care. In choosing forecasting models, the degree of judgment should be considered, and various approaches to modeling and sensitivity analysis should be tried. An excellent recent book on the principles to use in the choice and use of forecasting models is *Principles of Forecasting* [3]. This book summarizes knowledge from leading forecasting experts and from empirical studies across many fields and presents "hands-on and what to do and why" information.

Listed below are a few examples of some different forecasting models used for forecasting demand for health care services.

Kamentzky et al. [52] use least squares regression analysis to determine the demand for pre-hospital care in order to make ambulance staffing decisions. In the model they include demographic, operational and clinical variables that contribute to the types and levels of demand. Demographic variables are area population, area employment, persons per household, mean age, and ratio of blue collar to white collar workers, and indicators of social well-being such as median family income and percent of families with female heads. Operational variables include emergent cases, transport to hospitals, inter-hospital transport, standby, and volumes. Clinical variables include cardiac status, trauma, emergency or minor care. Using data from Pennsylvania, the authors find that the socio-economic, operational, and clinical variables are all significant in predicting unmet need, and they validate the model so that the transport system could be improved.

Kao and Tung [54] use demand forecasting for inpatient services in the British health service. They employ an auto-regressive, integrated moving average (*ARIMA*) time series model to forecast demand for inpatient services. The procedure for model development, parameter estimation, and diagnostic checking involves the use of deterministic trends with regular differencing between periods so that the basic trend changes from period to period. This model is stratified by patient service and month of year, so that monthly admissions and patient days can be forecasted by service and length of stay estimates can be made. Compared to actua1 data, the model produces forecast errors ranging from 21.5% (deviation from the predicted) in newborn nursery to 3.3% in psychiatry. The authors suggest that the demand forecasting system can be used for bed allocation and aggregate nurse planning.

Johansen et al. [51] demonstrate a model for forecasting intermediate skilled home nursing needs which combines elements of simple observational models and complex statistical approaches, and was utilization-based rather than population-based. The authors restrict their model to outpatient variables that were uniformly, clearly, and consistently collected and coded, including principal and secondary diagnoses, patient disposition, nature of admission, hospital size, metropolitan area, and marital status. Medical and demographic factors describe four risk categories into which patients could be assigned, indicating their overall risk for intermittent home care services. The authors first perform two-way tabulations on patients on the basis of these variables; then determine the predicted number of patients in each category using weighted averages. The expected cost per skilled nursing service is obtained by multiplying the expected number of patients in each category by the mean cost per patient. Sensitivity analyses determine the effects of changes in the health care system on these estimates. The authors determine the probability of need for service given the risk level of the patient, which ranges from a probability of 5% for a low-risk patient to 80% for a very high-risk patient. The authors note that this model incorporates easily observable characteristics, and provides good performance accuracy when compared with real data.

Kao and Poldadnik [53] describe adaptive forecasting of hospital census, demonstrating how institutional and exogenous variables can be used in forecasting models to improve accuracy longitudinally. The authors argue that such models should be analytically credible, yet simple and easy to use. In their model, the census on any given day is a function of a constant component, a linear trend factor, and random disturbances, which are minimized by a discounted least squares analysis. The authors then observe that, in addition to the basic pattern of census at many institutions, there are internal and external factors that could explain additional census variation. For example, renovations, holidays, and administrative actions may close units from time to time; utilization review programs could change length of stay; natural disasters or epidemics could change demand for a short time. The authors use tracking signals, rather than smoothing, to improve hospital forecasting and trigger different rates of parameter updating. In a case study, these techniques are used to improve forecasting decisions by including adjustment factors for holidays, adding, opening and closing nursing units, and unexpected events.

3.2. Patient scheduling

Controlling demand for services via scheduling can be very effective as a method of matching demand with the supply of services available and vice versa. Outpatients frequently dislike waiting for service, and consequently balk or renege on appointments if waiting time is considered excessive. Inpatients, likewise, are dissatisfied with slow, disruptive or bumped hospital service. Consequently, the problem of satisfying both patients and health care providers is a challenging one and most scheduling systems attempt to optimize the combined objectives of satisfaction of patients, satisfaction of physicians, and utilization of facilities in some weighted fashion. In many cases a better objective would be to optimize throughput and quality of outcomes.

Good patient scheduling has many benefits that include reduced staffing costs and reduced congestion in the hospital and clinics. Appropriate supply of personnel, facilities, equipment and services can be more effectively provided to meet the smoothed flow of demand. An area of benefit that is just beginning to be addressed is the improvement in quality of care (in addition to patient satisfaction) that comes from reduction of congestion via effective demand and supply scheduling. Quality is improved by providing the appropriate amounts and kinds of care at the appropriate times.

There are problems, however, in devising and implementing scheduling systems which meet the primary goals of minimizing numbers of staff and/or staff idle time (primarily physicians) and equipment idle time while maximizing or strongly satisfying patient needs. Some of these problems stem from inadequate information systems, many from resistance to change by staff, some from authorities who demand uniformity of approaches across institutions and others from failing to capture key linkages and system interactions because of the complexity of the core delivery processes. This last set of problems occurs more frequently in hospital inpatient settings in situations where complex progressive patient care is needed rather than in outpatient settings.

3.3. Outpatient scheduling

Effective scheduling of patients in doctors' offices or clinics for outpatient services is one of the earliest documented uses of operations research in improving health care delivery. Bailey [5] applies queueing theory to equalize patients' waiting times in hospital outpatient departments. He observes that many outpatient clinics are essentially a single queue with single or multiple servers. The problem then becomes one of building an appointment system to minimize patient waiting time and keeping the servers busy. The appointment system must be designed to have the inter-arrival times of patients somewhat smaller than their service time. Unfortunately, outside the laboratory, the service system ismore complicated. Some patients arrive late or not at all; some physicians arrive late; service times are not homogeneous but vary by the type and degree of illness; diagnostic equipment is not always available; there are unplanned arrivals of emergent patients and so forth. For these and other reasons many of the early outpatient scheduling models were not widely adopted.

However, more recent models and methodologies for effective outpatient scheduling show successful implementation. The three most commonly used systems involve variations on block scheduling, modified block scheduling and individual scheduling. In block scheduling, all patients are scheduled for one appointment time, for instance 9:00 AM or 1:00 PM. They are then served on a first-come-first-service (FCFS) basis. Clearly, this approach has long patient waiting times, high clinic congestion and minimal staff idle time. Furthermore, because many of these outpatients may have contagious diseases the likelihood of infecting other patients increases the longer these patients interact. Modified block scheduling breaks the day into smaller blocks (e.g. the beginning of each hour) and schedules smaller blocks of patients into those times. It has many of the characteristics of the block systems but patient waiting time is lowered and other bad quality effects are reduced. Block and modified block scheduling are in use in most of the world especially in those countries with national health care systems. On the other hand, individual scheduling systems schedule patients for individual times throughout the day often in conjunction with staff availabilities. If scheduled patient interarrival times (times between arrivals) are not significantly shorter than service times, patient waiting time is reduced and staff idle time can be kept small. However, these systems require much more information on patients' illnesses and needs, triaging may be necessary by the appointment scheduler, and unforeseen events can cause severe scheduling problems. In spite of these potential drawbacks, individualized outpatient scheduling systems are most widely used in the private sector in the United States.

The literature on outpatient scheduling is extensive beginning in the 1950s and peaking in the 1960s and 1970s. Since much of it is based on queueing or simulation, studies were done to determine parametric distributions for patient service times. Scheduling schemes to reduce patient waiting time, while not increasing physician idle time, were analyzed using these distributions as inputs. O'Keefe [70] gives a very good description of the waiting times, congestion, and bureaucracy in consultative clinics in the British Health Service. A modified block system is used. Using heuristic methods he shows that some improvement can be made in spite of overwhelming resistance to change and extensive system constraints. Satisfying the scheduling systems non-patient stakeholders (physicians and nurses) requires implementation of a policy that is *clearly suboptimal* for patients. The work is interesting in that it implicitly shows that to effect change in a bureaucratic system, it is essential to address and/or change the incentives of the stakeholders running the system.

Outpatient scheduling will require further refinement in the future, as the emphasis on this mode of care delivery continues to increase. Scheduling models need to include performance measures reflecting the costs and benefits for all participants. Segmentation of patients into categories with significantly different requirements for service can also enhance the performance characteristics of patient scheduling systems. Again, minimizing variation of patient times for service or waiting will have significant throughput improvement, waiting time reduction and service quality improvement because of the reduction in congestion and happier patients who will do less reneging or balking in appointments.

In clinics where emergent patients are reasonably frequent each day, the classification scheme must separate these patients from non-emergent other patients. Work by Shonick [87] for emergent patients in acute care general hospitals, and by other authors in other settings, demonstrates that a truncated Poisson distribution provides a good fit for the arrival process of such patients. An outpatient scheduling system, which considers the stochastic variation of emergency patients *separately* from the stochastic variation of no shows and late arrivals of scheduled patients, will better achieve minimal waiting time and minimal staff idle time.

3.4. Inpatient scheduling

There are three major dimensions of inpatient scheduling. First is the scheduling of elective admissions together with emergent admissions into appropriate units of the hospital each day (admissions, A). Second is the daily scheduling of inpatients to the appropriate care units within the hospital for treatment or diagnoses throughout their stay (transfers, T). Third is the scheduling of the discharges of patients to their homes or other care delivery institutions (discharges, D). Clearly, these scheduling activities (ATD) are linked and depend upon many characteristics of the patients and hospital. The models used for inpatient scheduling are more complex and require more data and better information systems than those for outpatients. Many different methodologies are proposed involving queueing models as represented by Markov and semi-Markov processes, mathematical programming, heuristic and expert systems, and simulation. There are also less formal modeling approaches more traditionally associated with rules-of-thumb and charting models.

Because of the complexities of inpatient scheduling problems and because of relatively poor internal forecasting and information systems, most hospitals use informal or ad hoc methods. Consequently, neither the size of the facilities, staffing, nor facility utilization are well planned, resulting in inefficiencies caused by peaks and valleys of occupancy as noted earlier. The valleys create a situation of excess labor and underuse of facilities. The peaks create congestion and, because of difficulties of finding appropriately trained personnel on short notice, at typical wages, often lead to patient dissatisfaction, lower quality, more adverse events and higher operating costs. Those problems can occur throughout the institution, involving physicians, residents, nurses, aides, and ancillary, support and administrative services personnel. On the other hand, analytic inpatient scheduling can ameliorate many of these problems and improve effective and efficient (optimizing) use of hospital resources.

As with outpatient scheduling, the inpatient scheduling literature began to appear in the early 1950's and peaked in the 1960's and 1970's. However, there has been a resurgence of interest and work this decade. Most of the studies on admission scheduling divide the patients into two categories: waiting list and emergency. Furthermore, most of these studies only cover admissions to a single service in the hospital (such as surgery, obstetrics, pediatrics or another single ward). The idea underlying many of these earlier scheduling systems is to compute the expected number of available beds or surgery slots for the next day (or 1onger). The schedule system would then reserve a block of beds for the emergent patients randomly arriving in the next 24 hours and then fill the remaining beds or slots from the waiting list of patients for elective admission. Typically, the amount of reserve beds or slots for emergency will be based on the means and variances or probability distribution of their arrival patterns (again usually a truncated or compound Poisson would be used) and on some measure of over run of demand such as 95% or 99% of the emergent demand would be satisfied daily or over some longer period. This variation on the classic inventory control problem is usually solved by simulation and/or queueing analytic methods.

In computing the anticipated bed availability for the next day, many authors attempt to estimate the length of stay of current patients and then forecast expected discharges. Most of the studies do not look at the hospital as a total system in that there may be other bottlenecks in the institution such as radiology, laboratory, personnel staffing, physician availabilities or transport which are adding unnecessary days to length of stay or causing other bed utilization effects. The most common scheduling role is to compute the number of beds or dedicated OR rooms or slots needed to accept a given portion of emergent patients and then to fill any remaining available OR slots or beds with waiting list patients. Unfortunately, because of pre-assigned beds and/or slot times to the different physician specialties, a large amount of artificial variation exists in most scheduling systems. Indeed, these systems do not smooth arrivals evenly over Monday through Friday and throughout each day. But fortunately, recent work in a few locations is showing that changing some old established rules and behaviors leads to significant improvement in costs, quality, throughput and revenues for both physicians and hospitals [65,66].

Also as input variability is reduced, better progressive care, better bed planning (capacity) decisions, personnel scheduling decisions and care delivery decisions follow. And as cost pressures continue to grow, more effective patient scheduling methods will be needed to balance and plan staffing, facilities, equipment procurement and services. Much more research and applications need to be studied to link these systems for even higher quality, lower cost care.

3.5. Work force planning and scheduling

The management of human resources is a major activity in health care organizations. Staffing costs usually represent the majority of the operating budget. Like many service organizations the ability to match staffing resources to a fluctuating demand directly affects operating efficiency and the quality of service. This is why, as stated several times earlier, the management of demand arrivals is the first order of business and often requires changes to the way the medical staff currently works. But the development of innovative approaches to the organization and management of nursing and other human resources holds great promise for further cost savings in the delivery of health services.

Although the planning and scheduling of health care personnel is not conceptually different than that of other personnel (one needs the right persons in the right places at the right times) there are several factors that make the problem in health care more complex. First, there is the interrelation among various highly trained and skilled personnel that must be available at the appropriate times for different patients. These personnel include different specialty categories of nurses, therapists, physicians, medical technicians and others. Staffing must be available 24 hours a day on all days. Personnel have preferences and requests for types of schedules and working conditions. Many function as relatively independent professionals with regard to the level and scope of tasks. Second, it is frequently difficult to measure the quality of work done hourly as it pertains to successful patient outcomes except where there may be adverse events. This measurement difficulty presents problems in determining the mix of types and skill levels of personnel that are really needed to obtain a given level of quality. Third, for most personnel categories there are 'flat' organizational structures with few career paths available. As a consequence, human resource management must continually cope with ways to maintain personnel satisfaction and enjoyment to retain highly capable individuals over the period of many years, even decades, or face the high costs of absenteeism, turnover, and general dissatisfaction. Indeed, many debates about professional nursing activities are direct outgrowths of basic nurse staffing and workload problems.

Most of the research in staffing and scheduling for health care organizations focuses on nursing. However, personnel availability and utilization in the laboratory, emergency department, respiratory therapy, HMO's, and other locations have also been examined. Hershey and colleagues [45] conceptualize the nurse staffing process as a hierarchy of three decision levels which operate over different time horizons and with different precision. These three decision levels are called corrective allocations, shift scheduling, and workforce planning. Corrective allocations are done daily. Shift schedules are the days-on days-off work schedules for each nurse for four to eight weeks ahead. Workforce plans are quarterly, semiannual, or annual plans of nursing needs by skill level. On any given day within a shift, the staff capacities among units may be adjusted to unpredicted demand fluctuations and absenteeism by using float, parttime, relief, overtime, and voluntary absenteeism. These corrective allocations depend upon the individuals' preferences, their availabilities, and capabilities. Shift scheduling is the matching of nursing staff availabilities to expected workload among units on a daily basis for a four to eight week period in the future. For each employee days on and off, as well as shift rotation, are determined. The individual's needs and preferences must be considered to bring about high personnel satisfaction.

The above two scheduling levels are tactical, in that they concern the utilization of personnel already employed within the organization or hired on a temporary basis from outside with their known mix of specializations and experiences. Workforce planning is the long-term balance of numbers and capability of nursing personnel among units obtained by hiring, training, transferring between jobs, and discharging. Because of the time lags involved, workforce-planning actions must be taken at least yearly to meet anticipated long-term fluctuations in demand and supply. Very few studies address this decision level. However, it is obvious that the more that patient demand can be forecasted and smoothed, i.e. the more that workload peaks and valleys can be eliminated, the better the workloads can be balanced for nursing personnel. Furthermore, the interdependence of the three levels must be recognized to bring about systematic nurse staffing improvements. Each level is constrained by available resources, by previous commitments made at higher levels, and by the degrees of flexibility for later correction at lower levels. Therefore, each decision level is strongly dependent on the other two. For optimal performance, one level cannot be considered in isolation. The final component of the model is the coordination of staffing management activities with other departments. For example, if any personnel group is short staffed, other groups bear a greater burden.

The earliest OR work on work force planning and scheduling in hospitals began with measuring the needs of patients for various types of care. Over time, such needs have come to include physical, hygienic, instructional, observational, emotional, and family counseling needs of patients. These types and amounts of care are quantified in patient classification systems and then related to the hours of different skilled personnel needed to meet them. These formal or informal models are needed to make corrective allocations. However, the more that arrivals can be smoothed throughout the week, these corrective allocations are less variable and less needed.

Longer term workload forecasting (one to two months) by skill level is needed for shift scheduling. Most forecasting in use merely extrapolates recent experience using adjustments for seasonal and week-end variations. Often the workload forecasting models used are simple moving averages, but occasionally regression and ARIMA time series models have been used [44] use a multiple regression approach to predict nursing labor hour requirements by ward, shift, day of the week and month of the year [75] also used multiple regression models to predict daily and weekly laboratory workloads for scheduling purposes. Other forecasting models and applications were discussed earlier in this chapter.

Effective shift scheduling (i.e., meets the health care needs of patients and the preferences of nurses at minimal cost) is a complex problem that attracts the interest of operations researchers. The earliest and simplest scheduling model is the cyclic schedule. This schedule repeats a fixed pattern of days on and off for each nurse indefinitely into the future. This type of schedule cannot easily adjust for forecasted or de facto workload changes, extended absences, or the scheduling preferences of individual nurses. Such rigid schedules place heavy demands on the corrective allocations and workforce planning levels. Hence, corrective allocation must be extremely flexible and workforce planning must more precisely forecast long term workforce needs to avoid excessive staffing [45].

The most commonly used shift scheduling method in practice is "self" scheduling where the nurses participate in their scheduling, usually through the head nurses and with some simple computer interfaces [57]. The nurses prefer this approach because it gives them some control over their schedules whereas some computer based algorithmic programs have often failed to consider their specific needs and preferences appropriately. The downside of this approach is that the actual scheduling of dozens of persons to meet the needs of a wide variety and wide severity of patients on different shifts and wards for many days into the future is a very complex and very large combinatorial problem. The human mind(s) cannot comprehend this level and amount of complexity and the resulting self-based schedules are far from optimal for patients or for the institutional care consistency objectives. In terms of complexity, the problem is analogous to letting the space astronaut team fly the Shuttle by hand from the start to the return. Consequently as we look farther and farther for true low-cost high-quality patient-centered care we will find that complexity in management decisions needs to be assisted by cutting edge solution techniques and sophisticated technological advances.

In Stockholm, Sweden (and many other Scandinavian cities) over 15,000 home health workers deliver care to tens of thousands of patients in their homes. Previously this scheduling was done by hand and because of the complexity of the number and locations of homes to visit, the numbers and specialty skills of care workers and the GIS routes through the highways and byways of the cities, the chosen routes were often poorly designed with many errors and missed assignments, unfair to some workers, more costly and unresponsive to the client's needs [26], developed optimization models and tools using mathematical programming and scheduling rules so that these workers deliver the care needed when needed. With their operations research model called LAPS CARE, system operational efficiency was increased 10–15% at an annual savings of $30–45 million.

4. Medical management and biomedicine

The contributions of operations research methodologies to disease prevention and clinical decision-making constitute a large and growing area of both health services research and operations research. This area is a hybrid that draws upon the mathematics and structural analysis of operations research and its solution approaches including optimization, stochastic processes, influence diagrams and simulation, as well as a deep knowledge of biological, economic, and sociological aspects of patient care. This section will review medical management in two areas. First is the use of *decision analysis and dynamic influence diagrams* to aid in the structuring and support of medical decisions. Second is *performance improvement*. In this area, operations research methodologies that improve the accuracy of diagnoses, the ability to diagnose under uncertainty, and the performance of testing or treatment strategies are reviewed. This area is particularly relevant to current concerns about quality of care and practice efficiency.

4.1. Decision analysis and dynamic influence diagrams

One of the first principles of approaching a decision in which there is risk and uncertainty is to determine the attributes, structure, and outcomes of those decisions, along with their concomitant probabilities. Decision trees and dynamic influence diagrams are often used to show probabilities, outcomes, chance nodes, and decision nodes for complex problems, such as thyroid irradiation treatment during childhood or coronary artery disease treatment. These models have been used in numerous health services research articles. The key part of this process of decision analysis is identification of critical nodes or those decision variables which are important to outcomes or which the decision-maker wants to modify. An example of the use of dynamic influence diagrams in decision analysis is given by Hazen [43]. In this paper he uses dynamic influence diagrams to structure and analyze a chain of decisions as to whether or not a patient should proceed to total hip replacement surgery. In this model back stepping loops can occur in that once a decision is made it may be necessary to revisit that decision or other decisions in the future before moving forward again. Decision influence diagrams are a network of looping, continuous, recycling decision processes. See Fig. 3.

In this dynamic influence decision process, the decision to be made was a choice between total hip arthroplasty (THA) or no surgery at all, that is, conservative management. The objective in making this decision is to calculate the optimal expected costs and quality adjusted life years (QALYS) under each choice. Quality adjusted life years have been proposed for use to measure the length of a person's life, adjusted for the quality experienced during that remaining lifetime. For example, 20 years experience in a state of health that is only half as desirable as an ideal state of health is in terms of QALYS only valued at 10 years. Many variables may be included in such a model: age, sex, mobility, and/or other functional, social, demographic, and racial characteristics of the patient. For illustration Hazen included only race, age, and sex. The use of quality adjusted life years for the objective was important because an older person undergoing THA may not have more expected years of life relative to not doing surgery but the quality of life going from American College of Rheumatology functional class III to functional classes I and II can be considerable and quite possibly well worth the cost. In his example Hazen used Cox stochastic trees to forecast the progression to death and its functional stages for a 85 year old white male and for a 60-year-old white female given no intervention. Each of these persons currently is in ACR class III and needs to choose between THA or conservative management. If the man chooses THA, his quality of life would be in ACR class I for about 2.9 years, followed by class II for about 1.4 years, followed by class III for 0.06 years and then death from other causes. For the woman, she would be in class I for nine years, class II for five years in class III for seven years. Considering all of

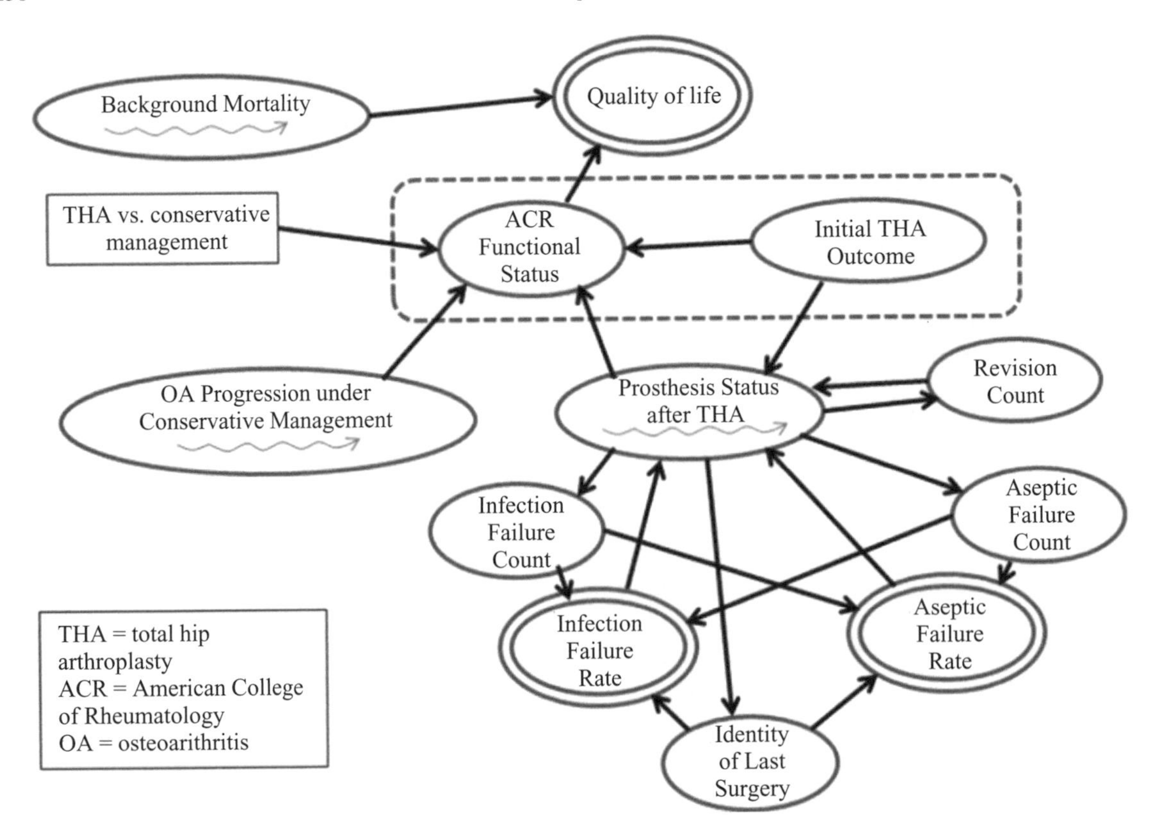

Fig. 3. A dynamic influence diagram for model of the choice between THA and conservative management. Source: Hazen, 2004 [Fig. 24-7].

the costs of surgery weighed against the increased quality of life and the longer nursing home costs of conservative management in later years, THA would be the better decision for both persons and indeed would also result in significant cost savings for the woman over her remaining lifetime due to reduced time in nursing home.

In another decision analysis model using multi-attribute utility theory, Simon [88] considers the decision needed to be made by a patient who has been diagnosed with prostate cancer and must choose among treatments (surgery, external beam radiation, brachytherapy, and dual radiation) or do nothing. The model uses up-to-date data collected from the medical literature to compute probabilities regarding the likelihood of death and other side effects for each of the treatments or for doing nothing. Next the model must incorporate the patient's individual preferences regarding length of life and quality of life for different states of health in view of the possible side effects (impotence, incontinence and toxicity). These preferences are closely related to QALYS. With this data entered, the model evaluates each treatment alternative and compares the results for the particular patient. This model is available to any potential patient with prostate cancer at http://soarthroughlife.com to evaluate the patient's choices based on the patient's own data and preferences.

In any decision analysis study it is essential to perform sensitivity analysis, where the parameters, particularly *ex ante* probabilities of chance events, are varied to determine the effect on the resultant decision to either errors in data or uncertainty itself. For example, one could vary the input data in either of the models by Hazen or Simon to analyze how the choices might change over a range of variation in the input data. Indeed, sensitivity analysis is used in almost all operations research modeling whenever any of the input data or variables have some uncertainty.

Also in a decision analysis study it is necessary to identify ambiguous outcomes as a result of some medical interventions. For example although death itself is a clearly identified state, it is not always clear that the decision in question can be implicated in a death which is proximal to the decision. This ambiguity is the basis for so-called severity correction or risk adjustment for mortality. Of course as more and more data is gathered from more and more subcategories of patient characteristics, it becomes easier to make inferential statements about the statistical validity of outcomes relating to the intervention. Beyond mortality, however, other indicators, such as life expectancy, quality of life, satisfaction, morbidity, or complications, are sometimes difficult to determine and ambiguous to structure. For these reasons sensitivity analysis plays an even greater role. The current state of the decision analysis literature regarding outcomes has improved considerably so that most articles now clearly identify and, appropriately define outcomes as indicated in the examples above. An early and still useful and readable book on clinical decision analysis is [93].

4.2. Performance improvement

Medical decision *performance improvement* applications are seen in several areas. The first is in improving diagnostic accuracy for chronic and/or acute conditions. An example of work done in this area is given by Rubin et al. [86] using a Bayesian network to assist mammography interpretation. Interpreting mammographic images and making correct diagnoses is challenging even to experienced radiologists. The accuracy of the correct diagnoses is limited by both the quality of the images and by the accuracy of the interpretations. False-negative and false positive interpretations are not uncommon and lead to different follow-up and treatment decisions. In a sense false-negative interpretations are worse because of delaying cancer treatment and leading to higher morbidity and mortality. But false positives have their own risks because patients without cancer undergo unnecessary biopsy causing anxiety and increased medical costs. The American College of radiology developed BI-RADS that is a lexicon of mammogram findings and the distinctions that describe them. The authors have built a Bayesian network model that represents the probabilistic relationships among BI-RADS findings combined with other patient risk factors to improve interpretations and decisions. Their evidence suggests that this Bayesian network model can help to reduce variability and improve overall interpretive performance in mammography. Many other diagnostic areas have been addressed over the past few decades including gastrointestinal diseases, neurological diseases and others where there are multiple possibilities for choices and decisions must be narrowed down based on evidence of highest probability and likelihood.

A second application area concerns improving the performance of testing strategies. This area frequently uses tree structuring and network modeling, but involves analysis aimed at optimization or efficiency/effectiveness improvement. An early example to improve the performance of testing strategies in the 1980s was done by Schwartz et al. [86] for screening blood for the HIV antibody and making decisions affecting blood donor acceptance. At the time the work was done, limited knowledge was available about the biology, epidemiology and early blood manifestations of HIV. Furthermore the initial and conditional sensitivities and specificities of enzyme immunoassays and Western blot tests had wide ranges of errors. Finally, nothing was then known of the effectiveness of registries, counseling of donors, self reporting of donors sexual and drug injection activities and related educational programs. A Bayesian decision tree model, with the decisions probabilistically based on which screening test to use and in what sequence, was used to minimize the number of HIV infected units of blood and blood products entering the nation's blood supply at an acceptable cost. The model was used at a meeting of an expert panel of the National Heart Lung and Blood Institute to inform the panelists who were deciding which blood screening protocol to use at all blood screening centers in the United States. The model provided several outputs: 1. Expected number of infected units entering the blood supply during a specific period of time, 2. Expected number of uninfected units discarded or wasted during that period of time, 3. Expected number of uninfected donors falsely notified, 4. Expected cost per donated unit for the screening regimen being evaluated, 5. Incremental cost and incremental number of wasted units for different screening regimens.

The third application is in the treatment of diseases. Of all areas of operations research applications in health care delivery, this area is one of the fastest growing. These disease treatment decision support models are usually based in optimization, artificial intelligence, and computer science/management information systems and provide decision support to the physician for improved treatment procedures and treatment decisions. However, many clinicians still hesitate to use some of these models for diagnosis or treatment even though they have demonstrated better outcomes. Of course, there are many possible reasons why some innovations are rapidly adopted while others may diffuse slowly or only stay in the research mode. It is a goal of present and future research to study this clinician-model interface process in order to understand the dynamics of adoption and diffusion. As this knowledge grows, operations research-based knowledge systems will become more useful to the practicing physician.

In spite of adoption difficulties, there are some good examples of where operations research has contributed significantly to treatment outcomes. An example of the use of operations research in the reduction of the costs of treatment of prostate cancer and improvement in the quality of outcomes using brachytherapy (the placement of radioactive "seeds" inside a tumor) is given by Lee and Zaider [61]. Alternatives to brachytherapy are do nothing, have surgery, have external beam radiation therapy or use dual radiology (brachytherapy and external beam). The objectives of all of the treatments are to minimize cancer-related mortality while maximizing removal of cancer cells and minimizing damage to healthy cells and other organs in proximity. The current practice of doing the brachytherapy is for physician/technicians to map the location and extent of the tumor using ultrasound, study these maps over a period of several days and then determine where to place the radioactive seeds. Unfortunately by the time of the procedure some of the other organs as well as the prostate had shifted somewhat in the patient and because seed placement is in millimeters, a good plan a few days before is often not so good at procedure time. A real time analysis that could quickly analyze the actual situation and optimally choose placements in the prostate from the thousands of possible locations, millimeters apart, to minimize damage to healthy tissue and organs and maximize the death of the cancerous cells was needed. Using a real time computer driven nonlinear mathematical programming model linked to real time imaging procedures, Lee and Zaider not only achieved these medical objectives in brachytherapy, they also reduced direct surgical costs by $5,600 per patient and noted large indirect cost savings and quality improvement from fewer complications from impotence, incontinence and toxicity and leading to a higher quality of life faster.

Two other papers focus on radiotherapy treatment for cancer using mathematical optimization techniques. Holder [48] uses linear programming for intensity modulated radiotherapy treatment, IMRT. The vast majority of these treatment plans currently are designed by clinicians through intelligent trial and error. However, it is becoming essential to use optimization for extremely complicated and complex plans. Indeed, the complexity and capabilities of IMRT has rapidly proceeded beyond the scope of human comprehension and future improvements in technology will only increase this degree of complexity. For more in-depth study of this area, go to http://www.trinity.edu/aholder/HealthApp/oncology/ for a depository of recent papers and a list of interested researchers.

[27,28] developed optimization tools for radiation treatment planning in the MATLAB programming environment. Their optimization tools apply in both the intensity modulated radiation therapy environment and/or the three-dimensional conformal radiotherapy environment. In both of these papers the objective is to deliver a specified dose to the target area (above a minimum and below a maximum level of dosage) and spare or minimize damage to surrounding healthy tissue and nearby critical body structures and organs.

4.3. Screening for disease

The introduction of and improvements in tests that detect diseases have resulted in advances in medical diagnosis and disease detection – the first step in disease treatment or prevention. These tests may be applied to an individual (individual screening) or to large subsets of the population (mass screening). These two cases present different modeling problems because the objectives of the decision makers frequently differ, and the constraints and parameters affecting the decisions may vary. For example, in mass screening control and treatment, the objective may be to minimize the prevalence of a contagious disease in the population or subpopulations subject to resource constraints, compliance levels and other population-based constraints. For an individual, the objective may be to prolong life (or the quality of life) and the constraints may be related to the individual's ability or willingness to pay, the individual's characteristics and history and the individual's life style and environment. In each case the decision makers are also usually different persons, e.g., the public health official or HMO director for mass screening and the patient or patient's physician for individual screening.

The decision maker must consider several factors in choosing a screening protocol. First, screening programs have to be designed in light of the tradeoff between the testing cost, which increases both with the frequency of test applications and with the accuracy of the test used, and the testing benefits to be achieved from detecting the disease in an earlier stage of development. Second, such a design must determine which kind of testing technology should be used, as different technologies may have different reliability characteristics (false positive and false negative levels) and costs. Third, the frequency of testing must be decided. Fourth, in the case of mass screening because different subpopulations may have different susceptibility to the disease, the problem of optimal allocation of a fixed testing budget among subpopulations must be considered. Fifth, behavioral problems of attendance at the testing location and compliance with treatment after disease discovery must be included in the analysis.

Direct quantifiable costs of mass screening and control of infectious diseases are those of the labor and materials needed to administer the testing and control programs and indirect costs involving the inconvenience and possible discomfort necessitated by the test, the cost of false positives which entails both emotional distress and the need to do unnecessary follow-up testing, the risk of physical harm to the individual (e.g., the cumulative effect of X-ray exposure or harm from unnecessary surgery) and the costs of disruption to the social fabric of the area, region or nation. These costs must be considered relative to the benefits to be gained by the reduction in disease prevalence and its subsequent cost savings from less treatment in the future and the increase in the overall health and quality of life of the population.

4.3.1. Epidemic control of contagious and other population-wide diseases

We know with probabilistic certainty that the world will be facing a major deadly viral pandemic in the not too distant future just as we know with probabilistic certainty that certain geographic regions will be facing major earthquakes, hurricanes and or tornadoes. The problem is we do not know when or what magnitude an impact one of these phenomena will have. Operations researchers study all of these phenomena along with substantive experts who understand the physical nature of the phenomena in order to build and analyze models that minimize the impact on society. Indeed, in the case of pandemics, work is currently being done at the macro level to determine what responses government, business, nonprofits and other key organizations should be taking to minimize the prevalence, rates of incidence, severity and societal disruptions of the pandemic disease or the diseases caused by bioterrorist attacks [56,60,62].

In the last two decades, epidemic control models have been developed for the detection, treatment and control of HIV and AIDS in populations and/or subpopulations. Models have also been developed for diarrheal diseases, hepatitis A, B, nonA-nonB, tuberculosis, syphilis, malaria, measles, influenzas and other infectious diseases. Brandeau [12] describes various operations research approaches and methods to screen, treat and control these types of infectious diseases. Some of these methods include cost effectiveness analysis, linear and integer programming, simulation, numerical procedures, optimal control methodologies, nonlinear optimization, and heuristic approaches. The methods used depend upon the characteristics of the epidemic populations involved and the constraints and parameters available for analysis. Some infectious diseases cause death directly where as others may lead to the introduction of other opportunistic deadly diseases. Depending upon the disease and its manifestation, it may be controlled by vaccination, quarantine, prevention or other public health methods. Decision makers must choose among the different control methodologies, screening methodologies and public safety issuesusually with limited budgets and other competing societal objectives. Zaric and Brandeau [95–97] present models for the control of HIV in populations. Kaplan [55] has also done extensive work in the control of HIV among intravenous drug users through needle sharing and other modeling methods. Kaplan's work has successfully been applied to HIV control in New Haven Connecticut and New York City as well as other locales. Larson [59] has also modeled epidemic control for pandemic influenza. Nigmatulina and Larson [69] discuss government imposed and voluntarily selected control interventions. These interventions involve the implementation and timing of non-pharmaceutical strategies such as travel restrictions, social distancing, quarantine and improved hygiene. The models used necessarily had to consider human behavioral change, disease dynamics and iterative feedback over time. They show that pandemic influenza control is very complex because of these characteristics, but there are ways of mitigating the severity and coping with the spread through the populations. In another study Finkelstein et al. [29], present ways to empower individuals and families in the event of pandemic influenza.

In some countries, mass screening protocols and disease control for non-contagious, as well as contagious diseases, have been established for national health programs. In the U.K, Davies and Brailsford [11] have constructed simulation software to screen for and treat diabetic retinopathy. The software model is flexible so that it is possible to test a wide range of screening scenarios and intervention strategies. The value of screening and control is reduction of damage to tissues leading to blindness, end stage kidney failure and limb amputations. The authors also discussed other screening models in the operations research and medical literature. Also in the UK mass screening protocols are used for the early detection of cervical and other cancers in national programs intended to reduce the prevalence of the disease and save lives.

In the US Paltiel et al. [74] constructed a state transition simulation model to treat asthma in populations such as members of an HMO or other managed care program. The model forecasts asthma related symptoms, acute exacerbations, quality adjusted life expectancy, health-care costs and cost-effectiveness. The authors' intent is to reduce asthma manifestations, improve life quality and reduce costs of care. Similar models could be constructed for the control of other subpopulation-wide diseases such as obesity, smoking and diabetes and managed care organizations or national programs.

4.3.2. Screening and control of non-contagious diseases for an individual

Models of screening programs for an individual frequently incorporate information on the disease's progression and then try to minimize expected detection delay (the time from disease incidence until its detection) or maximize the lead time (the time from detection by screening until self-detection or until symptomatic). Characteristically, these models take a longitudinal time frame for the individual, because an individual, through his/her lifetime, is subject to different conditional probabilities of incurring the disease. Thus, screening schedules are determined sequentially by utilizing prior testing results, or simultaneously for an entire lifetime, such as every xyears. A common example would be a physician telling a patient he or she should be screened every x years for prostate, breast, cervical or colorectal cancer depending on his or her age and other conditions.

Using the etiology and progress of a disease and its relationship to screening effectiveness, the reliability of test and the lead time gained from detection can be modeled as a function of the state of the disease as well as the time since the disease's incidence. Eddy [24], well aware of the complexity of relationships among these reliabilities, the disease development, and prognosis of breast cancer, developed the most comprehensive breast cancer screening model available by focusing on two attributes that carry information about the effectiveness of the screening tests: the mammogram interval and the patient's age. By modeling these two factors as random variables, Eddy was able to derive analytical expressions for the sensitivity (true-positive rate) and specificity (true-negative rate) of test procedures, utilizing repeatedly a Bayesian statistical approach. The design of screening strategies to optimally allocate fixed resources, however, is only briefly discussed by Eddy. He also uses the basic model to evaluate screening for other cancers, such as colorectal and cervical, as well as non-cancerous, non-contagious diseases. Eddy's work is very important as it was implemented by health agencies in national policy recommendations for screening intervals based on the individual's age, sex and prior histories. Eddy [25] gives a good exposition on the importance of screening, the critical factors and parameters necessary for screening models and a comprehensive sensitivity analysis of his model under various assumptions and parameters. The work of [83] mentioned earlier, on building a Bayesian network to assist mammography interpretation is also applicable in the screening process for raising the mammography test accuracy.

4.3.3. Computational biology and biomedicine

The most exciting new research area for operations researchers in healthcare, and potentially the most revolutionary area for change, is in computational biology, bioinformatics and medical applications. This area is pushing the knowledge base of operations research in mathematical programming, data mining, stochastic models and simulation to its theoretical and application limits and beyond. In genomics and proteomics the data bases are so huge, often measured in terabytes, and the network linkages describing the molecular phenomena so complex that new modeling techniques, algorithmic solution capabilities and data mining approaches must be developed by the operations research community and others [39], give an excellent concise review and illustrate the many needs to be filled by operations research in solving problems in computational biology. Abbas and Holmes [1] provide an earlier more in-depth review for operations researchers of some of the same areas in bioinformatics and point out the need for more research in these applications. Examples of some of the work being done in this area are given in the special issues: *INFORMS Journal on Computing* (*2004, 16: 4*) and the *Annals of Operations Research* (*2006, 148: 1*). The key challenge is to discover what information lies in the genome and how to use that information for medical and societal advantages. For example, we are already uncovering information on the building of proteins, actions of viruses, subsections of the DNA strand causing certain genetic diseases and the use of DNA structure in anthropology, forensics and genealogy. These discoveries are leading to new drug discoveries, new understanding of human evolution and genetic mutations, the chemical and physical functions of DNA subsets and disease treatments for genetic and viral diseases.

Earlier in this chapter operations research based responses to problems of prevention, amelioration and/or treatment of major pandemics have been discussed. But at the micro level dealing with the specific viruses involved in possible pandemics work is also ongoing. For example [14], using a Markov chain model for deriving the distribution properties of palindromes, have discovered that the SARS virus contains an exceptional number of 22 nucleotide bases long palindromes. Other studies in bioinformatics had suggested that palindromes could play a major part in the viral packaging, replication and defense mechanisms of the SARS type viruses. This work is an example of sequence alignment within the DNA bases.

Sequence alignment algorithms are also used to detect whether two or more DNA subsequences are evolutionarily related and what chemical and physical functions they possess. They can also be used to detect mutations in the genome that lead to genetic disease. And they are also used to construct phylogenetic trees that relate biological families and their divergences. The value of the study of phylogenetic trees is to construct the genealogical ties between organisms and to estimate the time of divergence between organisms since they last shared a common ancestor. This knowledge can be used in the study of gene evolution, population subdivisions, analysis of mating systems, paternity testing, environmental surveillance and the origins of diseases that have transferred species such as the transfer of SIV (simian immunodeficiency virus) to HIV (human immunodeficiency virus) in the 1930s well before it appeared on the human scene in the 1970s and 1980s. Some recent work by operations researchers Gusfield et al. [40], have extended phylogenetic trees modeling to phylogenetic networks modeling. This extension to networks is necessary as other research has shown that evolution is not hierarchical (due to recombination, horizontal gene transfer and other events). These authors develop new algorithmic and combinatorial results to gain insight into the structure of these networks.

Another very important area of molecular and computational biology is a study of protein folding, simulation and structure prediction. This is important because the structure of a protein greatly influences its function. This knowledge is useful to help determine the chemical structure of drugs needed to counter protein malfunctions also known as "targeted therapy" Stanton and MacGregor Smith [91], have shown that the native state of a protein seems to be close to the geometry of a Steiner tree and prove that the Steiner tree provides a lower bound on the protein's energy. The study of protein energy is valuable because it relates to the forces that drive the protein folding.

5. System design and planning

5.1. Planning and strategy

All organizations with long-term goals are involved with planning and strategy. This planning may take the form of supply chain structure and management, of what technologies to use, of aggregate planning for workforce, facilities and cash flow capacities, of financing options, of location analysis and of the many other factors and variables necessary for long-term operations.

In *most* industrially developed nations and in many developing nations, health care system-wide design and planning occurs principally at the federal or regional level. For the developed nations, with the exception of the United States, the interplay between history, culture, economics, politics, and other factors result in similar strategies for providing universal access and cost control, including some form of social insurance, common fee schedules, annual budgetsor salaries for all providers and formal or informal national budget caps. To counter the economic costs of these health care systems, each country engages in some types of strategic choices such as limits on accessibility, waiting lines for appointments, limits on purchase and deployment of technologies, drug formularies, only approved procedures, insurance premiums, co-pays and deductibles and other demand/supply restrictions. Operations research is often used in optimizing the planning and making the strategic choices needed to deliver care to the citizens.

A mathematical programming methodology that has seen much use in evaluating organizational performance among a group of similar types of organizations is data envelopment analysis (DEA). This methodology considers common multiple inputs and multiple outputs for each organization and finds the optimal combination of inputs and outputs that yield the greatest organizational performance. Usually this performance involves measures of efficiency and/or effectiveness (such as more and/or better outputs per input or the use of less inputs per output) and shows which of the organizations are performing optimally and which can be improved by realigning their mix of services and utilization of their inputs. The organizations that are performing optimally receive the highest efficiency score of one and the less efficient organizations a score of less than one. Using these scores an efficiency frontier is computed. The inefficient utilization of resources is represented by deviations from this frontier. For an inefficient organization to improve it must reduce and realign its inputs and/or increase its outputs to achieve the frontier. An excellent example of the use of this methodology is given by Ozcan et al. [72]. These authors use DEA to analyze the organizational performance of a group of community mental health centers. In doing this analysis they also develop efficiency measures for improving productivity in behavioral health care.

5.2. Technology assessment and adoption

As noted earlier in this chapter, because technology (new procedures, new devices, new drugs and their greater intensity of use) is the primary driving force in the rise of health care costs, the federal and regional design and planning processes largely determine the types and levels of facilities and technologies and frequently (perhaps implicitly) the levels of health care manpower and levels of services received by the population. For example, the United Kingdom, Australia and Canada have asked the question, "What additional values will these new technologies provide for us and at what cost"? To answer this question health-care systems in these three countries have implemented a quantitative model, called an incremental cost-effectiveness model, to determine whether their national health systems should adopt new technologies or new drugs when they become available.

Cost effectiveness analysis(CEA) and cost benefit analysis(CBA) studies are available in Gold et al. [37]. CEA is the ratio of net health care costs divided by the net health care effects from using a particular health care intervention. The net costs of health care include direct health care and medical costs for any given condition to which are added the costs of adverse side effects of any treatment and from which is subtracted any costs from reduced morbidity, since these are the savings which health care accrues from the prevention of disease. Net health care effectiveness is the increase in life years which result from the treatment to which are added the increased number of years gained from the elimination of morbidity. The number of life years lost to side effects is then subtracted. These years are frequently adjusted for quality of life (quality-adjusted life years, or QALY). The ratio of net costs to net effects is the cost effectiveness ratio.

CBA, on the other hand, goes farther and sets a monetary value on these net effects and then seeks to determine if the value of the benefits outweigh the net costs. However, this value setting process requires assignment of monetary value to life, which is frequently a controversial topic. Despite this shortcoming, several methodologies of life valuation such as willingness to pay and human capital consumption and production have been developed.

So using a cost-effectiveness approach to making technology choices, the United Kingdom, Australia and Canada have establish the following process. After the efficacy of a new technology/drug has been established, the incremental cost-effectiveness model given by this formula:

$$\frac{\textit{Incremental Cost of the New Vs. Existing Technologies}}{\textit{Incremental Effectiveness of the New Vs. Existing Technologies in QALYS}}$$

where QALYS = Quality Adjusted Life Years.

This formula is used to determine whether this *ratio* of the costs of the new technology/drug with its benefits to those of the existing technology/drug per additional QALY derived from the new technology/drug does or does not exceed some preset value/cost for an additional quality adjusted life year. In this manner the appropriate governmental or independent agency determines whether the new health-care technology/drugs contribute to the efficient use of national health-care resources. For example, in the United Kingdom in September 2001, the governmentally designated agency, The National Institute for Clinical Excellence, reviewed 17 new pharmaceutical products. Ten of the 17 pharmaceutical products were approved for use. Their decisions for the approved drugs appeared to be based on the cost of an additional QALY to be not more than about 30,000 British pounds. So that drugs that could deliver an additional quality adjusted life year for less than 30,000 pounds were approved and the others were not [6]. These countries have resorted to this incremental cost-effectiveness model to help control the costs of national health-care because, as also mentioned earlier, new health-care technologies, procedures and pharmaceuticals are largely cost increasing and must yield sufficient benefits to justify the incremental costs. In operations research other models are also available, besides the incremental cost-effectiveness model, to evaluate the value of new technologies. These other models take into account multiple objectives, additional constraints and multiple outcomes, including side effects, over longer time frames. As more countries attempt to control the rapidly rising cost of health care, more and more attention will have to be given to paying only for those technologies that deliver the most cost-effective health care to the populations.

5.3. Regionalization of services and technologies

Operations research modeling and analysis has been used in other strategic planning applications such as supporting decisions concerning regionalization, health districting and the expansion and contraction of services. Earlier mention has been made about the implementation of strategic plans to combat pandemics and bioterrorist attacks.

Regionalization of health care services is an important component of system planning and is common in countries with national health-care systems. In the US regional decisions are often made by large multi-institutional systems such as Kaiser Permanente, Henry Ford, Intermountain, and Cleveland Clinic health systems, and by the federal VA, PHS and DOD health systems. However, the operations research methodologies which underlie regionalization are robust and can be useful for the operation of multi-institutional systems, distribution of high technology equipment, location of facilities, allocation of resources, aggregate planning and in other health care issues which could be useful in all health systems.

Because regionalization is frequently sought to improve the cost or quality of a health care system through more effective distribution of services, regionalization questions are often optimal clustering problems (the decision maker attempts to partition the set services so that some objective is optimized) or resource allocation problems (the central authority must plan for and allocate scarce resources to regions or districts).

Bonder [8] describes a very complex discrete event simulation model of an entire large geographically and populous healthcare region. This model was developed for the Military Health System in the United States. In any region there are always a large number of capacity, organizational, resource allocation and process change decisions. The model simulates the flow of individual patients through the entire health care system, as they are being diagnosed, treated and rehabilitated. The model can be used to ask questions and build scenarios for many strategic and tactical issues such as: how many hospitals and clinics are required and where should they be located, how many personnel of what specialties are needed, what is the optimal flow of patients through a reconfigured system.

At the national planning level Rizakow et al. [81], develop a decision support system, AIDSPLAN, which is a spreadsheet model to plan for the resources needed for *HIV/AIDS* related services in the United Kingdom. The model incorporates demand forecasting by patient categories, care protocols and resource and budget needs for central and local planners in the British National Health Service. It can also be used with the planning efforts of earlier math programming balance of care (BOC) models incorporated in micro-computer software to determine resource needs and allocations for entire health service regions and districts [7,10,18,89].

As mentioned earlier in this chapter, the admission of emergency department patients is often in conflict with admissions of elective patients in hospitals that are already at or near capacity. This situation was occurring in Nottingham, England [11], constructed a large system dynamics model to study the flow patients through the hospitals and other health services in this large region. The model exposed the bottlenecks that were occurring and allowed the researchers to examine alternative scenarios to improve the patient flows to hospitals at the regional level. With this analysis and with the analysis from a companion discrete event simulation model, the health authorities were able to make changes that better utilized the regional resources and met the needs of the population in the region.

5.4. Location of facilities

Location of health care delivery facilities and services has much in common with the location aspects of many types of facilities or services which have a geographically dispersed customer base, and where there is a need to be close enough to customers for ease of access and/or speed of access, as well as a need for low cost of site location and operations. Health care facilities and services are often subject to public control laws and, in the case of emergency vehicle locations where there are maximum response time requirements, the locations may need to balance closeness to customers and hospital facilities.

Siting or location problems usually fall into one of five categories with somewhat distinctive characteristics:

1. The first category is the regionalization of health care facilities (see earlier section).
2. The second category is the opening or removal of a single facility such as an acute care hospital or a central blood bank that needs to be geographically close to its customer bases. Here the customers are the patients and their physicians, and (to a lesser extent) hospital employees. Generally, mathematical programming or heuristic approaches are used to determine optimal or near-optimal locations. Major consideration is given to the current location of similar institutions in the region.
3. The third category is the location of ambulatory neighborhood clinics that are primarily used for routine outpatient medical and/or surgical care and for preventive care. Again, proximity to

patients is an important criterion in the location decision, as are network linkages to the general and specialized hospitals in the region. The location of health maintenance organization facilities surgery centers, diagnostic centers such as CT-scanner centers and polyclinics fall into this category. Sometimes network mathematical programming is used for this analysis. For example, in order to locate ambulatory medical service centers for the independently living elderly, a p1anning strategy advocated by [19] incorporates the concept of aggregate activity spaces used by the target population in the criteria for determining the facility location. This approach is particularly suited to services for the elderly, who tend to restrict activity to familiar areas of the community. A similar idea could be used for the location of pediatric health service centers near schools and/or recreation areas.

4. The fourth category comprises the location of specialized long-term care facilities. The primary criteria for these location decisions are not so much closeness to customer bases but costs of site acquisition and construction, cost of operation, and (to some extent) speed of access to acute care facilities. The types of facilities involved in this category are nursing homes, psychiatric hospitals, skilled nursing facilities, and rehabilitation centers.
5. The fifth category of health care location problems is the site locations for emergency medical services (EMS). This problem involves determination of the number and placement of locations, number and types of emergency response vehicles and of personnel. This problem is similar to the location of fire stations' equipment and crews, in which speed of response is a primary criterion. Speed of response includes distance to the problem occurrence location, but also the distance from the occurrence location to the treatment facility. In this latter regard, the problem differs from firestations, where the occurrence location and the treatment location coincide. For example, if the health care treatment location is near the edge of a populated region, it is probably not optimal to locate the EMS at the midpoint of the region or close to the treatment center, whereas it may be optimal to locate a firestation there. The EMS location problem has received much attention from operations researchers. It is rich in problem structure, having sufficient technical complexity yet minimal political and sociological constraints. The primary methods used to solve this problem are mathematical programming, queueing analysis and simulation. The solutions may then be modified heuristically, to satisfy non-quantitative constraints.

[30] combine a deployment model with varying fleet sizes to determine the appropriate level of ambulance service. The Computerized Ambulance Location Logic (CALL) simulation program combines the Hooke-Jeeves optimum seeking search routine with an EMS queueing model [31], enhance the CALL approach by adding a contiguous zone search routine that relocates all deployed vehicles sequentially to zones contiguous to each vehicle's starting location. Individual and cumulative vehicle response times are then determined until a cumulative minimum value is identified. Model outputs include demand for hospital emergency services, ambulance utilization and workload, mean response time, probability of all vehicles being idle, distribution of response time, mean response time by zone and dispatch guidelines. Objective criteria used to evaluate site location alternatives include service equity, fleet size, and workload equity.

In a thorough review of the methodologies used for determining the location of health care facilities, Daskin and Dean [21], review three important models: the location set covering model, the maximal covering model and the P- median model. These models comprise the core methodologies used for location planning in health care. Depending upon the primary objectives of the location facilities problem: accessibility, adaptability and/or availability of the services for "customers" in the problem, one methodology may be better than the others.

Although most location problems in the literature and involve locating facilities geographically [58], use location analysis to determine the minimum number of fields of view to read a PAP test in a cytological sample. By minimizing the number of fields of view the time needed to analyze each sample is minimized. This particular problem differs from geographic facility location problems in that instead of looking at a few hundred location possibilities there are thousands or tens of thousands of such points to be considered. Also this problem is complicated by the fact that in addition to choosing the locations (fields of view) a routing problem must be optimally solved as the microscope is moved from one field of view to the next. The authors develop efficient heuristic solutions to this set of problems.

Verter and La Pierre [2] construct mathematical programming location models for the optimal location of facilities to deliver preventive services. The goal is to maximize the patients' participation in the prevention programs. They develop algorithms to solve derivative sub-problems and applied their models to locate public health centers in Fulton County, Georgia, USA, and to locate mammography-screening centers in Montreal, Quebec, Canada.

In another project [17], mixed-integer programming is used to locate Traumatic Brain Injury (TBI) units optimally in an existing region of Veterans Administration health centers. It was not financially or physically possible to locate full service TBI units at all Veterans Administration health centers. Consequently, in order to make treatment as accessible as possible within budget, it was necessary to find those locations that minimized the total patient costs for treatment, lodging and travel, as well as costs associated with diverting or displacing the use of other services provided by the facility. The authors then apply this analysis to help locate these treatment centers in the six Florida-based VA medical centers in Veterans Integrated Services Network Region 8.

Pezzella et al. [76] provide an example of health service districting. In this paper, the authors develop a model by which local health departments in Italy are assigned into regional health structures. Dimensions of the analysis include an analysis of the demand for health services based on demographic, socio-economic, and geographical information, interviews with experts and surveys of special disease populations, and an analysis of available hospital services, which are considered in the proposed mathematical model for optimal districting. The authors note previous attempts to perform such regionalization by set partitioning, generalized assignment models, location and allocation models, and other linear programs. The authors use a linear program which has two objectives: to minimize the average distance of individuals from the nearest center, which improves access, and to minimize the deviation between proposed and existing districting which improves political acceptability. The model achieves the objectives by assigning hospitals to nuclei and then building reduced graphs in such a way that these distances are minimized. The authors apply the model to a case study of the Cosenza province in Italy and discuss two formulations of the optimal districting solution.

Another example of a regionalization question involving the location of facilities, the regionalization of CT scanners, is addressed by Bach and Hoberg [4]. The authors consider total cost per year of a regional system of CT scanner operation, cost per scan, utilization levels and average and maximum distance travelled by patients. They use a linear programming model that considers the total cost of operations for the CT scanner system as the sum of transportation costs (determined by patient travelling) and operational costs, such as staffing, supplies and facility support. The operational costs include fixed, threshold, and variable costs. The objective of the program is to minimize total cost. The authors apply the model to the Baden-Wurttemberg region in Germany. They consider a number of alternatives and rank-order them on the basis of total cost. They find that an increase in the number of CT scanners in a regional system does not necessarily increase the total cost of operation due to decreased travel costs.

Pierskalla [80] considers the supply chain problem of delivering blood and blood products to the hospitals and clinics in a region in a timely manner meeting all of the regional needs at minimum cost.

Table 3
Decisions and models used in blood banking applications

Decisions to be made	Models use to aid these decisions
Determining number, size, functions performed and locations of Regional and Community Blood Centers 1. Number and Sizes 2. Locations	1. Econometric models for economies of scale yielding optimal number, sizes and functions to be performed at the RBC and CBCs 2. Mathematical programming location-allocation models to determine the optimal cost effective locations of the RBC and CBCs and the allocations of blood drawing areas and sites to supply the centers and the hospitals served by the centers
Scheduling of donor drawing sites, amounts and locations weekly and monthly	Mathematical programming scheduling models for balancing supply needs of whole blood to meet forecasted demands for blood products
Forecasting demands for blood products	Statistical models to build the demand distributions by blood type at each HBB and aggregated to their CBC and forecasting models to project future demands
Determining optimal inventory levels of blood products at the RBC, CBCs and HBBs	Stochastic dynamic programming and statistical and simulation models to build Cobb-Douglas response surfaces to determine optimal inventory level equations for each location
Determining optimal shipping routes to send blood products daily from centers to HBBs	Mathematical programming transportation models
Determining transshipment rules to move outdating blood products to HBBs with higher probabilities of their use and to move blood products from one HBB with lower demands to another that has a higher probability of shortages	Simulation models to construct optimal transshipment rules by creating optimal response surfaces and using multiple regression
Determining optimal blood issuing policies for crossmatching	Simulation models were used to determine under what conditions the policy "first (oldest) in first out" – FIFO, or the policy "last (youngest) in first out" – LIFO, was optimal

Using many operations research techniques, questions addressed include: how many community blood centers should there be in the region, what donor areas and transfusion services should be assigned to each, what blood banking functions should be performed at the centers or the hospitals and how overall supply and demand should be coordinated. There are strategic facility location questions to be answered and tactical operational issues to be resolved in order to minimize the total system costs and meet all the needed demands. These tactical issues involved optimally collecting blood from donors, producing multiple blood components, setting and controlling inventory levels, allocating blood to hospitals and clinics, scheduling delivery to multiple sites and making optimal decisions about issuing, cross matching, and cross match releasing blood and blood products. Algorithms and models are presented to decide how many blood banks to set up, where to locate them, how to allocate hospitals to the banks, and how to route the supply operation of vehicles so that the total system costs are minimized, and the hospital needs are met. With data from blood centers throughout the US [16], demonstrate significant economies of scale within operating areas (such as laboratories, storage and administration) in central blood banks. Combining these results with actual transportation costs data, Or and Pierskalla [71] evaluate site location and vehicle scheduling in the Chicago metropolitan area. Table 3 illustrates some of the many decisions and methodologies used in solving the supply chain problem in blood banking.

5.5. *Capacity planning and analysis*

Many studies are conducted at the institutional level to plan the addition, expansion or contraction of services and facilities. In health care, this problem is complicated by the interdependence among services and among institutions created by criss-crossing physician privileges, patient co-morbidities, unknown levels of latent demand in the community, and potential creation of demand by changing the numbers and types of attending physicians. These and other factors must be considered in planning capacity.

There are essentially two types of capacity planning approaches. The first is de novo planning for new facilities that are to be established in a region or community. For this type of planning is necessary to have forecasted the patterns of demands, the costs of constructing and operating new facilities with its appropriate technologies and workload levels and any actions by competitors. This planning should also take into consideration any economies of scale or scope in the size and/or operation of the new facilities and the ease or difficulty of allowing for future expansion or contraction.

The second planning approach concerns the addition to or modification of the capacity of existing facilities. This type of planning is generally more difficult than de novo planning because it is first necessary to make certain that the existing capacity is managed optimally. Frequently it is the case that new capacity is added at significant expense but better throughput analysis and management of the existing capacity would easily have met the increasing demands on the institution. Earlier in his chapter it was discussed how smoothing the various streams of demand arrivals would not only improve throughput but also open up more capacity for future demands. The example shown was from the Cincinnati Children's Hospital Medical Center where improved management allowed the hospital to avoid the construction of 102 additional beds to meet increasing needs with savings of more than $100 million in construction costs (see Exhibit 1).

There are also other demand side strategies to use to optimize the utilization of existing facilities. These strategies could involve deleting or eliminating certain services or procedures that are excessively costly or excessively disruptive to the treatment of patients or with developing complementary services that would relieve the congestion and utilization of existing services. There are also supply side strategies that can be used to improve the management of capacity. Many of these were discussed earlier in the need for optimizing the performance of ancillary and administrative services, work shift allocations and scheduling, cross training of employees, effective use of part-time employees at peak times and optimal transfer and discharge planning. Once the current utilization of capacity is optimized the planning for expansion and other modifications of existing facilities can proceed somewhat in the matter as that done for de novo planning.

Green [37] gives an excellent review of the many problems and issues which must be considered in capacity planning and management in hospitals. She also gives examples of where operations research techniques and approaches can provide substantial benefit in improving capacity utilization. She covers issues of emergency room delays in triaging, how many hospital beds are actually needed to meet demands and occupancy, the impact of seasonality and the organizational structure on utilization, issues such as staffing and cross-training and allocation of that human capacity among competing patient groups. Unfortunately for many reasons, many hospital managers do not have the capability to perform these analyses even though they are acutely aware of their need to use their resources more efficiently and effectively.

In another review article Smith-Daniels et al. [90] also report on operations research approaches and capacity analysis problems for hospitals and other healthcare delivery institutions.

Schneider [85] examines the question of how the consolidation of obstetric services among hospitals might affect the case load and profitability of hospitals in three communities. He models three factors: comparability of services, patient load redistributions, and financial measures. Comparability of services determines if closures of services in some locations changes the overall regional level of service as measured by staffing, bed requirements, number of delivery rooms, and outcomes measures (including still births, neonatal mortality, percent primary of Caesarian sections, and percent of breach deliveries). Patient load redistribution examines how the underlying patient volume is redistributed among remaining units after some units close and how this affects the service at related institutions. Financial analysis determines how direct service-specific and marginal cost sare used to determine the net savings under closure conditions and the costs of increased services at remaining units that increase in volume. The author finds that most hospitals in the three communities face significant losses on existing obstetric services, that five of seven hospitals would improve financial performance if their obstetric services closed, and that if one obstetric service were closed per community, overall costs would be reduced by 7–15% with comparable levels of service quality.

The opening of new services is also addressed. Romanin-Jacur and Facchin [82] examine the effect of opening an independent pediatric semi-intensive care unit in a pediatric hospital. The unit would have its own rooms, staff, and instruments and be devoted to the care of severely ill patients. The question they raise is one of distribution of current capacity, in which the question is the reallocation of beds from the general ward to the new unit rather than addition to total capacity. The authors consider several classes of case arrival sources, including urgencies from the floors and the surgical ward, emergent admissions, and planned admissions. Each class is modeled with Poisson inter-arrival times for all services, except planned surgical operations that are deterministic. Using length of stay from historical data, a simulation model is used to determine the optimal number of beds for the unit. The authors present a staffing schedule to optimize nurse distribution, based on optimal number of beds.

An important and frequently encountered question in service planning is whether a new service can improve productivity, quality, or cost performance in such a way that it is a desirable addition to other services offered by an institution or a health care system. In some early studies Hershey and Kropp [23] and Denton et al. [46] used operations research techniques to resolve the question of whether it is more productive at high quality for physicians to use physicians' assistants and nurse practitioners in their practices. The answer was a clear yes but that initially costs might rise due to increased physician supervision time as the PAs and NPs learned the practice processes.

6. Conclusions

The value of operations research concepts, methods and approaches to health care decision-making has been demonstrated many times over and can and will play an even greater role in our attempts to manage future growth in costs, use of technologies, improvement in quality of care and management of problems of access to care. Many examples have been given of this value in this chapter. In some of these examples, millions of dollars of costs have been saved or revenues enhanced. In others the savings were smaller but quality improvements were often significant, technologies utilized more successfully, patient and/or provider satisfaction higher and access to care available and more timely. The examples shown are but a small subset of the large number of operations research applications accomplished in health care organizations to date.

References

[1] A.E. Abbas and S.P. Holmes, Bioinformatics and Management Science: Some Common Tools and Techniques, *Operations Research* **52**(2) (2004), 165–190.

[2] L.H. Aiken, S.E. Clarke, D.M. Sloane, J. Sochalski and J.H. Silber, Hospital Nurse Staffing andPatient Mortality, Nurse Burnout, and Job Dissatisfaction, *JAMA* **288**(16) (23/30 October 2002), 1987–1993.

[3] J.S. Armstrong, *Principles of Forecasting*, New York, Kluwer Academic Publishers, 2001.
[4] L. Bach and R. Hoberg, A Planning Model for Regional Systems of CT Scanners, *SocioEconom Planning Sci* **19** (1985), 189–199.
[5] N.T.J. Bailey, *The Mathematical Theory of Infectious Disease and Its Applications*, London, Charles Griffin and Co. Ltd, 1975.
[6] S. Birch and A. Gafni, The 'NICE' Approach to Technology Assessment: An Economics Perspective, *Health-Care Management Science* **7** (2004), 35–41.
[7] D. Boldy, The Relationship Between Decision Support Systems And Operational Research: Health Care Examples, *European J Oper Res* **29** (1987), 1128–1134.
[8] S. Bonder, Changing Health Care Delivery Enterprises, in: *Building a Better Delivery System: A New Engineering/Health Care Partnership*, P.P. Reid, W.D. Compton, J.H. Grossman and G. Fanjiang, eds, Washington, D.C.: National Academies Press, 2005, pp. 149–152.
[9] C. Born, M. Carbajal, P. Smith, M. Wallace, K. Abbott, S. Adyanthaya, A. Boyd, C. Keller, J. Liu, W. New, T. Rieger, B. Winemiller and R. Woestemeyer, Contract Optimization at Texas Children's Hospital, *Interfaces* **34**(1) (2004), 51–58.
[10] T. Bowen and P. Forte, The Balance of Care Microcomputer System. *Proc. 2nd Internat. Conf. of Systems Science in Health and Social Service for the Elderly and Disabled*, Curtin University of Technology, Perth, Australia, 1987.
[11] S.C. Brailsford, V.A. Lattimer, P. Tarnaras and J.C. Turnbull, Emergency and On-Demand Health Care: Modeling a Large Complex System, *Journal of the Operational Research Society* **55**(1) (2004), 34–42.
[12] M.L. Brandeau, Allocating Resources to Control Infectious Diseases, in: *Operations Research and Healthcare: a Handbook of Methods and Applications*, Chapter 17, M.L. Brandeau, F. Sainfort and W.P. Pierskalla, eds, Boston, Kluwer Academic Publishers, 2004, pp. 695–720.
[13] M.L. Brandeau, F. Sainfort and W.P. Pierskalla, *Operations Research and Healthcare: a Handbook of Methods and Applications*, Boston, Kluwer Academic Publishers, 2004.
[14] D.S.H. Chew, K.P. Choi, H. Heider and M.-Y. Leung, Palindromes in SARS and Other Coronaviruses, *INFORMS Journal on Computing* **16**(4) (2004), 331–340.
[15] Cincinnati Children's Hospital Medical Center, A CFOs Perspective: improved patient flow and placement Boosts Capacity, *Staff Bulletin* **45**(5) (2009).
[16] M.A. Cohen, W.P. Pierskalla and R. Sassetti, Economies of Scale in Blood Banking, in: *Competition in Blood Services*, G.M. Clark, ed., New York, American Association of Blood Banks Press, 1987, pp. 25–37.
[17] M.J. Côté, S.S. Siddhartha, W.B. Vogel and D.C. Cowper, A Mixed Integer Programming Model to Locate Traumatic Brain Injury Treatment Units in The Department of Veterans Affairs: A Case Study, *Health Care Management Science* **10**(3) (2007), 253–267.
[18] I.L. Coverdale and S.M. Negrine, The Balance of Care Project: Modelling the Allocation of Health and Personal Social Services, *J Oper Res Soc* **29**(11) (1978), 1043–1054.
[19] E.K. Cromley and G.W. Shannon, Locating Ambulatory Care For The Elderly, *Health Services Res* **21** (1986), 499–514.
[20] D.M. Cutler, Technology, Health Costs and NIH. Harvard University and NBER paper presented at the NIH Roundtable on the Economics Biomedical Research, October, 1995.
[21] M.S. Daskin and L.K. Dean, Location of Health Care Facilities, in: *Operations Research and Healthcare: a Handbook of Methods and Applications*, (Chapter 3), M.L. Brandeau, F. Sainfort and W.P. Pierskalla, Boston, Kluwer Academic Publishers, 2004, pp. 43–76.
[22] R. Davies and S.C. Brailsford, Screening for Diabetic Retinopathy, in: *Operations Research and Healthcare: a Handbook of Methods and Applications*, (Chapter 19), M.L. Brandeau, F. Sainfort and W.P. Pierskalla, Boston, Kluwer Academic Publishers, 2004, pp. 493–518.
[23] R.T. Denton, A. Gafni, B.G. Spencer and G.L. Stoddart, Potential Savings from the Adoption of Nurse Practitioner Technology in the Canadian Health Care System, *Socio-Econom Planning Sci* **17** (1983), 199–209.
[24] D.M. Eddy, Screening for Cancer: Theory, Analysis and Design. Englewood Cliffs, NJ, Prentice-Hall, 1980.
[25] D.M. Eddy, A Mathematical Model for Timing Repeated Medical Tests, *Medical Decision Making* **3**(1) (1983), 45–62.
[26] P. Eveborn, M. Rönnqvist, H. Einarsdóttir, M. Eklund, K. Lidén and M. Almroth, Operations Research and Improves Quality and Efficiency In Home Care, *Interfaces* **39**(1) (2009), 18–34.
[27] M.C. Ferris, R. Einarsson, Z. Jiang and D. Shepard, Sampling Issues for Optimization in Radiotherapy, *Annals of Operations Research* **148** (2006), 95–115.
[28] M.C. Ferris, J. Lim and D. Shepard, Optimization Tools for Radiation Treatment Mining in MatLab, in: *Operations Research and Healthcare: a Handbook of Methods and Applications*, (Chapter 30), M.L. Brandeau, F. Sainfort and W.P. Pierskalla, eds, Boston, Kluwer Academic Publishers, 2004, pp. 775–806.
[29] S. Finkelstein, S. Prakash, K. Nigmatulina and R. Larson, Empowering Individuals And Families in the Event of a Flu Pandemic. Working paper, Operations Research Center, Massachusetts Institute of Technology, Cambridge, MA 02139, 2008.

[30] J.A. Fitzsimmons and R.S. Sullivan, Establishing the Level of Service for Public Emergency Ambulance Systems, *Socio-Econom Planning Sci* **13** (1979), 235–239.

[31] J.A. Fitzsimmons and B.N. Srikar, Emergency Ambulance Location Using the Contiguous Zone Search Routine, *J Oper Management* **2** (1982), 225–237.

[32] J.A. Fitzsimmons and M.J. Fitzsimmons, *Service Management: Operations, Strategy, and Information Technology*, Third edition. New York, McGraw-Hill, Inc, 2001.

[33] B.E. Fries, Bibliography of Operations Research in Health Care Systems: An Update, *Operations Research* **27**(2) (1979), 408–419.

[34] V. Gascon is to. and W.P. Pierskalla, (1996). Health Care Systems, in: *Encyclopedia of Operations Research and Management Science*, Gass, S. and Harris, C. eds, Boston, Kluwer Academic Publishers, 1996, pp. 273–275.

[35] S.I. Gass and C.M. Harris, eds, *Encyclopedia of Operations Research and Management Science*, Second Edition, Springer, 2000.

[36] E.J. Gaucher and R.J. Coffey, *Total Quality and Healthcare: From Theory to Practice*, San Francisco, Jossey-Bass Publishers, 1993.

[37] M.R. Gold, J.E. Siegel, L.B. Russell and M.C. Weinstein, eds, *Cost-Effectiveness in Health and Medicine*, Oxford University Press, USA, 1996.

[38] L.V. Green, Capacity Planning and Management in Hospitals, in: *Operations Research and Healthcare: a Handbook of Methods and Applications*, (Chapter 2), M.L. Brandeau, F. Sainfort and W.P. Pierskalla, eds, Boston, Kluwer Academic Publishers, 2004, pp. 15–42.

[39] H.G. Greenberg, A.G. Holder, M.-Y. Leung and R. Schwartz, Computational Biology and Medical Applications, *ORMS Today* **36**(3) (2009), 34–39.

[40] D.M. Gusfield, S. Eddhu and C. Langley, The Fine Structure of Galls in Phylogenetic Networks, *INFORMS Journal On Computing* **16** 2004, 459–469.

[41] T. Hanne, T. Melo and S. Nickel, Bringing Robustness to Patient Flow Management Through Optimized Patient Transports and Hospitals, *Interfaces* **39** (May–June 2009), 241–255.

[42] M.B. Harrington, Forecasting area-wide demand for health care services: A critical review of major techniques and their application, *Inquiry* **14** (1977), 254–268.

[43] G.B. Hazen, Dynamic Influence Diagrams: Applications to Medical Decision Modeling, in: *Operations Research and Healthcare: a Handbook of Methods and Applications*, (Chapter 24), M.L. Brandeau, F. Sainfort and W.P. Pierskalla, eds, Boston, Kluwer Academic Publishers, 2004, pp. 613–638.

[44] F.T. Helmer, E.B. Opperman and J.D. Suver, Forecasting nursing staffing requirements by intensity-of-care level, *Interfaces* **10** (1980), 50–59.

[45] J. Hershey, W. Pierskalla and S. Wandel, Nurse Staffing Management, in: *Operational Research Applied to Health Services*, D. Boldy, ed., London, Croon Helm, 1981, pp. 189–220.

[46] J.C. Hershey and D.H. Kropp, A Re-Appraisal of the Productivity Potential and Economic Benefits of Physician's Assistants, *Medical Care* **17** (1979), 592–606.

[47] R.M. Hogarth and S. Makridakis, Forecasting and planning: An evaluation, *Management Science* **27**(2) (1981), 115–138.

[48] A. Holder, Radiotherapy Treatment Design And Linear Programming, in: *Operations Research and Healthcare: a Handbook of Methods and Applications*, (Chapter 29), M.L. Brandeau, F. Sainfort and W.P. Pierskalla, eds, Boston, Kluwer Academic Publishers, 2004, pp. 741–774.

[49] Institute of Medicine, *To Err Is Human*, Washington, DC, The National Academies Press, 1999.

[50] Institute of Medicine, Ann Page ed., *Keeping Patients Safe: Transforming the Work Environment of Nurses*, Washington, DC, The National Academies Press, 2004.

[51] S. Johansen, S. Bowles and G. Haney, A model for forecasting intermittent skilled nursing home needs, *Res Nursing Health* **11** (1988), 375–382.

[52] R.D. Kamentzky, L.J. Shuman and H. Wolfe, Estimating need and demand for pre-hospital care, *Operations Research* **30** (1982), 1148–1167.

[53] E.P.C. Kao and F.M. Pokladnik, Incorporating exogenous factors in adaptive forecasting of hospital census, *Management Sciences* **24** (1978), 1677–1686.

[54] E.P.C. Kao and G.G. Tung, Forecasting demands for inpatient services in a large public health care delivery system, *Socio-Economic Planning Sciences* **14** (1980), 97–106.

[55] E.H. Kaplan, Economic Evaluation and HIV Prevention Community Planning: a policy analyst perspective, in: *Handbook of Economic Evaluation of HIV Prevention Programs*, D.R. Holtgrave, ed., New York, Plenum Press, 1998.

[56] E.H. Kaplan and L.M. Wein, Decision Making for Bioterror Preparedness: Examples from Smallpox Vaccination Policy, in: *Operations Research and Healthcare: a Handbook of Methods and Applications*, (Chapter 20), M.L. Brandeau, F. Sainfort and W.P. Pierskalla, Boston, Kluwer Academic Publishers, 2004, pp. 659–694.

[57] D.L. Kellogg and S. Walczak, Nurse Scheduling: From Academia to Implementation or Not? *Interfaces* **37**(4) (2007), 355–369.

[58] G. Laporte, F. Semet, V.V. Dadeshidze and L.J. Olsson, A Tiling And Routing Heuristic for the Screening Of Cytological Samples, *Journal of the Operational Research Society* **49** (1998), 1233–1238.
[59] R.C. Larson, Revisiting R_0, The Basic Reproductive Number for Pandemic Influenza. Working paper, Operations Research Center, Massachusetts Institute of Technology, Cambridge, MA 02139, 2008.
[60] E.K. Lee, S. Maheshwary, J. Mason and W. Glisson, Decision Support System for Mass Dispensing of Medications for Infectious Disease Outbreaks and Bioterrorist Attacks, *Ann Oper Res* **148** (2006), 25–53.
[61] E.K. Lee and M. Zaider, Operations Research Advances Cancer Therapeutics, *Interfaces* **38**(1) (2008), 5–25.
[62] E.K. Lee, T. Easton and K. Gupta, Novel Evolutionary Models and Applications To Sequence Alignment Problems, *Annals of Operations Research* **148** (2006), 167–187.
[63] M. Lipsitch, S. Riley, S. Cauchemez, A.C. Ghani and N.M. Ferguson, Managing and Reducing Uncertainty in an Emerging Influenza Pandemic, *The New England Journal of Medicine* **361**(2) (2009), 112–115.
[64] E. Litvak, P.I. Buerhaus, F. Davidoff, M.C. Long, M.L. McManus and D.M. Berwick, Managing Unnecessary Variability in Patient Demand to Reduce Nursing Stress and Improve Patient Safety, *Journal on Quality and Patient Safety* **31**(6) (2005), 330–338.
[65] E. Litvak, Optimizing Patient Flow By Managing Its Variability, in: *Front Office to Front Line: Essential Issues for Health Care Leaders*, S. Berman, ed., Oakbrook Terrace, IL, Joint Commission Resources, 2005, pp. 91–111.
[66] M.L. McManus, M.C. Long, A. Cooper, J. Mandell, D.M. Berwick, M. Pagano and E. Litvak, Variability in Surgical Caseload and Access to Intensive Care Services, *Anesthesiology* **98** (2003), 1491–1496.
[67] M.L. McManus, M.C. Long, A. Cooper and E. Litvak, Queuing Theory Accurately Models the Need for Critical Care Resources, *Anesthesiology* **100** (2004), 1271–1276.
[68] National Academy of Engineering and Institute of Medicine, in: *Building a Better Delivery System: A New Engineering/Health Care Partnership*, P.P. Reid, W.D. Compton, J.H. Grossman, and G. Fanjiang eds, Washington, D.C.: National Academies Press, 2005.
[69] K.R. Nigmatulina and R.C. Larson, Living with influenza: Impacts of government imposed and voluntarily selected interventions, *European Journal of Operational Research* **195**(2) (2008), 613–627.
[70] R.M. O'Keefe, Investigating Outpatient Department: implementable policies and qualitative approaches, *J Oper Res Soc* **36** (1985), 705–712.
[71] I. Or and W.P. Pierskalla, A Transportation Location-Allocation Model for Regional Blood Banking, *AIIE Transactions* **11**(2) (1979), 86–95.
[72] Y.A. Ozcan, E. Merwin, K. Lee and J.P. Morrissey, Benchmarking Using DEA: The Case of Mental Health Organizations, in: *Operations Research and Healthcare: a Handbook of Methods and Applications*, (Chapter 7), M.L. Brandeau, F. Sainfort and W.P. Pierskalla, Boston, Kluwer Academic Publishers, 2004, pp. 169–189.
[73] Y.A. Ozcan, Quantitative Methods in Health Care Management. San Francisco: Jossey Bass, 2005.
[74] A.D. Paltiel, K.M. Kuntz, S.T. Weiss and A.L. Fuhlbrigge, An Asthma Policy Model, in: *Operations Research and Healthcare: a Handbook of Methods and Applications*, (Chapter 26), M.L. Brandeau, F. Sainfort and W.P. Pierskalla, eds, Boston, Kluwer Academic Publishers, 2004, pp. 659–694.
[75] C.Y. Pang and J.M. Swint, Forecasting staffing needs for productivity management in hospital laboratories, *J Medical Syst* **9** (1985), 365–377.
[76] F. Pezzella, R. Bonanno and B. Nicoletti, A System Approach to Optimal Health-Care Districting, *European J Oper Res* **8** (1981), 139–146.
[77] W.P. Pierskalla, Examples Of Operational Systems Engineering Applications Relevant to Traumatic Brain Injury Care, Chapter 4 in *Systems Engineering To Improve Dramatic Brain Injury Care in the Military Health System*. National Academy of Engineering And Institute of Medicine. Washington, DC. The National Academies Press, 2009.
[78] W.P. Pierskalla and D.J. Brailer, Applications of Operations Research in Health Care Delivery, in: *Handbooks in OR and MS*, S.M. Pollock, ed., Elsevier Science B.V, 1994, 6 (pp. 469–505).
[79] W.P. Pierskalla, Sunrise Hospital. Teaching case study at the Department of Operations and Technology Management. UCLA Anderson Graduate School of Management. Los Angeles, California, 1999.
[80] W.P. Pierskalla, Supply Chain Management of blood Banks, in: *Operations Research and Healthcare: a Handbook of Methods and Applications*, (Chapter 5), M.L. Brandeau, F. Sainfort and W.P. Pierskalla, Boston, Kluwer Academic Publishers, 2004, pp. 103–146.
[81] B. Rizakow, J. Rosenhead and K. Reddington, AIDSPLAN: A Decision Support Model for Planning the Provision of HIV/AIDS – related Services, *Interfaces* **21**(3) (1991), 117–129.
[82] G. Romanin-Jacur and P. Facchin, Optimal Planning for a Pediatric Semi-Intensive Care Unit Via Simulation, *European I Oper Res* **29** (1982), 192–198.
[83] D.L. Rubin, E.S. Burnside and R. Shachter, A Bayesian Network to Assist Mammography Interpretation, in: *Operations Research and Healthcare: a Handbook of Methods and Applications*, (Chapter 27), M.L. Brandeau, F. Sainfort and W.P. Pierskalla, eds, Boston, Kluwer Academic Publishers, 2004, pp. 695–720.

[84] P. Santibáòez, M. Begen and D. Atkins, Surgical block scheduling in a system of hospitals: an application to resource and wait list of management in a British Columbia health authority, *Health-Care Management Science* **10**(3) (2007), 269–282.
[85] D. Schneider, A Methodology for the Analysis of Comparability of Services and Financial Impact of Closure of Obstetrics Services, *Medical Care* **19**(4) (1981), 393–409.
[86] J.S. Schwartz, B. Kinosian, H. Lee and W.P. Pierskalla, Strategies for Screening Blood for HIV Antibody: Use of a Decision Support System, *Journal of American Medical Association* **264**(13) (1990), 1704–1710.
[87] W. Shonick, Understanding the Nature of the Random Fluctuations of the Hospital DailyCensus: An important health planning tool, *Medical Care* **10**(2) (1972), 118–142.
[88] J. Simon, Decision Making with Prostate Cancer: A Multiple Objective Model with Uncertainty, *Interfaces* **39** (May-June 2009), 218–227.
[89] P. Smith, Large-Scale Models and Large-Scale Thinking: The Case of the Health Services, *Omega, International Journal Management Science* **23**(2) (1995), 145–157.
[90] V.L. Smith-Daniels, S.B. Schweikhart and D.E. Smith-Daniels, Capacity Management in Health Care Services: Review and Future Research Directions, *Decision Sciences* **19** (1988), 889–919.
[91] C. Stanton and J.M. MacGregor Smith, Steiner Trees and 3-D Macromolecular Conformation, *INFORMS Journal On Computing* **16** (2004), 470–485.
[92] V. Verter and S.D. Lapierre, Location of Preventive Healthcare Facilities, *Annals of Operations Research* **110**(1) (2002), 123–132.
[93] M.C. Weinstein, *Clinical Decision Analysis*, Philadelphia, Saunders, 1980.
[94] Wikipedia. at http://en.wikipedia.org/wiki/Main_Page.
[95] C.S. Zaric and M.L. Brandeau, Optimal Investment in a Portfolio of HIV Prevention Programs, *Medical Decision Making* **21** (2001), 391–408.
[96] C.S. Zaric and M.L. Brandeau, Resource Allocation for Epidemic Control over Short Time Horizons, *Mathematical Biosciences* **171** (2001), 33–58.
[97] C.S. Zaric and M.L. Brandeau, Dynamic Resource Allocation for Epidemic Control in Multiple Populations, *Mathematical Medicine and Biology* **19** (2002), 235–255.

William P. Pierskalla, Ph.D., is a Distinguished Professor Emeritus of Decisions, Operations and Technology Management in the Anderson Graduate School of Management at UCLA. He is also the Ronald A. Rosenfeld Professor Emeritus, The Wharton School, University of Pennsylvania. He was Dean of the John E. Anderson Graduate School of Management at UCLA. He holds the A.B. in Economics and M.B.A. degrees from Harvard University, an M.A. in mathematics from the University of Pittsburgh and a M.S. in statistics and a Ph.D. in operations research from Stanford University. His current interests include operations research, operations management, issues of global competition and the management and delivery aspects of health care delivery. Dr. Pierskalla is a member of the National Academy of Engineering (USA). He was President of the International Federation of Operational Research Societies. He is on the Editorial Advisory Boards of *Production and Operations Management, Encyclopedia of Operations Research & Management Science*, *International Transactions in Operational Research*, *Journal of the Operational Research Society* and *Health Care Management Science Journal* and has served on many other editorial boards. He was recently Vice President for Publications of the Institute for Operations Research and Management Sciences. He was President of the Operations Research Society of America, and is a past Editor in Chief of *Operations Research.* He is the 1989 recipient of the George E. Kimball Medal for distinguished service to the Operations Research Society of America and to the field of Operations Research and the 2005 INFORMS President's Award given to work that advances the welfare of society. Previously he was the Deputy Dean for Academic Affairs, the Director of the Huntsman Center for Global Competition and Leadership, Executive Director of the Leonard Davis Institute of Health Economics and the Chairman of the Health Care Systems Department at the Wharton School of the University of Pennsylvania. Prior to his positions at Wharton, he was on the faculties of Northwestern University, Southern Methodist University and Case Institute of Technology and has worked at Westinghouse Electric Corporation. He is a current board member of the Phoenix Health Systems Corp. He was a board member of member of the Archibald Bush Foundation (chairman 2002–2007), the Griffin Funds, the Northern Trust Bank of California, the iRise Corporation, Northern Wilderness Adventures Inc. and the Office Tenants Network Corporation. He has consulted to many business, educational and governmental organizations. He has given numerous lectures and seminars at Universities and organizations in the North and South Americas, Europe, Australia and Asia and has over fifty refereed articles in mathematical programming, transportation, inventory and production control, maintainability and health care delivery.

Information Knowledge Systems Management 8 (2009) 277–297
DOI 10.3233/IKS-2009-0143
IOS Press

Chapter 16

Engineering healthcare as a service system

James M. Tien and Pascal J. Goldschmidt-Clermont
E-mail: jmtien@miami.edu

Abstract: Engineering has and will continue to have a critical impact on healthcare; the application of technology-based techniques to biological problems can be defined to be technobiology applications. This paper is primarily focused on applying the technobiology approach of systems engineering to the development of a healthcare service system that is both integrated and adaptive. In general, healthcare services are carried out with knowledge-intensive agents or components which work together as providers and consumers to create or co-produce value. Indeed, the engineering design of a healthcare system must recognize the fact that it is actually a complex integration of human-centered activities that is increasingly dependent on information technology and knowledge. Like any service system, healthcare can be considered to be a combination or recombination of three essential components – people (characterized by behaviors, values, knowledge, etc.), processes (characterized by collaboration, customization, etc.) and products (characterized by software, hardware, infrastructures, etc.). Thus, a healthcare system is an integrated and adaptive set of people, processes and products. It is, in essence, a system of systems which objectives are to enhance its efficiency (leading to greater interdependency) and effectiveness (leading to improved health). Integration occurs over the physical, temporal, organizational and functional dimensions, while adaptation occurs over the monitoring, feedback, cybernetic and learning dimensions. In sum, such service systems as healthcare are indeed complex, especially due to the uncertainties associated with the human-centered aspects of these systems. Moreover, the system complexities can only be dealt with methods that enhance system integration and adaptation.

1. Healthcare as an engineering focus

Healthcare refers to the treatment and management of illness, and the preservation of health through services offered by the medical, dental, pharmaceutical, clinical laboratory sciences, nursing, and allied health professions. Healthcare embraces all the goods and services designed to promote health, including "preventive, curative and palliative interventions, whether directed to individuals or to populations" [29].

Clearly, engineering – the application of technical, scientific and mathematical knowledge to help design and implement materials, structures, machines, devices, systems, and processes that can achieve a desired objective – has and will continue to have a critical impact on healthcare. Indeed, as identified in Exhibit 1, every engineering discipline or technology has potential applications to biology; a number of such "technobiology" examples (i.e., through the application of technology-based techniques to biological problems) are cited and briefly described. (More specifically, technolobiology is to be differentiated from "biotechnology" which is about the application of biology-based techniques to technological problems; such techniques include neural networks, genetic algorithms and systems biology.) The Exhibit 1 technolobiology examples highlight the technological focus; they include biomedical, chemical, electrical, environmental, industrial, material and mechanical devices, approaches, and processes.

An overarching engineering approach that underpins many of the Exhibit 1 examples concerns addressing each biological problem from a systems perspective. In this regard, Grossman [5] has identified several disruptive engineering innovations that could change the way healthcare is organized, paid for,

Exhibit 1. Engineering healthcare: Technobiology examples

Discipline	Examples	Scope
Biomedical	1. PillCam 2. Neurostimulator 3. Hypothermia 4. Stem Cells from Adult Cells 5. Personalized Medicine	1. Swallowed pill can capture 50K gastrointestinal images 2. Nerve stimulation to treat migraine headaches, etc. 3. Lowering body temperature to 91.5 degrees to stem harmful chemical reactions when oxygen is restored following cardiac arrest 4. Employ 4 embryonic genes to induce stem cell growth 5. Tailor medicine through genetic profiling chips/sensors
Chemical	1. Tissues 2. Diagnostic 3. Microcyn	1. Regenerative medicine: engineering induced pluripotent stem (iPS) cells to create skin, muscle, bone, cartilage, fat, blood vessel, nerve, heart, liver, bladder, kidney, etc. 2. Tests that identify gene variations which can predict Lou Gehrig's disease, Parkinson's, Alzheimer, etc. 3. Electronically charged, super-oxidized water-based solution that attacks proteins in infectious agents of a wound, reducing need for antibiotics
Electrical	1. Bioimaging 2. Robotic 3. Bioinformatics 4. Ultrasound	1. High-definition laparoscope for colonoscopies, etc. 2. Automated assist in walking, moving, etc. 3. Large scale analysis of data for drug discovery, etc. 4. Focused-ultrasound surgery on fibroid tumors, prostates
Environmental	1. Sunshine Vitamin 2. Hearing Pill	1. Sunlight spurs body's production of vitamin D which can reduce instances of cancer, autoimmune disease, high blood pressure, heart disease, and diabetes 2. Naturally occurring substance called N-acetylcysteine (NAC) helps prevent hearing loss due to loud noise by helping body produce more glutathione
Industrial	1. Evidence-Based Protocols, Including False-Discovery-Rate 2. Adaptive Clinical Trials 3. E-Care 4. Concierge Care 5. Preventive Care 6. Personalized Care	1. Data mining and analysis of past treatments can point to effective protocols, including minimization of false positives linking diseases and DNA genes 2. Design and success criteria adjusted as clinical results are obtained 3. Integrated digital records and wearable wireless devices 4. VIP/premium services 5. Biomarkers/diagnostic tools allow for predictive care 6. Genomics-based adaptive, customized care
Material	1. Nanoparticle Medicine 2. Drug Delivery 3. Surgical Tape	1. Focused cancer treatment by targeting special nanoparticles which attach to cancerous cells 2. New drug delivery material with timed release 3. Biodegradable elastic polymer to close incisions or cuts
Mechanical	1. Haptics 2. Exoskeleton 3. Prosthetic 4. Artificial Disc 5. Asthma Mitigation	1. Sensing/manipulating of objects through touch 2. External anatomical feature that supports/protects a body 3. Orthopedic or bionic device for mobility impaired 4. Replaced neck disc, resulting in less pain and swelling 5. Alair System uses radio-frequency energy to warm the airway in asthma patients; keeps muscles from constricting

and delivered, including precision diagnostics and therapies (i.e., evidence-based medicine), advances in information/communication technologies (i.e., personal health record) and new business models (i.e., overcoming the cottage-industry structure and the dysfunctional reimbursement and regulatory framework). Continuing in the same vein, the contents of this paper are primarily focused on applying systems engineering to healthcare. More specifically, it is augured in Section 2 that healthcare is, almost by definition, a service (i.e., not an outcome of manufacturing, agriculture, construction, or mining). Moreover, healthcare should be regarded as a system that should be both integrated (Section 3) and adaptive (Section 4). The complexity of the healthcare service system is considered in Section 5, followed by several concluding insights in Section 6. The purpose of viewing healthcare as a complex service system is, of course, to be able to employ the range of methods that could make such a system efficient (i.e., meeting demand with minimum cost) and effective (i.e., producing the right service at the right time for the right consumer). Finally, it should be stated that the paper builds on both a presentation by one of the authors at a recent healthcare workshop [26] and a recent paper on complex service systems [20].

2. Healthcare as a service

As detailed in Tien and Berg [21–24], the importance of the services sector cannot be overstated; it employs a large and growing proportion of workers in the developed nations. As reflected in Exhibit 2, the services sector includes a number of large industries; indeed, services employment in the US is at 82.1 percent, while the remaining four economic sectors (i.e., manufacturing, agriculture, construction, and mining), which together can be considered to be the physical "goods" sector, employ the remaining 17.9 percent. Healthcare – which employs 10.8% of the US workforce – is, of course, one of the largest industries in the services sector. Yet, as Tien and Berg [23] augur, engineering research and education have not followed suit; the majority of research is still manufacturing- or hardware-oriented and degree programs are still in those traditional disciplines that were established in the early 1900s. On the other hand, medical research and education are somewhat more sensitive to the services need of healthcare; for example, evidence-based protocols are becoming more prevalent in the practice of medicine. Nevertheless, Hipel et al. [6] maintain that services research and education deserve more attention and support in this 21st Century when the computer chip, the information technology, the Internet and the flattening of the world [3] have all combined to make services – and services innovation – the new engine for global economic growth.

What constitutes the services sector? It can be considered "to include all economic activities whose output is not a physical product or construction, is generally consumed at the time it is produced and provides added value in forms (such as convenience, amusement, timeliness, comfort or health) that are essentially intangible..." [14]. Implicit in this definition is the recognition that services production and services delivery are so integrated that they can be considered to be a single, combined stage in the services value chain, whereas the goods sector has a value chain that includes supplier, manufacturer, assembler, retailer, and customer. Alternatively, services can be considered to be knowledge-intensive agents or components which work together as providers and consumers to create or co-produce value [8].

Unfortunately, the US healthcare system is a good example of a people-intensive service system that is in disarray. It is the most expensive and, yet, among the least effective system for a developed country; a minority of the population receives excellent care, while an equal minority receives inadequate care [12]. This situation is not due to a lack of well-trained health professionals or to a lack of innovative technologies; it is due to the fact that it is based on a fragmented group of mostly small, independent providers driven by cost-obsessed insurance companies – clearly, it is, at best, a non-system [16]. As a consequence, an integrated and adaptive healthcare system must be designed and implemented, one requiring the participation and support of a large number of stakeholders (i.e., consumers, doctors,

Exhibit 2. Scope and size of U.S. employment

Industries	Employment (M)	Percent
Trade, Transportation & Utilities	26.1M	19.0%
Professional & Business	17.2	12.6
Health Care	14.8	10.8
Leisure & Hospitality	13.0	9.5
Education	13.0	9.5
Government (Except Education)	11.7	8.5
Finance, Insurance & Real Estate	8.3	6.1
Information & Telecommunication	3.1	2.2
Other	5.4	3.9
SERVICES SECTOR	**112.6**	**82.1**
Manufacturing	14.3	10.3
Construction	7.5	5.5
Agriculture	2.2	1.6
Mining	0.7	0.5
GOODS SECTOR	**24.7**	**17.9**
TOTAL	**137.3**	**100.0**

Source: *Bureau of Labor Statistics,* April 2006.

hospitals, insurance companies, etc.). For example, patients must take increased responsibility for their own healthcare in terms of access and use of validated information.

In the remainder of this introductory section on services, it would be helpful to highlight three overarching influences. First, the emergence of e(lectronic) services is totally dependent on information technology; they include, as examples, medical records, financial services, banking, airline reservation systems, and consumer goods marketing. As discussed by Tien and Berg [22], e-service enterprises interact or "co-produce" with their customers in a digital (including e-mail and Internet) medium, as compared to the physical environment in which traditional or bricks-and-mortar service enterprises interact with their customers. Similarly, in contrast to traditional services which include low-wage "hamburger flippers", e-services typically employ high-wage earners and services that are more demanding in their requirements for self-service, transaction speed, and computation. In regard to data input that could be processed to produce information that, in turn, could be used to help make informed service decisions, it should be noted that both sets of services rely on multiple data sources; however, traditional services typically require homogeneous (mostly quantitative) data input, while e-services increasingly require non-homogeneous (i.e., both quantitative and qualitative) data input. Paradoxically, the traditional service enterprises have been driven by data, although data availability and accuracy have been limited (especially before the pervasive use of the Universal Product Code – UPC – and the more recent deployment of radio frequency location and identification – RFLID – tags). Likewise, the emerging e-service enterprises have been driven by information (i.e., processed data), although information availability and accuracy have been limited, due to a data rich, information poor (DRIP) conundrum [19].

Consequently, while traditional services are based on economies of scale and a standardized approach, electronic services emphasize economies of expertise or knowledge and an adaptive approach. Another critical distinction between traditional and electronic services is that, although all services require decisions to be made, traditional services are typically based on predetermined decision rules, while electronic services require real-time, adaptive decision making; that is why Tien [19] has advanced a decision informatics paradigm, one that relies on both information and decision technologies from a real-time perspective. High-speed Internet access, low-cost computing, wireless networks, electronic sensors and ever-smarter software are the tools for building a global services economy. Thus, in e-commerce, a sophisticated and integrated service system combines product (i.e., good and/or service) selection,

Exhibit 3. Services versus manufactured goods

Focus	Services	Goods
Production	*C*o-Produced	*P*re-Produced
Variability	*H*eterogeneous	*I*dentical
Physicality	*I*ntangible	*T*angible
Product	*P*erishable	"*I*nventoryable"
Objective	*P*ersonalizable	*R*eliable
Satisfaction	*E*xpectation-Related	*U*tility-Related
Life Cycle	*R*eusable	*R*ecyclable
OVERALL	*CHIPPER*	*PITIRUR*

order taking, payment processing, order fulfillment and delivery scheduling into a seamless system, all provided by distinct service providers; in this regard, it can be considered to be a system of – different – systems.

The second influence on services is its relationship to manufacturing. The interdependences, similarities and complementarities of services and manufacturing are significant. Indeed, many of the recent innovations in manufacturing are relevant to the service industries. Concepts and processes such as cycle time, total quality management, quality circles, six-sigma, design-for-assembly, design-for-manufacturability, design-for-recycling, small-batch production, concurrent engineering, just-in-time manufacturing, rapid prototyping, flexible manufacturing, agile manufacturing, distributed manufacturing, and environmentally-sound manufacturing can, for the most part, be recast in services-related terms. Thus, many of the engineering and management concepts and processes employed in manufacturing can likewise be employed to deal with problems and issues arising in the services sector.

Nonetheless, there are considerable differences between goods and services. Tien and Berg [22] provide a comparison between the goods and services sectors. The goods sector requires material as input, is physical in nature, involves the customer at the design stage, and employs mostly quantitative measures to assess its performance. On the other hand, the services sector requires information as input, is virtual in nature, involves the customer at both the production and delivery stages, and employs mostly qualitative measures to assess its performance. Of course, even when there are similarities, it is critical that the co-producing nature of services be carefully taken into consideration. For example, in manufacturing, physical parameters, statistics of production and quality can be more precisely quantified; on the other hand, since a services operation depends on an interaction between the recipient and the process of producing and delivering, the characterization is necessarily more subjective and different.

A more insightful approach to understanding and advancing services research is to explicitly consider the differences between services and manufactured goods. As identified in Exhibit 3, services are, by definition, co-produced; quite variable or heterogeneous in their production and delivery; physically intangible; perishable if not consumed as it is being produced or by a certain time (e.g., before a flight's departure); focused on being "personalizable"; expectation-related in terms of customer satisfaction; and reusable in its entirety. On the other hand, manufactured goods are pre-produced; quite identical or standardized in their production and use; physically tangible; "inventoryable" if not consumed; focused on being reliable; utility-related in terms of customer satisfaction; and recyclable in regard to its parts. In mnemonic terms and referring to Exhibit 3, services can be considered to be "chipper", while manufactured goods are a "pitirur".

Although the comparison between services and manufacturing highlights some obvious methodological differences, it is interesting to note that the physical manufactured assets depreciate with use and time, while the virtual service assets are generally reusable, and may in fact increase in value with repeated use and over time. The latter assets are predominantly processes and associated human resources that build on the skill and knowledge base accumulated by repeated interactions with the service receiver, who is involved in the co-production of the service. Thus, for example, a surgeon should get better over time, especially if the same type of surgery is repeated. Indeed, clinical productivity increases for an average physician, from the dawn of a career to almost the end of a career, with a slight slowing down towards the end. Likewise, while most US physicians practice at a financial loss over the first few years, they progressively improve their financial standing over the course of their career.

In services, automation-driven software algorithms have transformed human resource-laden, co-producing service systems to software algorithm-laden, self-producing services. Thus, extensive man-power would be required to manually co-produce the services if automation were not available. Although automation has certainly improved productivity and decreased costs in some services (e.g., telecommunications, Internet commerce, etc.), it has not yet had a similar impact on other labor-intensive services like healthcare. However, with new multimedia and broadband technologies, some hospitals are customizing or personalizing their treatment of patients, including the sharing of electronic records with their patients.

A third critical influence on services is the computationally-driven move towards mass customization. "Customization" implies meeting the needs of a customer market that is partitioned into an appropriate number of segments, each with similar needs (e.g., Amazon.com targets their marketing of a new book to an entire market segment if several members of the segment act to acquire the book). "Mass customization" implies meeting the needs of a segmented customer market, with each segment being a single individual (e.g., a tailor who laser scans an individual's upper torso and then delivers a uniquely fitted jacket). And "real-time mass customization" implies meeting the needs of an individualized customer market on a real-time basis (e.g., a tailor who laser scans an individual's upper torso and then delivers a uniquely fitted jacket within a reasonable period, while the individual is waiting). To a large extent, one could argue that healthcare is, almost by definition, a real-time mass customized service; however, at the present time, healthcare is not computationally-driven and therefore not cost-effective.

It is interesting to note that in regard to customization and in relation to the late 1700s, the US is in some respects going "back-to-the-future"; thus, advanced technologies are not only empowering the individual but are also allowing for individualized or customized goods and services. For example, e-education reflects a return to individual-centered learning [18], much like home schooling in a previous century. Moreover, when mass customization occurs, it is difficult to say whether a service or a good is being delivered; that is, a uniquely fitted jacket can be considered to be a co-produced service/good or "servgood". The implication of real-time mass customization, then, is that the resultant, co-produced "servgood" must be carried out locally, although the intelligence underpinning the co-production could be residing at a distant server and delivered like a utility. As a conseqence, while manufacturing jobs have already been mostly relocated overseas (with only about 10.3 percent of all US employees still involved in manufacturing) and service jobs (which now comprise about 82.1 percent of all US jobs) are beginning to be relocated overseas, real-time mass customization should help stem job outflow, if not reverse the trend. In this regard, real-time mass customization should be regarded as a matter of national priority. (It should be noted that while manufacturing jobs are decreasing and at 10.3 percent of all jobs, manufacturing, as a proportion of the gross domestic product, has remained about constant at 25 percent.)

Clearly, healthcare needs to transition from being a traditional (although high-wage) service to an electronic-based service industry, one relying on digital media for such activities as real-time access to patient records. (Some digitally-based medical approaches need further assessment and improvement; thus, while robotic surgery is quite helpful in the repair of small nerves and blood vessels, its overall efficacy is still under debate – nevertheless, as robotic surgery is further refined, it will undoubtedly become a standard technique in the surgeon's arsenal of tools.) Additionally, healthcare must adopt some of the methods that have enabled manufacturing to be efficient (e.g., reduced cycle time, improved quality, etc.), while focusing on service effectiveness (e.g., maintaining a high standard of co-production, meeting consumer expectation, etc.). Most importantly, healthcare must be adaptive and must customize their treatments to the needs of their patients, ranging from evidence-based protocols to "servgood" or personalized medications.

3. Healthcare as an integrated system

A service system like healthcare is actually an integration or combination of three essential components – people, processes and products. In particular, people can be grouped into those demanding services (i.e., consumers, users, patients, buyers, organizations, etc.) and those supplying the services (i.e., suppliers, providers, clinicians, servers, sellers, organizations, etc.); although sometimes ad hoc, processes are primarily procedural (i.e., standardized, evolving, decision-focused, network-oriented, etc.) and/or algorithmic (i.e., data mining, decision modeling, systems engineering, etc.) in structure; and products can be physical (i.e., facilities, sensors, information technologies, etc.) or virtual (i.e., e-commerce, simulations, e-collaboration, etc.) in form.

Given the co-producing nature of services, it is obvious that people constitute the most critical component or element of a service system. In turn, because people are so unpredictable in their values, behaviors, attitudes, expectations, and knowledge, they invariably raise the complexity of a service system. Moreover, the multi-stakeholder – and related multi-objective – nature of such systems serve to only intensify the complexity level and may render the system to be indefinable, if not unmanageable. Human performance, social networks and interpersonal interactions combine to further aggravate the situation. While people-oriented, decision-focused methods are further considered in Section 4, it is interesting to note that sometimes systems are too big to manage or, alternatively, to let fail. Thus, although in the 2008 economic disaster, the US Federal Government allowed Lehman Brothers to fail, it could not let either the insurance conglomerate American International Group or the giant Citigroup holding company go bankrupt. In fact, federal regulators across the globe are now – in 2009 – trying to ensure that such disasters do not happen again, perhaps by breaking up too-big-to-fail international firms so that they could fit and operate within national borders.

Processes which underpin system integration include standards, procedures, protocols, and algorithms. By combining or integrating service processes, one could, for example, enhance a "one-stop shopping" approach, a highly desirable situation for the consumer or customer. Integration of financial services has resulted in giant banks (e.g., the above-mentioned Citigroup); integration of home building goods and services has resulted in super stores (e.g., Home Depot); and integration of software services has resulted in complex software packages (e.g., Microsoft Office). Integration also enhances system efficiency, if not its effectiveness. For example, the radio frequency location and identification (RFLID) tag – or computer chip with a transmitter – serves to integrate the supply chain. However, as supply chains become more electronically integrated and interdependent, cyber security becomes more problematic [2].

In regard to service-related products, one can group them into two categories. First, there are those physical products or goods (e.g., autos, aircrafts, satellites, computers, etc.) which, as indicated in Section 2, enable the delivery of effective and high-quality services (e.g., road travel, air travel, global positioning, electronic services, etc.). Second, there are those more virtual products or services, including e-commerce.

Exhibit 4. System Integration: Dimensions

Dimension	Definition	Characteristics	Elements
Physical	Degree of Systems Co-Location	Natural	Closed; Open; Hybrid
		Constructed	Goods; Structures; Systems
		Virtual	Services; Simulation; E-Commerce
Temporal	Degree of Systems Co-Timing	Strategic	Analytical; Procedural; Political
		Tactical	Simulation; Distribution; Allocation
		Operational	Cognition; Visualization; Expectation
Organizational	Degree of Systems Co-Management	Resources	People; Processes; Products
		Economics	Supply; Demand; Revenue
		Management	Centralized; Decentralized; Distributed
Functional	Degree of Systems Co-Functioning	Input	Location; Allocation; Re-Allocation
		Process	Informatics; Feedback; Control
		Output	Efficiency; Effectiveness

More importantly and as detailed in Exhibit 4, service system integration can occur over the physical, temporal, organizational and functional dimensions. Physical integration can be defined by the degree of systems co-location in the natural (i.e., closed, open, hybrid), constructed (i.e., goods, structure, systems) or virtual (i.e., service, simulated, e-commerce) environment. An urban center's infrastructures (e.g., emergency services, health services, financial services, etc.) are examples of a constructed environment. Over time and with advances in information technology and the necessity for improved efficiency and effectiveness, these infrastructures have become increasingly automated and interlinked or interdependent. In fact, because the information technology revolution has changed the way business is transacted, government is operated, and national defense is conducted, the US President [28] singled it out as the most critical infrastructure to protect following 9/11. Thus, while the US is considered a superpower because of its military strength and economic prowess, non-traditional attacks on its interdependent and cyber-underpinned infrastructures could significantly harm both the nation's military power and economy. Clearly, infrastructures, especially the information infrastructure, are among the nation's weakest links; they are vulnerable to willful acts of sabotage, if not invasions of privacy. Moreover, as indicated earlier, this interdependency contributed significantly to the 2008 economic disaster or recession. Recent efforts at imbuing infrastructures with "intelligence" make it increasingly feasible to address the safety and security concerns, allowing for the continuous monitoring and real-time control of critical infrastructures.

Temporal integration can be defined by the degree of systems co-timing from a strategic (i.e., analytical, procedural, political), tactical (i.e., simulation, distribution, allocation), and operational (i.e., cognition, visualization, expectation) perspective. Expectation, for example, is a critical temporal issue in the delivery of services. More specifically, since services are to a large extent subject to customer satisfaction and since, as Tien and Cahn [25] postulated and validated, "satisfaction is a function of expectation," service performance or satisfaction can be enhanced through the effective "management" of expectation. When applied to healthcare, however, it may be difficult, if not impossible, to manage a patient's expectation under certain emergency situations.

Organizational integration can be defined by the degree of systems co-management of resources (i.e., people, processes, products), economics (i.e., supply, demand, revenue), and management (i.e., centralized, decentralized, distributed). In regard to management integration, Tien et al. [27] provide a consistent approach to considering the management of both goods and services – by first defining a value chain and then showing how it can be partitioned into supply and demand chains, which, in turn, can be appropriately managed. Of course, the key purpose for the management of supply and demand chains is to smooth-out the peaks and valleys commonly seen in many supply and demand patterns, respectively.

Moreover, real-time mass customization occurs when both supply and demand chains are simultaneously managed. The shift in focus from mass production to mass customization (whereby a service is produced and delivered in response to a customer's stated or imputed needs) is intended to provide superior value to customers by meeting their unique needs. It is in this area of customization – where customer involvement is not only at the goods design stage but also at the manufacturing or co-production stage – that services and manufacturing are merging in concept [23], resulting in a "servgood". The simultaneous, real-time customized management of both the supply and demand chains is further considered in Section 5.

Functional integration can be defined by the degree of systems co-functioning in regard to input (i.e., location, allocation, re-allocation), process (i.e., informatics, feedback, control), and output (i.e., efficiency, effectiveness). From an output perspective, for example, it is obvious that a system should be about integrating and enhancing efficiency and effectiveness, the twin pillars of productivity. However, it should be noted that efficiency is mostly related to the manner in which the supply chain has been designed for optimal operation, while effectiveness is mostly related to the manner in which the demand chain has been responsive to consumer needs.

Again, healthcare – as a service system – must be integrated in regard to people, processes and products, as well as over the physical, temporal, organizational and functional dimensions. It is obvious that designing an efficient and effective healthcare system is not easily accomplished; socialistic systems like Sweden's cost too much, while capitalistic systems like the US's are both high cost and unfair. New design approaches are required. The information technology revolution has permitted the analysis part of system design to be largely undertaken by computers; it allows for a simulated and collaborative redesign process to occur – until a satisfactory design is achieved which meets specified performance (e.g., morbidity, mortality, cost, etc.) criteria. The resultant and integrated healthcare system must be a comprehensive, interoperable system of systems. Perhaps the best example of an integrated healthcare system is that proposed by Goldschmidt-Clermont et al. [Undated]; based on the autonomic computing initiative, they propose an autonomic healthcare system that combine the existing hospital information technology with operational processes to bring down the barriers among different specialties and to improve the quality of care being provided. As a final point, it should be noted that the human body is itself an amazingly integrated system of systems, one that should not be perturbed by surgeries and other intrusive treatments; indeed, the clinical specialist that should command the highest salary is one who focuses on the body as a system of systems.

4. Healthcare as an adaptive system

Because a service system is, by definition, a co-producing system, it must be adaptive. Adaptation is a uniquely human characteristic, based on a combination of three essential components – decision making, decision informatics, and human interface. (Indeed, designing a healthcare system is about making decisions or choices about the system's characteristics or attributes.) Exhibit 5 provides a framework for decision making. To begin, it is helpful to underscore the difference between data and information, especially from a decision making perspective. Data represent basic transactions captured during operations, while information represents processed data (e.g., derivations, groupings, patterns, etc.). Clearly, except for simple operational decisions, decision making at the tactical or higher levels requires, at a minimum, appropriate information or processed data. Exhibit 5 also identifies knowledge as processed information (together with experiences, beliefs, values, cultures, etc.), and wisdom, in turn, as processed knowledge (together with insights, theories, etc.). Thus, strategic decisions can be made with knowledge, while systemic decisions can be made with wisdom. Unfortunately, for the most part,

Exhibit 5. System Adaptation: Decision Making Framework

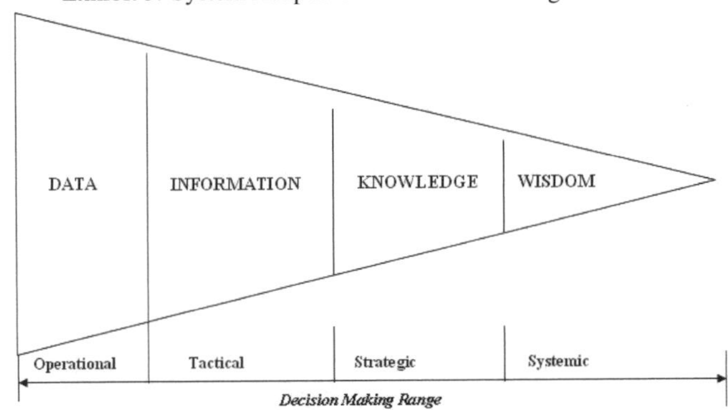

Exhibit 6. System Adaptation: A Decision Informatics Paradigm

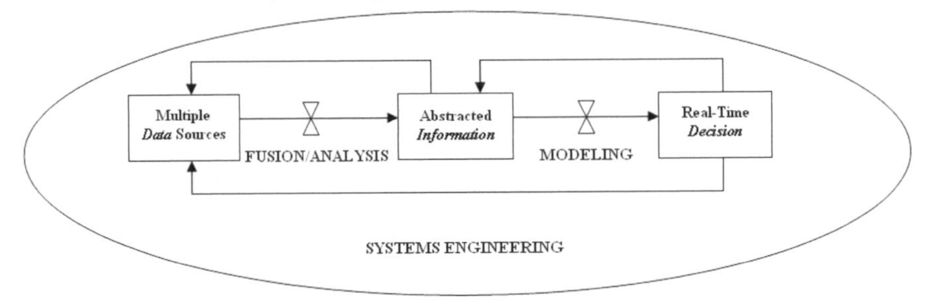

the literature does not distinguish between data and information; indeed, economists claim that because of the astounding growth in information – really, data – technology, the US and other developed countries are now a part of the global "knowledge economy". Although electronic data technology has transformed large-scale information systems from being the "glue" that holds the various units of an organization together to being the strategic asset that provides the organization with its competitive advantage, the US is far from being a knowledge economy. In the continuum of data, information, knowledge, and wisdom, the US – together with other advanced economies – is, at best, at the beginning of a data rich, information poor (DRIP) conundrum, as identified in Section 2.

The fact remains that data – both quantitative and qualitative – need to be effectively and efficiently fused and analyzed in order to yield appropriate information for informed or intelligent decision making in regard to the design, production and delivery of goods and services, including healthcare. As depicted in Exhibit 6, the nature of the required real-time decision (regarding the production and/or delivery of a service) determines, where appropriate and from a systems engineering perspective, the data to be collected (possibly, from multiple, non-homogeneous sources) and the real-time fusion and analysis to be undertaken to obtain the needed information for input to the modeling effort which, in turn, provides the knowledge to identify and support the required decision in a timely manner. Clearly, methods must be developed that can fuse and analyze a steady stream of non-homogeneous (i.e., quantitative and qualitative) data – this is especially true for healthcare, where quantitative data from monitoring devices must be complemented with the patient's qualitative assessments before the clinician can recommend an appropriate treatment. The feedback loops in Exhibit 6 are within the context of systems engineering; they serve to refine the analysis and modeling steps.

Continuing with the decision informatics paradigm in Exhibit 6, it should be noted that decision modeling constitutes the information-based modeling and analysis of alternative decision scenarios;

they include operations research, decision science, computer science, industrial engineering and, more recently, business analytics. At present, decision modeling methods suffer from two shortcomings. First, most of the available – especially optimization – methods are only applicable in a steady state environment, whereas in the real-world, all systems are in transition. (Note that steady-state, like average, is an analytical concept that allows for a tractable, if not manageable, analysis.) Second, most of the available methods are unable to cope with changing circumstances; instead, we need methods that are adaptive so that decisions can be made in real-time, as is required in most healthcare situations. Thus, non steady-state, adaptive decision methods are required. More importantly, real-time decision modeling is not just about speeding up the models and solution algorithms; it, like real-time data fusion and analysis, also requires additional research and development.

The systems engineering methods implicit in Exhibit 6 concern the integration of people, processes, and products from a systems perspective; they include electrical engineering, human-machine systems, system performance and system biology. Again, the real-time nature of co-producing services – especially human-centered services that are computationally-intensive and intelligence-oriented – requires a real-time, systems engineering approach. Ethnography, a branch of anthropology that can help identify a consumer's unmet needs, is being used to spot breakthrough product and service innovations. Another critical aspect of systems engineering is system performance; it provides an essential framework for assessing the decisions made – in terms of such issues as satisfaction, convenience, privacy, security, equity, quality, productivity, safety and reliability. Similarly, undertaking systems engineering within a real-time environment will require additional thought and research.

Human interface is another essential element of an adaptive service system; it is actually a critical tool in systems engineering. Such interface could include the interactions between and among humans and software agents, machines, sub-systems, and systems of systems. Human factors constitute a discipline that deals with many of these interactions. However, another critical interface concerns how humans interact with data and information. In developing appropriate human-information interfaces, one must pay careful attention to a number of factors. First, human-information interfaces are actually a part of any decision support model; they structure the manner in which the model output or information is provided to the decision maker. Cognition represents the point of interface between the human and the information presented. The presentation must enhance the cognitive process of mental visualization, capable of creating images from complex multidimensional data, including structured and unstructured text documents, measurements, images and video. Second, constructing and communicating a mental image common to a team of, say, clinicians and nurses could facilitate collaboration and could lead to more effective decision making at all levels, from operational to tactical to strategic. Nevertheless, cognitive facilitation is especially necessary in operational settings which are under high stress. Third, cognitive modeling and decision making must combine machine learning technology with a priori knowledge in a probabilistic data mining framework to develop models of, say, a nurse's tasks, goals, and objectives. These user-behavior models must be designed to adapt to the individual decision maker so as to promote better understanding of the needs and actions of the individual, including adversarial behaviors and intents.

More importantly and as detailed in Exhibit 7, service system adaptation can occur over the monitoring, feedback, cybernetic and learning dimensions. Monitoring adaptation can be defined by the degree of sensed actions in regard to data collection (i.e., sensors, agents, swarms), data analysis (i.e., structuring, processing, mining), and information abstraction (i.e., derivations, groupings, patterns). Data are acquired by sensors, which could be in the form of humans, robotic networks, aerial images, radio frequency signals, and other measures and signatures. In regard to patients, for example, sensors which

Exhibit 7. System Adaptation: Dimensions

Dimension	Definition	Characteristics	Elements
Monitoring	Degree of Sensed Actions	Data Collection	Sensors; Agents; Swarms
		Data Analysis	Structuring; Processing; Mining
		Information Abstraction	Derivations; Groupings; Patterns
Feedback	Degree of Expected Actions	Standardized	Pre-Structured; Pre-Planned
		Procedural	Policies; Standard Operating Procedures
		Algorithmic	Optimized; Bayesian
Cybernetic	Degree of Reactive Actions	Deterministic	Known States; Deterministic Actions
		Dynamic	Known State Distributions; Dynamic Actions
		Adaptive	Unknown States; Adaptive Actions
Learning	Degree of Unstructured Actions	Cognition	Recognition-Based; Behavioral
		Evidence	Information-Based; Genetic
		Improvisation	Experience-Based; Evolutionary

monitor their vital signs are essential, as are verbal inputs from the patients themselves. More recently, data warehouses are proliferating and data mining techniques are gaining in popularity. However, no matter how large a data warehouse and how sophisticated a data mining technique, problems can occur if the data do not possess the desirable attributes of measurability, availability, consistency, validity, reliability, stability, accuracy, independence, robustness and completeness.

Moreover, in most situations, data alone are useless unless access to and analysis of the data are in real-time or at least in a meaningful time frame. In developing real-time, adaptive data processors, one must consider several critical issues. First, as depicted in Exhibit 6, these data processors must be able to combine (i.e., fuse and analyze) streaming data from sensors and other appropriate input from knowledge bases (including output from tactical and strategic databases) in order to generate information that could serve as input to operational decision support models and/or provide the basis for making informed decisions. Second, as also indicated in Exhibit 6, the type of data to collect and how to process it depend on what decision is to be made; these dependencies highlight the difficulty of developing effective and adaptive data processors or data miners. Further, once a decision is made, it may constrain subsequent decisions which, in turn, may change future data requirements and information needs. Third, inasmuch as the data processors must function in real-time and be adaptable to an ongoing stream of data, genetic algorithms, which equations can mutate repeatedly in an evolutionary manner until a solution emerges that best fit the observed data, are becoming the tools of choice in this area.

Feedback adaptation can be defined by the degree of expected actions based on standardized (i.e., pre-structured, pre-planned), procedural (i.e., policies, standard operating procedures), and algorithmic (i.e., optimized, Bayesian) approaches. In general, models underpin these approaches. As an example, Kaplan et al. [7] have developed a set of complex models to demonstrate that the best prevention approach to a smallpox attack would be to undertake immediate and widespread vaccination. Unfortunately, models, including simulations, dealing with multiple systems are still relatively immature and must be the focus of additional research and development. Such system of systems models are quite complex – especially in regard to a possible misalignment of the underlying system objectives – and will require a multidisciplinary approach.

Cybernetic adaptation can be defined by the degree of reactive actions that could be deterministic (i.e., known states, deterministic actions), dynamic (i.e., known state distributions, dynamic actions), or adaptive (i.e., unknown states, adaptive actions). Cybernetics is derived from the Greek word "kybernetics", which refers to a steersman or governor. Within a system, cybernetics is about feedback (through evaluation of performance relative to stated objectives) and control (through communication, self-regulation, adaptation, optimization, and/or management); thus, cybernetic adaptation refers to actions that are undertaken based on an assessment of the feedback signals and then taking corrective steps to control the system so as to achieve the desired system objectives. A system is defined by state variables that are known in a deterministic manner (resulting in deterministic feedback or cybernetic actions); that are known in a probabilistic or distributional manner (resulting in dynamic feedback or cybernetic actions); or that are unknown (resulting in adaptive feedback or cybernetic actions). As an example, autopilots – which are programmed to deal with deterministic and dynamic situations – can, for the most part, take off, fly and land a plane; yet, usually two human pilots are also on the plane, just in case an unknown state occurs and the adaptive judgment of a human pilot is required. Clearly, a trained human – like a clinician or surgeon – is still the most adaptive controller, although machines are becoming more 'intelligent' through adaptive learning algorithms.

System control is perhaps the most critical challenge facing designers of multiple, interrelated systems or system of systems (SoS). Due to the difficulty, if not impossibility, of developing a comprehensive SoS model, either analytically or through simulation, SoS control remains an open problem and is, of course, uniquely challenging for each application domain. Moreover, real-time control – which is required in almost all application domains – of interdependent systems poses an especially difficult problem. The cooperative control of an SoS assumes that it can be characterized by a set of interconnected systems or agents with a common goal, which unfortunately is not the case with most public-private healthcare systems. Classical techniques of control, optimization and estimation could be used to create parallel architectures for, as an example, coordinating numerous sensors. However, many issues dealing with real-time cooperative control have not been addressed, even in non-SoS structures. For example, one issue concerns the control of an SoS in the presence of communication delays among the SoS sub-systems.

Finally, learning adaptation can be defined by the degree of unstructured actions based on cognition (i.e., recognition-based, behavioral), evidence (i.e., information-based, genetic), and improvisation (i.e., experience-based, evolutionary). Learning adaptation is mostly about real-time decision making at the operational level. In such a situation and as indicated earlier, it is not just about speeding up steady-state models and their solution algorithms; in fact, steady-state models become irrelevant in real-time environments. In essence, it concerns reasoning under both uncertainty and severe time constraints. The development of operational decision support models must recognize several critical issues. First, in addition to defining what data to collect and how they should be fused and analyzed, decisions also drive what kind of models or simulations are needed. These operational models are, in turn, based on abstracted information and output from tactical and strategic decision support models. The models must capture changing behaviors and conditions and adaptively – usually, by employing Bayesian networks – be responsive within the changing environment. Second, most adaptive models are closely aligned with evolutionary models, also known as genetic algorithms; thus, they function in a manner similar to biological evolution or natural selection. Today, computationally-intensive evolutionary algorithms have been employed to develop sophisticated, real-time pricing schemes to minimize traffic congestion [17], to enhance autonomous operations in unmanned aircrafts, and to determine sniper locations in modern day warfare (e.g., in Iraq). Third, computational improvisation is another operational modeling approach that can be employed when one cannot predict and plan for every possible contingency. (Indeed, much of what happened on 9/11 was improvised, based on the ingenuity of the responders.) Improvisation involves learning by re-examining and re-organizing past knowledge in time to meet the requirements of an unexpected situation; it may be conceptualized as a search and assembly problem, influenced by such factors as time available for planning, prevailing risk, and constraints imposed by prior decisions [9]. The rise of cloud computing – whereby the vast array of machines (including laptops and smartphones) can be connected to data and algorithms almost anytime and anywhere – is becoming an essential tool to computational decision making, including improvisation.

Exhibit 8. Complex service systems: Healthcare system considerations

System stages	Healthcare system considerations	Critical methods	
		Integrative	Adaptive
1. Purpose	Stakeholders; Triaging; Business Model	√	√
2. Boundary	Spatial; Temporal; Interdependent	√	√
3. Design	Robust; Efficient; Effective	√	√
4. Development	Models; Scalability; Sustainability	√	√
5. Deployment	Risk; Uncertainty; Unintended Consequences	√	√
6. Operation	Flexible; Safe; Secure	√	√
7. Life Cycle	Predictable; Controllable; Evolutionary	√	√

Again, healthcare – as a service system – must be adaptive in regard to decision making, decision informatics, and human interface, as well as over the monitoring, feedback, cybernetic and learning dimensions. At all levels of healthcare decision making, there are a spectrum of possible methods that can be utilized, ranging from adopting adaptive – instead of randomized – medical trials, to autonomous control, to virtual-touch tools, to genetic algorithms, to improvisation, all able to cope with imprecision, uncertainties and partial truth [31]. As an example, shared or informed decision making is becoming more popular and, as a result, patients are electing to have fewer surgeries for clogged arteries (when they are informed that, except for reducing chest pains, drugs are just as effective as angioplasty surgeries – with balloons and stents – in preventing heart attacks and death), prostate cancer (when they are informed that 97 percent of men with prostate cancer die of some other cause), and herniated discs (when they are informed that the outcomes are the same when they have surgery or not). Moreover, the methods can be used to process information, take into account changing conditions, and learn from the environment; thus, they are adaptive and, to a large extent, responsive to a data stream of real-time input. In a fully integrated and adaptive system of systems (SoS), each system must be able to communicate and interact with the entire SoS, without any compatibility issues. On a less global scale, personalized medicine development [1] and delivery [11] reflect healthcare adaptation at its finest.

5. Healthcare as a complex system

Service systems can indeed be complex, requiring both integrative and adaptive approaches to deal with their complexity. There are a number of ways of identifying the complexity of a system [15], especially a service system. Exhibit 8 lists seven system stages that underpin the complexity of a healthcare service system and that require integrative and adaptive methods to mitigate, if not to handle, the complexity.

First, the system's purpose is hard to define, given the many stakeholders (i.e., patients, clinicians, insurers, etc.) involved, the multiple objectives (i.e., wellness care, emergency care, acute care, etc.) of each stakeholder, and the overarching business models (i.e., revenues, expenditures, endowments, etc.). How one combines all these divergent viewpoints into a consistent and viable purpose is an almost impossible task. Second, the system's boundary is, at best, ill-defined and shifting; the spatial (i.e., offices, clinics, homes, hospitals, etc.), temporal (i.e., schedules, activities, resources, etc.), and interdependent (i.e., infrastructures, supply chains, demand chains, etc.) relationships are difficult to ascertain. Third, the system's design must be robust (i.e., to insure reliability, quality, integrity, etc.), efficient (i.e., to minimize cost, inventory, waste, etc.), and effective (i.e., to maximize usefulness, satisfaction, pervasiveness, etc.). Fourth, the system's development must be based on models (i.e., gedanken experiments, simulations, networks, etc.), scalability (i.e., multi-scale, multi-level, multi-temporal, etc.), and sustainability (i.e., over time, space, culture, etc.). Fifth, the system's deployment must be with minimal risk (i.e., morbidity,

Exhibit 9. Complex service systems: Supply integration and demand adaptation research

Supply integration	Demand adaptation: Fixed	Demand adaptation: Flexible
Fixed	Unable To Manage Price Established (At Point Where Fixed Demand Matches Fixed Supply)	Demand Chain Management (DCM) Product Revenue Management Dynamic Pricing Target Marketing Expectation Management Auctions
Flexible	Supply Chain Management (SCM) Inventory Control Production Scheduling Distribution Planning Capacity Revenue Management Reverse Auctions	Real-Time Customized Management (RTCM) Customized Bundling Customized Revenue Management Customized Pricing Customized Modularization Customized Co-Production Systems

co-morbidity, mortality, etc.), uncertainty (i.e., unexpected attitude, behavior, performance, etc.), and unintended consequences (i.e., delays, bad side effects, deteriorating vital signs, etc.). Sixth, the system's operation must be flexible (i.e., agile, transparent, redundant, etc.), safe (i.e., with minimal natural accidents, human failures, unforeseen disruptions, etc.), and secure (i.e., with minimal system viruses, system crashes, privacy intrusions, etc.). Seventh, the system's life cycle must be predictable (i.e., in regard to inputs, processes, outcomes, etc.), controllable (i.e., with appropriate sensors, feedback, cybernetics, etc.), and evolutionary (i.e., with learning capabilities, timely recoveries, intelligent growth, etc.).

System complexity can also be characterized by a simple two-by-two, supply versus demand, matrix [27]; Exhibit 9 provides an insightful understanding of supply chain management (SCM, which can occur when demand is fixed and supply is flexible and therefore manageable), demand chain management (DCM, which can occur when supply is fixed and demand is flexible and therefore manageable), and real-time customized management (RTCM, which can occur when both demand and supply are flexible and therefore manageable or allowing for real-time mass customization). Exhibit 9 identifies several example SCM, DCM and RTCM methods. The literature is overwhelmed with SCM findings (especially in regard to manufacturing), is only recently focusing on DCM methods (especially in regard to revenue management), and is devoid of RTCM considerations, except for a recent contribution by Yasar [30].

Exhibit 10 contains an RTCM application: two SCM methods – capacity rationing (CR) and capacity extending (CE) – and two DCM methods – demand bumping (DB) and demand recapturing (DR) – are combined to deal with the customized management of, as illustrations, either a goods problem concerned with the rationing of equipment to produce classes of goods or a services problem concerned with the rationing of nursing staff to co-deliver classes of services. More importantly, in a 2-class customized management of the {CR, CE, DB, DR} problem and employing an incremental analysis or greedy algorithm solution approach, Yasar [2005] has shown that:

- the profit from simultaneously applying {CR, DB} $\geqslant$ the profit from sequentially applying {CR, DB};
- the more customized management methods employed, the more robust or stable the profit;
- the smaller the initial capacity, the more profit is impacted by the customized management methods;
- the profit from applying {CR, CE, DB, DR} $\geqslant$ the profit from applying {CR, CE, DB} $\geqslant$ the profit from applying {CR, CE} or the profit from applying {CR, DB} $\geqslant$ the profit from applying {CR} $\geqslant$ the profit from applying {first come, first served}; and
- the {CR} application is equivalent to a single period {newsvendor} problem.

Exhibit 10. Examples of real-time customized management of supply and demand chains

Real-time customized management methods	Goods example Rationing of equipment to produce classes of products	Services example Rationing of nursing staff to co-deliver classes of services
Supply Chain Management		
– Capacity Rationing (CR) – Capacity Extending (CE)	– CR of equipment – CE of equipment (e.g., outsourcing, overtime)	– CR of nurses – CE of nurses (e.g., outsourcing, overtime)
Demand Chain Management		
– Demand Bumping (DB) – Demand Recapturing (DR)	– DB of customer orders – DR of customer orders	– DB of nursing services – DR of nursing services

Extending the 2-class to an n-class customized management of the {CR, CE, DB, DR} problem and employing a greedy algorithm and simulated approximation solution approach, it can be shown that:

– the same findings and insights can be obtained as in the case of the 2-class problem;
– the profit from an n-class problem $\geqslant$ the profit from an $(n-1)$-class problem; and
– the greater the n value, the more robust or stable the profit.

Additionally, extending the n-class customized to a real-time customized management of the {CR, CE, DB, DR} problem and employing an adaptive, non-parametric regression of successive differences (in incoming data) solution approach, it can be shown that:

– the same findings and insights can be obtained as in the case of the n-class customized management problem;
– the profit from real-time customized management $\geqslant$ the profit from just customized management; and
– the fewer the number of customized management methods employed, the greater is the sensitivity of profit to real-time solutions.

In sum, it has been shown that the real-time, simultaneous application of customized management methods to both the supply and demand chains yields significant system efficiency, if not effectiveness. However, solving these real-time problems requires solution approaches – namely, greedy, incremental or simulated algorithms – that transcend the steady-state approaches that are currently available. Greedy algorithms are relatively straightforward: they are shortsighted in their approach in that they make decisions on the basis of information at hand without worrying about the effect that these decisions may have in the future; they are computationally-oriented; and they are usually quite time efficient. Obviously, they do not guarantee optimality in the classical or mathematical programming sense, but then optimality is a difficult, if not meaningless, concept to ascertain in a constantly changing, real-time environment.

Returning to Exhibit 9, it should be emphasized that it is in the RTCM or fourth quadrant of the exhibit that both system integration (as reflected in the SCM methods) and system adaptation (as reflected in the DCM methods) are combined and dealt with simultaneously. Thus, a combined integration and adaptation research effort is synonymous to a real-time customized management (RTCM) activity, which can only occur when both demand and supply are flexible and thereby allowing for real-time mass customization. This fourth quadrant also highlights the complexity involved in designing a service system that is at once both integrated and adaptive. Clearly, healthcare is an example of such a complex system. Finally, it should be noted that electronic data processing underpins nearly all aspects of integration and adaptation, especially in regard to healthcare [10].

6. Concluding insights

The previous sections have demonstrated the importance of considering healthcare from a systems engineering perspective. In essence, healthcare is in general a people-intensive service system. Moreover, in order to be an efficient and effective system, it must be, respectively, an integrated and adaptive system, all of which adds to the complexity of the service system. As indicated throughout the paper, there are many areas where new and additional methods are required to define, model and solve an aspect of the healthcare system. Much research remains to be undertaken.

A number of other insights can be ascertained from an integrated and adaptive view of healthcare services. First, as noted earlier, electronic-based medical records constitute the glue that should keep the healthcare system integrated and adaptive. Unfortunately, most medical records – including patient data, drug prescriptions, laboratory diagnostics, clinician reports, and body scans – are still in manual folders and, as a consequence, difficult to access, fuse and analyze. More recently, Microsoft and Google, respectively, launched HealthVault and Health for consumers to store and manage their personal medical data online, and Wal-Mart is allowing its intranet to serve as a repository for the health histories of its more than one million staff members. While patients have a legal right to obtain their medical records from doctors, hospitals, and testing laboratories, it is indeed a tedious and overwhelming process due to the fact that the records are not in electronic form. Nevertheless, sharing such electronic records with new medical providers and third-party services should make it easier to cut waste, eliminate red tape, coordinate care, spot adverse drug interactions, reduce repeat or ineffective tests, allow for medication reminders, and track vital signs. Indeed, as part of the 2009 economic stimulus package, the U. S. is mounting a massive effort to modernize healthcare by making all health records standardized and electronic within five years, a monumental task given that only about 17% of the 800,000 clinicians employ computerized records. Moreover, personal data residing on Microsoft, Google or Wal-Mart server grids or clouds do raise significant privacy concerns. At present, the Health Insurance Portability and Accountability Act (HIPAA) only requires doctors, hospitals and third-party payers to not release information without a patient's consent. Of course, HIPAA's requirements could be broadened and new rules could be enacted that give consumers stronger protection and legal recourse if their records are leaked or improperly shared for other than its intended purpose.

Second, as real-time healthcare decisions must be made in an accelerated and co-produced manner, the human service provider (e.g., clinician) will increasingly become a bottleneck; he/she must be supported by a smart robot or software agent. For example, the clinician could use a smart alter ego or agent – sometimes called a virtual personal assistant – which could analyze, and perhaps fuse, all the existing and incoming e-mails, phone calls, Web pages, x-rays, drug prescriptions, and medical examinations, and assigns every item a priority based on the clinician's preferences and observed behaviors. It should be able to perform an analysis of a message text, judge the sender-recipient relationships by examining an organizational chart and recall the urgency of the recipient's responses to previous messages from the same sender. To this, it might add information gathered by watching the clinician via a video camera or by scrutinizing his/her calendar. Most probably, such a smart agent would be based on a Bayesian statistical model – capable of evaluating hundreds of user-related factors linked by probabilities, causes and effects in a vast web of contingent outcomes – which can infer the likelihood that a given decision on the software's part would lead to the clinician's desired outcome. The ultimate goal is to judge when the clinician can safely be interrupted, with what kind of message, and via which device. In time, smart agents representing both providers and consumers will become the service co-producers; they will employ decision informatics techniques and cloud computing to accomplish their tasks. It should be noted that smart agents may never be appropriate for certain situations, especially, as examples, where a nuanced patient behavior is critical or when a catastrophic surgical consequence is on the balance. Obviously, these situations require direct patient-clinician interaction or co-production, perhaps assisted by smart agents – with access to databases and algorithms that are a part of cloud computing – which can help in the identification of alternative diagnoses and treatments.

Third, perhaps the best example of an integrated and adaptive service system is the evolving Web 2.0. It is user-built, user-centered and user-run. In other words, it is a social network for integration – including collaboration and communication – of activities (e.g., eBay, Amazon.com, Wikipedia, Twitter, MySpace, Friendster, LinkedIn, Plaxo, etc.), entertainment (e.g., Facebook, Ning, Bebo, Second Life, World of Warcraft, etc.), searches (e.g., Google, Yahoo, MSN.com, Bing, etc.), and knowledge computation (e.g., Wolfram Alpha). Unfortunately, the integrated web, while being a somewhat successful e-commerce platform, is unable to interpret, manipulate or make sense of its content. On the other hand and with the encoding of web pages in a semantic web format, the evolving web will be able to allow for the above mentioned smart or decision informatics supported agents to undertake semantic analysis of user intent and web content, to understand and filter their meaning, and to adaptively respond in light of user needs. The Semantic Web, then, could be an ideal complex service system where integration and adaptation will constitute the basis for its functionality. However, several obstacles must be overcome before reaching full functionality. For example, semantic standards or ontologies – such as the Web Ontology Language (OWL) – must be established so as to maintain compatible and interoperable formats; at present, health care and financial services companies are each developing their own ontology. Indeed, a healthcare system of systems (SoS) also needs a common ontology to allow for new system components to be appropriately integrated into the SoS without a major effort, so as to achieve higher capabilities and performance than would be possible with the component systems as stand-alone systems. Of course, the healthcare ontology must be transdisciplinary – beyond a single disciplinary – in scope; with such an ontology, healthcare may indeed exist as a social network of patients, clinicians, insurers and other related providers.

Fourth, as a critical aspect of complexity, modern systems of systems are also becoming increasingly more human-centered, if not human-focused; thus, products and services are becoming more personalized or customized. Certainly, services co-production implies the existence of a human customer, if not a human service provider. The implication is profound: a multidisciplinary approach must be employed for, say, healthcare – it must also include techniques from the social sciences (i.e., sociology, psychology, and philosophy) and management (i.e., organization, economics and finance). As a consequence, researchers must expand their systems (i.e., holistic-oriented), man (i.e., decision-oriented) and cybernetic (i.e., adaptive-oriented) methods to include and be integrated with those techniques that are beyond science and engineering. For example, higher patient satisfaction can be achieved not only by improving service quality but also by lowering patient expectation. In essence, as stated by Hipel et al. [6], systems, man and cybernetics is an integrative, adaptive and multidisciplinary approach to creative problem solving; it takes into account stakeholders' value systems and satisfies important societal, environmental, economic and other requirements in order to enhance the decision making process when designing, implementing, operating and maintaining a system or system of systems to meet societal needs in a fair, ethical and sustainable manner throughout the system's life cycle. Interestingly, an adaptive, human-centered (i.e., human-to-human) system that functions in real-time is the Twitter social network, based on easy-to-use, 140-character bursts of constant chatter which can inform and engage a participant with an intensity that cannot be replicated offline.

Fifth, perhaps the most critical US healthcare issue is, as alluded to earlier, the universal access of patients to healthcare. Payers – particularly private insurances – have nearly eliminated access of at-risk individuals to healthcare providers, by not allowing them to enroll in their insurance programs. (At the extreme, only the very healthy and relatively young individuals are able to purchase a private insurance plan.) Thus, a huge access problem is created for the uninsured, which solution is to go to the emergency room, at a time where severity of illness is already advanced and costly and where treatment must be provided at no cost. A vicious subsidization cycle ensues whereby individual insurance premiums sky-rocket, mainly to pay for the care of individuals who are at-risk and unable to get insurance or who cannot afford the insurance premium. Indeed, by employing the technobiology approach of systems engineering to remedy the US healthcare is what is required in order to equilibrate the insurance imbalance and to make it an efficient and effective system. In this regard, payment for care should be more weighted to output or value provided than to input or activity undertaken [13]. Additionally, such manufacturing techniques as cross-training and multi-use of facilities can enhance both efficiency and effectiveness. Furthermore, contrary to a widely-held belief, waste is not a necessary by-product of excellence. All of these issues must be taken into consideration as the US Congress seeks to reform healthcare; it must integrate public plans (e.g., Medicare and Medicaid) with a plethora of private plans (that are neither affordable nor portable) in order to achieve healthcare coverage for all its residents.

Sixth, a final insight concerns the customization or personalization of medical treatments through advances in genetics, proteomics and metabolomics. Most common illnesses will eventually be preventable; the challenge is to know which prevention effort will be most effective for a given individual. Employing markers of risk (e.g., gene variants, blood levels of a protein moiety, etc.) may allow for the targeting or personalization of preventive measures in a highly cost-effective way. In this manner, humans can be sheltered from chronic illnesses and pandemics, and remain fully functional until an advanced age (say, 100), beyond which survival is genetically limited. Thus, healthcare is indeed a service, one that can be personalized and that can enhance the quality – and length – of an individual's life.

References

[1] M.G. Aspinall and R.G. Hamermesh, "Realizing The Promise of Personalized Medicine", *Harvard Business Review* **85**(10) (2007), 108–117.

[2] N. Donofrio, Editor, *Global Innovation Outlook: Security and Society*, Armonk, NY: IBM Corporation, 2008.

[3] T.L. Friedman, *The World Is Flat: A Brief History of the Twenty-First Century*, New York, NY: Farrar, Strauss & Giroux, 2005.

[4] P.J. Goldschmidt-Clermont, C. Dong, N.M. Rhodes, D.B. McNeill, M.B. Adams, C.L. Gilliss, M.S. Cuffe, R.M. Califf, E.D. Peterson and D.A. Lubarsky, Undated, "Autonomic Care Systems for Hospitalized Patients", Submitted for publication in *Academic Medicine.*

[5] J.H. Grossman, Disruptive Innovation in Health Care: Challenges for Engineering, *National Academy of Engineering: The Bridge* **38**(1) (2008), 10–16.

[6] K.W. Hipel, M.M. Jamshidi, J.M. Tien and C.C. White, The Future of Systems, Man and Cybernetics: Application Domains and Research Methods, *IEEE Transactions on Systems, Man, and Cybernetics Part C* **30**(2) (2007), 213–218.

[7] E.H. Kaplan, D.L. Craft and L.M. Wein, Emergency Response to A Smallpox Attack: The Case for Mass Vaccination, *Proceedings of the National Academy of Sciences* **99**(16) (2002), 10935–10940.

[8] P. Maglio, S. Srinivasan, J. Kreulen and J. Spohrer, Service Systems, Service Scientists, SSME, and Innovation, *Communications of the ACM* **49**(7) (2006), 81–85.

[9] D. Mendonca and W.A. Wallace, Studying Organizationally-Situated Improvisation in Response to Extreme Events, *International Journal of Mass Emergencies and Disasters* **22**(2) (2004), 5–29.

[10] C. Meyer, The Convergence of Information, Biology, and Business: Creating an Adaptive Health Care System, *National Academy of Engineering: The Bridge* **38**(1) (2008), 26–32.

[11] S. Mitragotri, Recent Developments in Needle-Free Drug Delivery, *National Academy of Engineering: The Bridge* **38**(2) (2008), 5–12.

[12] National Academies, 2006, *Engineering the Health Care System*, Washington, DC: National Academies Press.

[13] M.E. Porter and E.O. Teisberg, *Redefining Health Care: Creating Value-Based Competition on Results*, Boston, MA: Harvard Business School Press, 2006.
[14] J.B. Quinn, J.J. Baruch and P.C. Paquette, Technology in Services, *Scientific American* **257**(6) (1987), 50–58.
[15] W.B. Rouse, Complex Engineered, Organizational and Natural Systems, *Wiley InterScience Online: Systems Engineering* **10**(3) (2007), 260–271.
[16] W.B. Rouse, Health Care As A Complex Adaptive System: Implications for Design and Management, *National Academy of Engineering: The Bridge* **38**(1) (2008), 17–25.
[17] J.M. Sussman, Intelligent Transportation Systems in a Real-Time, Customer-Oriented Society, *National Academy of Engineering: The Bridge* **38**(2) (2008), 13–19.
[18] J.M. Tien, Individual-Centered Education: An Any One, Any Time, Any Where Approach to Engineering Education, *IEEE Transactions on Systems, Man, and Cybernetics Part C: Special Issue on Systems Engineering Education* **30**(2) (2000), 213–218.
[19] J.M. Tien, Towards A Decision Informatics Paradigm: A Real-Time, Information-Based Approach to Decision Making, *IEEE Transactions on Systems, Man, and Cybernetics, Special Issue, Part C* **33**(1) (2003), 102–113.
[20] J.M. Tien, On Integration and Adaptation in Complex Service Systems, *Journal of Systems Science and Systems Engineering* **17**(4) (2008), 385–415.
[21] J.M. Tien and D. Berg, Systems Engineering in the Growing Service Economy, *IEEE Transactions on Systems, Man, and Cybernetics* **25**(5) (1995), 321–326.
[22] J.M. Tien and D. Berg, A Case for Service Systems Engineering, *Journal of Systems Science and Systems Engineering* **12**(1) (2003), 13–38.
[23] J.M. Tien and D. Berg, On Services Research and Education, *Journal of Systems Science and Systems Engineering* **15**(3) (2006), 257–283.
[24] J.M. Tien and D. Berg, A Calculus for Services Innovation, *Journal of Systems Science and Systems Engineering* **16**(2) (2007), 129–165.
[25] J.M. Tien and M.F. Cahn, *An Evaluation of the Wilmington Management of Demand Program*, Washington, DC: National Institute of Justice, 1981.
[26] J.M. Tien and P.J. Goldschmidt-Clermont, On Designing An Integrated and Adaptive Healthcare System, *Engineering A Learning Healthcare System: A Look to the Future*, Washington, DC: Institute of Medicine, 2009.
[27] J.M. Tien, A. Krishnamurthy and A. Yasar, Towards Real-Time Customized Management of Supply and Demand Chains, *Journal of Systems Science and Systems Engineering* **13**(3) (2004), 257–278.
[28] US President, *Executive Order on Critical Infrastructure Protection*, Washington, DC: The White House, 16 October 2001.
[29] World Health Organization Report (WHO), *Why Do Health Systems Matter,* Geneva, Switzerland: World Health Organization, 2000.
[30] A. Yasar, *Real-Time and Simultaneous Management of Supply and Demand Chains*, Ph.D. Thesis, Troy, NY: Rensselaer Polytechnic Institute, 2005.
[31] L.A. Zadeh, The Evolution of Systems Analysis and Control: A Personal Perspective, *IEEE Control Systems Magazine* **16**(3) (1996).

Dr. James M. Tien received the BEE from Rensselaer Polytechnic Institute (RPI) and the SM, EE and PhD from the Massachusetts Institute of Technology (MIT). He has held leadership positions at Bell Telephone Laboratories, at the Rand Corporation, and at Structured Decisions Corporation (which he co-founded in 1974). He joined the Department of Electrical, Computer and Systems Engineering at RPI in 1977, became Acting Chair of the department, joined a unique interdisciplinary Department of Decision Sciences and Engineering Systems as its founding Chair, and twice served as the Acting Dean of Engineering. In 2007, he joined the University of Miami as a Distinguished Professor and Dean of its College of Engineering. Dr. Tien's areas of research interest include the development and application of computer and systems analysis techniques to information and decision systems. He has published extensively, been invited to present numerous plenary lectures, and been honored with both teaching and research awards, including being elected a Fellow in IEEE, INFORMS and AAAS and being a recipient of the IEEE Joseph G. Wohl Outstanding Career Award, the IEEE Major Educational Innovation Award, the IEEE Norbert Wiener Award, and the IBM Faculty Award. He is an Honorary Professor at a number of non-U.S. universities. Dr. Tien is also an elected member of the US National Academy of Engineering.

Dr. Pascal J. Goldschmidt-Clermont received his medical degree from the Universite Libre de Bruxelles and completed residency and fellowship training in Brussels at Erasme Academic Hospital and in the United States at The Johns Hopkins University. Following his training at Hopkins, he served as an associate professor in the university's Department of Cell Biology and Anatomy, Department of Pathology, until 1997. He became director of cardiology at The Ohio State University College of Medicine and Public Health, where he established the Heart and Lung Research Institute and a heart hospital. He joined the Duke University Medical Center faculty in 2000 and served as chief of Duke's Division of Cardiology before becoming chairman of the Department of Medicine. Dr. Goldschmidt-Clermont's research interests concern the application of genomics and cell therapy to the prevention, diagnosis and treatment of coronary artery disease. He became senior vice president for medical affairs and dean of the University of Miami Leonard M. Miller School of Medicine in 2006, where he has established the International Medicine Institute, The Miami Institute for Human Genomics, and the Interdisciplinary Stem Cell Institute. He also serves as CEO of the University of Miami Health System (UHealth). In 2008, Dr. Goldschmidt received the inaugural Jay and Jeanie Schottenstein Prize in Cardiovascular Sciences from the Ohio State University Heart and Vascular Center.

Information Knowledge Systems Management 8 (2009) 299–309
DOI 10.3233/IKS-2009-0144
IOS Press

Chapter 17

Process engineering: A necessary step to a better public health system

David A. Ross
E-mail: dross@phii.org

Abstract: With its primary focus on community health, the public health system focuses on intervention and prevention of disease and injury to protect entire populations. As a federation of city, county and state entities operating independently under a complicated array of local, state and federal laws, public health can best be understood as a complex adaptive system. The dynamic nature of this system and the need for public health agencies to relate and respond to numerous stimuli in terms of new regulations, changing health status, emerging threats and shifting policy, can mask the commonality of underlying business processes performed within the public health sector. Heightened demand for interoperable, adaptive information systems across the broader US health system necessitates the recognition of this commonality and highlights the need for comprehensive analysis and understanding of these core business processes. In turn, this analysis paves the way for public health to apply proven systems engineering techniques to streamline, automate and facilitate those processes. Here, we look at the nature of the public health system and the evolution of a purpose-built methodology for process engineering within public health. We also present a case study based on the application of the methodology to develop requirements for public health laboratory information management systems.

1. Overview

In the US the entities referred to as the "health system" are actually a combination of personal care services and population (public) health services acting independently, and at times in unison, in pursuit of health goals established at all levels of government and private industry. Reforming the nation's health system requires a more systems-oriented view of all components of the health system, including those of public health. Although public health shares many challenges with health care, it is a poorly understood component of the US health system. At its core, the role of public health has a primary focus on the health of population and the community. This involves interventions that protect an entire population, rather than individuals. Additionally public health focuses on the prevention of disease and injury prior to problems occurring, rather than to the treatment of existing problems [10]. Analysis of the business processes that make up public health will be needed to rationalize where and how the population-focused public health authority interacts with the health care delivery sector. This requires a good understanding of the nature of public health as it is practiced in this country.

Our nation's public health system is actually a federation of city, county and state public health entities acting under local law carrying out similar services under a web of formal and informal collaborative agreements to act as a system of services. Because of its federated nature, it is not a command and control system. Rather, public health agencies relate and respond to numerous stimuli (e.g., laws, outbreaks, political mandates, etc.), and apply a range of knowledge, skills and abilities to a constantly changing environment. Thus, the public health system is best understood as a complex adaptive system.

1389-1995/09/$17.00

1.1. *Public health as a complex adaptive system*

Public health, and the health system at large, behave like complex adaptive systems because they are non-linear and dynamic in nature; are composed of independent agents; the rules of the various agents are not uniform and therefore likely to conflict; the agents of the system learn and adapt; learning leads to self organizing behavior; and there is no single point of control [7]. Public health agencies function within a dynamic community environment, often acting through the professional judgment of staff in reaction to local events. In doing so, they learn as individuals and as organizations. Public health is not hierarchically organized beyond the state level, and in many locales not beyond the city or county level of government. The state and local legal basis of public health means that the particular business rules governing actions may change from locale to locale. By these measures, public health is itself a complex adaptive system operating within the larger health system.

1.2. *A program-centered view*

Public health programs cover a broad range of activities. Most often, public health responsibilities are expressed in terms of health goals, such as assuring all children are appropriately immunized, preventing HIV infection, assuring that TB patients are treated appropriately, or in terms of broad purpose, such as conducting infectious disease surveillance. As a result, public health practitioners tend to work in function- or program-specific silos of information and activity. Unfortunately, this functional or goal-based view of public health does little to explain *how* the work of public health is accomplished, should be accomplished, or could be accomplished, in order to achieve greatest effectiveness or efficiency.

This blinkered view, along with the continuous learning and adaptation of public health agencies to changing health status and the emergence of new health threats (i.e., emerging infectious diseases, such as novel H1N1; and bioterrorism threats, including biological, chemical and radioactive agents) disguises the underlying pattern of activities common to all public health agencies. Yet key findings from the CDC's Public Health Emergency Preparedness Cooperative Agreement show a promising trend toward a more common set of capabilities among disparate public health agencies. These capabilities include systems that enable the agencies to receive and evaluate reports of urgent health threats 24/7/365 (all state health departments now have this capability, up from only 12 in 1999); a 33 percent increase in the number of public health laboratories able to detect biological and chemical agents; public health laboratories in all states that can quickly communicate with clinical laboratories; response plans, documentation and training in key preparedness areas; and participation of all states in the Health Alert Network, which enables critical public health information to be rapidly disseminated and exchanged.

Even with the recognition that public health is grappling with the same issues across the nation – and trending in the same direction, in terms of emerging capabilities and requirements – the underlying activities that address these issues are *only now beginning to be recognized as coherent business processes able to be found in any public health agency*. And it should be noted that, despite our dynamic society and the evolving nature of health threats, many of the business processes of public health remain relatively stable. This makes them ideally suited to the application of systems engineering concepts, which offer a logical pathway to defining a system of activities that can be more readily monitored and measured to produce reliable outputs – in this case, better public health.

2. Organization and evolution of public health services

Today's public health system aspires to delivering essential services but must do so through a maze of local, state and federal funding and through a rather complex array of local, state and federal laws [1].

At the federal level, the Food and Drug Administration (FDA) regulates drugs, medical devices, food and drugs, and the Centers for Disease Control and Prevention (CDC) acts with the State Department to maintain quarantine at the borders. With those exceptions, most public health law is local, with legal authority resting with state and county governments. In some states, the state public health agency has authority over all local health departments and public health services. In other states, the authority for public health intervention rests completely with the county government. And, in a few states there is a hybrid of state and local authority.

Public health agencies also vary from locale to locale in the breadth of services offered at the local level. For example, in some states it is common to find public health agencies that deliver personal primary health care services in addition to population-based services, while in other states personal care services are handled by the private medical community and through networks of health care centers and safety net clinics.

Historically, public health services have evolved when new technologies, such as a vaccine, offer the opportunity to create greater population health protection. With each new technical advance has come a new program to promote it. Consequently, public health agencies are often explained in terms of their categories, that is, in terms of having an immunization program or an HIV prevention program or a restaurant inspection program. The industry known as public health more closely resembles a collection of subsidiary companies or standalone divisions – so-called "stove pipes" – than a system of interrelated parts. Rarely is public health described as a system of services organized to optimize community health status – even though that is the stated goal of public health.

3. Understanding the public health system

In 1988, the Institute of Medicine framed public health as having three essential or core functions: population health assessment, assurance that legally mandated services are delivered, and health policy development [1]. In response to this, the public health community developed a more specific view of its work through a listing of ten essential services: monitor health status, diagnose and investigate health problems and hazards, inform and educate about health threats, mobilize community partnerships, develop policies and plans, enforce laws and regulations, link people to needed personal health services, assure competent public and personal health care workforce, evaluate effectiveness, accessibility and quality, and research for new solutions to health problems [3]. All of these services are focused on population health.

3.1. Population health

Kindig and Stoddart [2] define population health as "the health outcomes of a group of individuals, including the distribution of such outcomes within the group." It is the population focus that distinguishes many public health activities from those found in the personal health care delivery system. Population health looks beyond the individual, the focus of the medical care delivery system, by measuring and assessing the many factors that affect health on a population-level, such as disease vectors, environment, social structure, resource distribution, food supplies and, of course, infectious agents. Population health emphasizes the importance of social determinants of health, the interaction of people and their environment and broad economic factors that ultimately play a large role in health status [9]; public health programs, therefore, seek to improve the health of an entire population.

As we have discussed, understanding population focus is key to understanding the public health component of the health system. Each programmatic area within this population focus, as outlined in the essential public health services listed above, represents a complex interaction of individuals with their physical and social environments; for example, environmental protection, food safety, infectious disease prevention and outbreak intervention, and even chronic disease prevention and health promotion.

Attaining population health improvement goals requires an understanding of the dynamic nature of this interaction among individuals, their environments, and the providers of health services. As mentioned above, the health system overall (and the public health component within this complex system) can be viewed as an array of actors relating to an array of stimuli best understood as a complex adaptive system [7]. Driven by its population health focus, public health stimulates change in the larger health system in many ways; for example, through community health assessment activities such as Mobilizing for Action through Planning and Partnerships (MAPP), developed by the National Association of County and City Health Officials (NACCHO).

Through this program, public health agencies work in strategic partnership with their communities to assess community health in four areas: Community Themes and Strengths (where are we now, and what are our health assets); Local Public Health System (a "report card" on the delivery of essential public health services); Community Health Status (measures and prioritizes community health and quality of life issues); and Forces of Change (threats and opportunities represented by upcoming legislation, technology changes, etc.). Through this and similar population health-focused activities, public health agencies inform the overall health system with a well-developed picture or snapshot of the risk factors most responsible for adverse health effects.

On the national health policy front, data used to monitor health status stimulates national health policy analysis. For example, the National Health and Nutrition Examination Survey (NHANES), a program of the CDC's National Center for Health Statistics (NCHS), conducts studies that combine interviews and physical examinations to assess the health and nutritional status of adults and children in the United States.

Thus public health provides community, state and national information sets – population health data – that become the basis for legislative or community action, which in turn may impact personal health care delivery services. By the same token, public health also reacts to changes brought on by the health care system. For example, when evidence from clinical research indicated that screening for cervical cancer would reduce cancer mortality, public health agencies were prompted to develop screening awareness campaigns.

4. Need for process description

As we have seen, public health agencies at all levels of government address their population focus largely through a disease or problem orientation. Services are also frequently funded on a disease or categorical basis, which leads to isolated programs of activity. These isolated programs often replicate a set of activities that could, in fact, be shared services, if public health agencies chose to view their work as a comprehensive system of services.

Unfortunately, there has been within the public health sector a bias against seeing their work in terms of a 'business'. This bias, although it arises from an altruistic instinct to serve the broader good of the community, has tended to prevent public health agencies from adopting and benefiting from the organizational, technological and process-improvement advantages that have developed in the competitive crucible of the for-profit sector.

Until recently, public health has not recognized the importance of understanding and documenting its business processes. For example, prior to CDC's National Electronic Disease Surveillance System (NEDSS) initiative, infectious disease data were reported case by case to disease-specific program registries and slowly compiled to produce state and national estimates of disease prevalence and incidence. The disease-specific approach to this surveillance required duplicative reporting processes and programs and failed to acknowledge the underlying commonality of the surveillance business process.

In the face of threats of bioterrorism, emerging infectious diseases, and a growing awareness that health status is influenced by factors beyond the control of health care providers, the public health industry is now charged with seamlessly supporting and integrating a full range of functional islands. Numerous national organizations and initiatives have arisen in support of this effort. For example, the CDC's Public Health Information Network (PHIN) works nationally to improve the electronic information exchange capacity of public health by establishing standards, and defining functional and technical requirements for interoperable public health information systems. PHIN activities support public health integration into the Nationwide Health Information Network (NHIN). Established in 2004 by the Office of the National Coordinator for Health Information Technology (ONC), NHIN provides a set of conventions for nationwide health information exchange. These standards include technical, policy, data use and service level agreements, and other requirements for secure data exchange and interoperable communication of health information among those involved in supporting health and healthcare.

In this era of heightened demand for interoperability, public health must build information systems capabilities that link across public health programs as well as extending to external health system partners – essentially *enterprise information systems* [8] that capture, integrate and analyze data from multiple sources. The requirement for such large-scale integration of information makes it critical for public health agencies to understand their core business processes, and to embrace methodologies for streamlining and improving these processes. This is possible only if the business processes of public health are thoroughly described and understood to be common across all agencies, despite the sector's federated nature.

This evolving information mission, and the use of information systems arising from an enterprise approach to core population health surveillance, outbreak response, and event remediation, has provoked a discussion and explication of the work of public health in terms of core business processes [6]. This has led the Public Health Informatics Institute (the Institute) to define an approach to business process definition that incorporates practice-based subject matter experts, thereby bridging the public health body of experience and population health focus with the best practices of business process improvement and information systems design.

Public health information systems must be able to adapt rapidly to the evolving needs of policy makers, scientists and citizens. In order to do so, information system requirements must be based on a comprehensive understanding of the business processes they will automate and facilitate. Thus, the objectives and tasks within a process must be measurable, operators and business risks must be explicit, etc. To this end, the Institute's methodology guides representatives and stakeholders of key practice components through a managed collaborative study of activities, to produce consensus-based business process models upon which new enterprise information systems can be built [5].

5. A new approach

The Institute's collaborative approach to defining requirements for an information system necessitates an acceptance of the core principle that the business of public health is not unique to each locale. Due to differences in state law, health agencies have varying structures for how work is done. However, all public health agencies have similar problems and information needs that arise from the business processes they have in common.

Public health agencies have typically approached the development of information systems on an independent program-specific basis, without cross-functional or inter-agency planning, and without due consideration of underlying business processes. This approach results in disparate information systems with high development costs, which nonetheless fail to adequately support the work of the agency. System requirements developed collaboratively, based on a common model of business processes, lead to systems that are interoperable, provide optimal support for public health functions, and reduce development costs to individual agencies through leveraging shared resources.

A key principle of good system design, although a relatively new concept in the public health sector, is the practice of putting the logical before the physical. This is accomplished through conducting a thorough examination of agency workflow prior to, and supporting the development of, physical system requirements. Public health is no less – and possibly more – susceptible to the appeal of a new technology or sales pitch than businesses in other sectors. It is important for public health agencies to embrace technology advances, in order to meet the policy-driven timeline and obligation to become fully participating members of the emerging integrated health system. But an informed assessment of these advances requires an understanding of how they support the goals and work of agencies. This understanding, in turn, is based on a solid analysis of the underlying business processes that make up the work, in order to develop a logical model of the agency's operations.

Early engagement of stakeholders will ultimately increase user interest in and acceptance of the final product. It will also lead to a solution that better meets the needs of users, and one that reflects proven best practices. A collaborative approach to articulating the components of each business process and representing them graphically leads to a much deeper joint understanding of public health. It defines explicitly what is known about the business processes. It also enables agencies to see how others do the same processes, which leads to insights into how these processes may be improved at different sites. It is a powerful tool for describing and understanding the work of public health within the profession as well as to outside partners.

The approach used by the Institute is known as the *Collaborative Requirements Development Methodology*. It consists of three phases, familiar in the realm of commercial information system development (if not always applied in sequence), but relatively new to the public health sector.

These phases are: business process analysis, business process redesign, and system requirements definition. The first phase looks at how the organization's work is performed, and produces documentation of core business processes. Business process redesign focuses on how the work *should be* performed, and documents ways in which processes can be restructured to improve efficiency. In the final phase, requirements are developed based on the redesigned business processes, to describe how information systems should be built to support the work most effectively. In the work of the Institute, it has been determined that, while the resulting set of business processes and the attendant system requirements may be tailored to meet individual agency needs, they are fundamentally common to all public health organizations. This is a key finding in advancing acceptance of repeatable systems engineering practices within the public health sector.

5.1. Business process analysis

As practiced by the Institute, business process analysis makes use of two graphical tools to model the work, context diagrams and task flows, as well as a business process matrix, which is useful in

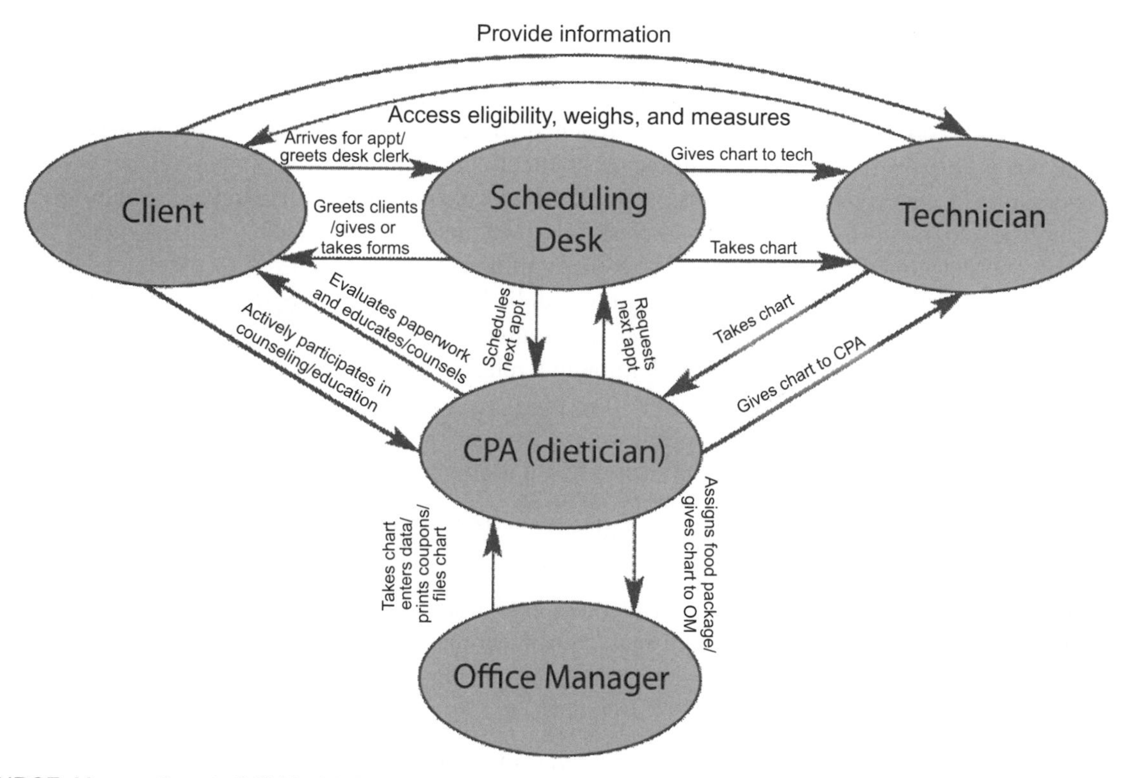

SOURCE: Monroe County (MI) Health Department (Director of Community Health Jamie Leizerman & Health Officer Dr. Rebecca Head)

Fig. 1. Context Diagram: Depicts the entities and information exchanges of a typical public health intake and enrollment process, in context of a specific program.

maintaining a consistent approach to defining business processes. These tools enable a wide variety of stakeholders, including senior management, front-line public health workers, and information technology staff, to understand and actively participate in the business process analysis.

5.2. *Context diagrams*

Reflect the relationships and boundaries that exist between the entities involved in a given process, and depict the exchanges of information among them, within the context of that process. These diagrams are key to helping public health stakeholders define their work, establishing the beginning and end of each business process, in a way that serves to facilitate analysis of their workflows. Context diagrams provide the foundation for all of the other activities of the analysis project.

5.3. *Task flow diagrams*

Like standard flowcharts, depict a single direction of information flow (beginning to end) through a process. The activities, represented as rectangles, show the tasks which must be performed, as well as identifying the resources needed. Decision points, symbolized by diamonds, indicate junctures at which the information flow may be terminated or diverted within the process, depending on different task outcomes. As the name indicates, task flow diagrams help stakeholders to visualize the flow of

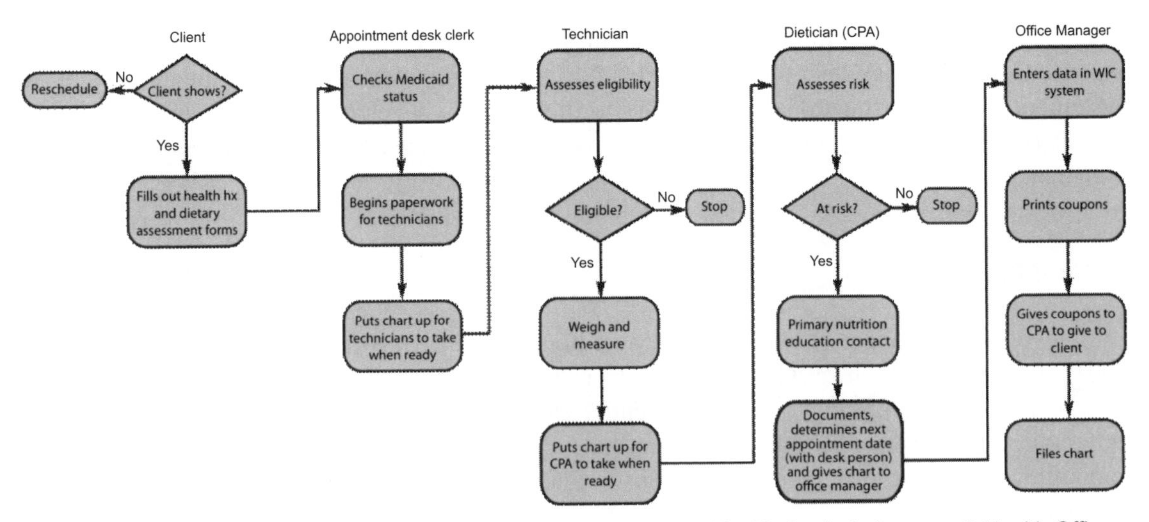

SOURCE: Monroe County (MI) Health Department (Director of Community Health Jamie Leizerman & Health Officer Dr. Rebecca Head)

Fig. 2. Task Flow Diagram: Depicts the flow of information through activities and decision points within the same process represented in the context diagram in Fig. 1.

information through the process, so that they can readily see areas where tasks may be combined, simplified or eliminated to streamline the process. They also highlight potential bottlenecks due to insufficient data or authority at decision points, and show where the process is subject to terminate in an incomplete state. Again, this visual modeling of processes has proven especially valuable in working with those public health practitioners who have the most information about the processes and their desired outcomes, but the least experience with business process improvement methodologies.

A **business process matrix** is a table that is used to show the components that characterize each business process. The matrix is used to define the goals, objectives, triggers, inputs, outputs, business rules and outcomes for all of the business processes. This is helpful in maintaining a consistent approach to process definition across an organization, and facilitates standardizing the granularity of the master list – the key to effectively using the results of business process analysis as a foundation for the redesign and requirements definition phases [5].

5.4. *Business process redesign*

Inefficiencies within a business process are revealed by identifying the *value-added* tasks – e.g., those tasks necessary for the completion of the process. A sequence of value-added tasks makes up the value chain for the process. The quality improvement goal of business process redesign is to maximize the percentage of tasks that actually comprise the value chain. Tasks that do not add value to the process are candidates for redesign or removal in order to improve efficiency. Within the process, non-value-added activities that cannot be changed are likely targets for automation during the requirements definition phase [5].

5.5. *Requirements definition*

Requirements for a public health information system describe the way in which the system supports the work of the organization. Only when the business processes have been defined (and redesigned where necessary) is it possible to *engineer* an information system that meets the functional needs of the organization. This may take the form of defining what is required to inform evaluation of an existing system, or to develop functional and design specifications for developing a system in-house; either way, it ensures that the functionality of the resulting system will be based on the actual workflow needs of the organization [5].

6. Case study

Many of the challenges of public health were highlighted during the bioterrorism events in the fall of 2001, in various public health labs. These labs provide diagnostic testing, disease surveillance, applied research, laboratory training, and other essential services. Clinicians, hospitals, emergency responders, and public health officials at local, state and federal agencies rely on the rapid, accurate, and complete communication of information from the labs to diagnose, treat, prevent, and control diseases and other public health threats.

Despite their important role in ensuring public health, prior to the end of 2001, funding for developing or updating information systems had been extremely limited. As a result, during the anthrax crisis, many of these labs struggled to meet heightened information needs armed with inadequate and outdated paper-based tracking and surveillance methods, along with obsolete computers, spreadsheet programs, and basic database software programs that were not automated or networked. This situation led to a unique collaboration, supported by the Robert Wood Johnson Foundation, for using the Collaborative Requirements Development Methodology to define requirements for a laboratory information management system that would advance the capacity of the labs to respond to bioterrorism and other public health threats [4].

6.1. Participants

In September 2002, the Institute formed a requirements definition collaboration with the Association of Public Health Laboratories (APHL) and representatives from 16 public health labs from across the country.

6.2. Products and outcomes

Although the public health laboratories had not previously collaborated on the development of information system requirements, and participants were widely dispersed throughout the country, use of the Institute's methodology enabled the group to produce a comprehensive requirements document that was released in November of 2003 for all public health labs across the country to use.

The document provided a conceptual framework that described the work performed in a public health laboratory, through detailed descriptions of 16 core business processes and the relationships between them. On the basis of this framework, over 500 laboratory information system requirements were documented, spanning the defined business processes. The document was designed to enable public health labs to easily modify the requirements to meet the needs of their individual labs, choosing a subset of processes, or deleting any processes not under their specific jurisdictions.

The document also included an explanation of the database interfaces required to link laboratory information systems with other relevant system databases, as well as a delineation of vendor-related requirements specifications commonly found in requests for proposals (RFPs). This served to facilitate the implementation of specific projects by providing a foundation for the formation of comprehensive vendor requests.

In a second phase of the project, the requirements were refined to create a set of logical design specifications that offers a framework for future development initiatives, ensuring that public health laboratory information systems will have the high degree of interoperability and capacity necessary for mutual assistance in a crisis situation.

Users of the requirements document have reported that they were able to develop and/or implement their information systems more efficiently. Some labs have used the document to develop RFPs to identify and evaluate commercially available systems, to ensure that these systems would meet the needs of their labs. Other labs have worked collaboratively to build a system based on open source technology, and have used the requirements document in the design phase of their development efforts. However it has been used, the labs report that the work has resulted in information systems that are much more comprehensive and robust than they would have been able to attain without using the methodology [4].

7. Conclusion

It has been illustrated with the lab project, as well as with other projects currently in development, that systems engineering concepts can be used to improve the public health system. Thoughtful planning in the development of information systems will assist public health in developing the cohesive, interoperable information systems required in the complicated public health environment. If these information systems can support a multitude of work processes, public health can more readily cross organizational boundaries within departments, and more importantly, across agencies through all layers of government, in order to better perform their work.

Systems engineering concepts are especially powerful in the public health sector when agencies come together to work collaboratively. Working collaboratively has the additional benefit of helping to increase the informatics knowledge of the public health workforce. This increased knowledge is important for the future success of information systems development within public health, as the rate of success is increased with the participation of a range of stakeholders in this endeavor.

References

[1] Committee for the Study of the Future of Public Health Division of Health Care Services Institute of Medicine, *The Future of Public Health*. Washington, D.C.; National Academy Press, 1988.

[2] D. Kindig and G. Stoddart, What is Population Health? *American Journal of Public Health* **93**(3) (March 2003), 380–383.

[3] Public Health Functions Steering Committee, *Public health in America, fall 1994*. Available online at http://www.health.gov/phfunctions/public.htm. Accessed June 2, 2009.

[4] Public Health Informatics Institute, *The LIMS Project: Summary of Evaluation Findings*. Decatur, GA: Public Health Informatics Institute, 2007.

[5] Public Health Informatics Institute, *Taking Care of Business: A Collaboration to Define Local Health Department Business Processes*, Decatur, GA: Public Health Informatics Institute, 2006.

[6] D. Ross and A. Hinman, Public health informatics, in: *Public Health & Preventive Medicine*, (15th edition), R.B. Wallace and N. Kohatsu, eds, New York: McGraw Hill Medical, 2008, pp. 49–54.

[7] W. Rouse, Managing Complexity: Disease Control as a Complex Adaptive System, *Information Knowledge Systems Management* **2**(2) (June 2000), 143.

[8] D.M. Strong and O. Volkoff, A Roadmap for Enterprise System Implementation, *Computer* **37**(6) (2004), 22–29.

[9] R.B. Wallace, Public health and preventive medicine: Trends and guideposts, in: *Public Health & Preventive Medicine*, (15th edition), R.B. Wallace and N. Kohatsu, eds, New York: McGraw Hill Medical, pp. 49–54.

[10] W. Yasnoff, P. O'Carroll, D. Koo, R. Linkins and E. Kilbourne, Public Health Informatics: Improving and Transforming Public Health in the Information Age, *Journal of Public Health Management & Practice* **6**(6) (November 2000), 67.

Dr. David Ross directs the Public Health Informatics Institute, a program of the Task Force for Global Health, which is affiliated with Emory University. The Institute supports public health practitioners in improving their use of information and information systems to achieve greater impact on community health. He received his Doctor of Science degree in applied math and operations research from The Johns Hopkins University. His career spans health care research and administration, environmental health research, and public health and medical informatics consulting. He served in scientific and senior management roles at the Centers for Disease Control and Prevention (CDC), retiring as a commissioned officer of the US Public Health Service in 1998. He also worked as an executive with a leading health information technology firm implementing clinical information systems. He served on the Institute of Medicine's (IOM) core committee for the evaluation of the U.S. government's global HIV/AIDS PEPFAR program, the IOM panel recommending the research agenda for public health preparedness, is a commissioner on the Certification Commission for Health Information Technology (CCHIT) and advises the World Health Organization's Health Metrics Network Technical Working Group.

Information Knowledge Systems Management 8 (2009) 311–339
DOI 10.3233/IKS-2009-0145
IOS Press

Chapter 18

Engineering responses to pandemics

Richard C. Larson and Karima R. Nigmatulina
E-mail: rclarson@mit.edu

Abstract: Focusing on pandemic influenza, this chapter approaches the planning for and response to such a major worldwide health event as a complex engineering systems problem. Action-oriented analysis of pandemics requires a broad inclusion of academic disciplines since no one domain can cover a significant fraction of the problem. Numerous research papers and action plans have treated pandemics as purely medical happenings, focusing on hospitals, health care professionals, creation and distribution of vaccines and anti-virals, etc. But human behavior with regard to hygiene and social distancing constitutes a first-order partial brake or control of the spread and intensity of infection. Such behavioral options are "non-pharmaceutical interventions." (NPIs) The chapter employs simple mathematical models to study alternative controls of infection, addressing a well-known parameter in epidemiology, R_0, the "reproductive number," defined as the mean number of new infections generated by an index case. Values of R_0 greater than 1.0 usually indicate that the infection begins with exponential growth, the generation-to-generation growth rate being R_0. R_0 is broken down into constituent parts related to the frequency and intensity of human contacts, both partially under our control. It is suggested that any numerical value for R_0 has little meaning outside the social context to which it pertains. Difference equation models are then employed to study the effects of heterogeneity of population social contact rates, the analysis showing that the disease tends to be driven by high frequency individuals. Related analyses show the futility of trying geographically to isolate the disease. Finally, the models are operated under a variety of assumptions related to social distancing and changes in hygienic behavior. The results are promising in terms of potentially reducing the total impact of the pandemic.

1. Introduction

An outbreak of pandemic influenza has the potential to be more disastrous than a nuclear exchange between two warring nations. Historical examples, such as the 1918–19 "Spanish Flu" that killed over 40 million people, have demonstrated how catastrophic the flu can be. Influenza pandemics have occurred intermittently over centuries, and experts agree that the next pandemic is only a matter of time. At the writing of this chapter there is a novel flu strain – A(H1N1), commonly referred to as the "Swine flu" – circulating through the globe and sparking fears that it may mutate and become a deadly killer. While medical advances over the past century have been significant, we still don't have a simple cure for the flu, and when a severe flu virus emerges, it can spread quickly throughout the world causing a pandemic. Such a disaster would not only place extraordinary and sustained demands on the public health and medical care systems, but would also burden the providers of essential services and strain the operations of all businesses. The U.S. federal government projects that up to 40% of the US population may be absent from their daily routines for extended periods as a result of illness or care-giving responsibilities. High rates of worker absenteeism could in turn affect critical infrastructure, including the operations of water treatment facilities and power plants, while efforts to slow the spread of disease could limit the availability of food. A pandemic could impact all sectors of society. The US National Intelligence Council's 2020 Project "Mapping the Global Future" identified a flu pandemic as the single most important threat to the

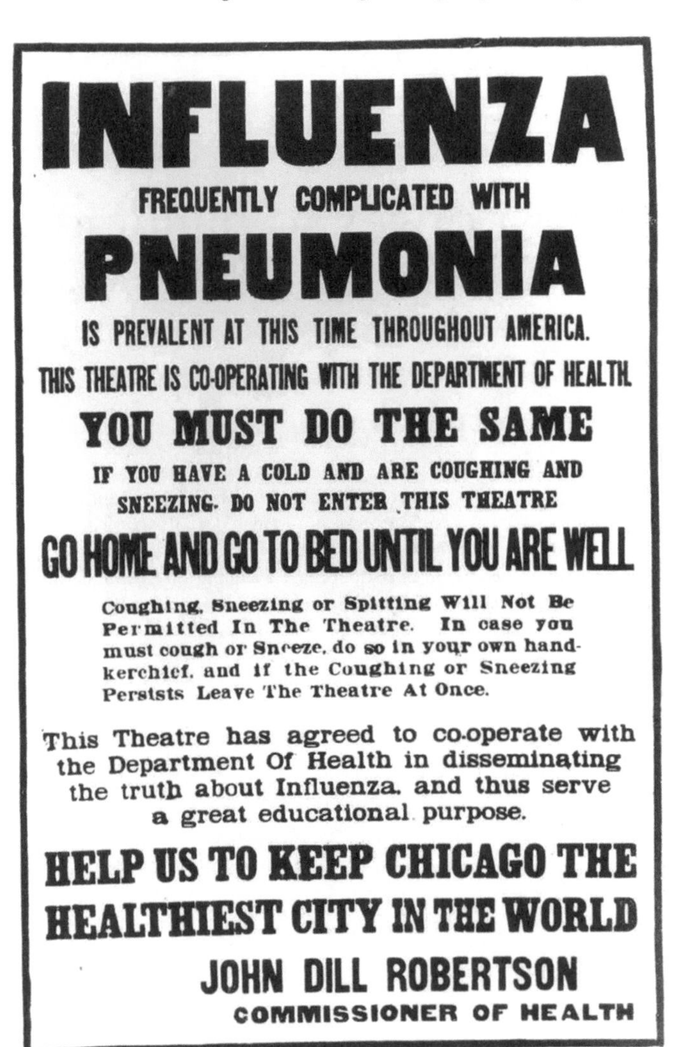

Posted in Chicago, 1918.
http://1918.pandemicflu.gov/pics/posters/Chicago_Poster_1918.jpg.

global economy [28]. It is for these reasons, and more – discussed below – that we select **influenza** pandemics as our focus in a chapter entitled, *Engineering Responses to Pandemics.*

A common definition of "engineering' is as follows: *"The application of scientific and mathematical principles to practical ends such as the design, manufacture, and operation of efficient and economical structures, machines, processes, and systems."* [1] In engineering the response to a pandemic, we need to use "scientific and mathematical principles" to design processes and systems to mitigate the seriousness and consequences of the flu and to create a total system response to it.

A standard engineering approach towards pandemic flu has been to tackle obvious more traditional engineering problems. These problems range from "optimizing" vaccine and anti-viral distribution and stockpiling strategies, to hospital surge capacity analysis, to developing solutions to supply chain

[1] http://www.answers.com/topic/engineering Cited July 9, 2009.

disruptions that are almost guaranteed in a pandemic. See, for example work by [5,8,25]. However, a broad engineering mindset allows going beyond the study of isolated subsystems and well-defined operational problems to develop models of disease spread and – to some extent – control. Understanding disease dynamics to help anticipate the impact of the infection would in turn help develop more applicable preparedness and response plans. *The key here:* The disease dynamics are partly under our individual and collective control. Any engineered system in anticipation of the flu must take this into account.

Pervasive pandemic preparedness at all levels will be essential in mitigating the flu, but many current plans – especially at the state level in the U.S. – lack details and implementation logistics, often skirting the complex issues. Some unknowns including the virulence, morbidity and speed of transmission of the viral strain hamper precise planning. Since there is no way to test run a pandemic, policy makers must often rely on mathematical models to guide their decision making and evaluate "what-if" scenarios. These models can help systematically to gauge the effectiveness of medical and government imposed interventions, medical measures as well as social distancing and hygiene behavioral changes. Understandably, the epidemiology community has done the majority of the work in the area of pandemic transmission modeling.

The "Engineering" for systems problems as complex as pandemic influenza needs to encompass many aspects of the problem, drawing on ideas and methods not only from traditional engineering, but also from the management sciences and – especially – the social sciences. Human behavioral response to pandemic flu is a first-order characteristic of any realistic model of flu progression. Highly stylized mechanistic problem formulations, sometimes derisively labeled 'toy problems,' are not applicable in these settings. But that is not to say that simplicity is bad *per se*. Albert Einstein said, "*Keep it simple but not too simple*!" The idea is to simplify the analysis, but only to the point that needed insights from the analysis are retained.

With pandemic influenza, we are dealing with a worldwide problem involving decisions by literally billions of people. Initially the physics of flu transmission is governed by the inherent purely scientific properties of the novel flu virus. These properties relate to aerosol flu in-air latency time in rooms and other closed places, half-life of flu virus particles on various surfaces, efficiency of infectivity (i.e., ease of passing the virus from person to person and creating a newly infected person), levels of morbidity and mortality by age and other population descriptors, etc. But once the flu has emerged and is recognized as a danger, myriad decision makers come into play. These include governments at all levels – local, regional and federal – that initiate steps in response to the flu. These steps can be medical, such as supporting research leading to a new vaccine, or managerial, such as convening various stakeholders and starting to execute a flu response plan. These plans contain many elements, including steps to limit human-to-human interactions that may otherwise accelerate the propagation of the virus. Examples of governmental steps to reduce virus transmission include the prohibition of certain public events, the closing of schools, quarantining and forced self-isolation. Simultaneously with government-mandated steps, individuals within the population begin to change their behavior, perhaps seeing fewer people on a day-to-day basis, washing hands more frequently, coughing into their elbows, not shaking hands or kissing upon greetings, wearing face masks, etc.

Both governmental 'top-down' and individual 'bottom up' behavioral changes can affect dramatically the propagation properties of the flu, and ultimately the total number of people who will become infected. Beforehand, no one knows exactly how these steps will play out. Added to this complexity is the fact that flu viruses mutate continuously. A mild virus in June may become a lethal virulent virus in October. No one knows how these mutations will evolve. Thus, we have a complex stochastic global system with unknown emergent properties, yet demanding timely informed decisions by decision makers at all levels [41]. Risks are high. Do nothing and the flu may infect over 40 percent of the population and kill tens of millions. Or, take steps believed to reduce levels of infection, and one disrupts daily lives, the economy, children's education, etc., but likely reduces the severity of the flu pandemic.

We believe that mathematical models that are simple, but not too simple, can add significant insight into what to do in the case of a pandemic flu. This is the classic paradigm in engineering science, the use of mathematical models for circuit design, for bridge building, for creating mechanical devises, etc. But we are humble in face of the flu, as the dynamics are always changing, and no model will be anywhere near perfect. For pandemic flu, there are no known equivalents to Newton's laws of physics or Kirchoff's circuit laws. All current models are flawed. But we can rely on data from past pandemics and axiomatic reasoning to develop models to obtain decision insights. That is our goal. We recommend that the word "optimal" be avoided when analyzing pandemic flu since (1) the disease dynamics are *a priori* unknown and emergent; (2) the existence of numerous stakeholders precludes the existence of an uncontested single objective function; and (3) there exists no uncontested set of constraints.

This chapter will describe models that provide insight into disease transmission dynamics. Several important epidemiological concepts including the basic reproductive number – R_0 will be discussed. A basic understanding of transmission dynamics makes very clear the impact that human behavior has on the spread of infection. A public well educated about the infection and regularly updated on the extent of infection spread will react and alter their daily behavior in attempts to protect themselves from becoming ill. The resulting behavioral changes have the potential to 'mitigate' the outbreak. This chapter will show that peoples' behavior is a first-order effect and must be included in any engineered design for a flu preparedness and response system.

We recognize that, in writing this chapter, we are addressing at least two different audiences with two distinctly different cultures. The two professional groups – engineering and medicine – are quite different culturally and in other ways. We see this chapter as primarily engineering-oriented with considerable input from the medical research community, especially epidemiology. The engineering approach gives rise to the references to Kirchoff's Laws, Newtonian physics, etc. The idea is that there are a few fundamental laws of nature in the domain you are studying, and – as any engineer would attempt to do – you try to design a good system utilizing these laws. Much of the medical community focuses on 'evidence-based medicine,' often with the bar set very high in terms of randomized controlled experimentation. But this research paradigm is very difficult with pandemic influenza, a world-wide occurrence only a few times per century. We will attempt to address these cultural differences and explain how our modest contribution fits into the bigger picture.

2. Background: What is a pandemic?

Influenza pandemics are usually associated with high morbidity, excess mortality as well as economic and social disruptions. As defined by the World Health Organization (WHO), influenza pandemics arise when:

1. A "novel" influenza virus subtype, to which the general population has no pre-existing immunological protection, emerges.[2]
2. The virus infects humans and causes serious illness.

[2]This also implies that no vaccine is available at the onset of the outbreak.

3. It spreads efficiently amongst people with sustained chains of transmission.

Once such an event starts and reaches a certain level of local or regional spread, continued worldwide spread of the virus is considered inevitable especially given the highly interconnected nature of today's world.

From the year 2000 until early 2009, the most discussed strain of flu with pandemic potential was H5N1, also referred to as the "Avian Flu". This virus has infected birds in over 35 countries becoming endemic in Southeast Asia and has resulted in the deaths, through illness and culling, of over 200 million birds across Asia. The H5N1 virus has been reported to have infected 436 people in 15 countries, resulting in 262 deaths [76]. This subtype has not yet shown an ability to transmit efficiently between humans, but many caution that it is important to maintain a high level of vigilance because another strain may cause the next pandemic.

In late April 2009 in Mexico these warnings became reality. H1N1, a viral strain referred to as the "swine flu" was identified and began to spread to other countries. While the estimated death toll at time of writing (July 2009) has been more consistent with expectations for seasonal flu, the socio-economic losses are significant [41]. The WHO has already declared the H1N1 strain as a full-fledged pandemic even though the death toll has remained at seasonal flu levels. Since viral mutations are almost impossible to predict, at the writing of this chapter, it is too early to tell what total costs the world will incur as a result of this virus, but already this strain has highlighted the importance of pandemic preparedness at all levels. At this point, antiviral medications such as Tamiflu are effective for the H1N1 strain, but it is very unclear whether the virus will develop resistance to the drugs or if our infrastructure will be sufficient to administer the limited antiviral stockpiles rapidly enough. Sufficient vaccine doses require 6–9 months of production time, as a result even with a virus that emerged in the spring we are naked against a fall wave of the flu.

The lack of vaccines does not need to spell out a doomsday scenario because *even without medical interventions regular people have the ability to decrease the cumulative amount of flu transmission through behavioral change*. Often this point is overlooked by models that inherently assume that individuals maintain their behavior throughout the entire outbreak regardless of its severity. Furthermore, some epidemiologists argue that while behavioral changes do indeed decrease the burden of infection at the peak of the pandemic, they don't change the cumulative number of people who become ill over the entire outbreak [54]. Using mathematical models we argue the overall effectiveness of non-pharmaceutical interventions (NPIs) and demonstrate the potential control the population can have over disease dynamics.

3. Modeling approaches

The types of models that have been used to describe the spread of infection range from basic deterministic differential equations to detailed stochastic agent-based models. The basic compartmental models are contained within a series of three 1930's papers by W.O. Kermack and A.G. McKendrick [31–33]. This most prominent epidemiology modeling approach is based on dividing the host population into several compartments based on their status with respect to the disease. A set of partial differential equations then describes the transfer rate of individuals from one compartment to the next. For more on compartmental models refer to *Mathematical Epidemiology*, Allen L.J.S., Springer, 2008.

Many recent models incorporate information about social network structures in order to understand the impact of social mixing patterns. Network models can range from simple lattice and random mixing networks, to small-world graphs or incredibly detailed social networks where nodes represent people, and edges represent specified relationships or interactions. These networks provide a backbone for stochastic Monte Carlo models that simulate how an infection could spread from one source node to the rest of the population. These studies have shown that the degree, 'betweenness' and farness of nodes alter disease dynamics [6]. The most computationally intensive agent-based stochastic simulation models have been used to "play out" more specific scenarios [11,14,43].

The simulation models include an incredibly detailed level of granularity, while many compartmental models assume inter-connected sets of homogeneous groups within the population. Any one model may be most applicable in a given setting, depending on the question that is being addressed. In general, an insightful model should provide a balance of the extreme of simplified abstraction that makes the model virtually useless in practice and the other extreme of meticulous detailed complexity that is time consuming, difficult to verify while giving the appearance of accuracy and completeness, but providing little intuition. The models presented later in this chapter attempt to achieve this sort of balance.

4. R_0, the basic reproductive number

In virtually all epidemiological models one of the most commonly referred to parameters is R_0. The *basic reproductive number* – R_0, is defined to be the expected number of secondary infections produced by a typical index case in a completely susceptible population [69]. As the population of susceptibles is depleted, the generation-specific reproductive number, $R(t)$, is called the *effective reproductive number*. $R(t)$ is the mean number of secondary infections that will result from each newly infected individual in generation t.

Policy makers often refer to the reproductive number to guide their decision making process. It appears that one of the reasons for the popularity of R_0 is that it is somewhat intuitive. An infection can grow in a fully susceptible population if and only if $R_0 > 1$ [23]. This well-established statement can be somewhat misleading because an $R_0 > 1$ does not guarantee that a disease will take off. Usually, a value of 2 for R_0 is thought to result in a doubling of the number newly infected with each generation of the flu. But consider a population where half of the population – group 1 – because of behavioral and immunological reasons, will spread the virus to 4 people if infected, while the other half – group 2 – never spreads the virus. By some definitions of the reproductive number, we have an R_0 of 2. If the first person to get infected is a member of group 2 the virus dies out right away. This is an example of a case where $R_0 >$ 1, but the disease dies out after the index case more than half of the time. We can write an equation from which we can compute the exact value for the self-extinction probability, which we will call P_E. For our simple example, we can write

$$P_E = (1/2) + (1/2)P_E^4.$$

The logic is this: P_E is equal to 1/2, due to the 50% chance that patient zero will infect no others, plus (1/2) times the probability that each of the four people infected under the second possibility for patient zero will themselves spawn an infection process that dies out – each independently and each with probability P_E. The numerical solution to this equation is $P_E = 0.543$. So, we have a feasible situation in which R_0 is 2.0 and yet 54.3% of the "epidemics" die out very quickly on their own. There is no exponential growth, obviously, for such cases.

As described by Heesterbeek [20], $R_0$was conceived in Germany by demographers in the 1880's and formalized in 1925 to model the progression of a country's population. The original R_0 was defined to be the average number of female offspring born to one female over her entire life. For the year 1879, this number for Germany was estimated by Richard Bockh to be 1.06. The time scale was decades and the system was in approximate equilibrium. With an influenza epidemic, the time scale is in days and weeks and nothing approximating equilibrium exists. To the contrary, the system is characterized by markedly changing parameter values as society copes daily with the influenza's evolution. Over the last three decades, epidemiologists have adopted the R_0 concept and applied it to a variety of diseases, some of which (e.g., malaria) exist in a type of quasi-equilibrium similar to that of population demographics. But the original demographic motivation and near steady state environment supporting R_0simply do not exist in a dynamic influenza epidemic situation. In summary, R_0 and its successor $R(t)$ as fixed-trajectory concepts in rapidly evolving infectious disease epidemics are of limited value at best.

We often hear epidemiologists attach to an infectious disease a given number for R_0, as if that number characterizes some constant of nature, independent of anything else. One might hear, "Consider an infectious disease with R_0 equal to 3.14159, etc., etc." One mathematical researcher even calls R_0 the "... one parameter that (almost) does it all" [29]. For the H1N1 swine flu in circulation as of this writing, the WHO (World Health Organization) has estimated R_0 for H1N1 to be between 1.4 and 1.6. The very form of the statement implies that R_0 exists as a defined constant of the H1N1 flu, independent of the contextual social and physical environments in which the disease is developing. But disease environments play a significant role in determining the numerical value for R_0 and for subsequent values of $R(t)$. Our own research into tracking of H1N1 has shown that fitting exponential growth curves to the daily numbers of confirmed cases of H1N1 demonstrates that statistical estimates of R_0 vary widely among states and among countries [18]. Yet, many authors discussing R_0 describe it as if there is one correct numerical value, worldwide, and discrepancies in estimated values are usually attributed to statistical noise and reporting errors. Even in demography, where quasi steady-state operation supports use of the R_0 concept, human behavior demonstrates that the birth rate defined R_0 is far from an immutable constant. In Germany today, more than a century after the first estimate of Germany's R_0, the current R_0 is estimated to be about 0.70, a 33 percent drop from Bockh's 1879 estimate of 1.06. Worldwide, the demography interpretation of R_0 today varies by a factor of seven, from over 3.5 daughters per female (Mali and Niger) to under 0.5 (Hong Kong). In demography, we see that the numerical value of R_0 depends strongly on social and environmental context. It is not a constant of nature. So too in infectious disease applications we should expect R_0 to depend on context. In influenza, as in demography, the numerical value of R_0 depends strongly on the societal situation in which it is embedded. In some existential sense then, R_0 does not exist as a number independent of context.

The consensus definition of R_0 states that it is the mean value of a random variable. As in all probabilistic situations, the mean of a random variable conveys some useful information. But expressing the mean in terms of other more fundamental quantities can yield additional insights. Suppose I come face to face with λ people on a day that I am infectious but asymptomatic. We select the Greek letter lambda (λ) since in modeling analyses it often refers to frequency of occurrence, such as the daily frequency of interacting with other people. Many people who become infected with the flu have one such day before they feel and appear sick, and not being able to identify these people is what makes eradication of the flu so difficult. Define an 'indicator variable' as follows:

$$X_i = \begin{cases} 1 \text{ if person } i \text{ becomes sick as a result of exposure to me} \\ 0 \text{ if person } i \text{ does not become sick as a result of exposure to me} \end{cases}$$

Now, we let *NI* be defined to be the number of people I will infect on this day. *NI* can be written as simply counting the indicator variables,

$$NI = X_1 + X_2 + X_3 + \ldots = \sum_{i=1}^{\lambda} X_i$$

Suppose for example $\lambda = 50$ and that all X_i's are 0 except for X_9, X_{18} and X_{45}, each being equal to one. In that case, I have infected 3 of the 50 individuals that I have come face to face with on this day. Now, at any given level of intensity of face-to-face contact, there is a probability p that I will pass the infection on to the person I am facing. Sometimes p is called the "transmission probability." We can now write an expression for the mean number of people I will infect on this day. It is simply the mean of

$$NI = X_1 + X_2 + X_3 + \ldots = \sum_{i=1}^{\lambda} X_i,$$

which equals λp. We thus have a simple expression for R_0, and that is

$$R_0 = \lambda p. \tag{1}$$

Flu is an infectious respiratory disease, spread by human contacts. Reduce human contacts, and reduce prevalence of the flu. By writing $R_0 = \lambda p$, we have expressed R_0 in terms of two other parameters, each of which we can control to some extent. We have a fighting chance of reducing R_0, perhaps a little, perhaps even to below 1.0, the critical value to assure that the disease dies away rather than grows exponentially. In the sense of this discussion, R_0 indeed does not exist as a separate quantity. It is a function of both the inherent properties of the given virus *and* the population's behavioral responses to it.

How do we control λ and p? One reduces λ simply by reducing the number of face-to-face contacts we have each day. If a parent is shopping for groceries, rather than following the European tradition of daily shopping, perhaps one switches to weekly shopping, or, better yet, to groceries delivered to one's door. If you manage a team of employees, rather than have face-to-face meetings during a flu emergency, have conference calls instead, with many workers telecommuting. Many companies have already created comprehensive pandemic flu plans that include telecommuting, reduced face-to-face encounters and even increased minimum desk spacing between workers. The desk spacing idea relates more to the parameter p, the probability that any given face-to-face contact will result in a new infection. How else can we reduce p? Wash hands with hot water and soap several times daily. Do not shake hands during greetings with colleagues. Cough or sneeze into your elbow, not into the open air or your bare hand. Be careful not to touch surfaces that might have recently been contaminated with flu virus. Encourage your city's large employers to stagger work hours, so that public transportation subways and busses are less crowded during now-stretched-out rush hours. Even run the subways and busses with windows opened. The key here is that R_0 is a direct function of social context and human behavior, behavior that can be altered to reduce the numerical value of R_0.

Reducing the number and intensity of human-to-human contacts has been called "social distancing." It is a key control parameter in any engineered response to the flu. Social distancing has roots over centuries, often as a type of group evolutionary survival mechanism. In rural India in the 19th and early 20th Centuries, subsistence farm families who lived closely together in villages but who worked separate land plots outside of the villages, left the villages and lived separately on their land whenever they heard from a trusted messenger that 'a plague' was 'in the vicinity.' They returned to their village homes once the signal was given that the risk of plague had subsided, the duration of the distancing typically being about two weeks.[3] While this policy seemed to work well for rural subsistence farmers, we may well ask, "What is the analogue to the movement to the land in our highly-networked interconnected Western style of life?" We are not self sufficient and we rely on others to provide virtually all essential services and products for living. Given all the interconnected networks upon which we rely, is social distancing itself, in the simple ways in which we can do it, sufficient to control the evolution and penetration of a flu pandemic? This question is a major challenge when addressing response to pandemic flu.

Of course there are limitations to our analysis. The causal model creating infection is more complex than just counting the numbers of face-to-face contacts. One can touch surfaces contaminated minutes or perhaps even hours before by individuals who we do not see face to face. If contaminated hands then touch one's mouth or eyes, infection can result. With SARS (Severe Acute Respiratory Syndrome), residents of a Hong Kong high-rise apartment complex became infected by a faulty sewage system, again not 'seeing' the infected person responsible for spreading the infection. But we believe that a model that counts the number of face-to-face contacts and includes the intensity of these contacts represents a valid primary mechanism for depicting how the disease propagates through the population. Adding complexities such as the two just cited does not alter the main conclusions of our arguments. Our approach is buttressed by findings of others. For instance, Riley et al. [58] credits reduction in the number of face-to-face contacts in Hong Kong as the primary cause for reduction in spread of SARS.

To see more about the complexities of using R_0 as an input value to guide policy, refer to a study by Meyers et al. They focus their study on SARS and illustrate that for a single value of R_0, any two outbreaks, even in the same setting, may have very different epidemiological outcomes [45]. While using $R(t)$or R_0 provides a computationally intuitive basis for describing disease dynamics, this approach neglects important complexities related to heterogeneities and uncertainties [9,34].

From an engineering point of view that is taken in this paper, expressing R_0 as the product of λ and p is good news. Both λ and p are controllable to some extent, so R_0 is controllable to some extent. Behavioral changes can reduce R_0 and as a result, reduce the chance that you or a loved one becomes infected with the flu.

5. Basic model

In this model one community is divided into several groups based on their daily social activity levels.[4] Since influenza spreads from one person to the next through social interaction it is important to know how much people interact amongst each other. We assume, as most other models, that face-to-face contact is the major method of influenza transmission.[5] We will presume that face-to-face social contacts

[3]This policy of Indian farm families was presented to the author by Dr. Nitin Patel whose father reported that tradition to him. Dr. Patel's father was born in 1909 and lived in the rural village of Karamsad, state of Gujarat, India. Once as a boy he had to leave the village with his family to avoid 'the plague.' Our hypothesis is that the terminology 'the plague' related to several different serious and sometimes fatal diseases and did not precisely refer to any specific plague such as the bubonic plague. (Paragraph and footnote taken from Larson [34].)

[4]The model presented is described by R.C. Larson in the paper titled "Simple Models of Influenza Progression Within a Heterogeneous Population" [34] and further elaborated on by K.R. Nigmatulina and R.C. Larson in a paper titled "Living with Influenza: Impacts of government imposed and voluntarily selected interventions" [52].

[5]Transmission of influenza occurs through respiratory emissions from sick individuals when talking, sneezing or coughing. These emissions enter the environment and can either come in direct contact with a well individual or are transmitted indirectly through an inanimate object. Within the context of our model we assume that the majority of transmission occurs during direct interaction.

within each community occur as a homogeneous Poisson process with rate parameters dependent on the level of social activity of the individual. Furthermore, the interaction between people in different groups is random and proportional to their activity levels. For the rest of the numerical calculations and simulations, unless otherwise noted, we will split the population of each community into three groups: high, medium and low activity persons. We will define:

λ_H– Average number of social contacts of a High activity person/day;
λ_M– Average number of social contacts of a Medium activity person/day;
λ_L– Average number of social contact of Low activity person/day;
N_H, N_M, N_L– Initial total populations of High, Medium and Low activity persons, respectively;
$N_H(t)$– Population of High activity persons active on day t;
$S_H(t)$– Number of High activity susceptible persons on day t;
$I_H(t)$– Number of High activity infective & asymptomatic persons on day t;
$R_H(t)$– Number of High activity recovered & immune persons on day t.

This notation continues in the same manner for the other populations, M and L. Let us clarify that throughout the remainder of this chapter we define one day as one generation of the infectious period of the virus. One day in the context of our model is closer to 2 to 3 actual 24-hour days.

The outbreak is initiated by one infectious individual who interacts normally with people on day 0. By the end of this day the initial seeder self-isolates, recovers or dies, and no longer infects any other individuals. Evidence of self-isolating behavior has been observed in practice [77] and reflects peoples' departure from the infectious category. On day one, the individuals recently infected from the index case interact normally and transmit the virus until they leave the infective group on day two. A recovered individual never reenters the susceptible population since people gain immunity if they survive the disease. This pattern continues for the rest of the outbreak.

From Larson's paper [34] we know that for a random person on day t the probability that the next interaction will be with an infected individual is:

$$\beta(t) \equiv \frac{\lambda_H I_H(t) + \lambda_M I_M(t) + \lambda_L I_L(t)}{\lambda_H N_H(t) + \lambda_M N_M(t) + \lambda_L N_L(t)}$$

$\beta(t)$ is the fraction of all interactions of infected people over the total number of interactions in the entire active population on day t. The number of people circulating on day t is all those who have not gotten sick as well as those who have gotten sick, but also recovered and reentered the population. Assume that d is the duration of the sickness from the beginning of infection until the individual can reenter the population and that h is the fraction of people who survive the virus and can reenter the population. Then,

$$N_H(t+1) = N_H(t) - I_h(t) + hI_H(t-d)^6$$

Assuming homogeneous susceptibility let:

p = probability that a susceptible person becomes infected, given contact with an infectious individual.

Using the knowledge that the number of interactions is Poisson distributed, we know that the probability that a random susceptible High activity person gets infected on day t is:

$$p_H^S(t) = \sum_{i=1}^{\infty} \frac{(\lambda_H)^i}{i!} e^{-\lambda_H} \left[\sum_{j=0}^{i} \binom{i}{j} \beta(t)^j (1-\beta(t))^{i-j} \left(1 - [1-p]^j\right) \right]$$

[6]Note, for $t - d < 0$, $I_j(t-d) = 0$ for all j.

Table 1
Parameters used as the base case for the research

Parameter name	Variable	Community A
Initial size of High activity group	N_H	100,000 ppl
Initial size of Medium activity group	N_M	100,000 ppl
Initial size of Low activity group	N_L	100,000 ppl
Rate of contact of High activity persons	λ_H	50 ppl/day
Rate of contact of Medium activity persons	λ_M	10 ppl/day
Rate of contact of Low activity persons	λ_L	2 ppl/day
Conditional probability of successful transmission	p	0.10
Duration of sickness from day of infection	d	9 days
Percent of people who recover & reenter population	h	98%

Table 2
The results of Yang-chih Fu's research on the distribution of the frequency of daily human contacts

Number of daily contacts	Number of respondents	Percent of respondents	Cumulative percentage
0–4	410	13.67	13.67
5–9	426	14.20	27.87
10–19	685	22.83	50.70
20–49	792	26.40	77.10
50–99	349	11.63	88.73
100+	338	11.27	100
Total	3,000	100.00	

which as shown in Larson can be simplified to [34]:

$$p_H^S(t) = 1 - e^{-\lambda_H \beta(t) p}$$

In Table 1, we present the base case parameter values that we continue to use throughout this paper to present the results of our modeling analysis based on the above formulations.

The average rates of contact, λ_H, λ_M, λ_L, in the different groups are based on the research done by Yang-chih Fu. Some of the best data on the frequency distribution of daily human contacts is a result of the survey conducted by Fu. He asked people in nine countries and 46 different settings: on average, about how many people do you have contact with in a typical day, including all those who you say hello, chat, talk or discuss matters with, whether you do it face-to-face, by telephone, by mail or on the Internet, and whether you personally know the person or not [12,13]? The results of the survey are shown in Table 2.

The results of this study are not perfectly suited for calibrating the activity level of people in our model because it includes human contacts that are not face-to-face such as the telephone and the Internet. While it is unclear exactly how many relevant contacts people have on a daily basis we can use the results of Fu's other study, which indicates that in Taiwan 83% of all daily contacts are face-to-face [12]. While it is unclear if these values are best suited to describe the United States, this data is very instructive and confirms that there is a significant amount of heterogeneity in the population.

Returning to the model, the proposed approach assumes that the contact rates per day remain constant even as members of the susceptible population become sick and leave the circulating population. In the context of standard compartmental models this is known as standard incidence. Let us also consider the mass action incidence model where as the number of active people decreases, we anticipate a reduced amount of overall social activity. In this alternative approach λ, the average number of daily contacts

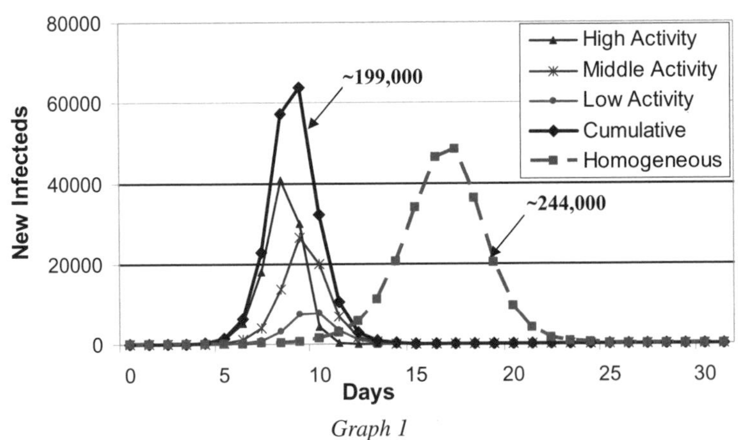

Graph 1

Comparing spread of infection between heterogeneously and uniformly active communities of 300,000 individuals.

per person, is proportional to the size of the remaining population in circulation. As shown by Larson in this case all λ's become time dependent. For example, $\lambda_H(t)$ – daily rate of social contact of a High activity person on day t. Let $N(t) = N_H(t) + N_M(t) + N_L(t)$, and then

$$\lambda_H(t+1) = \frac{\lambda_H(t)N(t+1)}{N(t)} = \frac{\lambda_H(0)N(t+1)}{N(0)}.$$

Thus we have,

$$p_H^S(t) = 1 - e^{-\lambda_H(t)\beta(t)p}$$

The cumulative number of infected individuals, as well as the infection peak, is higher for the standard incidence model.[7]

Let us focus on the mass action incidence model and the input values in Table 1. The expected infection transmission for the hypothetical heterogeneous community is compared to the disease dynamics in a similar homogeneous community in Graph 1. Notice that the virus spreads faster through a population with several activity levels when compared to a homogeneous community with an equivalent average activity level. Furthermore, the high activity individuals are the first to get infected. Practically all of the high activity people, 99.9% get infected while less than 25% of the low activity individuals get sick. As the number of high activity people is depleted by day 9, the total number of people getting sick also starts to diminish around the same time. Because of their behavioral characteristics[8], the high activity people are the drivers of influenza transmission.[9]

The imprecise, but widely accepted, definition of R_0 is the average number of people infected by the initial seeder in a fully susceptible population. For the heterogeneous and uniform communities, the expected number of daily contacts of a randomly selected person from either population will be the same. Thus using one interpretation, without more knowledge of the activity groups' dynamics, R_0 is identical in both instances. Relying singly on R_0would not have captured the possibility of these significantly

[7]For more on the comparison of the Standard Incidence and Mass Action models refer to thesis by Nigmatulina [53].

[8]The behavioral traits and not the biological propensity to shed the virus cause these individuals to be the drivers of infection.

[9]These qualitative results are supported by the findings of the real-time surveillance system at Boston's Children's Hospital. Children, compared to adults, have more contacts and increased vulnerability to be drivers of seasonal flu; particularly, preschoolers are seen as "hotbeds of infection" [50].

different outcomes. R_0 is meaningless and often misleading without knowledge of the societal structure of the underlying population. Graph 1 illustrates a fundamental flaw in the usage one averaging parameter such as R_0 (or $R(t)$) as the sole modeling factor.

Other types of heterogeneities also exist and can be similarly modeled. Diverse susceptibility levels and varying infectivity levels are just two more examples of heterogeneities present in the population. [10] In reality our population can be described by a complex combination of many different types of heterogeneities. When compared to heterogeneity in susceptibility and infectivity levels, diversity of activity levels is the most influential and easily observable type of heterogeneity. It is also a behavior that people have the ability to alter in the case of a pandemic.

6. Multi-community model

The basic model assumes that there is random mixing within the community, so that a randomly selected individual has a chance of encountering any other individual. While this isn't precisely true because often people interact within smaller social networks such as family, friends or colleagues, but it is still possible that an individual would have an unplanned encounter with a stranger at a grocery store, bus, movie theater etc. Yet this complete mixing assumption doesn't hold when describing people in two different cities. Thus the next step is to expand our one-community model to a multi-community structure and determine whether travel restrictions between communities have the potential to stop its spread.

Spatial complexity can be modeled through a loosely connected multi-community structure based on Monte Carlo simulation to model disease spread between cities. Consider a two community model – Community A and Community B – each has its own demographic and epidemiological composition. A and B are two communities – each with 300,000 people – with identical compositions: 100,000 people, respectively, in each activity level, high, medium and low. These populations are loosely connected by very few random daily travelers. A certain number of randomly selected people from each activity level j, T^j_{AB}, travel overnight from A to stay exactly one day in B before returning home the next night. In the base case $\mathrm{T}^j_{AB} = \mathrm{T}^j_{BA} = 2$, giving us a total of 12 travelers going back and forth between two communities. During a visitor's one-day stay in the adjacent community his interaction level is unchanged from what it was within his/her home community.

The outbreak is initiated with an infectious seed in Community A, and the disease propagates to other individuals within this community. Since travelers continue their movement between communities, eventually it is likely that one of the travelers becomes infected, thus he becomes the passageway for the transition of the infection from one community to another. There are 2 ways that Community B can get the infection:

1. An infected individual residing in A travels from A to B and infects people in Community B which instigates the outbreak in B (even though the traveler returns to A at the end of the day)
2. A susceptible individual residing in B travels from B to A and gets infected while visiting Community A. The newly infected individual returns home to Community B and becomes the initial spreader within his community.

[10] For details on modeling these types of heterogeneities refer to thesis by Nigmatulina, 2009.

The two processes compete to bring the pandemic to Community B. After the pandemic is in both populations, assume that the few individuals traveling back and forth, with or without the infection, will not change the disease dynamics in either of the communities.

This structure allows us to apply large population-based averaging techniques to model the infection spread within the community. At the same time, we use Monte Carlo simulation to model the stochastic person-to-person transmission of infection to reflect the intra community spread of infection. One question is: if the initial case occurs on day 0 within Community A, on average how quickly will it spread to an adjacent community?

The probability of the virus spreading to a new community changes with every generation of the flu. Recall that whenever we refer to a 'day' we imply one generation of the flu which is equivalent to approximately 2–3 actual 24-hour days. In order to find the probability that on day t at least one infectious individual from activity level j visits Community B, we can "identify" this random individual and find the probability that this traveler gets infected during day $t-1$. The probability that exactly k infected individuals of activity level j travel from A to B and bring in the virus on day t is:

$$p_j^{AB}(k,t) = \binom{T_{AB}^j}{k}\left(1 - e^{-\lambda_j^A \beta^A (t-1)p}\right)^k \left(e^{-\lambda_j^A \beta^A (t-1)p}\right)^{T_{AB}^j - k}$$

Thus the probability that none of day t travelers from A to B are infectious is:

$$\prod_j p_j^{AB}(0,t) = \prod_j \left(e^{-\lambda_j^A \beta^A (t-1)p}\right)^{T_{AB}^j}$$

Symmetrically, as long as $\mathrm{T}_{AB}^j = \mathrm{T}_{BA}^j$ for all j, the probability that a traveler from Community B gets infected and brings back home the infection on day t is the same. So $p_j^{AB}(k,t) = p_j^{BA}(k,t)$. Lastly the probability of having the infection enter for the first time on day i is:

$$P(i \text{ is the 1st day of infection in B}) = \prod_{t=0}^{i-1}\prod_j p_j^{AB}(0,t)p_j^{BA}(0,t) * \left(1 - p_j^{AB}(0,i)p_j^{BA}(0,i)\right)$$

Notice that the probability of never infecting a neighboring community is greater than 0, thus the expected time until the next community gets contaminated is infinity. Instead one can determine the probability that day t is the first day of infection entering into the neighboring community. These calculations show that the probability of infection spread is almost certain if the twelve travelers maintain their trips and if the virus is relatively transmissible amongst individuals. Furthermore, the high activity travelers are very likely to be infected during the peak times of the community outbreak.

These calculations are supported by historical examples demonstrating that one infected traveler is enough to infect a whole population. During the 1918–1919 flu, many Alaskan villages were completely devastated by influenza because the man who brought the villagers their mail also brought the flu [67]. In China's remote Shanxi province, the spread of the 1918 pandemic was traced to a single woodcutter, tramping from village to village [17]. In Canada, the virus wore the uniform of a stubborn Canadian Pacific Railways official who flouted quarantine, dropping off infected repatriate soldiers from Quebec all the way west to Vancouver [17]. Some of the only places to escape unscathed during the 1918 pandemic were 3 small islands completely shut off from the outside world; they even refused mail delivery [22]. On the mainland one successful case was a resort town in New Zealand, which went to the extreme of cutting itself off from the world by using a "rotating roster of shotgun-wielding vigilantes" [17].

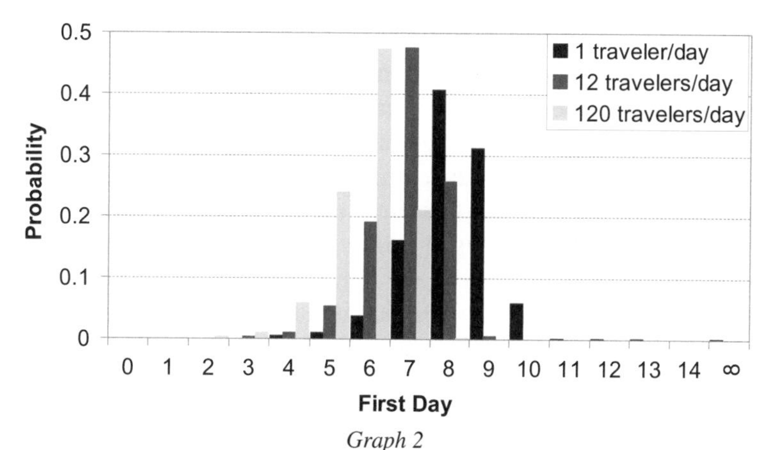

Graph 2
A histogram of the first day of infection spread in Community B that is adjacent to the source community. Even if the number of travelers is decreased from 120 to 1 person a day, influenza is still highly likely to spread.

7. Travel restrictions

During SARS, some governments enforced travel restrictions. Even simple travel advisories decreased the number of voluntary travelers to SARS-infected communities [2]. This suggests that travel patterns will change in the case of flu, so it is interesting to further consider the potential effect of travel restrictions. To model this, one can vary the number of travelers between the cities. For numerical calculations, change the number of travelers from the baseline number of 12 daily[11] travelers to between 1 and 120 daily travelers. In the case of one daily traveler, the person is a highly active individual. Realistically, highly active individuals are more likely to travel outside of their community than recluses. Notice that the direction of the traveler, whether it's A to B, or B to A, is not important.

Our results for a varied number of travelers are summarized in Graph 2. As the number of travelers increases, the infection becomes more likely to reach the adjacent community earlier. This suggests that Japan's plan to fly home all of its citizens in the event of a pandemic [63] may cause it to be one of the earlier countries to become infected. The startling finding is that even with one daily highly-active traveler between the two communities, the disease still spreads to the adjacent community with an incredibly high probability. This indicates that travel restrictions, unless 100% effective, will fail to stop geographical infection spread. During the outbreak, the number of sick grows exponentially while the restriction only decreases travel by a fixed factor. As a result, incomplete travel controls only delay the spread by one or two days, until the exponentially growing number of sick becomes high enough and any traveler is highly likely to become sick.

In order to stop the disease from moving into a neighboring city, all travel must be stopped and the intervention must be initiated early and sustained beyond the peak until the threat of the transition is small. Travel restrictions would be more burdensome when used in combination with other interventions and behavior changes that spread out the virus over a longer period. Lastly, once a travel restriction fails and an infected individual enters a fully susceptible town, the travel restriction becomes totally useless because it does not change the dynamics of the disease within the newly infected town.

It is almost impossible to completely stop the movement of people across borders. In the case of SARS, studies indicate that thermal screening and health declarations of travelers did not significantly

[11] Recall, "day" refers to one generation of the flu, equivalent to approximately 2–3 24-hour days.

stop the flow of determined travelers or the spread of SARS [2]. Within a matter of weeks in early 2003, SARS spread from the Guangdong province of China to rapidly infect individuals in some 37 countries around the world [64]. Overall, travel restrictions are expensive, almost impossible to implement and are often ineffective.

Taking the model a step further highlights that in today's very interconnected world the virus will spread very quickly to many geographical areas. Consider a fully interconnected three community model with one initially infected community and two neighboring susceptible communities. In this case the disease spreads almost concurrently to both of its adjacent communities. In the scenario where susceptible cities are connected to multiple sources of infection, the community experiencing a more severe outbreak will dominate infecting new cities. The number of commuters between nearby cities is high. Management consultants are examples of people who are likely to crisscross the world in the course of a week. This type of global connectedness could be catastrophic for emergency systems that, in a pandemic, would face the equivalent to 50 Hurricane Katrina's hitting the United States all at once. This scenario would leave no one immune and capable of helping out others; communities will have to fend for themselves. Current events support this finding; the rapid geographical spread of the swine flu in 2009 is an example. This suggests that, instead of controlling transmission between communities, managing the infection's spread within communities is likely to be the more effective strategy.

In summary, geographical isolation of the flu is almost impossible; reducing the prevalence – the number infected – within a given geographical region *is* possible.

8. Behavioral changes

When studying and modeling sexually transmitted diseases, especially HIV/AIDS, behavioral changes are often cited as the main factors determining transmission dynamics, but when it comes to modeling flu, behavior is almost always ignored. Few would argue that:

1) People will alter their behavior in a pandemic by becoming more aware of hygiene and decreasing their human contacts.[12]
2) Limiting the number of daily interactions and improving hygiene decrease transmission.

It is unlikely that society will implement severe measures as they did in 1918–1919 making it "unlawful to cough and sneeze" punishing violators with up to a year in jail [24]. However, even without forceful implementation people are likely to try to decrease their likelihoods of getting ill by improving hygiene related behaviors. Most people will not maintain their daily routines if they discover that there is a deadly disease attacking within their city, state, country or the world. Based on the information portrayed in the media, individuals will probably both limit their daily contacts and decrease the closeness of the remaining contacts. History has provided us with multiple examples of people responding to news of a disease by altering their daily behavior.

Recent statistical studies of the 1918 influenza pandemic in US cities have supported the hypothesis that early implementation of multiple non-pharmaceutical interventions could reduce transmission rates by 30–50% and lower the peak death rates by about 50% [3,19]. The timing and force of these interventions have been attributed as some of the main reasons for the variation of different cities' experiences [3].

[12]There are also potential negative behavior changes. An example is the worried well phenomenon where healthy people seek medical assistance because of their concerns about possibly being ill.

The array of outcomes ranges from the Philadelphia one hump epidemic curve lasting a month and a half with a peak excess death rate of over 250/100,000 population, to the St. Louis two-wave four-month experience with a peak excess death rate of less than 75/100,000 population [19]. The findings of these studies suggest that these interventions within cities helped save lives during the 1918–1919 pandemic, and may help save future lives.

Those who still doubt the relevance of behavioral changes, should consider the recent example of the social behavior changes that occurred during SARS. One survey indicates that during the SARS outbreak in Hong Kong 78% of the population covered their mouths while sneezing or coughing, 76% of individuals wore masks, 65% washed their hands after contact with possibly contaminated objects [42]. Economic factor studies in Hong Kong, Beijing, Singapore and Toronto indicate that there was a sharp drop in interactive social activities as restaurants and entertainment centers suffered sharp drops in clientele [55,57]. Specifically in Hong Kong, tourism was crippled in March when the WHO issued a rare warning for travelers to avoid Hong Kong and the Guangdong Province. As a result of weakening demand, airlines slashed more than a third of flights and hotels in Hong Kong reportedly were up to 90% empty [74]. In Singapore sales were down about 30% as people avoided stores and malls, some stores suffered up to 75% declines in sales [74]. It is clear that voluntary activities like tourism were strongly affected by fear of the disease. The resulting adverse economic impact in parts of East Asia was comparable with the 1998 financial market crisis [47,48,65]. It is apparent that many people took precautionary measures as a result, and the outcome in Hong Kong was the 90% decrease in the reported spread of other respiratory diseases [42]!

Similarly, in a more Western city of Toronto, during the SARS outbreak there was a reported drop of up to 71.5% in revenue per available hotel room for downtown Toronto. This translates into hotel occupancy rates in the range of 30% to 40%, instead of the seasonal 70% average [60]. At least five major citywide conventions were called off, contributing a loss of over 20,000 attendees, and this does not include the vast amount of individual-hotel convention businesses that were also cancelled [60]. The long list of voluntary behavior changes in Toronto due to SARS includes over 800 bus tours, music concerts, corporate travel, and school field trips [60]. All these examples are strong evidence that people will not maintain their daily actions. We know that the effect of these "soft" and self-imposed interventions was significant [66]. There are significant gaps in our knowledge of these behavior changes, but overlooking these behavior changes is indefensible.

Various interventions, both behavioral and technological, have been shown to decrease transmission of the flu. Improved hygiene, including hand washing and using alcohol-based hand sanitizer, has been shown to decrease the spread of influenza in controlled environments such as day cares, schools and nursing homes [10,44,59,75]. While there is no conclusive data regarding the effectiveness of surgical masks, there is some evidence indicating that wearing a mask will help prevent the infected from spreading it to the well by containing and slowing the speed of droplets [26]. There is evidence that shows that specialized air handling, which includes ventilation, HEPA filtering and exhaust fans, are effective in reducing potential aerosol transmission of influenza [37]. In addition, ultra-violet light, specifically UV-C, has the potential to disinfect air by inactivating virus-containing aerosols [71].

9. Data on behavior changes

The most relevant data for creating mathematical models on reactive behavior comes from SARS. SARS was first identified in China's southern province of Guangdong in November 2002. By February 26, 2003 Hong Kong officials reported their first case of SARS and no later than March 14, 2003 the

Table 3
Results of a telephone survey monitoring community knowledge, perceptions and practices during the SARS outbreak in Hong Kong in 2003 [35]

	Initial phase						Second phase				
Date of interview	3/21	3/22	3/23	3/24	3/28	4/1	4/8	4/11	4/24	5/12	All
New SARS cases on previous day	20	32	20	25	51	80	41	28	24	4	–
Perceived chance of infection (% very large/large)	3.9	9.2	8.8	11.1	14.3	12.4	7.0	7.1	7.3	4.7	8.7
Improved Hygiene											
Wearing a mask	11.5	16.7	7.7	16.7	66.9	84.3	87.3	87.7	93.9	85.4	64.3
Hand hygiene	61.5	66.7	63.7	80.3	94.1	95.1	93.7	94.2	94.5	95.9	86.9
Disinfecting home	–	–	–	36.4	56.8	69.4	72.2	80.0	83.5	73.1	70.1
Behavior											
Avoid going outside	28.2	28.2	31.9	36.4	50.0	57.1	62.4	58.7	47.3	36.3	45.8
Avoid crowded places	59.0	67.7	54.9	68.2	76.3	85.4	81.0	89.0	81.2	69.6	75.5
Avoid visiting hospitals	59.7	63.5	52.7	62.1	73.4	75.0	76.4	86.5	79.9	68.6	71.8
Avoid using public transportation	14.1	15.4	16.5	24.2	26.6	36.2	27.8	31.0	25.0	17.1	24.4
Avoid going to work	–	2.6	2.2	4.5	6.1	8.1	7.7	7.3	5.5	1.2	4.9
Not allow kids to go to school	–	–	–	12.5	35.7	38.1	31.0	36.7	39.6	16.3	31.6

virus reached Canada. Overall the virus spread to some 37 countries, with 8,096 known infection cases and 774 deaths.

Some of the best data on SARS comes from studies and surveys of Hong Kong. A large number of SARS cases in Hong Kong were first reported on March 10th in the Prince of Wales Hospital and continued until June 2nd [36]. On March 26th a second large scale outbreak occurred in Amoy Gardens [36]. As a reaction, on March 29th all classes were suspended [35]. On March 31st a large number of Amoy Gardens' residents were quarantined. On April 2nd the WHO issued a travel advisory warning for Hong Kong. Afterwards, the situation started to improve. Classes resumed in universities on April 14th and while secondary schools reopened in later April, primary schools stayed closed till May 12th or 19th. At the end of the outbreak a total of 1,755 SARS cases were recorded.

During that time phone surveys were conducted by several different research groups and all groups found that public health measures, such as wearing masks, frequent hand washing, avoidance of crowded places, disinfection of the living quarters, etc had been practiced by most of the Hong Kong population [35, 36,42]. In one of these studies, the progressions of the voluntary interventions throughout the outbreak were recorded. Through ten sequential telephone surveys 1397 adult Hong Kong residents were asked about their knowledge and perceptions of the disease, its risks and fatality as well as their susceptibility and practice of various interventions. In Table 3 one can find the results of this survey that are relevant to this research.

It is clear that the perceived chance of infection fluctuated with the number of people that became infected on the previous day. Furthermore, the various hygiene and behavioral measures implemented by the population are correlated to the number of new cases. In this study, the researchers found that the correlation between the number of cases and the fraction of the population participating in the intervention was high[13] for the initial, escalating phase of the outbreak that lasted through April 1st [35]. As the perceived chance of infection increased, more people started altering their behavior to reduce the likelihood of illness. From the experience of Hong Kong that is captured in this study, it is clear that people not only alter their behavior in the case of a disease outbreak, but the worse the outbreak, the

[13] r* is in the range of 0.85–0.97 for the different interventions.

more the population will react. The importance of timely, accurate, comprehensive information about the disease becomes vital in this scenario. The researchers conclude that "perceptions are important in determining preventative behaviors," and that policy makers should be aware of the importance of the public' reactions. Later in this chapter we will propose several approaches to including these human behaviors into our model.

10. Herd immunity: What it means in terms of total number infected

As mentioned before, there are many who agree that implementation of NPI's indeed does reduce the peak severity of the pandemic, in terms of maximum number infected at any time, and this is good for managing hospital surge capacity. But some also suggest that use of NPI's may only prolong the pandemic period, ultimately infecting as many people as would have been infected without use of NPI's [41]. Our modeling analysis and recent work of others [4,14,27,30] have shown that this need not be true. Given our model assumptions, with NPI's the total number infected is almost always less, sometimes significantly so.

We can demonstrate this property with a simple back-of-the-envelope analysis, invoking the concept of herd immunity. All else being equal, herd immunity occurs in a population when the infectious disease no longer grows exponentially, and starts to die out geometrically from generation to generation. Herd immunity occurs when the effective reproductive number drops to $R(t) = 1$, signifying that each newly infected person infects – on average – only one additional person. At this point in the evolution of the pandemic, no further exponential increase occurs. Usually herd immunity is achieved because a significant fraction of the population has become immune to the disease, either by vaccination or by having had the disease and being recovered and immune to further infection. Let us call$R(0) = R_0 > 1$. Recall from Eq. (1) that $R_0 = \lambda p$, where λ is the pre-intervention mean number of daily face-to-face contacts by a random member of the population, and p is the initial conditional probability of passing on the infection to the person in a random face-to-face contact. Define the "critical time" t_c such that $R(t_c) = 1$. The critical time is the time at which herd immunity is achieved.

Let's first do this without NPI's. At $R(t_c) = 1 = \lambda_{t_c} p_{t_c}$, we assume that the frequency of day-to-day contacts $\lambda_{t_c} = \lambda$ is unchanged during the pandemic.[14] Thus, for this equation to work, we need a reduction in p, so that $p_{t_c} < p$. We get this because some face-to-face contacts are recovered or vaccinated and now immune to further infection. Suppose at time t_c, the time of herd immunity, we have a fraction f of the population in state *R*, immune to re-infection, and the residual (1-f) still susceptible. For those who are still susceptible, the conditional probability of infection given exposure from a face-to-face contact remains unchanged at p. Thus $p_{t_c} = p(1-f)$. Then we must have $\lambda p_{t_c} = \lambda p(1-f) = 1$ or $f = (\lambda p - 1)/\lambda p = 1 - 1/R_0 > 0$. To see if this makes sense, we try $R_0 = \lambda p = 2$ and obtain $f = 1 - 1/2 = 1/2$. This makes sense: with $R_0 = 2$, one half of the population needs to be immune for herd immunity to occur. Other numerical examples are similarly intuitively appealing. (For additional discussion of herd immunity, consult any textbook on mathematical epidemiology such as Nelson and Williams [51, p. 627].)

Now, let's redo this exercise having $R_0 = \lambda p = 2$, but with NPI's. Suppose we alter daily behavior to reduce λ by a factor of $1/\sqrt{2}$, that is we have a new λ, call it λ', such that $\lambda' = \lambda/\sqrt{2}$, roughly a 30%

[14]This may be corrected in a more sophisticated analysis, as we adjust for the reduced population because some are either sick in bed or may have died. With a reduced population, we may wish to model the number of face-to-face daily contacts as reduced in accordance with the reduced circulating population.

reduction in daily contacts. Suppose by social distancing and hygienic steps we also reduce p by a factor of $1/\sqrt{2}$, defining a new p, call it p', such that $p' = p/\sqrt{2}$, which is roughly a 30% reduction in infection probability, given face to face contact. If we can all do that by invoking NPI's, then the new R_0, call it R_0', becomes $R_0' = \lambda' p' = (\lambda/\sqrt{2})(p/\sqrt{2}) = \lambda p/2 = 2/2 = 1$. That is, we can start the pandemic at herd immunity level by invoking NPI's at the beginning. If we could do that, the pandemic would never grow exponentially and would die off geometrically instead. This is most likely impossible in practice, since time is required for officials to observe and recognize a new and novel flu virus, one that could grow to epidemic and then pandemic levels. But the point remains: We individually and collectively have the power through self-selected behavioral changes to alter dramatically the course of the flu. To avoid a dangerous re-emergence, perhaps a 'second wave' after NPI's have squelched the first wave, these behavioral changes must be held in place until the threat of the flu is passed.

11. Modeling behavior changes

There has been very little progress in the field of quantitative health behavior modeling [72]. One of the main deterrents for quantitative modeling of human reactionary behavior is that it is difficult and there is no obvious solution or approach. This does not justify avoiding these models; behavior is a first order affect and has a strong impact on transmission dynamics. We have proposed several different methods for modeling human behavior changes. While it is almost impossible to verify their quantitative accuracy the principles are intuitive and qualitative results are insightful. In this section we will present one of our approaches to modeling behavior and its impact on transmission, for more of these models refer to Nigmatulina and Larson [52] or Nigmatulina [53].

There are several qualitative social behavior models that predict people altering their behavior given knowledge of a deadly infection. Coping responses affect human functions to moderate and decrease the negative impacts and stressors in life's circumstances [56]. Protection motivation theory, the transactional model of stress and coping, the health belief model (HBM) and behavior intention model (BIM) all indicate that individuals will attempt to assess their perceived risk or attitude towards the threat based on factors like threat severity and their vulnerability [66]. Combining threat assessment with perceived response efficacy and level of confidence in one's ability to react appropriately, individuals determine their intended and actual behavior [66]. This type of reactionary coping behavior was observed when HIV became more prevalent; people's sexual behavior became much more cautious. Similarly, with genetic diseases such as diabetes or heart disease, individuals with heightened risks alter their behavior.

For the development of the model, it is difficult to predict which kind of information people will use to assess their "perceived threat". Logical choices for evaluating susceptibility will be the virus' proximity to home and its virulence, while mortality and morbidity rates are likely to determine perceived severity. In the case of SARS in Hong Kong, it was clear that people reacted to the news of infection spread by altering their daily routines depending on the severity of the news as well as the number of earlier deaths and infections. Furthermore, the survey study of Singapore found that people who were more anxious about becoming sick, practiced more precautionary measures [57]. Within the context of the model presented in Section 5 the death rate for the disease is not specified, thus the number of infected individuals is the best gauge reflecting the community members' vulnerability and severity of the threat.

In order to incorporate behavior change into our model we use $\pi_X(t)$as a feedback parameter that indicates the "concern level" within Community X on day t. If $\pi_X(t) = 1$ then there is no anxiety or behavior change within the community, for $\pi_X(t) = 0$ the community practically shuts down. Here are a few examples of what the population could use to gauge their risk levels, to define their $\pi_X(t)$ and consequently alter their behavior.[15]

1. Initially, the only information available to people will be the experience of their own community. People may use the number of yesterday's new infections ignoring everything that happened before yesterday as a measure of their risk. We quantify this "memoryless" approach of evaluating the risk factor as:

$$\pi_X^1(t, C_1) = \left(1 - \frac{\text{Number of infected people in Community X from day } t-1}{\text{The total population in Community X}}\right)^{C_1}$$

   C_1 is an input representing the importance of yesterday's information. For $C_1 = 1$ the number of infected individuals is linearly correlated to the risk level. As C_1 grows, the relevance and impact of yesterday's news grows exponentially.[16]

2. The news media are likely to present the cumulative number of infections within the community, this is another possible data set that people may use to estimate their risk levels. The related concern parameter is $\pi_X^2(t)$:

$$\pi_X^2(t, C_2) = \left(1 - \frac{\text{Number of infecteds in Community X up to and including day } t-1}{\text{The total population in Community X}}\right)^{C_2}$$

   C_2 is another input which represents the strength of impact of this cumulative information. Note that C_1 will have a smaller impact than C_2.[17]

3. It is also clear that if a city's adjacent communities all get infected the level of concern within the city will be heightened to reflect the suffering of neighboring cities. We will not include this in the following model, but refer the reader to the previously mentioned works for incorporating this factor.

In reality each individual is likely to change his or her behavior using a combination of all three described approaches. Yesterday's information is likely to be the most prevalent in the mind of the community, but community residents are also likely to remember the events of the past several weeks and be aware of the experiences of their neighbors. In our model we can uniformly alter the actions of people within each group using

$$\pi_X(t, C_1, C_2) = \pi_X^1(t, C_1) * \pi_X^2(t, C_2)$$

as the overall feedback parameter for behavior change. The parameters that will reflect this concern level through altered behavior are λ and p.

Let us focus on λ. People in all activity levels are likely to decrease the number of contacts that they have on a daily level. It is likely that children will be kept at home, public transportation will be avoided,

[15]There is no evidence suggesting one level of time granularity for tracking behavior over another, we use the most analytically logical time step: one generation of the flu. Throughout this section when we use the term "day", we are referring to one generation of the flu, which corresponds to 2–3 actual days.

[16]The authors have not been able to find the application of the behavior forecasting models to predict general behavior changes in the case of pandemic flu, but we have found numerous examples of HBM used to estimate altered human interactions to reduce their risk for HIV infection. Studies in this area indicate that there may be non-linear relationships between the factors and the dependent variable, thus we allowed for this variability through the addition of the C parameters [62].

[17]Studies in this area indicate that there may be non-linear relationships between the factors and the dependent variable, thus we allowed for this variability through the addition of the C parameters.

entertainment activities such as shopping or going to the movies will be temporarily suspended, even the number of contacts within the office may decrease as conference calls replace face-to-face contacts [61]. All these behavior changes were observed during the SARS outbreak [74]. To model this decrease in contact rate over time we propose multiplying λ^j, the contact rate for a group of activity level j by, $\pi_X(t, C_1, C_2, C_3)$, the perceived level of concern. So,

$$\lambda^j(t) = \lambda^j \pi_X(t, C_1, C_2, C_3)$$

The results seen in Graph 3, compare two identical populations except that one solely relies on yesterday's information and the other uses cumulative information up to and including yesterday to assess their risk. For the "memoryless" group represented by the gray curve the peak of the epidemic is lowered compared to a 'do nothing' or 'stay the course' policy. Also, the cumulative number of infections is decreased compared to 'do nothing,' but the virus maintains its presence within the community for a long period requiring sustained vigilance. Realistically, people will use more than just yesterday's information to access their risk. By "remembering" the number of people who were infected prior to yesterday, the group represented by the black curve diminishes the prevalence of the virus much faster. This shows the potential effectiveness of social distancing in reducing the cumulative burden of the infection. The main difference in the two group behaviors is the intensity of the interventions in the declining half of the outbreak. In the black curve interventions are maintained at a high level until the infection is completely depleted. For the gray curve the intensity of the interventions decreases in the later half of the outbreak. The moral of this story: Stay vigilant throughout the risk period.

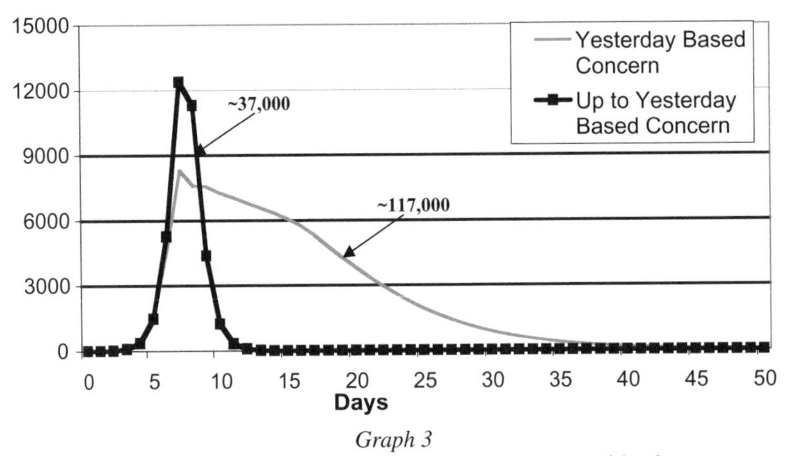

Graph 3
The impact of different types of behavior changes on the epidemic curve.

Now let's consider the human contact frequencies, the λ's, by different groups. The average number of interactions is likely to decrease, but it is unlikely that the λ's are going to change to the same degree for each activity level. Highly active people will be able to decrease their number of interactions dramatically, but less active people may be unable to sever their few, but vital ties to the community. For example, a politician may decide to cancel his/her campaign rally, stay at home and contact his office through telecommunication. On the other extreme, a retired handicapped grandmother whose only daily contact is with her grandson who brings her daily groceries, is not likely to change her pattern at all. This leads us to consider the scenario where only the highly active individuals, with many voluntary contacts, limit their daily contacts. The results are presented in Graph 4. Just changing the behavior of the highly

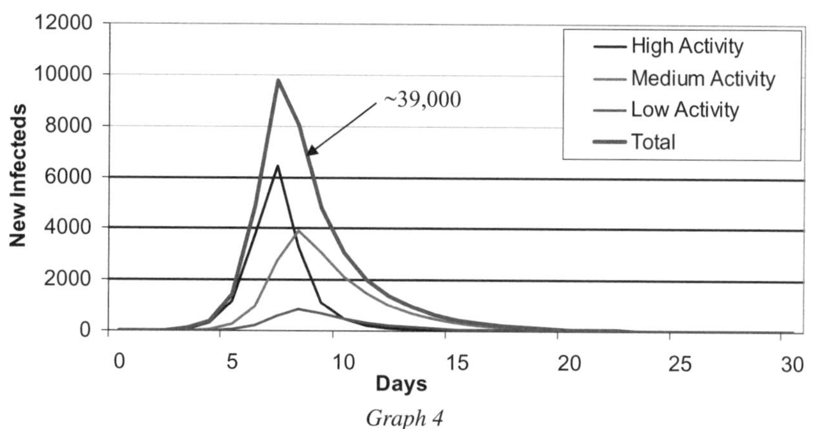

Graph 4

Infection spread within a community that reacts by social distancing only in the highly active group, to news over all previous days.

active individuals has a similar impact as decreasing the behavior of the entire community. If highly active individuals decrease their number of daily contacts by about 90% during the riskiest time, then a massive communitywide outbreak could be prevented. This result has multiple policy implications. It underlines the importance of closing schools since children have a high number of non-vital daily contacts within a school setting. All individuals who act as social focal points should decrease their average number of contacts, especially if this can be done without disrupting the community.

Overall, these models show the importance of including behavioral changes and their potential impact on disease transmission dynamics. From these models it becomes clear that the timing of behavioral changes and the behavior of the highly active people are some of the most important factors for transmission. Yet, the most important point is that behavioral changes such as limited social contact and improved hygiene must be included in future pandemic flu models, because they are first-order effects.

12. Tipping point boundary

In the case of an influenza pandemic, it is highly unlikely that any single intervention will be sufficient to stop the outbreak, but a combination of several measures may have the chance of halting the spread of infection. We demonstrated this above, reducing both λ and p by 30%, thereby reducing R_0 from 2.0 to 1.0. Hand hygiene measures are effective at slowing down transmission, but if the virus is highly virulent and has a reproductive number, $R_0 \approx 2$ or higher, hygiene improvements may be insufficient unless people also socially distance themselves. Many interventions that can be implemented within a community are not mutually exclusive, and need to be assessed and implemented together. In fact, the CDC has put out a document titled "Interim Pre-pandemic Planning Guidance: Community Strategy for Pandemic Influenza Mitigation in the United States. Early, Targeted, Layered Use of Nonpharmaceutical Interventions" discussing the importance of implementing multiple NPI's early on in the outbreak. We believe that this can be taken a step further; NPI's, as well as pre-pandemic low efficacy vaccines, antivirals, and other measures should all be considered and evaluated by modelers as bundles of interventions.

While we do not evaluate the interplay of these different interventions in this chapter, we do look at many of the interventions separately, and suggest an approach to presenting their combined efficacy. It is important to note that the effectiveness of the interventions will not be additive. For example, using alcohol based hand sanitizer is not going to be as incrementally beneficial to someone who already washes

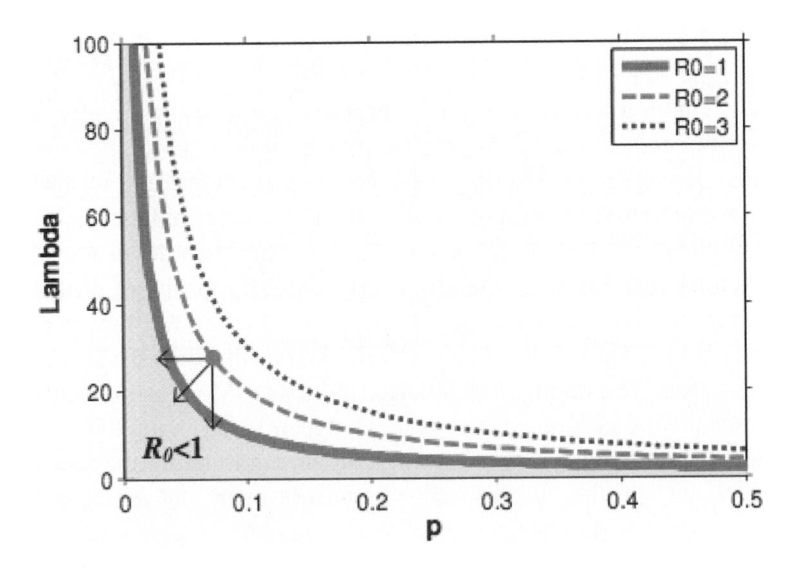

Fig. 1. The two dimensional tipping point boundary where $R_0 < 1$. To stop a pandemic, the set of interventions must decrease either λ or p or both to the gray area under the boundary.

his or her hands, but is still likely to be somewhat useful. Each additional measure will decrease the reproductive number until eventually R_0 may be below the pandemic causing threshold of 1. We propose creating a multidimensional "tipping point boundary" that illustrates what bundles of interventions are sufficient to lower the reproductive number to below 1. The effectiveness of various interventions will be on the different axes. All the points below the boundary will be combinations of interventions that will lead to disease extinction, and the points above are all the bundles of measures that will lead to exponential growth in the disease. All points precisely on the boundary have $R_0 = 1$, the herd immunity value.

Let us generalize the simple numerical example we did above, a simple two-dimensional illustration of the boundary concept. Recall we know that the reproductive number, $R_0 = \lambda p$, where λ is the average rate of contact and p is the conditional probability of infection. Both of these parameters are not disease-specific constants and can be altered through various hygienic, social distancing or even medical measures. In order to avoid an outbreak, the reproductive number needs to become less than 1, so the objective is to get to a scenario where as a result of all interventions $\lambda p < 1$. In Fig. 1 one can see the two-dimensional tipping point boundary. It is the thick solid line where $R_0 = 1$, and any points in the gray area under that boundary would cause a disease to die out in the population. Consider a flu strain that is comparable in virulence to the 1918–1919 pandemic[18] and, without any interventions, has an $R_0 = 2.0$. Thus without any interventions, the scenario can be described by a point on the dashed line in Fig. 1. In order to stop the transmission, the combination of NPI's and medical interventions needs to decrease either λ or p or both to the gray area, where $R_0 < 1$ and the virus will die out.

Our simple example can be extended to multiple dimensions, where each dimension represents a specific type of intervention rather than the aggregate. If developed, this type of tool would be tremendously helpful for decision makers who could test out their multiple intervention policies. We encourage future research in this area. Additionally, this illustration makes obvious that people, through NPI's, have the power to mitigate the outcome of the outbreak.

[18]The reproductive number for the 1918–1919 pandemic was estimated to be somewhere in the range of 1.8 to 3 [46].

13. Conclusions

Infectious diseases remain a leading cause of morbidity and mortality worldwide, with HIV, tuberculosis and malaria estimated to cause 10% of all deaths each year. Even the normal annual 'seasonal flu" in the USA kills an average of 36,000 people each year, comparable to the number lost in auto accidents. New pathogens continue to emerge in animal and human populations. Therefore, it is sensible to study the general implications of an infection propagation model in order to adopt broader, far reaching measures to strengthen the institutional, regulatory and technical capacity of the human health sector.

Even without a Kirchoff's Laws or a Newtonian physics of the flu, we hope that we have shown that simple models, some axiomatically derived and some based on empirical studies, can help us engineer a system for preparing for and responding to pandemic influenza. Much is now known, especially when we compare to our almost total lack of scientific knowledge in 1918, facing the infamous "Spanish Flu." We have emphasized human behavior as a key ingredient in mitigating the spread and effects of the flu. We took this track because the flu preparedness plans of many states treat pandemic flu as purely a medical issue. Their focus is on distribution of medicines such as anti-virals and vaccines, hospital surge capacity, coordinating a central command in emergency situations, and maintaining the health of health-care workers. While each of these is important, they are all responsive measures, all assuming that the physics of the spread of the disease is pre-ordained. We could not disagree more. We believe and hope that this chapter has shown that non-pharmaceutical interventions (NPI's), both government mandated and individually selected, may dramatically alter the course of the disease. This 'partial control' must be included, must be emphasized in any state or federal plan. This control is no less important than the flight controls that a pilot has for her aircraft or the dosage controls that an anesthesiologist has for his patient. All engineers understand the importance of controls, even partial ones, as NPI's are. But any engineered flu preparedness and response system must include them.

Catastrophes, natural disasters and terrorist attacks have all tested people's ability to cope with and adapt to extremely grim, demanding and dangerous circumstances. Whether through social distancing, cooperating and working together or relying on the help of others, people have demonstrated that they can adjust to various difficulties. An avian, swine or any other flu pandemic is not going to demolish our world. However, there is evidence that during SARS the losses that resulted initially were fueled and magnified by panic due to lack of public information and lack of guidance. Thus in order to minimize disruption, suffering and losses, the government must know how to win the trust and confidence of the population, calm the people, and organize and rally the public as a strategic partner in battling the disease.

Acknowledgements

Work on this chapter was supported by the Sloan Foundation of New York under a grant entitled, "*Decision-Oriented Analysis of Pandemic Flu Preparedness & Response*," and under a cooperative agreement with the U.S. Centers for Disease Control and Prevention (CDC), grant number 1 PO1 TP000307-01, LAMPS (Linking Assessment and Measurement to Performance in PHEP Systems), awarded to the Harvard School of Public Health Center for Public Health Preparedness (HSPHCPHP) and the Massachusetts Institute of Technology (MIT), Center for Engineering Systems Fundamentals (CESF). The discussion and conclusions in this chapter are those of the authors and do not necessarily represent the views of the Sloan Foundation, the CDC, the U.S. Department of Health and Human Services, Harvard or MIT. We thank Dr. Stan Finkelstein for helpful comments on an earlier draft.

References

[1] L.J.S. Allen, *Mathematical Epidemiology* (F. Brauer, P. van den Driessche and J. Wu, eds). New York: Springer, 2008.
[2] D.M. Bell, World Health Organization Working Group on Prevention of International and Community Transmission of SARS. Public health interventions and SARS spread, 2003. *Emerging Infectious Diseases.* Retrieved July 15, 2009 from http://www.cdc.gov/ncidod/EID/vol10no11/04-0729.htm, 2004.
[3] M.C.J. Bootsma and N.M. Ferguson, The effect of public health measures on the 1918 influenza pandemic in U.S. cities, *PNAS* **104**(18) (2007), 7588–7593.
[4] P. Caley, D.J. Philp and K. McCracken, Quantifying social distancing arising from pandemic influenza, *Journal of the Royal Society Interface* **5**(23) (2008), 631–639. doi:10.1098/rsif.2007.1197.
[5] S. Chick, H. Mamani and D. Simchi-Levi, Supply chain coordination and influenza vaccination. Retrieved July 15, 2009 from http://faculty.insead.edu/chick/papers/SCMFluv-OR-rev_v6.pdf, 2006.
[6] R.M. Christley, G.L. Pinchbeck, R.G. Bowers, D. Clancy, N.P. French, R. Bennett et al., Infection in social networks: Using network analysis to identify high-risk individuals, *American Journal of Epidemiology* **162**(10) (2005), 1024–1031. doi:10.1093/aje/kwi308.
[7] O.A.P. Diekmann, J.A.J. Heesterbeek and J.A.J. Metz, On the definition and computation of the basic reproductive ration R_0 in models for infectious diseases in heterogeneous populations, *Journal of Mathematical Biology* **28**(4) (1990), 365–382.
[8] A. Ekici, P. Keskinocak and J.L. Swann, Pandemic Influenza Response. Proceedings of the 40th Conference on Winter Simulation, in: *Winter Simulation Conference*, S. Mason, R. Hill, L. Mönch and O. Rose, eds, San Diego: The Society for Modeling and Simulation International, 2008.
[9] S. Eubank, H. Guclu, V.S.A. Kumar, M.V. Marathe, A. Srinivasan, Z. Toroczkai et al., Modeling disease outbreaks in realistic urban social networks, *Nature* **429** (2004), 180–184.
[10] A.R. Falsey, M.M. Criddle, J.E. Kolassa, R.M. McCann, C.A. Brower and W.J. Hall, Evaluation of a handwashing intervention to reduce respiratory illness rates in senior day-care centers, *Infection Control and Hospital Epidemiology* **20** (1999), 200–202.
[11] N.M. Ferguson, D.A.T. Cummings, S. Cauchemez, C. Fraser, S. Riley, A. Meeyai et al., Strategies for containing an emerging influenza pandemic in Southeast Asia, *Nature* **437**(7056) (2005), 209–214.
[12] Y.C. Fu, Measuring personal networks with daily contacts: A single-item survey question and the contact diary, *Social Networks* **27**(3) (2005), 169–186.
[13] Y. C. Fu, Contact diaries: Building archives of actual and comprehensive personal networks, *Field Methods* **19**(2) (2007), 194–217.
[14] T.C. Germann, K. Kadau, I.M. Longini, Jr. and C.A. Macken, Mitigation strategies for pandemic influenza in the United States, *PNAS* **103**(15), 5935–5940. doi: 10.1073/pnas.0601266103.
[15] L.M. Glass and R.J. Glass, Social contact networks for the spread of pandemic influenza in children and teenagers, *BMC Public Health* **8**(61) (2008). doi:10.1186/1471-2458-8-61.
[16] R.J. Glass, L.M. Glass, W.E. Beyeler and H.J. Min, Targeted social distancing design for pandemic influenza, *Emerging Infectious Diseases* **12**(11) (2006), 1671–1681.
[17] M. Greger, *Bird Flu: A virus of our own hatching.* New York: Lantern Books, 2006.
[18] S. Hashmi, M.A. Perches, S.N. Finkelstein and R.C. Larson, Estimating R_0 for A(H1N1) by State and Country. To appear, 2009.
[19] R.J. Hatchett, C.E. Mecher and M. Lipsitch, Public health interventions and epidemic intensity during the 1918 influenza pandemic, *PNAS* **104**(18) (2007), 7582–7587. doi:10.1073/pnas.0610941104.
[20] J.A.P. Heesterbeek, A brief history of R0 and a recipe for its calculation, *Acta Biotheoretica* **50**(3) (2002), 189–204.
[21] J.M. Heffernan, R.J. Smith and L.M. Wahl, Perspectives on the basic reproductive ratio, *Journal of the Royal Society Interface* **2**(4) (2005), 281–293.
[22] P.S. Herda, The 1918 influenza pandemic in Fiji, Tonga, and the Samoas, in: *New Countries and Old Medicine: Proceedings of an International Conference on the History of Medicine and Health*, L. Bryder and D.A. Dow, eds, Auckland: Pyramid Press, 1995, pp. 46–53.
[23] H.W. Hethcote, The mathematics of infectious diseases, *SIAM Review* **42**(4) (2000), 599–653.
[24] C. Hudson, Something in the air, *Daily Mail* (21 August 1999), 30–31.
[25] R.L. Itzwerth, C.R. MacIntyre, S. Shah and A.J. Plant, Pandemic influenza and critical infrastructure dependencies: Possible impact on hospitals, *Medical Journal of Australia* **185**(10) (2006), S70–S72.
[26] S. Inouye, Y. Matsudaira and Y. Sugihara, Masks for influenza patients: Measurements of airflow from the mouth, *Japanese Journal of Infectious Disease* **59** (2006), 179–181.
[27] T. Jefferson, R. Foxlee, C. Del Mar, L. Dooley, E. Ferroni, B. Hewak et al., Physical interventions to interrupt or reduce the spread of respiratory viruses: Systematic review, *British Medical Journal* **336** (2008), 77–80. doi:10.1136/bmj.39393.510347.

[28] W. Karesh and R.A. Cook, The human-animal link, *Foreign Affairs* **84**(4) (2005), 38–50.

[29] M. Keeling, The mathematics of diseases, *+plus magazine* **14** (2001).

[30] J.K. Kelso, G.J. Milne and H. Kelly, Simulation suggests that rapid activation of social distancing can arrest epidemic development due to a novel strain of influenza, *BMC Public Health* **9** (2009), 117. doi:10.1186/1471-2458-9-117.

[31] W.O. Kermack and A.G. McKendrick, A contribution to the mathematical theory of epidemics, *Proceeding of the Royal Society London* **115**(772) (1927), 700–721.

[32] W.O. Kermack and A.G. McKendrick, A contribution to the mathematical theory of epidemics: The problem of endemicity, *Proceeding of the Royal Society of London* **138**(834) (1932), 55–83.

[33] W.O. Kermack and A.G. McKendrick, A contribution to the mathematical theory of epidemics: Further studies of the problem of endemicity, *Proceeding of the Royal Society of London* **141**(843) (1933), 94–122.

[34] R.C. Larson, Simple models of influenza progression within a heterogeneous population, *Operations Research* **55**(3) (2007), 399–412.

[35] J.T.F. Lau, H. Tsui and J.H. Kim, Monitoring community responses to the ARS epidemic in Hong Kong: From day 10 to day 62, *Journal of Epidemiology and Community Health* **57** (2003), 864–870.

[36] J.T.F. Lau, H. Tsui, M. Lau and X. Yang, SARS transmission, risk factors, and prevention in Hong Kong, *Emerging Infectious Diseases* **10**(4) (2004), 587–592.

[37] Y. Li, G.M. Leung, J.W. Tang, X. Yang, C.Y.H. Chao, J.Z. Lin et al., Role of ventilation in airborne transmission of infectious agents in the built environment- a multidisciplinary systematic review, *Indoor Air* **17** (2007), 2–18.

[38] M. Lindholm, Stochastic epidemic models for endemic diseases: The effect of population heterogeneities, *Stockholm University Research Reports in Mathematical Statistics* **10** (2007).

[39] M. Lipsitch, C.E. Mills and J. Robins, Estimates of the basic reproductive number for 1918 pandemic influenza in the United States – implications for policy. *MIDAS, Models of Infectious Disease Agent Study.* Retrieved February 8, 2008 from http://www.ghsi.ca/documents/Lipsitch_et_al_Submitted%2020050916.pdf, 2007.

[40] M. Lipsitch, T. Cohen, B. Cooper, J.M. Robins, S. Ma, L. James et al., Transmission dynamics and control of severe acute respiratory syndrome, *Science* **300**(5627) (2003), 1966–1970. doi: 10.1126/science.1086616.

[41] M. Lipsitch, S. Riley, S. Cauchemez, A. Ghani and N.M. Ferguson, Managing and reducing uncertainty in an emerging influenza pandemic, *The New England Journal of Medicine* **361**(4) (2009), 112–115.

[42] J.Y.C. Lo, T.H.F. Tsang, Y.H.L. Leung, E.Y.H. Yeung, T. Wu and W.W.L. Lim, Respiratory infections during SARS outbreak, Hong Kong, 2003, *Emerging Infectious Diseases* **11**(111) (2005), 1738–1741.

[43] I.M. Longini, A. Nizam and S. Xu, Containing pandemic influenza at the source, *Science* **309**(5737) (2005), 1083–1087.

[44] S.P. Luby, M. Agboatwalla, D.R. Feikin, J. Painter, W. Billhimer, A. Altaf et al., Effect of handwashing on child health: A randomized controlled trial, *The Lancet* **366** (2005), 225–233.

[45] L.A. Meyers, B. Pourbohloul, M.E.J. Newman, D.M. Skowronski and R.C. Brunham, Network theory and SARS: Predicting outbreak diversity, *Journal of Theoretical Biology* **232**(1) (2005), 71–81.

[46] C.E. Mills, J.M. Robins and M. Lipsitch, Transmissibility of 1918 pandemic influenza, *Nature* **432** (2004), 904–906.

[47] MSNBC News Service, Record SARS deaths in Hong Kong. Retrieved April 15, 2003, from http://www. msnbc.com, 2003.

[48] MSNBC News Service, SARS hits airlines, Qantas cuts jobs. Retrieved April 9, 2003 from http://www.msnbc. com, 2003.

[49] I. Nasell, The threshold concept in stochastic epidemic and endemic models, in: *Epidemic models: Their structure and relations to data*, D. Mollison, ed., Cambridge: Cambridge University Press, 1995, pp. 71–83.

[50] L. Neergaard, Is it time to vaccinate more kids to stop flu's spread? Associated Press, October 5, 2005.

[51] K. Nelson and C.F.M. Williams, Infectious Disease Epidemiology: Theory and Practice, Jones & Bartlett Publishers, ISBN-13: 9780763728793, 2nd edition, 2006.

[52] K.R. Nigmatulina and R.C. Larson, Living with influenza: Impacts of government imposed and voluntarily selected interventions, *European Journal of Operational Research* **195** (2009), 613–627.

[53] K.R. Nigmatulina, Modeling and responding to pandemic influenza: Importance of population distributional attributes and non-pharmaceutical interventions (Ph.D. dissertation, Massachusetts Institute of Technology, 2009), 2009.

[54] H. Oshitani, Potential benefits and limitations of various strategies to mitigate the impact of an influenza pandemic, *Journal of Infection and Chemotherapy* **12** (2006), 167–171. doi:10.1007/s10156-006-0453-z.

[55] X. Pang, Z. Zhu, F. Xu et al., Evaluation of Control Measures Implemented in the Severe Acute Respiratory Syndrome Outbreak in Beijing, *Journal of the American Medical Association* **290**(24) (2003), 3215–3221.

[56] L.I. Pearlin, E.G. Menaghan, M.A. Lieberman and J.T. Mullan, The stress process, *Journal of Health and Social Behavior* **22**(4) (1981), 337–356.

[57] S.R. Quah and L. Hing-Peng, Crisis Prevention and Management During Outbreak, Singapore, *Emerging Infectious Diseases* **10**(2) (2004), 364–368.

[58] S. Riley, C. Fraser, C.A. Donnelly, A.C. Ghani, L.J. Abu-Raddad, A.J. Hedley et al., Transmission dynamics of the etiological agent of SARS in Hong Kong: Impact of public health interventions, *Science* (2003). doi:10.1126/science.1086478.

[59] L. Roberts, W. Smith, L. Jorm, M. Patel, R.M. Douglas and C. McGilchrist, Effect of infection control measures on the frequency of upper respiratory infection in child care: A randomized, controlled trial, *Pediatrics* **105** (2000), 738–742.
[60] M. Rosszell, SARS and its impact on tourism in Toronto, *Canadian Lodging Outlook and HVS International* (March 2003).
[61] M.Z. Sadique, W.J. Edmuns, R.D. Smith, W.J. Meerding, O. de Zwart, J. Brug et al., Precautionary behavior in response to perceived threat of pandemic influenza, *Emerging Infectious Diseases* **13**(9) (2007).
[62] B.L. Stiles and H.B. Kaplan, Factors influencing change behavior: Risk reduction for HIV infection, *Social Behavior and Personality* **32**(6) (2004), 511–534.
[63] Y. Shimbun, SDF planes to fly home Japanese stranded in event of flu pandemic. *Yomiuri Online*. Retrieved July 15, 2009 from http://www.yomiuri.co.jp/, 4 February 2009.
[64] R.D. Smith, Responding to global infectious disease outbreaks: lessons from SARS on the role of risk perception, communication and management, *Journal of Social Science and Medicine* **63**(12) (2006), 3113–3123.
[65] J.W. Schoen, SARS business impact spreading. In *MSNBC News Service*. Retrieved April 2, 2003 from http://www.msnbc.com.
[66] C. Tang and C. Wong, An outbreak of the severe acute respiratory syndrome: Predictors of health behaviors and effect of community prevention measures in Hong Kong, China, *American Journal of Public Health* **93**(11) (2003), 1887–1888.
[67] A. Underwood, Resurrecting a killer fly: A scientist explains why he re-created the lethal virus that killed millions in 1918 and what it can teach us about today's flu. Newsweek. 2005. Retrieved August 15, 2009 http://milkriverarchive.blogspot.com/2005/10/com-battle-against-poultry-flu.html, 7 October 2005.
[68] University of Twente, Netherlands, Health Communication. Retrieved July 15, 2009 from http://www.tcw.utwente.nl/theorieenoverzicht/Theory%20clusters/Health% 20Communication/, 2004.
[69] P. Van den Driessche and J. Watmough, Further notes on the basic reproduction number. In *Mathematical Epidemiology*, New York: Springer, 2008, pp. 159–178.
[70] H.W. Watson and F. Galton, On the probability of the extinction of families, *The Journal of the Anthropological Institute of Great Britain and Ireland* **4** (1875), 138–144.
[71] M.M. Weiss, P.D. Weiss, D.E. Weiss and J.B. Weiss, Disrupting the transmission of influenza A: Face masks and ultraviolet light as control measures, *American Journal of Public Health* **97** (2007), S32–S36.
[72] N.D. Weinstein and A.J. Rothman, Commentary: Revitalizing research on health behavior theories, *Health Education Research* **20**(3) (2005), 294–297.
[73] P. Whittle, *Probability* (pp. 124–125). Hoboken: John Wiley and Sons, 1976.
[74] P. Wiseman, SARS in Hong Kong behavior changes: Panic over illness has bigger impact than SARS itself. *USA Today*. Retrieved July 15, 2009 from http://www.usatoday.com, 13 April 2003.
[75] World Health Organization Writing Group, WHO. Nonpharmaceutical interventions for pandemic influenza, national and community measures, *Emerging Infectious Diseases* **12**(1) (2006).
[76] World Health Organization, WHO. Cumulative number of confirmed human cases of avian influenza A/(H5N1) reported to WHO. Retrieved July 15, 2009 from http://www.who.int/csr/disease/avian_influenza/country/en/, 2009.
[77] X. Zeng and M. Wagner, Modeling the effects of epidemics on routinely collected data, *Journal of the American Medical Informatics Association* **9** (2002), S17–S22.

Richard C. Larson received his Ph.D. from MIT where he is Mitsui Professor in the Department of Civil and Environmental Engineering (CEE) and in the Engineering Systems Division (ESD). He is currently founding director of the new Center for Engineering System Fundamentals. The majority of his career has focused on operations research as applied to services industries. He is author, co-author or editor of six books and author of over 85 scientific articles, primarily in the fields of urban service systems (esp. emergency response systems), queueing, logistics, disaster management, disease dynamics, dynamic pricing of critical infrastructures and workforce planning. His first book, Urban Police Patrol Analysis (MIT Press, 1972) was awarded the Lanchester Prize of the Operations Research Society of America (ORSA). He is co-author, with Amedeo Odoni, of *Urban Operations Research*, Prentice Hall, 1981 (republished in 2007). He served as President of ORSA, (1993–4), and INFORMS (2005), Institute For Operations Research and the Management Sciences. He has served as consultant to the World Bank, United Nations, Rand Corp., Kuwait Foundation for the Advancement of Science, Hibernia College in Ireland, Hong Kong University, the U.S. Department of Justice, American Airlines and various other corporations. With Structured Decisions Corporation (and its precedent companies – Q.E.D., ENFORTH and Public Systems Evaluation), Dr. Larson has undertaken major projects with the U.S. Postal Service, Citibank, American Airlines, the City of New York, Conagra, Diebold, BOC and other firms and organizations. Dr. Larson's research on queues has not only resulted in new computational techniques (e.g., the Queue Inference Engine and the Hypercube Queueing Model), but has also been covered extensively in national media. Dr. Larson served as Co-Director of the MIT Operations Research Center (over 15 years in that post). He is a member of the National Academy of Engineering and is an INFORMS Founding Fellow. He has been honored with the INFORMS President's Award and the Kimball Medal. He currently directs a research project on use of non-pharmaceutical interventions to combat pandemic flu and serves on the Institute of Medicine's Standing Committee on Medical Readiness and on its Board on Health Sciences Policy. From 1995 to mid 2003, Dr. Larson served as Director of MIT's CAES, Center for Advanced Educational

Services. Dr. Larson's position at CAES focused on bringing technology-enabled learning to students living on the traditional campus and to those living and working far from the university, perhaps on different continents. He was founder, with Glenn Strehle, of *MIT World.* http://mitworld.mit.edu. He is founding Director of LINC, Learning International Networks Consortium http://linc.mit.edu, an MIT-based international project that has held four international symposia and sponsored a number of initiatives in Africa, China and the Middle East. He recently started LINC's newest and largest initiative, BLOSSOMS, *Blended Learning Open Source Science or Math Studies*. http://blossoms.mit.edu.

Karima R. Nigmatulina is a Project Scientist in the disease modeling group at Intellectual Ventures located in Seattle, WA. In June 2009 she received her Ph.D. from MIT in Operations Research; her thesis was "Modeling and Responding to Pandemic Influenza: Importance of Population Distributional Attributes and Non-Pharmaceutical Interventions." A large portion of her doctoral research, done with her adviser Professor Richard Larson, is described or referenced throughout the chapter. While at MIT, Dr. Nigmatulina worked together with the MIT Emergency Preparedness Group to improve the university's preparedness for a pandemic. For her research in the area of pandemic influenza she received the first place award at the NAS Student Forum on Science and Technology Policy in 2008. Prior to MIT she received her B.S.E from Princeton University in Operations Research and Financial Engineering as well as four certificates from the Woodrow Wilson School of Public and International Affairs, Finance, Engineering and Management Systems, and Dance departments. Additionally, Dr. Nigmatulina is an early contributor to MIT BLOSSOMS, Blended Learning Open Source Science or Math Studies, offering interactive learning videos for high school math and science classes. http://blossoms.mit.edu. Her learning video is called, "Taking Walks, Delivering Mail: An Introduction to Graph Theory".

Information Knowledge Systems Management 8 (2009) 341–365
DOI 10.3233/IKS-2009-0146
IOS Press

Chapter 19

Understanding and enhancing the dental delivery system

Paul M. Griffin*
E-mail: pmg14@psu.edu

Abstract: Dental decay is the most prevalent chronic disease among both children and adults in the U.S. The Surgeon General's Report on Oral Health found that there had been marked improvement in oral health in many Americans over the last 50 years and that good oral health could be achieved by all Americans largely due to the presence of safe and effective interventions to prevent and control oral disease However, recent national data suggest that several disparities in dental care exist. In this chapter, we present a model of the dental health system as well as key differences with the general medical health system. We further discuss the major issues that the dental care delivery system will have to address in order to ensure that all Americans have access to effective interventions to prevent and control disease in an environment of decreasing supply of dentists per capita and potentially increasing demand. We then discuss strategies and policies to address these emerging issues in the context of this model. Finally, we conclude with suggestions on how engineering techniques could be used to improve the system.

1. Background

Dental caries is the most prevalent chronic disease among U.S. children and adults. It is also the most prevalent untreated disease [29,60]. Over 50% of youth have experienced dental caries by age 15 and this value increases to over 90% for adults by age 50 [29]. Dental disease is also costly. U.S. dental expenditures in 2006 were 91.5 billion dollars [20]. This amount was roughly 20% of that spent on physician and clinical professional services (Table 1).

The first ever Surgeon General's Report (SGR) on Oral Health in 2000 [75] found that there had been marked improvement in most American's oral health over the last 50 years and that good oral health could be achieved by all Americans largely due to the presence of safe and effective interventions to prevent and control oral disease [75]. Indeed analyses of national survey data indicate that this trend in improved oral health has continued from the 1990s to the present for all age groups with the exception of decay in primary teeth [29]). The SGR, however, also found that significant disparities in oral health status existed by race/ethnicity and income. Recent national data indicate that these disparities still exist (Tables 2 and 3).

Although lower income children have access to public dental insurance, dental utilization is significantly lower among these children compared to their higher-income counterparts. Among the very young, children from families with incomes exceeding 400% of the federal poverty level (FPL) were about 67% more likely to have a past year dental visit than children from families with incomes less than 100% of the FPL in 2005 (Table 4). Among elementary school aged children and youth, this comparison increases to 75% and 100%, respectively.

1389-1995/09/$17.00

Table 1
National health expenditures (billions) on dental and physician and clinical professional services and source of payment: Calendar years 2000–2006

Year	Dental professional services				Physician and clinical professional services			
	Total	Out of pocket (% of total)	Private insurance (% of total)	Public (% of total)	Total	Out of pocket (% of total)	Private insurance (% of total)	Public (% of total)
2000 (Levit et al., 2002)	60	26.9 (44.8)	30.1 (50.2)	2.8 (4.7)	286.4	33.2 (11.6)	136.7 (47.7)	95.2 (33.2)
2001 (Levit et al., 2003)	65.6	28.5 (43.4)	33.2 (50.6)	3.7 (5.6)	313.6	35 (11.2)	150.9 (48.1)	105.4 (33.6)
2002 (Levit et al., 2004)	70.3	30.9 (44.0)	34.8 (49.5)	4.5 (6.4)	339.5	34.3 (10.1)	166.9 (49.2)	114.8 (33.8)
2003 (Smith et al., 2005)	74.3	32.9 (44.3)	36.5 (49.1)	4.9 (6.6)	369.7	37.6 (10.2)	183.6 (49.7)	123 (33.3)
2004 (Smith et al., 2006)	81.5	36.1 (44.3)	40.5 (49.7)	4.9 (6.0)	399.9	40.0 (10.0)	194 (48.5)	138.3 (34.6)
2005 (Catlin et al., 2007)	86.6	38.3 (44.2)	43.1 (49.8)	5.2 (6.0)	421.2	42.5 (10.1)	203.3 (48.3)	148.5 (35.3)
2006 (Catlin et al., 2008)	91.5	40.6 (44.4)	45.3 (49.5)	5.5 (6.0)	447.6	46.2 (10.3)	219.7 (49.1)	153.1 (34.2)

*Sources of funding do not sum to 100% because did not include other private as funding category, which was included in total expenditures.

Table 2
Prevalence of any and untreated dental caries in permanent teeth and missing permanent teeth by family income status among dentate persons of various ages: NHANES 1999–2004

Age	Any (DMFT)		Untreated (DT)		Edentulism	
	< 100% FPL	> 200% FPL	< 100% FPL	> 200% FPL	< 100% FPL	> 200% FPL
6–11*	28.28 (2.28)	16.31 (1.33)	11.76 (1.74)	3.57 (0.66)		
12–19†	65.55 (1.40)	54.00 (1.49)	27.15 (1.99)	12.86 (1.33)		
20–64‡	91.48 (0.65)	91.19 (0.47)	39.26 (1.63)	20.56 (0.90)	9.28 (1.12)	2.35 (0.20)
65+§	83.47 (2.52)	95.53 (0.72)	33.22 (3.31)	14.22 (1.21)	44.19 (3.63)	17.25 (1.27)

*(Dye et al., 2004): Series 11: Tables 10 and 11.
†(Dye et al., 2004): Series 11: Tables 25 and 26.
‡(Dye et al., 2004): Series 11: Tables 40, 41, and 47.
§(Dye et al., 2004): Series 11: Tables 61, 62, and 68.

Table 3
Mean number of filled, decayed, missing, and decayed, missing and filled permanent teeth by family income status among dentate persons of various ages: NHANES 1999–2004

Age	DMFT		FT		DT		MT	
	< 100% FPL	> 200% FPL	< 100% FPL	> 200% FPL	< 100% FPL	> 200% FPL	< 100% FPL	> 200% FPL
6–11*	0.63 (0.06)	0.32 (0.03)	0.44 (0.03)	0.26 (0.03)	0.18 (0.03)	0.05 (0.01)	–	–
12–19†	2.88 (0.14)	2.28 (0.12)	2.17 (0.16)	1.94 (0.11)	0.62 (0.06)	0.30 (0.04)	0.09 (0.01)	0.04 (0.01)
20–64‡	10.22 (0.24)	10.30 (0.13)	4.56 (0.20)	7.87 (0.13)	1.51 (0.11)	0.48 (0.04)	4.15 (0.19)	1.95 (0.08)
65+§	17.30 (0.55)	18.15 (0.21)	4.10 (0.35)	10.24 (0.17)	1.01 (0.15)	0.29 (0.04)	12.19 (0.75)	7.61 (0.22)

*(Dye et al., 2004): Series 11: Table 12.
†(Dye et al., 2004): Series 11: Table 27.
‡(Dye et al., 2004): Series 11: Table 42.
§(Dye et al., 2004): Series 11: Table 63.

Adults from higher-income families are about twice as likely to report a past year dental visit than adults from lower-income families (Table 4). Adults and older adults in lower-income families may have no access to public dental insurance. A multivariate analysis of healthcare expenditures among lower-income persons with insurance found that for children, utilization did not differ by whether insurance was public (Medicaid/SCHIP) or private, whereas for adults, dental utilization was higher for those with

Table 4
% of U.S. popoulation reporting past year dental visit by age and income: Medial Expenditure Panel Survey

Age in years	Federal Poverty level	Year					
		2000	2001	2002	2003	2004	2005
2–5	< 100%	28.76	21.1	24.74	27.81	29.8	26.66
2–5	100%–199%	24.61	23.98	24.05	26.92	29.04	31.34
2–5	200%–399%	30.74	30.07	28.3	33.22	31.38	33.26
2–5	⩾ 400%	37.54	36.24	43.9	43.59	53.29	45.02
6–11	< 100%	35.33	32.68	38.81	41.36	42.92	42.71
6–11	100%–199%	40.44	43.03	43.85	42.62	47.79	45.74
6–11	200%–399%	56.1	54.79	58.42	63.01	63.32	59.13
6–11	⩾ 400%	72.03	77.04	72.19	74.52	76.07	75.95
12–19	< 100%	27.18	28.72	31.7	29.28	32.35	35.01
12–19	100%–199%	35.34	32.45	33.42	38.46	34.6	36.51
12–19	200%–399%	52.05	53.1	53.21	53.67	50.88	52.41
12–19	⩾ 400%	64.99	67.91	70.89	71.79	68.78	69.62
20–29	< 100%	22.81	22.26	20.82	23.72	20.38	20.84
20–29	100%–199%	23.21	24.12	25.7	25.48	25.85	29.63
20–29	200%–399%	31.34	32.81	33.85	34.3	32.39	35.25
20–29	⩾ 400%	38.54	45.7	46.07	45.52	48.63	43.31
30–39	< 100%	25.03	21.85	20.74	19.53	20.9	21.01
30–39	100%–199%	29.04	24.33	26.57	25.73	23.35	23.13
30–39	200%–399%	40.31	40.93	38.2	40.78	42.28	36.69
30–39	⩾ 400%	49.99	54.04	54.72	53.92	53.22	52.21
40–49	< 100%	30.04	24.09	21.32	20.6	23.37	21.21
40–49	100%–199%	32.37	30.72	28.33	27.06	29.72	25.62
40–49	200%–399%	41.08	42.29	41.59	42.17	40.71	39.8
40–49	⩾ 400%	54.31	55.91	59.13	59.4	56.52	57.12
50–59	< 100%	25.53	31.32	28.86	28.74	24.26	27.92
50–59	100%–199%	25.12	33.29	27.83	29.32	28.27	25.68
50–59	200%–399%	38.7	40.66	42.62	39.21	43.37	41.9
50–59	⩾ 400%	57.88	60.72	62.51	62.44	61.59	60.72
60–69	< 100%	22.49	27.63	33.67	28.73	31.93	27.09
60–69	100%–199%	30.06	29.38	32.18	28.44	34.25	30.52
60–69	200%–399%	38.97	43.57	41.41	42.9	40.09	42.63
60–69	⩾ 400%	58.64	58.21	58.57	62.19	61.05	62.41
70–79	< 100%	28.2	30.03	28.77	32.91	27.6	35.83
70–79	100%–199%	28.57	26.01	32.37	34.5	28.39	29.13
70–79	200%–399%	43.48	43.6	40.9	44.64	45.95	45.67
70–79	⩾ 400%	56.72	55.02	59.93	58.11	64.93	62.58
80+	< 100%	25.9	28.51	24.8	23.37	24.7	28.76
80+	100%–199%	24.77	32.54	28.43	29.6	28.03	27.94
80+	200%–399%	38.19	34.38	40.97	38.44	38.33	44.31
80+	⩾ 400%	50.39	46.96	53.4	55.42	43.28	46.61

private insurance. The difference in the findings for children and adults was attributed to the fact that Medicaid dental coverage for children is mandatory, whereas for adults it is optional [44]. Medicaid frequently only covers emergency dental care for adults [75] and it should also be noted that Medicare does not cover routine dental services.

The SGR also voiced concerns that the declining dentist to population ratio may decrease the capability of the dental workforce to meet the emerging demands of society and provide required services efficiently [75]. The number of active dentists per 100,000 U.S. resident population peaked at 60.2 in 1994 (Table 5 [5]). This value decreased to 59.0 in 2000 and is expected to further decline to 54.3 in

Table 5
Professionally active dentists per 100,000 U.S. resident population: ADA; US Department of Commerce*

Year	Dentists per 100,000 U.S. resident population
1991	59.9
1992	60.0
1993	60.1
1994	60.2
1995	60.0
1996	59.9
1997	59.3
1998	59.5
1999	59.2
2000	59.0
2005	58.0
2010	56.7
2015	55.5
2020	54.2

(Burt & Eklund, 1999, p. 34).

2020. This trend is largely attributable to a decrease in the number of students accepted into dental schools – the number of dental school graduates declined from a high of 5,756 in 1982 to a low of 3,778 in 1993 [5]. Since 1993 this value has been gradually increasing – in 2002 there were 4349 graduating dentists [59]. The increase in graduates, however, has not kept pace with the increase in population. The dentist to population ratio has steadily declined since 1994.

In addition, there has been a significant increase in potential demand for dental services due to the increase in both the number of adults with some natural teeth as well as the total number of natural teeth retained per adult, the relevant unit of treatment. Findings from the two most recent National Health and Nutrition Examination Surveys (NHANES tracks nationally representative indicators of health status over time, the two most recent rounds were conducted in 1988–1994 and 1999–2004) indicated that the number of adults with at least one natural tooth increased from 93.89% to 96.24% among adults, aged 20 to 64 years and from 66.10% to 72.78% among adults, aged 65+ [29]. There was also a significant increase in the mean number of retained teeth among dentate adults. As a result, the total number of teeth increased by over 600,000 (Table 6). Further evidence that the quantity of dental services demanded may exceed supply is that inflation in the price of dental services has outpaced that for physician services since 1997 (Fig. 1).

Thus, two major issues that the dental care delivery system will have to address are 1) ensuring that all Americans have access to effective interventions to prevent and control disease and 2) containing costs in an environment of decreased supply of dentists per capita and potentially increasing demand. This chapter describes the dental health system using a modified version of a model set forth by Andersen that is commonly used in health services research [7]. We then discuss strategies/policies to address these two emerging issues in the context of this model. Finally, we conclude with suggestions for needed research by engineers.

2. Dental care system

From a societal perspective, the goal of the dental care system (Fig. 2) is to maximize dental health outcomes (perceived and evaluated dental health status which in turn lead to enhanced quality of life)

Table 6
Increase in number of teeth: NHANES 1988–1984 to NHANES 1999–2004

Age	NHANES 1988–1994			NHANES 1999–2004			Change (000s)
	Population (000s)	Mean Teeth per person	Total Teeth (000s)	Population (000s)	Mean Teeth per person	Total Teeth (000s)	
6 to 11*	22,132	28.0	619,475	23,908	28.0	669,185	49,710
12 to 19†	27,812	27.9	776,511	31,062	27.0	839,606	63,095
20 to 34‡	59,525	27.0	1,604,794	54,108	27.4	1,481,477	−123,317§
35 to 49‡	52,319	24.5	1,283,385	60,472	25.6	1,548,688	265,303*
50 to 64‡	31,383	20.7	649,628	41,214	22.7	935,558	285,930*
65 to 74**	17,657	13.6	240,946	17,647	14.7	259,622	18,675
75+**	11,256	9.8	110,444	14,263	12.6	179,904	69,460††
ALL	222,084		5,285,183	242,674		5,914,039	628,856

*(Dye et al., 2004): Series 11 Table 12.
†(Dye et al., 2004): Series 11 Table 27.
‡(Dye et al., 2004): Series 11 Table 42.
§Difference in mean missing teeth per person statistically significant between surveys.
**(Dye et al., 2004): Series 11 Table 67 and 68.
††Mean number of teeth obtained by multiplying % dentate by mean number of teeth per dentate person. The difference between % dentate increased between surveys.

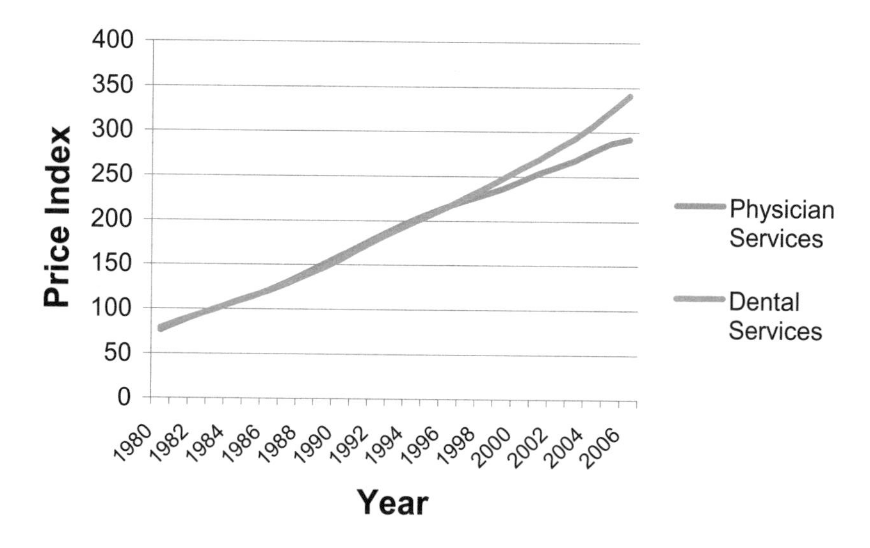

Fig. 1. Trends in consumer price index for physician and dental services [16].

within the constraints of available resources. The five basic components of the system – the environment (E), population characteristics (P), supply of dental personnel (D), individual dental health behaviors (B), and finally dental health outcomes (O) – are described below. This section elaborates this representation of the system and the following section discusses how it can be employed to enhance dental care access and outcomes.

2.1. Environment

The environment includes the dental delivery system as well as external factors not included in the other components that are exogenous to or beyond the control of the delivery system. Elements of the

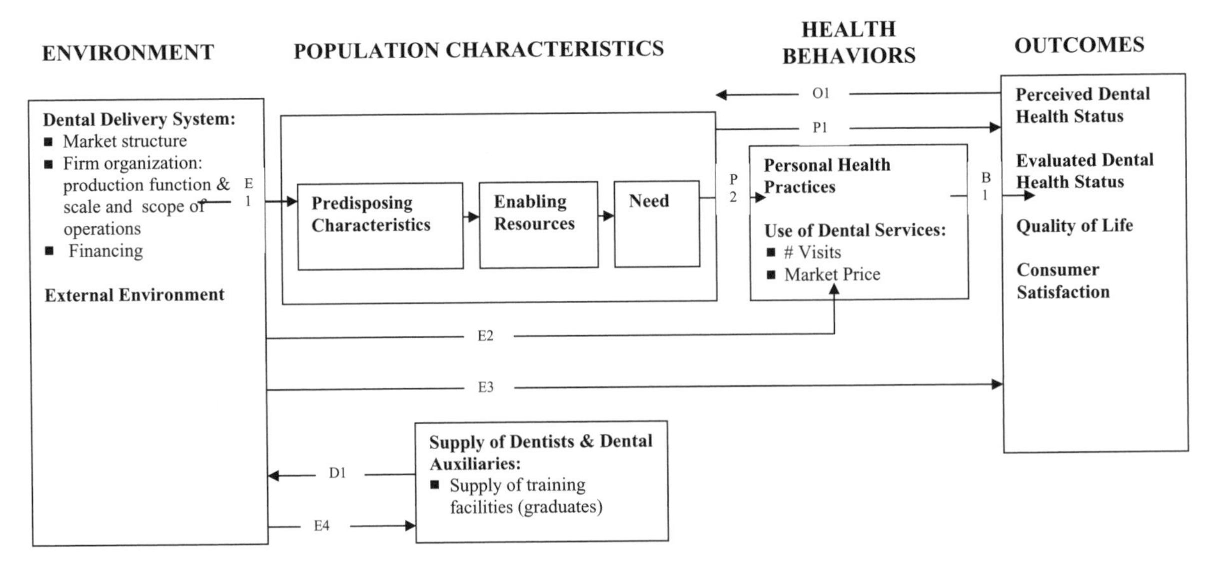

Fig. 2. Overview of dental care system.

dental delivery system include 1) the market structure in which dental firms operate; 2) the organization of individual dental firms, (e.g., production function, firm scale (output per firm), and scope (degree of specialization); and 3) available financing options for care.

Because much has been written on drivers of inefficiency in the medical care delivery system, throughout this section we will compare the dental delivery system to that in medical. It should also be noted that the dental profession has evolved parallel to, but separately from the medical profession. Medicine and dentistry have different educational, health care delivery, and payment systems. The dental market consist of thousands of small, independent firms – dental care is typically delivered in private dental offices [75] of which almost 90% have 2 or fewer dentists (68.7% sole practitioners, 19.6% 2 dentists, and 11.7% group practice). Dental practices tend to be more integrated in terms of ownership of equipment compared to medical, in which equipment may be owned by hospitals where physicians have privileges. About 92% of dentists own their practice whereas only 25% of physicians are solo practitioners or self employed [55].

The medical conditions treated by dentists are fairly narrow in scope. The majority of procedures delivered are to treat decay or gum disease. Dental offices are typically quite similar in the scope of services provided. About 80% of dentists are general practitioners compared to 40% in medical [75]. The remaining dentists serve as specialists in one or more of nine ADA designated specialty areas [75] and over 50% of these specialists are orthodontists. It is anticipated that in the future the ratio of general dentist to specialist will decrease from 4:1 to 3:1 [5]. As a general rule the same dental team is likely to provide care over the medical condition cycle – prevention, diagnosis and treatment, and management and control. In addition, the same dental team will likely deliver all specialty services (e.g., radiology, anesthesiology, and surgery) to the patient. Thus compared to medical care, dental care is more likely to have the following attributes [64]: 1) dedicated to one medical condition, 2) integrated in that for the same episode all services are likely to be provided by the same team; and 3) coordinated in that again the same team will provide care over the cycle of the dental condition.

The professional structure of dentistry, however, can limit competition. Whereas only 30% of doctors belong to their professional association, the American Medical Association, over 70% of dentists belong to the American Dental Association. This professional structure reinforces dentistry's leverage over the content of governmental legislation and regulations affecting the profession, thereby influencing the market for dental care [49]. As a result, there are both barriers to entry such as strict licensure requirements in some states and restrictions to allowing non-dentist professionals, e.g. dental hygienists, to practice without the supervision of a dentist. The result of the latter restriction would also impact the dental production function since a fixed input, the dentist, is required in the provision of virtually all dental services in most states.

Dental productivity as measured by real dental expenditures per dentist increased by 1.31% per annum from 1960 to 1998. Annual growth rates varied greatly over this time span equaling 3.95% from 1960–1974, −0.13% from 1974–1991, and 1.05% from 1991 to 1998 [12]. The negative growth rate from 1960 to 1974 may be attributable to a large supply of dentists that may have exceeded demand for dental care. The growth rate in dentist productivity outpaced that of the non farm business sector from 1960 to 1974 (2.8%) but lagged behind thereafter (1.2% from 1973 to 1979, 1.4% from 1979 to 1990, and 1.5% from 1990 to 2000) [17]. Major inputs into the dental production function include dentists, dental hygienists, dental assistants, office staff, equipment, and office space. One study found that output increased by the following amounts when the following inputs were increased by 10%: dentist hours 2.92%, hygienist hours 2.74%, dental assistant hours 1.28%, other staff hours 3.69%, and office space (which is also a proxy for equipment) 1.77% [5].

Dentistry also differs from medical in terms of billing codes. There are no uniformly accepted diagnostic billing codes and thus procedural codes are used for electronic billing [9,45]. Few dental offices keep electronic records and there is no standard record system [45].

Adults are less likely to have dental insurance than medical insurance – 55% versus 86% in 2001 [26]. Dental coverage was added to insurance plans well after other types of health services were covered. From 1967 to 1981 the percentage of adults with dental insurance increased from 2% to 38%. Thus, the addition of dental insurance occurred largely during a period of high inflation. Some have argued that this was the main reason for the increase in dental insurance coverage; as individuals were pushed into higher tax brackets, increased fringe benefits, e.g., dental insurance coverage, became more appealing [51]. This would suggest that dental insurance coverage would be more sensitive to taxes on employer contributions to health plans.

The percentage of dental care expenditures financed by private insurance, 50%, is quite similar to that in medical. Dental financing differs from medical in that a much smaller portion is financed by the government (about 35% of medical compared to 5% for dental; Table 3). For dental the gap in government financing is covered by out of pocket expenditures (about 45% for dental compared to about 10% for medical). Thus in dental there are two primary payers – private insurance companies and patient out of pocket expenditures. Insurance companies could conceivably have greater bargaining power than individual patients and thus it is possible that costs could be shifted from insurance companies to private patients. One constraint on shifting costs to private pay consumers would be that the demand for dental care is fairly price elastic [30,51]. The lack of consolidation among dentists (consolidation has occurred in medical in response to increased bargaining power of insurers) would suggest that either insurance companies do not have bargaining power or if they do, that the discounts in services provided to insured patients are being offset by costs of services provided to private pay patients. It is possible that consolidation of dental firms could increase if dental insurance coverage increased. Further evidence that dental insurance companies have not gained bargaining power is that dentists are still the party that determines the appropriateness of care. At present, billing codes to insurance companies are not by diagnosis but by procedure. Finally, more generous insurance coverage has a much larger impact on probability of a dental visit than the cost per patient [51].

Table 7
Percentage of service covered by dental insurance type of service: Source 2002 survey of employers providing dental insurance to employees (n = 1265)

% service covered	Preventive	Minot restorative	Major restorative
90 to 100	88.5%	10.0%	0.6%
80–89	1.4%	75.6%	9.6%
70 to 79	8.6%	6.1%	2.6%
60 to 69	0.7%	1.4%	15.7%
50 to 59	0.1%	6.5%	70.9%
40 to 49	0.7%	0.3%	0.6%
30 to 39	0.0%	0.1%	0.0%

Dental insurance plans differ from those for medical insurance. This is primarily due to the differences between demand for dental care and medical care. Dental incidents tend to be predictable and not catastrophic [18], typically don't constitute a major loss to the patient, are not infrequent, and typically are not beyond the control of the individual. Thus dental insurance may be more vulnerable to both moral hazard (presence of insurance leads to additional claims) and adverse selection (patients may time the purchase of dental insurance to when they have higher need). As a result dental insurance typically covers a predefined set of services and prevention as opposed to true insurance that covers unpredictable and catastrophic events. A 2002 survey of 1265 employers who provided dental insurance to their employees found that the median annual maximum amount covered was $1,500. The plans were also more likely to cover the full costs (90% to 100%) of preventive care (90% of respondents; Table 7) than the full costs of major restorative care (9.7%).

The gold standard study on the effect of dental insurance on utilization and expenditures was the Rand Health Insurance Experiment (HIE) conducted from 1974 to 1982. This is the most recent study that randomly assigned participants to difference insurance plans. Random allocation is necessary because of selection bias – sicker patients may be more likely to purchase insurance with lower co-pays and thus higher utilization under such plans may be attributable to differences in both patient health status and extent of coverage. It should be noted that the HIE did provide "catastrophic coverage" to all study participants. The maximum amount paid per year was $1,000, which translates to roughly $3,300 in 2008 year dollars. The HIE found there was a significant surge in demand during the first year of more generous coverage. The first-year response to cost sharing was nearly twice that in the second year [51]. The HIE found that the first year increase in demand for dental due to more generous insurance was greater than that for medical whereas in the second year onward demand was more responsive for medical than for dental. Dental expenditures rose by 46% when the copayment rate fell from 95% to 0% [51]. About 2/3 of the increase was attributable to an increase in the likelihood of visiting a dentist. The response for dental co-insurance, however, was more sensitive to income than was medical, i.e., there was a much larger reduction in utilization in response to lowering co-insurance amounts among lower income than among higher income groups [38].

The HIE found that levels of total dental disease (treated and untreated decay and missing teeth) did not vary by level of coinsurance [10]. Persons with a 95% coinsurance rate were more likely to have higher levels of untreated decay and lower levels of treated decay. One limitation of the HIE was that the time horizon (average enrollment period was 3.67 years) may have not been sufficiently long to capture the benefits of prevention. Subgroup analyses indicated that more generous insurance benefited those most in need of care – those with less education and higher levels of unmet treatment needs at baseline.

The external environment or exogenous variable would include the composition of the population in terms of race/ethnicity and age as well as community preventive programs (community water fluoridation,

Table 8
Prevalence of any and untreated dental caries in permanent teeth and missing permanent teeth by educational attainment among dentate persons of various ages: NHANES 1999–2004

	Any (DMFT)		Untreated (DT)		Edentulism	
Age	< HS*	> HS	< HS	> HS	< HS	> HS
20–64†	85.93 (0.90)	92.91 (0.41)	45.20 (1.87)	16.48 (0.75)	8.07 (0.76)	1.66 (0.28)
65+‡	83.73 (1.61)	97.04 (0.67)	26.16 (2.31)	14.30 (1.31)	43.32 (2.56)	13.65 (1.10)

*HS = high school.
†(Dye et al., 2004): Series 11: Tables 40, 41, and 47.
‡(Dye et al., 2004): Series 11: Tables 61, 62, and 68.

policies related to tobacco use, free or highly subsidized treatment programs and public education campaigns promoting oral health) and the regulatory environment (e.g., practice acts).

2.2. Population characteristics

Population characteristics primarily influence demand for dental care. Certain knowledge, values, and attitudes may predispose a person to seek dental care. For example, persons who value oral health more highly may be more likely to practice better oral hygiene at home as well as to consume higher levels of clinical preventive services. Similarly consumption of clinical preventive services may increase with increased knowledge as to the benefits of such services. Studies indicate that more educated adults are more likely to know of the benefits of dental sealants, proven to be effective in reducing dental disease [42], and that their children are more likely to have sealants [34]. Higher educational attainment is associated with higher levels of dental utilization. Adults, aged 25+ years with some college, were more than twice as likely to have visited a dentist in the past year as adults who did not complete high school (58.48% versus 20.72% [54]). This association held even after controlling for income; among adults with family incomes less than the Federal Poverty Level, those with greater than a high school education were more than twice as likely to have visited a dentist as those with less than a high school education (38.73% versus 15.3%) and among adults with family incomes equal to or exceeding 400% of the Federal Poverty Level −63.43% of those with greater than a high school education reported a past year dental visit compared to 38.73% of those with less than a high school education [54]. Higher dental utilization in turn may translate into lower levels of unmet dental treatment needs – adults who did not graduate from high school were about twice as likely to have untreated dental decay and more likely to have lost all their natural teeth as were adults with at least some college (Table 8).

Increased resources may also enable a person to both seek and receive more dental care. Dental utilization is strongly associated with income (Table 4). Adults in the highest income bracket are about twice as likely to have visited a dentist within the past year as those in the lowest bracket. Dentists are also more likely to locate in areas with higher average incomes [71] and thus income might enable demand by decreasing travel time for dental care as well as increasing one's ability to pay for dental care. Studies also indicate that among persons living in families with lower incomes consumption of free dental services decreases as the travel distance to a dentist increases [53]. Finally, we note that travel time to dentists may vary greatly by geographic region. This variation may be partially attributable to variation in per capita income.

Demand for dental care is more responsive to increases in income than is demand for medical care. Medical care is perceived as a necessity – the percentage increase for medical care resulting from a 10% increase in income is less than 10% whereas dental care is perceived to be a luxury good – the percentage increase for dental care resulting from a 10% increase in income is greater than 10%. Well designed econometric studies in the mid 1970s (when a greater percentage of dental expenditures were paid out of pocket) found that a 10% increase in income resulted in a 17% increase in dental expenditures and a 15% increase in dental visits [30].

Finally, population characteristics may influence perceived dental health, which in turn influences utilization of dental services. All other things being equal, dental utilization should be higher among those with a perceived need. There is also evidence that there is interaction between dental need and income in terms of their influence on demand. An analysis of Norwegian survey data found that the increase in demand for dental care due to income was lower among younger cohorts with less disease than for older cohorts with more disease [39].

2.3. Supply of dentists and dental auxiliaries

Supply of dental services will depend on labor supply and their productivity. Supply of dental personnel will depend on the number of training facilities for dentists and dental auxiliaries and their respective class sizes. In 2003 there were 56 accredited dental education programs in the United States [59]. As discussed earlier in this chapter there was a marked decline in dental school capacity in the 1980s and 1990s – seven dental schools closed resulting in a nationwide loss of approximately 600 graduates per year [59]. In response to the decrease in capacity, the number of graduates reached a 30 year low of 3,778 in 1993, a 34% decline from its peak in 1984. Since 1993 the number of graduating dentists has gradually increased, equaling 4,349 in 2002. It should be noted that there was fairly low demand for a dental education during the late 1980s and early 1990s (perhaps attributable to a perceived oversupply of dentists) – dental schools averaged only 1.2 applicants for each available position. By 2002, the number of applicants had increased by over 50% [59]. Decreasing dental school capacity typically takes about 10 years to influence current number of practicing dentists [18]. In response to the decrease in capacity in the late 1980s, the rate of growth of active dentists began to decline in the 1990s and the dentist to population ratio began to decrease around 1995.

In contrast to dental education, there has been an increase in allied dental education programs. From 1990 to 2003, the number of programs providing dental assistant training increased from 255 to 259 and from 202 to 266 for dental hygienists [59]. Total enrollment in dental hygiene schools increased from 9,309 in 1990 to 13,016 in 2002 [59]. The increase in enrollment in dental assistant training programs was not as large as that for dental hygienists. First year enrollment increased from 5,500 to 7,304 [59].

2.4. Health behaviors

Health behaviors (B in Fig. 2) include personal health practices and consumption of clinical care (quantity and price), the latter being a function of both potential supply and potential demand of dental services. Health behaviors in turn directly link to dental health outcomes such as perceived and clinically assessed dental health status.

Dentistry has highly effective interventions to prevent dental disease. The Surgeon General's Report attributed the remarkable improvement in oral health over the past half century to the strong science base for prevention of oral disease that has been developed and applied in the community, in clinical practice, and in the home [75]. In addition, preventive interventions in dentistry, especially those offered at the community level offer high value (defined as health outcome per dollar cost spent); both community water fluoridation and school-based-sealant programs that target children at higher risk for tooth decay typically have been shown to be cost-saving [74]. The report also stated that there was little doubt that widespread use of fluoride has been a major contributor to the secular decline in tooth decay. Recent

Table 9
Percentage of patients receiving selected dental services from private practitioners in the United States, by year*

Procedure	1959	19969	1979	1989	1999
Examination	20.1	27.8	30.1	42.8	45.4
Prophylaxis	19.9	25.5	24.9	38.6	37.2
Fluoride treatment	0.9	4.0	6.8	9.8	10.6
Amalgam, 1 surface	20.1	15.9	8.5	5.3	3.0
Amalgam, 2 surface	20.6	16.4	9.6	7.2	4.0
Crown	1.6	2.9	5.2	5.3	5.9
Root Canal	1.7	2.9	3.2	2.6	3.3
Extraction	13.0	9.8	5.4	4.9	1.7
Resin – Anterior	NA	NA	NA	4.9	4.2
Resin – Posterior	NA	NA	NA	1.9	4.8

*(Burt & Eklund, 1999, pg. 56).

meta-analyses indicate that both clinically and self applied fluoride reduce incidence of tooth decay by about 25% [37,52]. These values are similar to estimates of the effectiveness of community water fluoridation when using more recent data [15].

Dental sealants are another highly effective intervention to prevent tooth decay. Among children and youth, about 90% of tooth decay in the permanent teeth occurs in the chewing surfaces of the back teeth [25]. Dental sealants are 100% effective in preventing such decay if they are fully retained [58]. Recent meta-analyses indicate 60% effectiveness from 2 to 5 years after placement [2,74]. Whereas the use of fluoride likely has not changed greatly over the last 20 years, the use of dental sealants has. National surveys conducted in 1988–1984 and in 1999–2004 show that dental sealant prevalence among adolescent has doubled from 18% to 38% [29]. The decrease in tooth decay (almost 20% reduction in mean number of teeth affected per child [29]) among adolescents between these two surveys may be partially attributable to the increased prevalence of dental sealants.

Because of the decrease in dental disease, the dental services provided in clinical practice are transitioning from being primarily therapeutic to mostly preventive (Table 9). One study found that real per-patient annual dental expenditures among adults with a past year dental visit fell from $529.93 in 1987 to $467.29 in 1996 [14]. For children, real expenditures declined from $578.05 to $498.57 [76].

2.5. *Dental health outcomes*

Two measures of oral health collected in NHANES are the number of decayed, filled, and missing teeth (DMFT), which is collected clinically and self assessed oral health. DMFT reflects past treatment needs (MFT) and current unmet treatment needs (DT), which can also serves as a measure of access to care. Tooth decay is the most common childhood chronic disease and a sizable number of adults, over 25%, have decayed teeth in need of clinical treatment [29].

Self assessed oral health is a fairly good predictor of clinical dental status. Almost 40% of adults report the condition of their teeth and mouth as being fair or poor compared to excellent, very good, or good [11]. Among persons told by NHANES examining dentists to seek dental care for an oral condition other than poor hygiene within the next two weeks, 83% reported fair or poor oral health (Table 10). Among persons with no referral for unmet treatment needs, 84% reported good, very good, or excellent oral health. An analysis of NHANES 1988–1994 suggests that perceived need for dental care is higher than that for medical care – the proportion of adults reporting their general health as excellent or very good was 24.2 percentage points higher than the proportion reporting their dental health as excellent or

Table 10

Prevalence (Prev), sensitivity (sn) and specificity (sp) of oral health symptoms and treatment needs among adults aged 20 years and older – United States, 1999–2004

Need/ symptom	Adults, aged 20 to 44			Adults, aged 45 to 64			Adults, aged 65+		
	Prev	Sn	Sp	Prev.	Sn	Sp	Prev.	Sn	Sp
	% (se)			% (se)			% (se)		
Poor oral health*	36.87 (1.01)	–	–	36.87 (1.73)	–	–	38.34 (1.55)	–	–
Missing Teeth (>= 90th percentile)	12.83 (0.59)	70.68 (2.44)	68.72 (1.00)	14.19 (0.82)	65.56 (2.85)	61.01 (1.80)	11.06 (0.73)	50.63 (3.39)	63.28 (1.57)
Decay	29.91 (1.20)	64.17 (1.56)	74.85 (0.91)	23.35 (1.20)	73.12 (1.91)	67.64 (1.66)	19.46 (1.33)	67.58 (2.39)	68.87 (1.35)
Urgent†	3.91 (0.49)	85.73 (3.34)	–	2.59 (0.44)	87.31 (3.70)	–	1.97 (0.46)	77.57 (4.55)	–
Unmet‡	25.99 (1.04)	60.92 (1.77)	–	20.76 (1.13)	71.36 (2.09)	–	17.48 (1.25)	66.45 (2.56)	–
Gum disease (Perio)	24.27 (1.49)	58.68 (1.99)	70.19 (1.09)	26.67 (1.71)	65.61 (2.14)	66.75 (1.67)	20.84 (1.77)	54.23 (2.73)	66.00 (1.70)
Urgent	3.31 (0.51)	84.27 (3.49)	–	2.58 (0.50)	82.20 (4.42)	–	2.03 (0.45)	76.85 (5.92)	–
Unmet	20.96 (1.29)	54.63 (2.29)	–	24.09 (1.55)	63.83 (2.39)	–	18.81 (1.51)	51.79 (2.86)	–
Any	62.17 (1.83)	49.67 (1.34)	84.29 (0.88)	58.84 (3.08)	55.38 (2.20)	77.41 (1.86)	52.66 (3.08)	49.86 (2.07)	74.73 (1.57)
Urgent	4.48 (0.55)	81.90 (3.26)	–	3.27 (0.58)	85.13 (3.86)	–	2.99 (0.66)	74.06 (5.67)	–
Unmet	57.69 (1.61)	47.16 (1.50)	–	55.57 (2.83)	53.63 (2.34)	–	49.66 (2.73)	48.40 (2.28)	–
Any or MT	64.26 (1.71)	49.64 (1.30)	86.16 (0.88)	61.20 (2.99)	55.14 (2.11)	79.04 (1.92)	57.62 (2.75)	48.89 (1.94)	76.26 (1.66)
Any but OHI§	42.55 (1.46)	58.47 (1.45)	79.21 (0.91)	38.86 (1.81)	65.73 (1.90)	73.27 (1.59)	33.51 (2.30)	56.74 (2.06)	71.11 (1.49)
Urgent	4.43 (0.54)	82.86 (3.25)	–	3.16 (0.56)	84.62 (3.96)	–	2.88 (0.65)	73.09 (5.90)	–
Unmet	38.12 (1.22)	55.63 (1.68)	–	35.70 (1.65)	64.05 (2.04)	–	30.63 (1.96)	55.20 (2.10)	–
Oral pain	2.09 (0.28)	47.44 (4.49)	63.35 (1.03)	1.89 (0.30)	62.15 (8.30)	58.48 (1.67)	0.79 (0.22)	57.59 (12.39)	61.77 (1.55)

*Reported condition of mouth or teeth as fair or poor compared to good, very good, or excellent.

†Told to visit dentist within 2 weeks.

‡Told to visit dentist at earliest convenience.

§Oral Hygiene Index (OHI).

very good [67]. This deficit in perceived good oral health relative to perceived good general health may be more attributable to higher prevalence of oral disease or access issues rather than to differences in quality of care.

The presence of certain characteristics in the dental market suggests that competition in this market may be based more on cost per unit of quality (i.e., value) than in the medical market. Dental patients are likely to know their clinical status and they internalize both the benefit and a substantial share of the cost of their dental care. The patient may also be in a better position to evaluate the contribution of the dental provider because in contrast to medical, the same dental team is likely to have provided care both across services and over the cycle of the dental condition (from prevention to management and control of disease). In addition, the American Dental Association publishes the cost of various dental services by region of the country annually. Various websites have used this information to inform consumers of the prevailing rates of specific dental procedures in their region of the country.

2.6. Flow in dental care system

The environment influences population characteristics, health behaviors, health outcomes, and supply of dental personnel. For example, race/ethnicity can affect knowledge, values, and attitudes about oral health (E1 in Fig. 2), financing options in the dental delivery system as well as extent of community preventive services can influence use of dental services (E2), the dental delivery system will influence consumer satisfaction (E3), and the number of dental training facilities will be influenced by the current dental delivery system (E4). Population characteristics influence health behaviors and outcomes. For example predisposing factors and need will influence outcomes such as consumer satisfaction and dental health status (P1) and enabling resources will influence access to and utilization of clinical dental services (P2). Health behaviors influence oral health outcomes (B1). The supply of dental personnel will influence the dental delivery system (D1). Finally, dental health outcomes such as perceived dental health status will influence population characteristics such as perceived dental treatment needs (O1).

Given that the goal of the dental care system is to maximize oral health outcomes within resource constraints an important issue is the relative contribution of the various components of the system on oral health outcomes. Findings from a 1985 study by the World Health Organization examining the relationship between dental manpower systems and oral health status suggest that the dental care delivery system (availability of manpower and access to dental services) was not the primary determinant of oral health status. Instead, other factors such as oral health beliefs of the population, personal health practices, and the commitment of a country and its dental profession to implementing prevention activity were considered to be of equal or greater importance.

3. Strategies to improve the dental delivery system

The oral health delivery system works relatively well for the majority of Americans. Oral health has markedly improved over the last half century. Indeed even from the 1990s to 2000s improvements in oral health were realized among all age groups with the exception of the very young [29]. As a result the composition of dental services has shifted from being primarily restorative to primarily preventive. Certain characteristics also contribute to more efficient delivery (i.e., competition in dental is more likely to be based on value) than in medical. Dental patients may be better informed as to their clinical dental status, the prevailing costs of dental procedures in their region of the U.S., and the quality of their dental care (in that the same dental team is likely to have provided care both across services and over the cycle of the dental condition). In addition, in contrast to medical, consumers likely internalize not only the benefit of dental care but also a substantial share of the cost. Finally, unlike medical care, dental care is typically dedicated to one condition and care is both integrated across all services and coordinated over the condition cycle by the same dental team

Two issues that must be addressed, however, are containing costs and ensuring that all Americans have access to effective interventions to prevent and control dental disease. Because real dental expenditures, i.e. quantity of services, are decreasing while at the same time increases in dental costs are outpacing those in medical, it is likely that dental inflation is at least in part supply induced. In this section we describe potential strategies to increase supply of clinical dental service and reduce health disparities or alternatively to improve access among the underserved. We define access as every person who is in need of preventive or treatment services receives the appropriate care. Barriers to access may be either demand driven – lack of health insurance and lack of understanding and awareness of need for preventive oral health care – or supply driven – low dentist participation in Medicaid, shortage or mal-distribution of dentists, and restrictive state laws [61]. The optimal strategy to decrease disparities will depend on the supply of dental care relative to demand. Policies that address disparities by increasing demand (e.g., education/health promotion campaigns or increasing insurance coverage to subsidize the cost of dental care) will only be effective if there is sufficient dental capacity. Thus, increasing the supply of dental services may be effective in both containing costs and decreasing disparities.

3.1. Increasing supply in traditional practice model

From Fig. 2 we see that there are at least three ways we can increase the supply of dental services for the general population – increase the number of graduating dentists (which in turn requires an increase in the number of training facilities), increase dentist productivity, or substitute dental auxiliary and other medical professionals for dentists in the delivery of preventive services. One strategy potentially to increase the supply of dental services to higher risk populations would be to raise Medicaid reimbursements. Higher reimbursements could result in dentists substituting Medicaid patients for private pay patients (unlikely unless net profit per Medicaid patient exceeds that for private pay patients) or to reduce their consumption of leisure because of the increased marginal revenue from seeing Medicaid patients. Thus the impact of raising Medicaid fees should be influenced by how high the new Medicaid fee is relative to private pay fees and dentists' current consumption of labor and leisure.

3.1.1. Increasing number of dentists or productivity of dentists

Increasing dental school capacity is a fairly long term solution – it takes about 10 years for changes in dental school capacity to influence the current number of practicing dentists [18]. There are similarly constraints on increasing productivity in that there are likely diminishing returns to adding support personnel to the fixed input of dentists.

3.1.2. Substituting dental auxiliary and medical professionals for dentists

Changing the environment to allow substitute labor to provide prevention without a dentist may take less time to impact supply of dental care. Two options currently being utilized in some states to expand the scope of services provided by dental auxiliary for the purpose of providing preventive (and sometimes simple restorative) care to reach underserved populations are allowing dental hygienists to provide certain services in certain settings without the supervision of a dentist and developing a new class of dental provider, the dental therapist. In most states dental hygienists' scope of practice is determined by boards of dentistry. Many state practice acts restrict the delivery of preventive oral health care to dentists. In others, delivery may be limited by laws that restrict the types of procedures that can be performed by dental hygienists or by laws that define the extent of dentist supervision (i.e., whether dentist has to be on premises when services are delivered and whether dentist has to sign off on work performed prior to patient dismissal). In 45 states dental hygienists must be supervised by a dentist when delivering services in an office setting [33]. For alternative settings, however, 22 states allow dental hygienists direct access to patients and in 12 of these states Medicaid will directly reimburse dental hygienists for delivery of services. Expanding the scope of practice for dental hygienists may be attractive in that while there was little change in the number of dentists per capita from 1990 to 2001, the number of dental hygienists per capita increased by about 45% [77]). In addition, because there is a mal-distribution of dentists [5], delinking hygienists to dentists' supervision would allow hygienists to provide preventive services in dental shortage areas. Finally, to the extent that hygienists are equally as effective as dentists, substituting a lower cost input for a higher cost input would save societal resources. Pilot studies indicate that extended practice models are safe, effective, and successful in reaching the underserved [32].

Another proposed strategy creates a new class of dental provider, the dental health aide therapist (DHAT). The DHAT model has been used in New Zealand for about 37 years and in 52 other countries. DHATs are allowed to provide primary preventive services as well as routine fillings and extractions. The DHAT model has been adopted by the Alaska Native Tribal Health Consortium as well as the state of Minnesota. Furthermore, two states have proposals for DHATs far along in the legislative process.

Innovative programs that increase access to preventive and therapeutic oral health services for underserved populations such as the DHAT model have been endorsed by the American Public Health Association [6]. However, one study found that expanding the scope of dental auxiliaries was in itself insufficient to increase access among underserved. The presence of the following factors increased the likelihood that changing state dental practice laws would have an impact [61]: 1) Gaining the support of dentists, perhaps the most important factor; 2) Creating reimbursement mechanisms (e.g., via Medicaid); and 3) Providing formal referral mechanism. Events in Wisconsin suggest that changing Medicaid reimbursement policy can have a significant impact on access to preventive services among underserved. After the state changed its Medicaid policy to reimburse dental hygienists for preventive procedures delivered in schools, the number of schools with more than 50% of their students on free and reduced lunch served by a dental sealant program doubled [27].

Another strategy to increase supply of dental care is to allow medical professionals to provide screenings, education, basic preventive services, and dental referrals, especially to the very young and very old who are much more likely to have a medical than a dental encounter. National data indicate that there has been an increase in the number of young children who have experienced dental decay (treated or untreated) in their primary teeth from the 1990s to present [29]. It should be noted, however, that the increase was in treated rather than untreated decay. Several states have experimented with allowing primary care personnel to provide dental services such as screening for dental decay, fluoride varnish, parent education, and dental referrals to children. Pilot studies in North Carolina found that after a 2 hour training session, primary care providers were fairly accurate in their assessment of referral need for very young children –70% of children with cavities were referred and greater than 90% of children with no cavities were not referred [63]. Allowing Medicaid to reimburse primary care providers resulted in 40,000 dental visits among 200,000 very young Medicaid eligible children [66]. In addition, surveyed parents of children participating in the program rated their children's preventive dental care highly [66]. One of the major impediments to primary care providers referring very young children to dentists was difficulty in finding a dentist who would accept very young children participating in Medicaid [28].

Successful implementation of such programs requires training pediatric providers about oral health and providing financial incentives such as Medicaid and/or SCHIP coverage [56]. Thirteen states are now allowing Medicaid to reimburse medical doctors for providing fluoride varnish and at least twelve have oral health curricula or training for primary care providers.

3.1.3. Raising medicaid reimbursements

The last strategy we will discuss to increase supply, raising Medicaid reimbursement rates, specifically targets the supply of dental services directed to underserved populations. An analysis of 6 states found that raising Medicaid reimbursement levels as well as changing other Medicaid policies (i.e., easing administrative processes and involving state dental societies and individual dentists as active partners in program improvement) were associated with an increase in Medicaid utilization ranging from 33% to 76% [13]. The analysis also found that the rate increases on their own while necessary were not sufficient to improve utilization. Utilization among these lower income children after rate increases ranged from 32% to 43%, which is still below utilization among all privately insured children −57.5%. Increasing Medicaid fees can result in relatively large increases in total Medicaid expenditures because the state is paying for new children as well as a higher rate for children that were already accessing the system. In light of the current state fiscal environment it may be a daunting task for states to further raise Medicaid reimbursement levels.

3.2. Increasing demand in traditional practice model

Another way to reduce disparities would be to increase demand for preventive and restorative dental care among those at highest risk (e.g., lower income and racial/ethnic minorities). From Fig. 2, we see that two ways to do this would be 1) to change financing within the dental delivery system to enable those at higher risk to obtain dental care and 2) to target educational campaigns at higher risk groups on the importance of oral health as well as the effectiveness of prevention to predispose them to seek clinical care. Increasing access to preventive dental care among those at highest risk could conceivably reduce dental expenditures. Infants and toddlers with severe tooth decay may require care in a hospital operating room under general anesthesia. Analyses of state Medicaid dental claims for children less than 6 years of age found that in Louisiana 45% of Medicaid dental costs were spent on the 5% of children hospitalized [36] and in Iowa 25% of costs were spent on the 2% of children hospitalized [43]. There is also some evidence that adults with tooth decay and limited access to clinical care are receiving care in hospital emergency rooms.

3.2.1. Expanding public insurance

Comprehensive dental coverage for children is a mandatory benefit for Medicaid enrolled children. Expanding coverage among lower income families by raising the income threshold for Medicaid eligibility or by mandating dental coverage in separate programs covering the working poor, i.e., the State Children's Health Insurance Program (SCHIP [31]) could increase dental for dental services by "enabling" families to pay for dental services. Preliminary findings from a study on the effect of SCHIP provision of dental services in 18 states suggest that in those states where reimbursement rates were set at their private market equivalent SCHIP results in increased dentist participation as well as increased utilization [3]. Thus, expanding public insurance coverage will improve access if sufficient attention is also paid to increasing the supply of providers (e.g., increasing reimbursements to their market equivalent).

Most of the studies on the effect of expanding Medicaid/SCHIP coverage have been conducted among children. It should be noted, however, that compared to children, poor adults of working age are more

Table 11
Percentage of children with past year dental visits and mean number of visits among those who visited dentist (MEPS 2005) http://drc.hhs.gov/create_query.htm

Age	% with past year visit	Mean number visits| past year visit
0–3	12.53	1.5
4–11	55.16	1.9
12–19	52.04	3.1
20–49	39.21	2.1
50+	47.03	2.6

likely to have untreated decay and older poor adults are as likely (Table 1). Thus expanding adult Medicaid coverage to adults could also impact oral health disparities. As of 2006, four states did not cover dental care for adults and 18 offered very minimal services (emergency care or extractions only) [44].

3.2.2. Risk based interval between dental visits

Redistributing demand for dental services by risk status has the potential to both reduce disparities and increase dental capacity. One proposed strategy to accomplish this is to base the intervals between dental visits on individual patient risk, i.e., shorter intervals for higher risk and longer intervals for lower risk patients. At present for lower risk patients it is customary to schedule dental check-ups every 6 months. Indeed, current guidance for parents recommends that most children visit the dentist twice a year [4]. Among children over 4 years old with a past year dental visit, the average number of dental visits typically exceeds 2 (Table 11).

An evidence based review of dental recall periods recommended that for children younger than 18 years, the recall interval should be between 3 to 12 months depending on the child's risk status and up to 24 months for adults [57]. A recent study found that for low caries increments (0.65 to 1.5 annually) recall intervals could be extended to 2 years [72]. This value is well below the average annual increment reported in national U.S. surveys [29].

3.3. Refitting the delivery model

Some studies have suggested that in addressing access among the underserved, it may be more helpful to view the issue less as a problem of supply of dentists and more as a poor fit between the current practice model and those populations most in need of care [35,55]. Possible solutions to "improving the fit" could include changing the external environment, changing the delivery site to alternative settings where those with the most dental disease are likely to be, and raising the expectations of the underserved through education that emphasizes the importance of oral health as well as awareness of available interventions and their effect. The last option would not only "predispose" underserved populations to seek care in traditional clinical settings but also to seek care in alternative settings as well as to engage in healthy self behaviors. As discussed in the previous section, there are highly effective as well as cost-effective interventions delivered in clinical and community settings to prevent dental disease. Andersen hypothesized that environmental factors other than the traditional clinical dental delivery system could have a significant impact on oral health outcomes. We conclude this section with a brief discussion of three such approaches – fluoridation of community water supplies (changing the environment), school based dental sealant programs (changing the delivery site), and a state initiative (Access to Baby and Child Dentistry Program (ABCD) in Washington) and and American Dental Association Initiative (Community Dental Health Coordinator (CDHC)) that work at changing expectations as well as developing nontraditional delivery models.

3.3.1. Changing environment – community water fluoridation

Community water fluoridation has played an important role in the reductions in tooth decay (40%–70% in children) and of tooth loss in adults (40%–60%) [21]. This public health intervention also typically saves public health resources, i.e., it is cost saving [74]. One study documented that fluoridation reduces Medicaid expenditures [22]. Fluoridation was listed as one of the ten great public health achievements in the 20th century [23]. Currently 70% of the persons on public water systems receive water that is fluoridated nationally [24]. This value, however, varies greatly at the state level, ranging from less that 10% to nearly 100% of a state's population. Changing this from a local decision to federal mandate for water systems serving sizable populations would make this safe, effective, and resource-saving intervention available to more Americans.

3.3.2. Non-clinical delivery – school-based sealant programs

About 90% of decay in children and adolescents occur in the chewing surfaces of the back teeth [25, 50]. As previously discussed dental sealants are highly effective in preventing tooth decay in these specific teeth. To reach lower-income children who typically lack access to restorative (percentage of six to eight-year-olds with untreated tooth decay is over two times higher among lower-income children than among higher-income children [29]) and preventive care (% of eight-year-olds with at least one sealant is over two times higher for higher income children than for lower income children [29]) 35 states and 4 territories [8] sponsor school-based sealant programs. These programs typically provide dental screenings, oral health education, and referral for dental treatments as well as sealant application. The percentage of lower income children served by these programs is likely low. Only 20% of these children have sealants and most children likely received their sealants in a clinical setting rather than a school-based program. Evidence from Ohio, a state with a well established dental sealant program suggests that expanding school-based sealant programs to all schools where greater than 50% of school children are on the free and reduced lunch program would likely greatly reduce disparities in sealant prevalence and ultimately in dental decay. Expanding school-based sealant programs would also likely result in meeting one of the nation health goals (namely 50% of 8-year olds with a sealant; Health People 2010).

3.3.3. Changing expectations – ABCD Program and CDHC Initiative

One interesting example of a collaboration among health departments, local outreach agencies, Medicaid enrolled families, and dentists to increase dental utilization among the very young is the Access to Baby and Child Dentistry Program (ABCD) in Washington [1]. This program tries to increase both supply of and demand for dental care. Enrolled families are coached about the importance of early preventive dental care and the importance of keeping dental appointments, which results in lower no-show rates in ABCD practices. ABCD certified general dentists receive enhanced Medicaid reimbursements for select preventive and restorative procedures. Over the 10 years of the program's existence dental utilization among very young Medicaid children has increased from 21% to 37%.

Another initiative sponsored by the American Dental Association that will soon be piloted is the Community Dental Health Care Coordinator. This program will create a new class of dental provider, the CDHC, to link underserved populations with care in Federally Qualified Health Centers (FQHC). The number of FQHC has increased from 848 in 2002 to 1076 in 2007. About 75% of FQHC provide dental care. The CDHC will promote oral health in their community by 1) integrating oral health information into the community's culture, language, and value systems, 2) enrolling persons eligible for public insurance into the appropriate program, and 3) coordinating care to FQHC through making appointments and providing transportation if necessary. The CDHC will provide dental assessment, dental prophylaxes, topical fluoride, sealants, and temporary restorations under the remote supervision of a dentist. The CDHC will then link the patient to a FQHC dentist who will complete care.

4. "Engineering" dental delivery

In this section, we discuss opportunities for engineering to improve the dental delivery system in terms of containing costs and increasing access among the underserved. We focus on three research areas: 1) cost/comparative-effectiveness to determine what procedures should be provided as well as the most efficient mode of delivery, 2) resource allocation to ensure adequate future supply of dental care as well as reducing current disparities and 3) process improvement to minimize the resources used in delivering dental care. We discuss both needed research in each of these areas and how engineering techniques could be employed in conducting this research.

4.1. Cost-effectiveness and comparative-effectiveness analyses

Cost effectiveness analysis (CEA) allows decision makers to determine the most efficient way to prevent disease or promote health. CEA compares the net societal cost per unit of effectiveness (which typically is in terms of quality of life) for different interventions. Markov modeling is frequently used to model disease progression with and without the disease.

We will briefly discuss aspects somewhat unique to dental that may make mathematical modeling more complex than in other health areas before moving on to research needs. First, dental disease unlike most other medical conditions, can affect 28 different sites (teeth) that can transition from sound to diseased. Disease in one tooth is a function of circumstances related to the individual tooth as well as the oral environment. Thus the probability of disease is correlated among teeth because of a common risk factor, the oral environment, and that environment is subject to change if any one tooth becomes diseased. Because of the complexity of dental disease at present there are not good models of disease progression. Having accurate models to predict disease progression would also be useful to predict future prevalence, which is not only important for cost effectiveness analyses but also for determining future resource requirements, which will be discussed in the next section.

The presence of multiple disease sites may also increase the difficulty of comparing the cost effectiveness of interventions that prevent dental disease to interventions that prevent other medical conditions. The most common outcome metric used in CEA is the quality adjusted life year where a value of 1 indicates a year of perfect health and 0 indicates death. At present, there is not a good measure of the loss in quality adjusted life years attributable to tooth decay or gum disease. Attempts have been made to develop a quality adjusted tooth year, which is valuable in comparing oral health interventions, but is not easily converted to the common medical metric of quality adjusted life years.

One important comparative-effectiveness research question is what is the optimal mix of interventions to be delivered in school-based programs to prevent tooth decay? Sealants and fluoride varnish have been shown to be effective and both are used in school-based programs. A recent meta-analysis suggested that sealants are more effective but that there was insufficient evidence to derive an actual value for the increase in effectiveness [40]. Such information, as well as the relative costs is needed. Fluoride varnish does not require meticulous technique (i.e., can be delivered by non-dental professionals) and does not require a portable dental unit. Thus, under certain conditions fluoride varnish could be more cost-effective. In addition, little is known as to the additional benefit fluoride varnish would provide over sealants. Similar analyses should be conducted on the cost effectiveness of different sealant materials used in school settings. Glass-ionomer sealants, although less effective than resin-based sealants, could again be more efficient in certain schools because they do not require the tooth to be completely dry before sealant application. As a result, they can be applied without portable dental equipment and thus may be feasible in some small schools with insufficient power supply for such portable equipment. Finally, it is important to examine the cost-effectiveness of linking delivery of sealants with other preventive services (e.g., vision, hearing, asthma, and vaccines) in school settings.

Determining how to increase the access among underserved populations may also involve comparing the effectiveness of alternative delivery models. Indeed, comparing the effectiveness of various delivery models in preventing tooth decay in children was included as one of the Institute of Medicine's 100 priority topics for comparative effectiveness research [41]. One pressing research question is to determine whether an across the board increase (i.e., x%) in Medicaid dental reimbursements under the current practice model would be more efficient than changing the practice model for delivery of prevention by alternative personnel in alternative settings and using the savings from hiring less costly personnel to raise reimbursements for restorative procedures at an even higher rate (i.e., $>$ x%).

A model that integrates the dental health system into the total health care system is needed to evaluate the effectiveness of using the medical system to screen for dental disease and to provide basic preventive services. Available data suggest that a sizable percentage of the population has had either a past-year dental visit with no medical visit or a past-year medical visit but no dental visit. This would suggest that not only might medical venues present unique screening opportunities for dental disease but also that dental venues alternatively might prove attractive for screening for other health conditions. Oral tests now exist for a host of non-dental conditions including HIV and HCV. The association between periodontal disease and CVD and diabetes might also present an opportunity to refer persons with periodontal disease and without a regular source of health care for testing for these conditions. An integrated model would allow the accurate computation of the opportunity cost of diverting medical personnel away from delivering other interventions to promote health as well as the cost of diverting dental personnel away from providing dental care.

Further research is also needed to determine the cost-effectiveness of: 1) vaccines to prevent dental carries, 2) community water fluoridation versus school-based sealant programs in non-fluoridated communities surrounded by fluoridated communities, and 3) different materials for amalgams and/or crowns.

4.2. Resource allocation

Research is also needed on allocating resources more efficiently. For example, data envelopment analysis or stochastic production function analysis could be used to determine the most efficient combination of different classes of dental workers and capital in the delivery of dental care in different settings. In addition, statistical forecasting tools as well as simulation models could be used to estimate future demand for different types of dental care. As alluded to earlier, middle aged and younger adults today have less dental disease and will be more likely to retain their natural teeth than previous cohorts. While this will likely result in higher demand for preventive care in the future as today's adults grow older, it is unclear at present whether this phenomenon will also translate into higher probability of dental disease and thus higher demand for restorative care. Combining information on efficient production and future demand will also allow today's decision makers to implement policies to ensure an adequate long run supply of dental personnel. Such policies would include determining dental school capacity as well as capacity for other dental personnel and perhaps examining the impact of financial incentives on dentist's decision to substitute labor for leisure.

Engineering has tools that are uniquely suited to effectively and efficiently allocate resources to increase access among the underserved. For example the following are key engineering focus areas: 1) refining measurement of access, ii) developing location models for positioning providers with respect to the network and the population, iii) developing resource allocation models, and iv) managing resources with a particular focus on scarce medical personnel. We briefly describe each below.

Measurement of access is important in order to determine if populations are receiving adequate dental care, and this becomes the objective of any allocation model. A related issue is the measurement of disparities (or equity of care). However, there is no agreement about what access or equity means, let alone how to measure it. What is required is a socially responsible measure that is useful from a resource allocation perspective. Survey measures are what we will primarily need to be used (due to the cost of information) and comparing the tradeoff of accuracy of information with quantity is important for survey designs.

An important factor for improving access is determining the best location for where these services should be provided. The area of facility location is a well studied class of problems in engineering. In this case, the goal is to locate a number of facilities across a geographic network. Often times there are constraints that must be considered such as budgets and/or supply of dentists. Several optimization techniques such as mixed integer programming can be used to model such a system and determine the best locations. There are some unique issues when considering access, however. First, facility location objectives have typically been made up of factors that are easily measurable such as cost. As mentioned previously, developing a useful proxy for access can be a challenge. In addition, demand for oral health networks can be more difficult than demand for traditional facility location systems since it depends on a much wider variety of factors (patient travel time, income, alternatives, etc.).

Health care access is defined in a large part by available resources. The effective use of those resources can help to improve access to care. Tools for resource allocations often include mathematical programming as well as the use of production-functions to measure impact. Queuing techniques have also been used to look at health organizations, such as to determine capacity or staffing. Further research in this area would also help organizations plan their use of scarce resources including limited labor supply, although it is important to recognize that the health industry faces different kinds of customer service constraints than those in many manufacturing industries.

Finally, engineering models are required to help effectively increase the supply of oral health personnel or to more efficiently use current personnel Supply could be increased through incentives such as increasing wages (e.g. through increases in Medicaid reimbursement) and increased funding to dental schools as well as providing bonuses for working in rural areas. Another means for increasing supply is through allowing other personnel to perform certain procedures by the relaxing of dental practice acts. Practice acts define who can perform which services and hence protect the public interest and safety of patients.

4.3. Process improvement

Another important area where engineering models can help improve the dental delivery system is by improving the processes used in delivery. One way to do this is through technology such as remote monitoring or information sharing. Another approach is to apply techniques common in manufacturing and logistics systems such as lean delivery, improved scheduling, sharing resources, and capacity management.

Particular areas that need to be studied include determining the marginal productivity of dentists and auxiliary personnel, estimating the substitutability of health care professionals other than dentists for delivering preventative care, and developing new models of delivery (e.g., in a school-based sealant program, determining the scheduling of students through the system, the optimal staffing of dentists, hygienists, and auxiliary personnel, and the delivery approach (e.g., strict 4-handed method versus some other approach).

Ultimately, it is important to examine and understand the mathematical relationships among the various components of Fig. 2. Systems engineering and systems dynamics principals (such as structural equations modeling and agent-based simulation) can be used to try to increase the understanding. There are various policies that can be considered through systems modeling approaches. The authors have attempted to present a complete model of the dental health system, but there is still much work to do in determining the relative impact of each component on dental health outcomes as well as the relative costs of implementing change in each component.

References

[1] Access to Baby and Child Dentistry, (2009). Increasing access to care for young Medicaid-eligible children. Washington: ABCD Program. Available at: http://www.abcd-dental.org/pdf/overview.pdf, accessed July 2, 2009.

[2] A. Ahovuo-Saloranta et al., (2004). Pit and fissure sealants for preventing dental decay in the permanent teeth of children and adolescents. Cochrane Database Systematic Review. 3:CD001930.

[3] R.A. Almeida, I. Hill and G.M. Kenney, (2001). Does SCHIP Spell Better Dental Care Access for Children? An Early Look at New Initiatives. Washington, DC: The Urban Institute, 2000.

[4] American Academy of Pediatric Dentistry, (2009). Regular dental visits. American Academy of Pediatric Dentistry. Available at: http://www.aapd.org/ publications/brochures/regdent.asp, accessed July 2, 2009.

[5] American Dental Association, Future of Dentistry. Chicago: American Dental Association, Health Policy Resources Center, 2001.

[6] American Public Health Association, (2005). Support for the Alaska dental health aide and therapist and other dental health programs. APHA Annual Meeting, Philadelphia. Available from: http://www.apha.org/membergroups/newsletters/sectionnewsletters/oral/winter06/2485.htm, accessed July 2, 2009.

[7] R. Andersen, Revisiting the behavioral model and access to medical care: does it matter? *Journal of Health and Social Behavior* **36** (1995), 1–10.

[8] Association of State and Territorial Dental Directors, (2003). Best practice approaches for state and community oral health programs: School-based dental sealant programs. Available from: http://www.astdd.org/docs/BPASchoolSealantPrograms.pdf, last accessed July 2, 2009.

[9] H.L. Bailit, Health services research, *Advances in Dental Research* **17** (2002), 82–85.

[10] H. Bailit et al., Does more generous dental insurance coverage improve oral health? *Journal of the American Dental Association* **110** (1985), 701–707.

[11] L. Barker, P.M. Griffin and S.O. Griffin, (2008). Utility of self-reported oral health as a surveillance measure. Proceedings of 2008 International Association of Dental Research, Toronto, Canada. Abstract #1152. Available at: http://iadr.confex.com/iadr/2008Toronto/techprogram/abstract_107933.htm, accessed July 2, 2009.

[12] T. Beazoglou, D. Heffley, L.J. Brown and H. Bailit, The importance of productivity in estimating need for dentists, *J Journal of the American Dental Association* **133** (2002), 1399–1404.

[13] A. Borchgrevink, A. Snyder and S. Gehshan, (2008). The Effects of Medicaid Reimbursement Rates on Access to Dental Care. Washington, DC: National Academy for State Health Policy, 2008. Available at http://www.nashp.org/Files/CHCF_dental rates.pdf (accessed July 3, 2009).

[14] L.J. Brown, T.P. Wall and R.J. Manski, The funding of dental services among U.S. adults aged 18 years and older recent trends in expenditures and sources of funding, *Journal of the American Dental Association* **133** (2002), 627–635.

[15] J.A. Brunelle and J.P. Carlos, *Journal of Dental Research* **69** (1990), 723–727.

[16] Bureau of Labor Statistics, Databases, Tables and Calculators by Subject (Series SEMC01 and SEMC02). Washington: Bureau of Labor Statistics. Available at http://data.bls.gov/cgi-bin/srgate, accessed July 2, 2009.

[17] Bureau of Labor Statistics, Productivity change in the non-farm business sector. Washington: Bureau of Labor Statistics. Available at: http://www.bls.gov/, accessed July 2, 2009.

[18] B.A. Burt and S.A. Eklund, The dentist, dental practice, and the community. 5th ed. Philadelphia, PA: Saunders, 1999.

[19] A. Catlin et al., National health spending in 2005: the slowdown continues, *Health Affairs* **26**(1) (2007), 142–152.
[20] A. Catlin, C. Cowan, M. Hartman and S. Heffler, National health spending in 2006: a year of change for prescription drugs, *Health Affairs* **27**(1) (2008), 14–29.
[21] CDC, Ten great public health achievements, United States1900–1999, *MMWR- Morbidity and Mortality Weekly Report* **48**(12) (1999), 241–243.
[22] CDC, Water fluoridation and costs of Medicaid treatment for dental decay – Louisiana. 1995–1996, *MMWR- Morbidity and Mortality Weekly Report* **48**(34) (1999), 753–757.
[23] CDC (S.L. Tomar and S.O. Griffin) Achievements in public health, 1990–1999: fluoridation of drinking water to prevent dental caries, *MMWR- Morbidity and Mortality Weekly Report* **48**(41) (1999), 933–940.
[24] CDC, Populations receiving optimally fluoridated public drinking water – United States, 1992–2006, *MMWR- Morbidity and Mortality Weekly Report* **57**(27) (2008), 737–764.
[25] CDC National Center for Health Statistics, National Health and Nutrition Examination Surveys 1999–2004. Hyattsville, MD: National Center for Health Statistics. Available from: www.cdc.gov/nchs/nhanes.htm, accessed July 2, 2009.
[26] P. Cooper and R.J. Manski, Establishing the true effect of dental insurance on dental use. Proceedings of AcademyHealth Meeting 2005. 22; abstract no. 4054.
[27] M. Crespin, K. Ordinans and B.J. Tatro, Partnering to Seal-A-Smile a report on the success of Wisconsin school based dental sealant programs. Madison, WI: Childrens Health Alliance of Wisconsin, 2009.
[28] G.G. Dela Cruz, R.G. Rozier and G. Slade, Dental screening and referral of young children by pediatric primary care providers, *Pediatrics* **114**(5) (2004), e642–e652.
[29] B. Dye et al., Trends in oral health status, United States, 1988–1994, *Vital and Health statistics Series* **11**(248) (2007), 1–92.
[30] P.J. Feldstein, Financing dental care: an economic analysis. Lexington: Lexington Books, 1973.
[31] S.A. Fisher-Owens et al., Giving policy some teeth: Routes to reducing disparities in oral health, *Health Affairs* **27**(2) (2008), 404–412.
[32] J.A. Freed, D.A. Perry and J.F. Kushman, Aspects of quality of dental hygiene care in supervised and unsupervised practices, *Journal of Public Health Dentistry* **57**(2) (1997), 68–75.
[33] S. Gehshan, (2008). Dental workforce trends: opportunities for improving access. National Academy for State Health Policy. Available from: http://www.mainedentalaccess.org/docs/Maine%20Oral%20Health%20Task%20Force%203_08.ppt#24, Accessed July 2, 2009.
[34] H.C. Gift, S.B. Corbin and R.E. Nowjack-Raymer, Public knowledge of prevention of dental disease, *Public Health Reports* **109**(3) (1994), 397–404.
[35] D. Grembowski, A. Ronald and C. Meei-shai, A public health model of the dental care process, *Medical Care Review* **46**(4) (1989), 439–497.
[36] S.O. Griffin et al., Dental services, costs, and factors associated with hospitalization for Medicaid-eligible children, Louisiana 1996–1997, *Journal of Public Health Dentistry*, **60**(1) (2000), 21–27.
[37] S.O. Griffin, E. Regnier, P.M. Griffin and V.N. Huntley, Effectiveness of fluoride in preventing caries in adults, *Journal of Dental Research* **86**(5) (2007), 410–415.
[38] J. Gruber, (2006). The role of consumer copayments for health care: lessons from the RAND Health Insurance Experiment and beyond. National Bureau of Research (Prepared for the Kaiser Foundation. Available at: http://www.kff.org/insurance/upload/7566.pdf, accessed July 2, 2009.
[39] J. Grytten and D. Holst, Do young adults demand more dental services as their income increases? *Community Dentistry and Oral Epidemiology* **30** (2002), 463–469.
[40] A. Hiiri, A. Ahovuo-Saloranta, A. Norblad and M. Makela, (2006). Pit and fissure sealants versus fluoride varnishes for preventing dental decay in children and adolescents, *Cochrane Database Systematic Review* 4:CD003067.
[41] Institute of Medicine, Initial national priorities for comparative effectiveness research. Washington DC: Institute of Medicine, 2009.
[42] K. Jones et al., Reducing dental sealant disparities in school-aged children through better targeting of informational campaigns, *Preventive Chronic Disease* **2**(2) (2005), A21. Available at: http://www.cdc.gov/pcd/issues/2005/apr/04_0142p.htm, accessed July 2, 2009.
[43] M.J. Kanellis, P.C. Damiano and E.T. Mamany, Medicaid costs associated with the hospitalization of young children for restorative dental treatment under general anesthesia, *Journal of Public Health Dentistry* **60**(1) (2000), 28–32.
[44] L. Ku, Medical and dental care utilization and expeditures under Medicaid and private health insurance, *Medical Care Research Review* **66**(4) (2009), 456–471.
[45] J.R. Langabeer, Economic outcomes of an dental electronic patient record, *Journal of Dental Education* **72**(10) (2008), 1189–1200.
[46] K. Levit et al., Inflation spurs health spending in 2000, *Health Affairs* **21**(1) 2002, 172–181.
[47] K. Levit et al., Trends in U.S. health care spending, 2001, *Health Affairs* **22**(1) (2003), 154–164.
[48] K. Levit et al., Health spending rebound continues in 2002, *Health Affairs* **23**(1) (2004), 147–59.

[49] J. Lipscomb and C.W. Douglass, A political economic theory of the dental care market, *American Journal of Public Health* **72**(7) (1982), 665–675.
[50] M.D. Macek, E.D. Beltrán-Aguilar, S.A. Lockwood and D.M. Malvitz, Updated comparison of the caries susceptibility of various morphological types of permanent teeth, *Journal of Public Health Dentistry* **63**(3) (2003), 174–182.
[51] W.G. Manning, H.L. Bailit, B. Benjamin and J.P. Newhouse, The demand for dental care: evidence from a randomized trial in health insurance, *Journal of the American Dental Association* **110**(6) (1985), 895–902.
[52] V.C. Marinho, J.P. Higgins, A. Sheiham and S. Logan, Fluoride toothpastes for preventing dental caries in children and adolescents. *Cochrane Database Systematic Review* 1:CD002278, 2003.
[53] N.N. Maserejian, F. Tranchtenberg, C. Link and M. Tavares, Underutilization of dental care when it is freely available: a prospective study of the New England Children's Amalgam Trial, *Journal of Public Health Dentistry* **68**(3) (2008), 139–148.
[54] Medical Expenditure Panel Survey, Query retrieved from NIDCR CDC Data Query System http://apps.nccd.cdc.gov/dohdrc/dqs/entry.html, 2005.
[55] E. Mertz and E. O'Neil, The growing challenge of providing oral health care services to all Americans, *Health Affairs* **21**(5) (2002), 63–77.
[56] W.E. Mouradian, E. Wehr and J.J. Crall, Disparities to children's oral health and access to care, *Journal of the American Medical Association* **284**(20) (2000), 1625–2631.
[57] National Institute for Clinical Excellence, (2004). Dental recall, Clinical Guideline 19. London: National Collaborating Centre for Accute Care. Available from: http://www.nice.org.uk/nicemedia/pdf/cg019niceguideline.pdf, accessed July 2, 2009.
[58] National Institutes of Health, Consensus development conference statement: dental sealants in the prevention of tooth decay, *Journal of Dental Education* **48**(2) (1984), 126–131.
[59] L.M. Neumann, Trends in dental and allied dental education, *Journal of the American Dental Association* **135** (2004), 1253–1259.
[60] P.W. Newacheck et al., The unmet health needs of America's children, *Pediatrics* **105**(4) (2000), 989–997.
[61] L. Nolan et al., (2003). The effects of state dental practice laws allowing alternative models of preventive oral health care delivery to low-income children. Center for Health Services Research and Policy. School of Public Health and Health Services. The George Washington University Medical Center, Washington DC. Available from: http://www.gwumc.edu/sphhs/departments/healthpolicy/chsrp/downloads/oral_health_exec%20summ.pdf, accessed July 2, 2009.
[62] Oral Health America, (2003). Keep America smiling: The oral health in America 2003. Chicago: Oral Health America. Available at: http://www.oralhealthamerica.org/pdf/2003ReportCard.pdf, accessed July 2, 2009.
[63] K.M. Pierce, R.G. Rozier and W.F. Vann, Accuracy of pediatric primary care providers' screening and referral for early childhood caries, *Pediatrics* **109**(5) (2002), E82-2.
[64] M.E. Porter and E.O. Teisberg, Redefining health care: Creating value-based competition on results. Boston: Harvard Business School Press, 2006.
[65] R.G. Rozier, G.D. Slade, L.P. Zeldin and H. Wang, Parents' satisfaction with preventive dental care for young children provided by nondental primary care providers, *Pediatrics Dentistry* **27**(4) (2005), 313–322.
[66] R.G. Rozier et al., Prevention of early childhood caries in North Carolina medical practice: implications for research and practice, *Journal of Dental Education* **67**(8) (2003), 876–885.
[67] A.E. Sanders and G.D. Slade, Deficits in perceptions of oral health relative to general health in populations, *Journal of Public Health Dentistry* **66**(4) (2006), 255–262.
[68] C.R. Scherrer, P.M. Griffin and J.L. Swann, Public health sealant delivery programs: Optimal delivery and the cost of practice acts, *Medical Decision Making* **27**(6) (2007), 762–771.
[69] C. Smith et al., Health spending growth slows in 2003, *Health Affairs* **24**(1) (2005), 185–194.
[70] C. Smith et al., National health spending in 2004: recent slowdown led by prescription drug spending, *Health Affairs* **25**(1) (2006), 186–196.
[71] E.S. Solomon, Demographic characteristics of general dental practice sites, *General Dentistry* **55**(6) (2007), 552–558.
[72] E.H. Tan, P. Batchelor and A. Sheiham, A reassessment of recall frequency intervals for screening in low caries incidence populations, *International Dentistry Journal* **56** (2006), 277–282.
[73] Task Force on Community Preventive Services et al., The Guide to Community Preventative Services: What Works to Promote Health? New York: Oxford University Press, 2005.
[74] B.I. Truman et al., Reviews of evidence on interventions to prevent dental caries, oral and pharyngeal cancers, and sports-related craniofacial injuries, *American Journal of Preventative Medicine* **23**(1) (2002), 21–54.
[75] U.S. Department of Health and Human Services, Oral health in America: A report of the Surgeon General. Rockville MD: Department of Health and Human Services, 2000.
[76] T.P. Wall, L.J. Brown and R.J. Manski, The funding of dental services among U.S. children aged 2 to 17 years recent trends in expenditures and sources of funding, *Journal of the American Dental Association* **133** (2002), 474–82.

[77] P. Wing, M.H. Langelier, T.A. Continelli and A. Battrell, A dental hygiene professional practice index (DHPPI) and access to oral health status and service use in the United States, *Journal of Dental Hygiene* **79**(2) (2005), 1–10.

Paul Griffin is a professor in the Harold and Inge Marcus Department of Industrial and Manufacturing Engineering at Penn State University where he serves as the Peter and Angela Dal Pezzo Department Head. His research and teaching interests are in health and supply chain systems. In particular, his current research activities have focused on cost-effectiveness modeling of public health interventions, health logistics, health access and economic modeling, and supply chain coordination and control including pricing and contracting mechanisms.

Section 5: Perspectives

Information Knowledge Systems Management 8 (2009) 369–382
DOI 10.3233/IKS-2009-0147
IOS Press

Chapter 20

Integrated health systems

Stephen M. Shortell and Rodney K. McCurdy
E-mail: shortell@berkeley.edu

Abstract: Before meaningful gains in improving the value of health care in the US can be achieved, the fragmented nature in which health care is financed and delivered must be addressed. One type of healthcare organization, the Integrated Delivery System (IDS), is poised to play a pivotal role in reform efforts. What are these systems? What is the current evidence regarding their performance? What are the current barriers to their establishment and how can these barriers be removed? This chapter addresses these important questions. Although there are many types of IDS' in the US healthcare landscape, the chapter begins by identifying the necessary healthcare components that encompass an IDS and discusses the levels of integration that are important to improving health care quality and value. Next, it explores the recent evidence regarding IDS performance which, while generally positive, is less than what it could be if there were greater focus on clinical integration. To highlight, the chapter discusses the efficacy of system engineering initiatives in two examples of large, fully integrated systems: Kaiser-Permanente and the Veterans Health Administration. The evidence here is strong that the impact of system engineering methods is enhanced through the integration of processes, goals and outcomes. Reforms necessary to encourage the development of IDS' include: 1) the development of payment mechanisms designed to increase greater inter-dependency of hospitals and physicians; 2) the modification or removal of several regulatory barriers to greater clinical integration; and 3) the establishment of a more robust data collection and reporting system to increase transparency and accountability. The chapter concludes with a framework for considering these reforms across strategic, structural, cultural, and technical dimensions.

"The current care systems cannot do the job. Trying harder will not work. Changing systems of care will." [19]

1. Introduction

As described in many of the previous chapters, the US healthcare delivery system costs too much, is prone to too many errors and too much waste, and is simply not organized to address the challenges of delivering healthcare in the 21st century. As shown in Fig. 1, there is need for models and approaches that can address the incentives for change, the capabilities of providers to respond to the incentives, and the need for accountability and performance metrics to know how well the system is responding. One model that incorporates all three corners of the triangle is the integrated delivery system (IDS). The IDS model has been around for many decades. Evidence regarding its viability and superior performance is accumulating. Yet there remain many questions including why IDS' have not been more widely adopted across the country. This chapter addresses this central question and offers recommendations for more widespread implementation of integrated delivery systems. We begin, by defining IDS', describing their key elements, offering some examples, and reviewing the existing evidence on their performance.

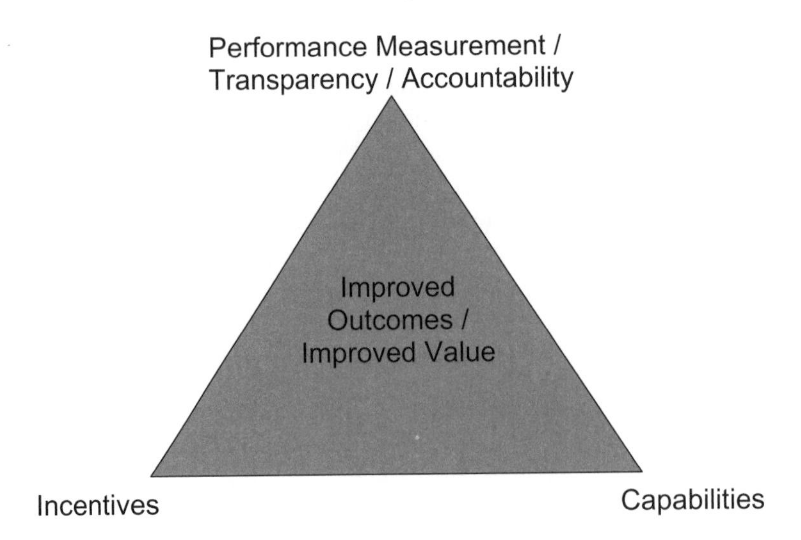

Fig. 1.

1.1. What are integrated delivery systems?

An IDS is a network of organizations that directly provides or arranges to provide a coordinated continuum of services to a defined population and is able and willing to be held accountable for the cost, quality and outcomes of care and, (with others), the health status of the population served [42]. This definition recognizes that not all components of the system may have a single central owner. Some components may involve various alliances and partnerships formalized through contractual relationships. The definition also emphasizes accountability for the cost, quality, and outcomes of care that are delivered. But it is also the IDS' responsibility to maintain and enhance the health of the population at large working with health departments, schools, city and regional planners, the business community, and others.

There are many different types of IDS. Examples include those in which the hospitals, physicians, and insurance products are owned or have exclusive contractual relationships with each other. Examples include Kaiser Permanente, Group Health Cooperative of Puget Sound, and the Veterans Administration (VA). In other cases, there is common ownership of hospitals and exclusive staff model relationships with physician organizations but without owned insurance plans. Examples include the Geisinger Clinic, the Billings Clinic, the Mayo Clinic, and the Cleveland Clinic. Other examples involve hybrid arrangements of owned hospitals but with both employed and non-employed physicians with and without owned insurance products. Examples include the Advocate Health System in Chicago, the Henry Ford Health System in Detroit, the Intermountain Health System in Salt Lake City, Utah, the Sharp Health System in San Diego and the Sutter Health system in Sacramento. Thus, it is best to consider IDS's as existing on a continuum based on the *scope* or number of different organizational entities involved (hospitals, physician organizations, nursing homes, home health centers, ambulatory surgery centers and so on) and the nature of the *economic / legal* relationship among the entities (owned vs. contractual).

1.2. Levels of integration

The *economic /legal* relationship represents the highest level of what we mean by an IDS. But whether such systems can deliver greater value to patients is a function of the extent to which they can actually provide "integrated" services to patients. Two types of integration are important – *functional* integration and *process* integration. Functional integration involves the extent to which support functions such as human resources, financial management, contracting, marketing, information systems, and related functions are coordinated across the operating units of the IDS. Process integration refers to the direct patient care activities that must be coordinated to form a unified whole experience for the patient. This has also been referred to as *clinical integration* [17,44]. While a certain amount of functional integration may be needed to provide a platform for clinical process integration to occur, it is the latter that is most important for achieving greater value. The failure of most IDS's to provide greater value over the past 15 years has been due to their over-emphasis on achieving functional and economic integration to the neglect of the clinical integration process. The greatest benefit but also the greatest challenges to IDS will come from the redesign of the work processes (i.e. clinical integration) as emphasized in Chapter 1.

2. A review of the evidence concerning integrated delivery systems

2.1. Integration and quality

The evidence suggests that integrated physician practices use more evidenced-based care processes, provide more preventive health services, and offer more health promotion programs for the populations they serve than non-integrated practices. Medical groups involve physicians practicing exclusively as either salaried employees of the group or as partners. The facilities are typically owned by the group and there is centralized administration and accountability. Independent Practice Associations (IPAs), on the other hand, are typically decentralized practices with physicians belonging as members typically via nonexclusive contracts. Using these definitions, a survey of 119 physician practices in California found that medical groups were more likely than IPAs to send reminders for mammograms, use diabetes disease management programs, contact patients who missed diabetic eye screenings, collect data on patients treated with beta-blockers after myocardial infarction, send reminders for pediatric well-child visits and/or immunizations, and collect data on patient satisfaction such as wait-times [32]. Also in California, Rittenhouse and Robinson [36] examined the use of care management processes in groups that serve predominately Medicaid patients finding that community clinics and hospital-based clinics used more care management processes for asthma and diabetes than IPAs. Using data from the National Study of Physician Organizations (NSPO), Schmittdiel et al. [41] found that medical groups were more likely to send reminders for preventive services than IPAs. In a related study, medical groups were four times more likely than IPAs to offer health promotion programs such as smoking cessation, stress management, weight loss and nutritional counseling [30]. In the first national longitudinal study of a cohort of 369 large physician practices, medical groups showed significantly greater improvement in the number of care management processes used for chronic illness care than IPAs [48]. In addition, research shows that physician groups that are vertically integrated with hospitals, multi-hospital systems, or health plans either by ownership or contractual arrangement, use more care management processes for patients with chronic illnesses and are more active in prevention and health promotion than physician owned groups [8,30]. In a national study to identify characteristics of high performing physician organizations, Shortell et al. [47] found that vertically-aligned groups were significantly more likely to score in the top quartile on indices for care management processes and health promotion than non-aligned practices.

Not surprisingly, due in part to the greater use of care management processes and preventive services, integrated physician groups perform better on quality and outcome measures such as HEDIS. In Mehrota et al.'s [32] study, medical groups scored significantly better than IPAs for the percent of enrolled female patients who had current mammograms and pap screenings, and for the percent of diabetic patients who had a current eye exam. Gillies et al. [16] developed composite indices for quality based on HEDIS measures to study the impact of physician group and health plan integration on outcomes. They examined the performance of 272 health plans and found that the greater the extent of network integration (defined as either a group or staff model), the higher the plan's performance for women's health screening, immunization rates, heart disease screening and diabetes screening. In Massachusetts, physician groups affiliated with a health care network scored better on 8 out of 12 HEDIS measures compared to non-affiliated groups [14].

Payment systems have also been used to operationalize integration. Shortell and Schmittdiel [46] studied the impact of prepayment incentives (e.g. capitation) on quality in large, multispeciality group practices compared to other groups of equivalent size. They found that the prepaid groups used more care management processes for asthma, congestive heart failure, depression and diabetes than large, but less integrated, physician organizations. In Minnesota, Keating et al. [24] examined 652 diabetic patients enrolled to 3 health plans to test for differences in 6 indicators of technical quality for diabetes care: HbgA1c, LDL, blood pressure control, and nephropathy consultations, eye exams, and foot exams. Patients whose physicians were fee-for-service had significantly lower quality scores than patients whose physicians were salaried.

Integrated physician organizations may also be better positioned to serve as "medical homes" – defined as providing primary first contact care and coordinating care across the entire spectrum of services that patients may need. Two studies examined the current infrastructure and internal capabilities of physician groups to serve as medical homes. Friedberg et al. [15] surveyed 412 physician practices specializing in adult primary care in Massachusetts. Network affiliation was associated with greater capabilities to provide feedback to physicians on patient satisfaction as well as to provide enhanced access for non-English speaking patients through on-site interpreters or bilingual clinic staff. Rittenhouse et al. [35] examined the extent to which large physician groups (greater than 20 physicians) were able to meet multiple criteria for serving as a medical home. They found that vertically integrated groups owned by hospitals or health plans had more capabilities currently in place to address physician-directed medical practice, care coordination, and quality and safety criteria of the medical home.

2.2. *Integration and costs*

There are fewer studies that attempt to examine the impact of integration on costs or efficiency in physician groups [50]. The evidence that is available, however, suggests that more integrated physician groups use fewer resources for the same level of services compared to non-integrated groups. Among Medicare patients in the top one-fifth of health care spending, beneficiaries enrolled in multispeciality or hospital-affiliated groups had lower overall costs than patients treated in smaller groups or solo practices [31]. Medicare patients in integrated delivery systems have fewer hospital days, fewer intensive care days, and less hospital and physician costs compared to other patients [49].

Further, in targeting high cost / high use veterans, the VA reduced clinic visits by 40%; hospital admissions by 63%; bed days by 60%; nursing home admission by 64% and nursing home bed days by 88% while improving overall quality of life (American Medical Group Practice Association, Conference Report, April 1, 2009). Also, recent data from the Medicare Physicians Group Practice Demonstration documented quality improvements while generating $50 million in savings over two years [51]. The key to understanding why the IDS' can achieve such results is they are able to create a *system of learning* on a scale that is not possible for other delivery models; particularly the fragmented small physician practices that still prevail in most parts of the United States.

2.3. Integration and systems engineering

The potential impact of system engineering initiatives on improving organizational performance is enhanced when the organization is highly integrated. Integration removes many of the potential barriers that more fragmented healthcare organization's face when deciding to invest in clinical information systems or quality improvement. Mehrota et al. [32] found that medical groups were more likely than IPAs to have an electronic medical record and to use quality improvement programs. In a national study of large physician practices, Robinson et al. [37] reported that IPAs had significantly less clinical IT capability overall than medical groups but that differences were more pronounced when focusing on specific IT capabilities. For example, they found that clinical IT adoption in IPAs was lowest for capabilities that required integration into the practice setting (e.g, decision support tools, electronic medical record, etc.). Adoption was higher for IT capabilities that could be hosted offsite, such as electronic registries, electronic prescribing, and email capabilities [37]. Friedberg et al. [15] found that network affiliation was associated with greater EMR capabilities and greater capacity to conduct quality improvement initiatives to improve patient satisfaction due to enhanced data collection capabilities. Physicians in larger, salaried groups (more than 50 providers) are significantly more likely to receive data on the quality of care provided to their patients, and to participate in quality improvement efforts, than their colleagues in smaller, non-salaried practices [2].

2.4. Examples of system engineering successes in integrated delivery systems

A closer look at two integrated delivery systems in particular, Kaiser-Permanente and the VA, offer valuable insight into the potential of systems engineering initiatives to improve quality and efficiency especially when conducted within large, integrated health delivery systems. Feachem et al. [12] compared health care cost and utilization data for the UK's National Health System (NHS) with that of Kaiser Permanente. The author's contend that, even though the NHS is more centralized from a payment system perspective, the system is more fragmented in terms of care delivery than Kaiser Permanente. They found that Kaiser Permanente performed better than the NHS in quality while the cost per beneficiary was roughly the same in both systems. The author's cited Kaiser's highly integrated system and investment in information technology as important attributes to its performance. Subsequent research identified efficiencies in hospital utilization as a main source of Kaiser Permanente's advantage. Specifically, bed-day use rates for elderly patients in the UK were almost four times higher than for Kaiser Permanente patients of the same age and acute care categories [18].

Jha et al. [21] examined the results of a system-wide reengineering effort in the VA. They compared the system's performance on multiple quality indicators to that of a national sample of Medicare fee-for-service patients. Baseline measures were calculated for the year prior to when reengineering efforts began. At baseline, the VA had consistently lower scores on quality indicators for prevention, acute care, and chronic care compared to the national sample. Internally, the researchers found that the VA had improved significantly on all nine indicators that it had monitored since baseline. In addition, the VA outperformed fee-for-service Medicare on 12 out of 13 indicators. The results led the authors to conclude: "We believe that the reengineering of VA health care, which included the implementation of a systematic approach to the measurement of, management of, and accountability for quality, was at the heart of the improvement." [21, p. 2224].

Asch et al. [1] analyzed medical records for 596 VA and 992 Medicare patients and measured 348 indicators of quality across 26 health care conditions. They categorized the indicators into four types of care: screening, diagnosis, treatment, and follow-up. They found that the VA performed substantially better across the entire spectrum of care. The difference in quality was particularly evident in indicators that had been identified previously by the VA for improvement. The greatest difference between the VA's performance and that of the national sample was associated with quality measures for procedures that tend to be underdocumented (e.g. counseling and education). The author's attributed this advantage to the VA's investment in an electronic medical record. However, not all of the variation could be contributed to documentation differences. The VA also outperformed the national sample in several areas where underdocumentation was not considered a problem (e.g. laboratory and radiology results) [1]. In addition, the VA has outperformed traditional fee-for-service Medicare on quality measures for the treatment of acute myocardial infarction in hospitals [33] and has been shown to provide better quality for diabetes care compared to commercial managed care plans [24]. In both of these studies, the authors attribute the VA's superior performance to its integrative care delivery system and reengineering efforts including: the implementation of a common EMR; the establishment and dissemination of national standards and best practices; the systematic collection, monitoring, and dissemination of quality data; and the alignment of payment incentives.

Much has been written about the inability to improve value in healthcare due to the lack of a business case for investing in quality or system engineering initiatives [26,34]. As Figure 2 portrays, IDS' are particularly well-suited, through advantages in scope and scale, to capitalize on the potential of systems engineering tools to improve healthcare value. As organizations become integrated, first horizontally across sectors, and then vertically between sectors, the applicability and feasibility of applying system engineering methods to achieve efficiency and lower costs increase due to the alignment of goals and incentives. Fully integrated organizational forms, combining physician, hospital, and payer components of the delivery system allow for the full spectrum of system engineering methods: system control, system analysis, and system design tools.

Statistical process control (SPC) and other system control methods allow for constant monitoring to ensure that performance remains within established limits. Patient wait times, personnel scheduling, and patient-level clinical variables are some examples of processes that are often monitored using system control methods. Hill Physician Medical Group, a large highly integrated independent practice association in California, has incorporated predictive modeling techniques to better manage patients with chronic illnesses [11]. Effective use of system control methods require the ability to collect and analyze data at the provider, care team, and organizational levels.

System analysis tools are often employed in order to evaluate the efficiency of established processes in accordance with established performance goals. By investing in clinical information technology and employing methods such as Deming's Plan-Do-Check-Act, vertically integrated systems such as Intermountain Health Care and Baylor Health System have significantly improved care coordination and patient outcomes during the critical transition from inpatient to outpatient care for patients with congestive heart failure [11].

System design tools such as quality functional deployment (QFD) deconstruct organizational and functional silos by incorporating the demands of various stakeholders into key processes. QFD establishes system-level performance goals based on stakeholder needs and identifies processes critical to the successful attainment of these goals. The VA's comprehensive reengineering effort cited earlier is a good example of how system design methods can guide process improvement to increase healthcare value. As organizational processes become integrated, the ability of systems engineering tools to improve health care value increases.

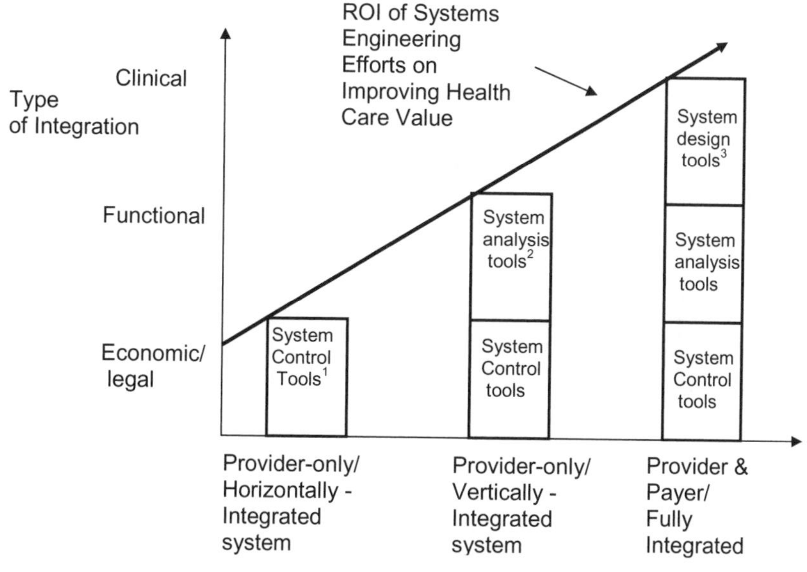

Notes:
1. Methods to monitor the performance of established processes within defined limits (e.g. statistical process control).
2. Methods to analyze the performance of established processes in order to improve efficiency, productivity, or value (e.g. Plan-Do-Study-Act).
3. Methods to design key processes in accordance with stakeholder demands (e.g. quality functional deployment).

Fig. 2.

3. Increasing the number of integrated delivery systems

The evidence that IDS' consistently outperform other health care delivery models is not conclusive. Nonetheless, the weight of the evidence suggests that IDS' have the greater capacity to redesign patient care processes. This is due to their greater use of team-based care, electronic health records, participation in formal ongoing quality improvement initiatives, and their ability to engage physicians in working for the overall organization's goals.

The question then becomes how might more IDS be encouraged to develop? We suggest that a combination of payment reform, modified regulatory and legal policies, and increased transparency and accountability are needed.

3.1. Payment reform

Most health care services such as hospital care, physician care, and nursing home care are paid separately in silos. Hospitals are paid by diagnostic related groups (DRGs); most physicians by fee-for-service and nursing homes by pre-established rates. There are no financial incentives for different parts of the system to work together on the patient's behalf.

A portfolio of payment reforms including total capitation, bundled payment, episode-of-care based payments, pay for performance, and care coordinator bonus payments could encourage greater integration. (See Table 1 for a summary) Congress on behalf of CMS' Medicare patients as well as private sector

Table 1
Evaluation of payment reform options

Reform option	Objective				
	Promote provider integration	Control costs	Improve quality	Political feasibility	Opportunistic feasibility
Full Capitation – Global Payment	***	***	**	–	*
Bundled Payment	**	**	**	**	**
Episode of Care Based Payment	**	**	**	**	*
Pay for Performance	*	*	**	***	**
Care Coordination Payment	*	*	**	**	**

Source: Adapted from: RE Mechanic and SH Altman (2009) Payment Reform Options: Episode Payment Is A Good Place to Start. Health Affairs, January 27, 2009, 28(1) Supplement: W267.
***High Potential.
**Good Potential.
*Low Potential.
–No Potential.

insurers could develop capitated payment rates for entire population of patients; episodes of care based capitated payment for selected chronic conditions; and bundled payments to hospitals and physicians for selected acute conditions. Each form of payment would require risk adjustment and local area cost of living and wage adjustments.

Total capitation would involve the establishment of a set dollar figure per patient per month for a pre-determined group of potential patients. This, in effect, establishes an overall budget for the IDS providing care to the given population. The most notable private sector example is Kaiser Permanente headquartered in Oakland, California with approximately nine million members enrolled in seven regions in the United States. The most notable public sector example is the VA headquartered in Washington D.C. with care provided to patients in 21 vertically integrated service networks (VISNs) around the country.

Capitation for all sources for a given population is only likely to work, however, when the delivery system is very tightly integrated as when hospitals are owned by the system or can exert major influence on other hospitals and the physicians are employed such as in the VA or in a exclusive relationship with the delivery system such as in Kaiser Permanente. The ability to redesign work care processes, eliminate waste and unwarranted complexity is more difficult when the hospitals and physicians are loosely coupled, and, therefore, are less capable of assuming overall risk for given population.

However, the federal government and private sector payers might be able to move toward total capitation over time through the use of episode care based payment for selected chronic conditions and bundled payments for selected acute conditions [28] For example, episode of care based payment might be developed for Diabetes and Asthma patients based on three years of previous risk adjusted cost and utilization data. Provided pre-determined quality criteria were met (for example, using the HEDIS or National Quality Forum Diabetes and Asthma Measures), providers could share in the savings. For an acute condition such as Coronary Artery Bypass Graft Surgery, Hip and Knee Replacements, a pre-determined risk adjusted payment might be established for the total care – hospitals, physicians, and other post hospitalization care – for the entire event constituting a "bundled" payment. Again, this could be initially based on three years of previous risk adjusted cost, utilization, and outcome data to establish the initial bundled rate. Provided that pre-established quality criteria were met, hospitals and physicians could share in any resulting savings.

Both episode-of-care based payment and bundled payment would provide incentives for hospitals and physicians to examine how care is currently being delivered, and to look for efficiencies and quality improvements that will enable them to provide more cost effective care. The key is to provide financial incentives for providers to become more *inter-dependent* in coordinating care for patients that transcends any one provider entity or setting alone.

In addition to paying for greater interdependence, CMS and private payers should also pay for results; that is, for achieving better outcomes and lower cost or more efficient utilization of resources. Existing pay for performance initiatives have primarily emphasized process indicators of quality such as preventive exams, diagnostic screening exams, lipid testing and results and blood sugar testing and results with less emphasis on outcomes or costs [38,39]. There have been small incremental improvements on these quality measures but not the "breakthrough" improvements desired. While some of the relative "under performance" may be due to the relatively small amount of financial incentives (generally on the order of two to three percent of physician annual income), a larger reason may be that many physicians are not yet organized in such a way that they can respond to the incentives in a more robust fashion. However, capitation, episodes-of-care based payment and bundled payment *combined with* some added payments for results may move more physicians (and hospitals) towards a more integrated delivery model to capture the rewards.

Third, physicians who choose to remain independent could be encouraged to take on greater responsibility for coordinating patient care by paying them a care coordination fee. Criteria would need to be established for physicians to serve as "personal or primary care coordinators" in return for the increased payment. Some examples of such criteria might be establishing a pre-determined volume of patients served; identifying a primary affiliated hospital and a list of physician referral partners; and the ability to share patient information across providers to monitor medication adherence and related data. In addition, or alternatively, physicians could sign up to be a personal primary care provider coordinator but the additional payment would depend on achieving certain pre-defined quality and cost results as previously discussed.

3.2. Modifying laws and regulations

The potential for hospitals and physicians to work more effectively together is currently restricted by prohibition against gainsharing [7,40]. Gainsharing prohibits hospitals from offering physicians financial assistance for use of electronic health records or other services. Such activities could be interpreted as inducement for physicians to admit patients to the hospital. However, hospitals can provide such assistance if the transaction meets certain clinical integration criteria such as the development of practice standards and protocols, investment of capital to purchase clinical information systems that provide quality and cost data at the provider level, and the establishment of a common medical director to provide oversight and coordinate patient care [7]. Gainsharing prohibition would need to be modified to allow hospitals and physicians to share savings that result from redesigning work processes under bundled payment arrangements.

IDS' require well functioning teams. Often the functioning team member is constrained by current practice laws restricting what nurse practitioners, physician assistants, pharmacists and others can do. This hampers the ability to redesign work that can result in a more cost-effective care. These laws should be changed to permit greater experimentation in the use of the different types of health care professionals. One approach would be the use of institutional licensure. Based on training standards and performance, the IDS as a whole, or a significant subcomponent for hospitals and physicians groups, would be licensed and held accountable for the care provided. In return, they would be permitted to make more flexible use of physician assistants, nurse practitioners and other health professionals. Another approach would be to license functions and activities based on people's competencies to perform rather than the degrees held or their job classification.

Anti-trust laws are another barrier to greater IDS formation. There is the concern that if various hospitals and physicians come together to form IDS' that such entities may dominate a given market. They become potential monopolies increasing prices and driving up costs. This is a legitimate concern as recent evidence suggests that hospital mergers, acquisitions, and consolidations have resulted in price increases with no or little evidence of quality improvement [9]. However, it is important to note that with CMS as the major payer moving to more capitation, episode of care based payment, bundled payments and payment based on results, it would be difficult for even the largest dominant IDS in a market to exert undue leverage given that Medicare patients are the largest single source of hospital revenue.

3.3. *Increasing transparency and accountability*

IDS' can also be promoted by expanding requirements for increased transparency and accountability for quality, cost, and service performance. CMS working with AHRQ should take the lead in building on the current annual quality report using measures approved by the National Quality Forum (NQF). These include ambulatory measures related to prevention, coronary artery disease, heart failure, diabetes, asthma, depression, prenatal care and quality measures addressing overuse and under-use [20, p. 69] It would also include Hospital Quality Alliance measures on coronary artery syndromes, heart failure, pneumonia, smoking cessation, surgical infection prevention, and various patient communication and patient experience measures. Measures of cost and resource use would also be reported. These data would be reported for the nation along with regional and state breakdowns and, where feasible, down to the individual IDS and medical practice site levels. Making such data visible and easily accessible will enable all stakeholders – CMS, Medicare patients, and providers to make more informed choices. Over time, private sector insurers will also report such data as a condition of participation in insurance exchanges. This will permit all employees and purchasers of care to be able to compare the performance of providers for purposes of making more informed choices. If these data reveal the superior performance of IDS, as some current data suggest, then one might expect the migration of patients to such systems. The competitive response on the part of others will be to form their own version of an IDS through the development of larger physician practices, and networks, physician-hospital organizations (PHOs) and related forms of practice comprising Accountable Care Organizations (ACOs) [13,43].

Much of the above, however, depends on the greater adoption and use of electronic health records (EHRs) by hospitals and physicians. Currently, only a small percentage of hospitals and physicians have fully functional EHRs [3,4,22]. Even larger practices have a relatively small number of EHR capabilities [37]. The Obama administration has allocated $19 billion for the adoption and implementation of EHRs in hospital and physician practices. The concern is that most of these funds will go to the purchase of hardware and software rather than to technical assistance to providers for first reassessing how care might be better delivered. Work process redesign needs to precede the implementation of electronic health records recognizing that these are, after all, only the tools to facilitate more cost-effective care. Although larger IDS' such as Kaiser Permanente, Inter-Mountain, the VA and others have already implemented EHRs, most hospitals and physicians have not. It will be important to target a significant portion of the information technology funds to assist such providers in adopting EHRs and adjusting to the short run loss of productivity that usually results [6].

Table 2
Framework for facilitating the development of IDS'

Strategy	Structure	Culture	Technical
– Strategic Priority for DHHS and CMS – Strategic Priority for Hospital and Physician Leaders	– That Link Hospitals, Physicians and Other Providers – That Facilitate Learning – Exchange of Information and Knowledge	– Move from Organization and Provider Centric to Patient and Family Centric – More from Individual Provider Autonomy to Collaborative Teams and Shared Decision-Making with Patits and Families	– Interoperable Electronic Health Records – Continuous Quality Improvement and Work Redesign Methods – Packaged Interventions Such as Chronic Care Model

4. Concluding framework

IDS's are likely to play a central role in the reform of the nation's health care system. New payment incentives, transformed legal and regulatory policies, and expanded data collection, analysis, and public reporting capabilities will encourage the development and spread of more IDSs of various forms. One way to think about how these factors might interact is to consider them in terms of *strategic, structural, cultural, and technical dimensions* (see Table 2). At the national policy level, the Department of Health and Human Services (DHHS) must make creating greater value a top strategic priority of the government and designate CMS to play a leadership role. At the operational level, hospital and physician leaders must do the same. Structures then need to be created that enable hospitals and physicians to work more effectively together in response to reformed payment systems which will encourage such collaboration. Some potentially viable structures are Accountable Care Organizations (ACOs) including multi-specialty group practices, revitalized physician-hospital organizations, virtual organizations based on naturally occurring physician referral networks and hospital relationships, and the development of interdependent physician organizations which link together small physician practices [13,43]. Such structures will provide greater opportunities for learning and the exchange of information and knowledge.

A major barrier to creating these structures is ingrained cultures. Specifically, there is need to move from an organization-centered and profession-centered culture to a patient-centered culture. Too often, the effort to redesign work processes in the name of patients tends to be dominated by the needs of the health care organizations and the professionals providing care. Instead, patients and their families need to be the first and primary sources of input in how they wish to receive care, taking into the account not only documented medical needs but also patient preferences. Particular attention needs to be paid to the growing cultural and linguistic diversity of the country calling for new cultural and linguistic skills in communicating with patients and families. Further, there needs to be a shift from a culture that emphasizes individual professional autonomy to collective teamwork among professionals and shared decision making between teams of professionals, patients, and their families. Finally, the technical tools to redesign patient care work processes must be made available. These include electronic health records with sufficient functionality, continuous quality improvement work process redesign methodologies, and the implementation of "package" interventions such as the chronic care model [52]. All four – strategy, structure, culture, and techniques – must be aligned to maximize the potential of IDS' and related forms to increase the quality and outcomes of care and moderate the rate of growth of costs of care for all Americans.

References

[1] S. Asch, E. McGlynn, M. Hogan, R. Hayward, P. Shekelle, L. Rubinstein et al., Comparison of quality of care for patients in the Veterans Health Administration and patients in a national sample, *Annals of Internal Medicine* **141**(12) (2004), 938–045.

[2] A. Audet, M. Doty, J. Shamasdin and S. Schoenbaum, Measure, learn, and improve: Physicians' involvement in quality improvement, *Health Affairs* **24**(3) (2005), 843–853.

[3] D. Blumenthal, Stimulating the Adoption of Health Information Technology, *New England Journal of Medicine* **360**(15) (2009), 1477–1479.

[4] D. Blumenthal and J. Glaser, Information technology comes to medicine, *New England Journal of Medicine* **356** (2007), 2527–2534.

[5] P. Budetti, S. Shortell, T. Waters, J. Alexander, L. Burns, R. Gillies et al., Physician and health system integration, *Health Affairs* **21**(1) (2002), 203–210.

[6] B. Chaudhry, J. Wang, S. Wu, M. Maglione, W. Mojica, E. Roth et al., Systematic Review: Impact of Health Information Technology on Quality, Efficiency, and Costs of Medical Care, *Annals of Internal Medicine* **144**(10) (2006), 742–752.

[7] L. Casalino, The Federal Trade Commission, clinical integration, and the organization of physician practice, *Journal of Health Politics, Policy, and Law* **31**(3) (2006), 569–585.

[8] L. Casalino, R. Gillies, S. Shortell, J. Schmittdiel, T. Bodenheimer, J. Robinson et al., External incentives, information technology, and organized processes to improve health care quality for patients with chronic diseases, *Journal of the American Medical Association* **289**(4) (2003), 434–441.

[9] A. Cueller and P. Gertler, Strategic integration of hospitals and physicians, *Journal of Health Economics* **25** (2006), 1–28.

[10] T. Emswiler and L. Nichols, Baylor Health Care System: High-performance Integrated Health Care. The Commonwealth Fund. Available at http://www.commonwealthfund.org/~/link.aspx?_id=621C6DDD08D74CCB933D64B0F98A4C52&_z=z, 2009.

[11] T. Emswiler and L. Nichols, Hill Physicians Medical Group: Independent Physicians Working to Improve Quality and Reduce Costs. The Commonwealth Fund. Available at http://www.commonwealthfund.org/Content/Publications/ Case-Studies/2009/Mar/Hill-Physicians-Medical-Group-Independent-Physicians-W orking-to-Improve-Quality-and-Reduce-Costs.aspx, 2009.

[12] R. Feachem, N. Sekhri and K. White, Getting more for their dollar: A comparison of the NHS with California's Kaiser Permanente, *British Medical Journal* **324** (2002), 135–143.

[13] E.S. Fisher, M.B. McCleim, J. Bertko et al., Fostering Accountable Health Care: Moving Forward in Medicare, *Health Affairs*, **28**(1) (27 January 2009), Supplement: W219–W231.

[14] M. Friedberg, K. Coltin, S. Pearson, K. Kleinman, J. Zheng, J. Singer et al., Does affiliation of physician groups with one another produce higher quality primary care? *Journal of General Internal Medicine* **22**(10) (2007), 1385–1392.

[15] M. Friedberg, D. Safran, K. Coltin, M. Dresser and E. Schneider, Readiness for the patient-centered medical home: Structural capabilities of massachusetts primary care practices, *Journal of General Internal Medicine* **24**(2) (2008), 162–169.

[16] R. Gillies, K. Chenok, S. Shortell, G. Pawlson and J. Wimbush, The impact of health plan delivery system organization on clinical quality and patient satisfaction, *Health Services Research* **41**(4, part 1) (2006), 1181–1199.

[17] R. Gillies, S. Shortell, D. Anderson, J. Mitchell and K. Morgan, Conceptualizing and measuring integration: Findings from the health systems integration study, *Hospital and Health Services Administration* **38**(4) (1993), 467–489.

[18] C. Ham, N. York, S. Sutch and R. Shaw, Hospital bed utilisation in the NHS, Kaiser Permanente, and the US Medicare Programme: Analysis of routine data, *British Medical Journal* **327** (2003), 1257.

[19] Institute of Medicine, *Crossing the Quality Chasm: A New Health System for the 21st Century*, Washington DC: National Academies Press, 2001.

[20] Institute of Medicine, *Rewarding Provider Performance: Aligning Incentives in Medicare*, Washington DC: National Academies Press, 2007.

[21] A. Jha, J. Perlin, K. Kizer and R. Dudley, Effect of the transformation of the Veterans Affairs Health Care System on the quality of care, *New England Journal of Medicine* **348**(22) (2003), 2218–2227.

[22] A. Jha, T. Ferris, K. Donelan, C. DesRoches, A. Shields, S. Rosenbaum et al., How Common are Electronic Health Records in the United States? A Summary of the Evidence, *Health Affairs* **25** (Web exclusive) (2006), w496–w507.

[23] N. Keating, M. Landrum, B. Landon, J. Ayanian, C. Borbas, R. Wolf et al., The influence of physicians' practice management strategies and financial arrangements on quality of care among patients with diabetes, *Medical Care* **42**(9) (2004), 829–839.

[24] E. Kerr, R. Gerzoff, N. Krein, J. Selby, J. Piette, J. Curb et al., *Diabetes care quality in the Veterans Affairs Health Care System and commercial managed care: The triad study* **141**(4) (2004), 272–281.

[25] C. Kim, D. Williamson, C. Mangione, M. Safford, J. Selby, D. Marrero et al., Managed care organization and the quality of diabetes care: The translating research into action for diabetes (triad) study, *Diabetes Care* **27**(7) (2004), 1529–1534.

[26] S. Leatherman, D. Berwick, D. Lies, S. Lewin, F. Davidoff, T. Nolan et al., The Business Case for Quality: Case Studies and an Analysis, *Health Affairs* **22**(2) (2003), 17–30.

[27] R. Li, J. Simon, T. Bodenheimer, R. Gillies, L. Casalino, J. Schmittdiel et al., Organizational factors affecting the adoption of diabetes care management processes in physician organizations, *Diabetes Care* **27**(10) (2004), 2312–1316.

[28] H. Luft, *Total Cure: The Antidote to the Health Care Crisis*, Cambridge, Massachusetts: Harvard University Press, 2009.

[29] S. McMenamin, H. Schauffler, S. Shortell, T. Rundall and R. Gillies, Support for smoking sessation interventions in physician organizations, *Medical Care* **41**(12) (2003), 1396–1406.

[30] S. McMenamin, J. Schmittdiel, H. Halpin, R. Gillies, T. Rundall and S. Shortell, Health promotion in physician organizations: Results from a national study, *American Journal of Preventive Medicine* **26**(4) (2004), 259–264.

[31] Medicare Payment Advisory Commission, Assessing alternatives to the sustainable growth rate system. Retrieved April 24, 2009, from www.medpac.gov/documents/Mar07_GSR_mandated_report.pdf, 2007.

[32] A. Mehrotra, A. Epstein and M. Rosenthal, Do integrated medical groups provide higher-quality medical care than IPAs? *Annals of Internal Medicine* **145**(11) (2006), 826–833.

[33] L. Petersen, S. Normand, L. Leape and B. McNeil, Comparison of use of medications after acute myocardial infarction in the Veterans Health Administration and Medicare, *Circulation* **104**(24) (2004), 2898–2904.

[34] P. Reid, W. Compton, J. Grossman and G. Fanjiang, *Building a Better Delivery System: A New Engineering/Health Care Partnership*, Washington DC:National Academies Press, 2005.

[35] D. Rittenhouse, L. Casalino, R. Gillies, S. Shortell and B. Lau, Measuring the medical home infrastructure in large medical groups, *Health Affairs* **27**(5) (2008), 1246–1258.

[36] D. Rittenhouse and J. Robinson, Improving quality in Medicaid: The use of care management processes for chronic illness and preventive care, *Medical Care* **44**(1) (2006), 47–54.

[37] J. Robinson, L. Casalino, R. Gillies, D. Rittenhouse, S. Shortell and S. Fernandes-Taylor, Financial incentives, quality improvement programs, and the adoption of clinical information technology, *Medical Care* **47**(4) (2009), 411–417.

[38] M. Rosenthal, B. Landon, K. Howitt, H. Song and A. Epstein, Climbing up the pay-for-performance learning curve: Where are the early adopters now? *Health Affairs* **26**(6) (2007), 1674–1682.

[39] M. Rosenthal and R. Dudley, Pay-for-performance: Will the latest payment trend improve care? *Journal of the American Medical Association* **297**(7) (2007), 740–744.

[40] W. Sage, Legislating delivery system reform: A 30,000-foot view of the 800-pound gorilla, *Health Affairs* **26**(6) (2007), 1553–1556.

[41] J. Schmittdiel, S. McMenamin, H. Halpin, R. Gillies, T. Bodenheimer, S. Shortell et al., The use of patient and physician reminders for preventive services: Results from a national study of physician organizations, *Preventive Medicine* **39**(5) (2004), 1000–1006.

[42] S. Shortell, D. Anderson, R. Gillies, J. Mitchell and K. Morgan, Building integrated systems - the holographic organization, *The Healthcare Forum Journal* **36**(2) (1993), 20–26.

[43] S. Shortell and L. Casalino, Health care reform requires accountable care systems, *Journal of the American Medical Association* **300**(1) (2008), 95–97.

[44] S. Shortell, R. Gillies, D. Anderson, K. Erickson and J. Mitchell, *Remaking Health Care in America: Building Organized Delivery Systems*, (1st ed.), San Francisco: Jossey-Bass, 1996.

[45] S. Shortell, R. Gillies, D. Anderson, K. Erickson and J. Mitchell, *Remaking Health Care in America: The Evolution of Organized Delivery Systems*, (2nd ed.), San Francisco: Jossey-Bass, 2000.

[46] S. Shortell and J. Schmittdiel, Prepaid groups and organized delivery systems: Promise, performance, and potential, in: *Toward a 21st century health system*, A. Enthoven and L. Tollen, eds, San Francisco: Jossey-Bass, 2004, pp. 1–21.

[47] S. Shortell, J. Schmittdiel, M. Wang, R. Li, R. Gillies, L. Casalino et al., An empirical assessment of high-performing medical groups: Results of a national survey, *Medical Care Research and Review* **62**(4) (2005), 407–434.

[48] S. Shortell, R. Gillies, J. Siddiqve, L. Casalino, D. Rittenhouse, J. Robinson and R. McCurdy, Improving Chronic Illness Care: A Longitudinal Cohort Analysis of Large Physician Organizations, *Medical Care* **47**(9) (2009), 932–939.

[49] J. Sterns, Quality, efficiency, and organizational structure, *Journal of Health Care Finance* **37**(1) (2007), 100–107.

[50] L. Tollen, *Physician Organization in Relation to Quality and Efficiency of Care: A Synthesis of Recent Literature*, The Commonwealth Fund, 2008.

[51] M. Trisolini, The Medicare Physician Group Demonstration: Lessons Learned on Improving Efficiency and Quality in Health Care. New York: The Commonwealth Fund, 2008.

[52] E. Wagner, B. Austin and M. Von Korff, Improving Outcomes in Chronic Illness, *Managed Care Quarterly* **4**(2) (1996), 12–25.

Stephen M. Shortell, Ph.D., M.P.H.M.B.A. is dean of the School of Public Health, the Blue Cross of California Distinguished Professor of Health Policy and Management, and Professor of Organizational Behavior at the School of Public Health and the Haas School of Business at the University of California-Berkeley. Dr. Shortell received his undergraduate degree from the University of Notre Dame, his masters degree in public health from UCLA, and his Ph.D. in the behavioral sciences from the University of Chicago. A leading health care scholar, Dr. Shortell has done extensive research identifying the organizational and managerial correlates of quality of care and of high performing health care organizations. He is currently conducting research on the evaluation of quality improvement initiatives and on the implementation of evidence-based medicine practices in physician organizations. He is an elected member of the Institute of Medicine and has received many awards including the distinguished Baxter-Allegiance Prize for his contributions to health services research, the Gold Medal Award from the American College of Healthcare Executives for his contributions to the health care field, and the Distinguished Investigator Award from the Association for Health Services Research. His most recent book (with colleagues) is entitled *Remaking Health Care in America: The Evolution of Organized Delivery Systems*. During 2006–07 he was a Fellow at the Center for Advanced Study in the Behavioral Sciences at Stanford.

Rodney K. McCurdy MHA is currently a doctoral student in Health Services and Policy Analysis at the University of California-Berkeley. He received a bachelor degree in business administration from the University of Maryland and a masters of health administration degree from Baylor University. He served 20 years as a healthcare administrator in the United States Air Force where he obtained the rank of Major and held a variety of leadership positions. His current research is associated with the National Study of Physician Organizations, a joint Berkeley, UC-San Francisco, and University of Chicago project. His research interests include the application of organizational theory to health care including effects of physician-hospital integration strategies and healthcare networks on quality and access. In addition, he is a consultant for strategy and business development to Sutter Health, a large multi-hospital system in Northern California. He is a Fellow with the American College of Health Care Executives and a member of both the Healthcare Financial Management Association and AcademyHealth.

Information Knowledge Systems Management 8 (2009) 383–414
DOI 10.3233/IKS-2009-0149
IOS Press

Chapter 21

Academic health centers

Fred Sanfilippo
E-mail: fredsanfilippo@emory.edu

Abstract: Academic Health Centers (AHCs) are comprised of academic, hospital, and clinical practice components that play a key role in healthcare delivery by their special ability to identify and implement improvements in outcomes, safety, cost-benefit, and satisfaction. They do this by utilizing a wide range of academic and clinical health professionals and disciplines to provide cutting-edge, highly specialized patient care as well as disproportionate uncompensated care in communities nationwide; to identify the effectiveness of different diagnostic and therapeutic approaches through clinical research; to foster new discoveries in biomedical science and technology and their clinical application; and to educate future generations of health professionals who apply these improvements.

As the traditional homes of innovation in health and healing through research, and as the major sites of implementing change through education, AHCs have been at the forefront of improving healthcare. To successfully improve the effectiveness and efficiency of healthcare delivery, it is critical that AHCs continue to serve as uniquely integrated models for improving quality and value through novel approaches in education, research, and service.

1. The academic health center: Introduction and background

1.1. Definition and models

There is no hard and fast definition of an AHC. The generally agreed upon definition – and the one used by the Association of Academic Health Centers (AAHC) – identifies AHCs as degree-granting institutions that include a medical school, at least one other health professional school, and affiliation with a teaching hospital or health system [55]. However, for several reasons there is a broad diversity of models under this or any current definition of AHCs.

First, the relative balance among the missions of healthcare, education, research, and community service at AHCs varies substantially. This can range from those institutions (often state supported) that are focused primarily on training physicians and other healthcare professionals, to those at research universities with a major interest and capability for discovery, to those affiliated with large clinical delivery systems more oriented to provide healthcare.

Second, in addition to the more than 130 medical schools that form the core of each AHC, there is a wide range in the number and type of other health professional schools and programs that are part of individual AHCs. Many AHCs include schools of nursing, public health, dentistry, pharmacy, allied health, veterinary medicine, and/or optometry, among others [1].

Third, the teaching hospital or health system affiliated with an AHC may range in size and complexity from a single on-site, university-owned hospital to a complex system of multiple independent hospitals and clinics with wide geographic dispersion that in some cases even extends to different states and countries.

1389-1995/09/$17.00

Fourth, the manner in which the staff of physicians as well as the nurses, dentists, pharmacists, and other health professionals, practice in their AHC can vary significantly. The organizational structure of clinical practices can be not-for-profit, for-profit, partnerships, or other corporate models involving individuals and groups. In addition, the relationship with the university and/or hospital partner can range from a loose affiliation, to being owned or controlled by either or both under one corporate umbrella.

Finally, the relationship among AHC components may range from a single unified model under one governance and management structure to a loose affiliation among the schools, hospitals, and practices [30].

With so much variation among AHCs in the structure and function of their component units and relationships to each other, it is not surprising that it is commonly said, "If you've seen one academic health center, you've seen one academic health center."

1.2. History and evolution

1.2.1. Creation of the AHC: the Flexner report

The AHC model of university-based schools and departments affiliated with hospitals and clinical practices has a relatively short and narrow history in the United States dating back 100 years to the work of Abraham Flexner and the impact of his landmark report in 1910 [20]. Supported by the Carnegie Foundation for the Advancement of Teaching, Flexner's report, "Medical Education in the United States and Canada," summarized the findings from his personal visits to all 175 medical schools then in the U.S. and Canada, which clearly described the unsatisfactory state of physician training at most of them. In many cases, students were selected simply on the basis of their ability to pay for training without regard to prior education or experience. Teaching was largely by apprenticeship with physicians who had neither university affiliation nor background in the scientific basis of disease, and whose methods of practice varied widely in terms of diagnostic and therapeutic decision-making.

In his report, Flexner discussed the best practices to be emulated from model programs at a handful of schools, especially Johns Hopkins, which had been established in the 1880s as the first research university in the nation. Its medical school, organized by the noted pathologist Dr. William Welch, was developed using the German model of teaching medicine based on science. The "Hopkins Model" of medical education and clinical practice was grounded in evidence-based scientific methods and the use of full-time educators, scientists, and physicians as faculty.

The impact of Flexner's report cannot be overstated. His public crusade to change medical education as the basis for addressing the significant national dissatisfaction with healthcare delivery became headline news around the country. Within a few years, more than 50 medical schools were closed. Moreover, Flexner's influence with private foundations led to financial incentives for medical schools that chose to emulate the academic Hopkins model.

As a result of the dramatic changes in medical education resulting from Flexner's work, the practice of American medicine quickly transitioned from largely a skill-based trade to a knowledge-based profession. Translation of newly discovered scientific findings to clinical practice accelerated markedly. The treatment of disease based on a standard use of medical and surgical intervention quickly followed suit, in contrast to what had often been a random or anecdotal mix of allopathic, homeopathic, naturopathic, and chiropractic approaches. In addition, the development of public health as a scientifically based discipline – focused on disease prevention – took hold as Welch subsequently went on to form the first school of public health in the world at Hopkins in 1918.

1.2.2. Evolution of AHCs

Following the transformation of medical education and practice, and the creation of public health as an academic discipline, biomedical research and discovery increased substantially through the first half of the 20th century. This "new model" of medical education had a profound impact on the growth of medical research. In particular, a wide range of novel drugs, along with new medical and surgical approaches for many diseases, was developed and began to offer many more options that significantly improved health outcomes. To enhance this growth in biomedical science and technology, the federal government began to support basic biomedical research after World War II with the establishment of the National Institutes of Health (NIH) and its substantial extramural funding programs [23]. This increased support for basic and clinical research dramatically accelerated the number of research faculty at many medical schools.

As the understanding of basic mechanisms and manifestations of health and disease increased, the importance of teaching scientific method and application did as well. By the 1950's, the profession of medicine based on scientific knowledge was in full bloom, and AHCs were expanding nationwide.

Following these fundamental changes in the educational and scientific basis for healthcare, ensuing changes in the cost and reimbursement for healthcare have had a profound influence on the clinical practice of medicine [14], along with the very nature of AHCs. The expanding complexity and scope of scientific discovery, and its application to education and practice required AHCs to find ways to subsidize the increased expense of personnel, facilities, and technology for education and research. Clinical revenue became a major means for supporting the academic missions along with fundraising, especially at private institutions, and state support at public ones. The enactment of Medicare and Medicaid in the 1960's provided additional sources of federal and state funding for clinical reimbursement, and contributed to the enormous growth in the number of clinical faculty at AHCs that followed suit. However, by the late 1960's overall expenditures for healthcare had already begun to become a serious national problem. As stated by then President Nixon on July 11, 1969, "Unless action is taken within the next two or three years ... we will have a breakdown in our medical system."

During the 1970s, the increasing shortage of primary care physicians, along with perceived local economic and healthcare service benefits, were major factors leading to the creation of several new AHCs across the country. Most of these were formed by creating state-sponsored medical schools that became affiliated with pre-existing community hospitals and private practices. Likewise, to enhance their strong integrated healthcare practices, new AHCs were developed at the Mayo Clinic with creation of its medical school in 1972, and more recently at the Cleveland Clinic through its affiliation with medical schools at Ohio State University and subsequently Case Western Reserve University.

With increasing financial pressures on clinical income to help support AHC activities (see next section), many AHCs in the 1990s were forced to re-assess the cost-benefit and organizational alignment of their healthcare enterprise. To mitigate financial risk, some universities loosened their hospitals/health system relationship by divesting ownership (e.g., University of Minnesota, Georgetown), while others strengthened their relationship through changes in management and governance (e.g., Johns Hopkins, University of Pennsylvania) [27]. The benefit of hindsight to date suggests that the latter strategy of increasing rather than diminishing organizational alignment had a greater benefit in improving academic and clinical productivity of the AHC. With the increasing operational and financial complexity and interdependence of the component units of AHCs, there has been an increasing trend over the past decade to align management and governance structures across the clinical and academic components (see below).

The turn of the millennium has brought with it the aging of the baby boomers and the conclusion by many that a significant shortage of physicians is impending. After several years of debate, the Association of American Medical Colleges (AAMC) took the position in 2006 of recommending a significant increase in the number of medical students trained in the United States [2,3]. The controversy around this will be discussed in a later section of this chapter, but a major impact has been an increase in the number of new medical schools being developed to meet the perceived need, which in turn is again resulting in the creation of new AHCs.

1.3. Funding: Sources and uses

The funding models for AHCs vary significantly according to their mission emphasis, public vs. private status, and their organizational structure and alignment. The cost of educating health professionals has risen dramatically in the past 10–20 years, with medical student education having the greatest increase due to rising use and cost of technology as well as faculty and staff salaries [2,3]. Nursing education has also become a challenge, largely because the significant increases in compensation and relative shortages of nurses in practice have put significant pressure on the cost and availability of nursing faculty [19].

Direct sources for funding the education of health professionals include tuition, endowment income, and state subsidies, especially at public institutions. Shortfalls in these sources from the academic units of AHCs are usually addressed by funds flow from the clinical units. Thus, the alignment between organizational components has a significant impact on the ability of the AHC to support educational activities. A recent example of this impact was seen at the University of Utah medical school, where reduced state and federal support resulted in an announced reduction of the 2009 entering class size by 20% [8].

For those AHCs heavily engaged in basic biomedical research, the unfunded overhead of externally sponsored research typically approaches 10–25% of expenditures, representing a significant expense that is not covered by indirect cost recovery [50]. For those with large research expenditures that can exceed $100M, this becomes a significant financial challenge [22]. Support for this shortfall comes largely from fundraising, technology transfer, and clinical income subsidy. As with educational activities, funding from the clinical units to cover research shortfalls is highly dependent upon the organizational alignment of each AHC.

Over the past 20 years, clinical revenue has been largely tied to reimbursement for physician encounters and medical procedures, rather than health outcomes and value. Healthcare expenditures have risen dramatically as a result of many factors (discussed below and in other chapters), and attempts by payers to control costs have focused primarily on volume pricing and "managing" care delivery, rather than improving the quality or value of the care provided. "Managed care" provided by health plans quickly moved to financial management of expenses, often by negotiating discounted payments to providers – sometimes below their costs – and by administratively limiting services to patients. This had the perverse impact of moving healthcare from a highly personalized professional service to essentially a commodity. For AHCs, the impact of these factors on clinical revenue has varied dramatically depending upon their local market and the size and scope of the care they provide, which together are what mostly determine patient mix and payer mix. Based on these factors, some AHCs, especially those with a significantly large local market share, have generated significant clinical margins, while others have not.

In terms of expenses, the growth of highly specialized care and newly developed options for treatment and diagnosis have added disproportionate costs at AHCs, which have been the major providers of such services. Moreover, as the providers of last resort in many communities, and offering the widest range of clinical options for training students and residents, AHCs typically provide a significant and disproportionate share of uncompensated care in communities, especially those without public hospitals

Table 1
The Value Proposition of AHCs: Community and Societal Benefits

Healthcare
– Broad range of services
– Sub-specialists
– Experimental treatments
– Referrals to other AHCs
Education
– Quality and quantity of physicians
– Nurses, dentists, other professionals
– Biomedical scientists
– New, evolving healthcare disciplines
Research
– Basic biomedical mechanisms
– Translational, applied research
– Technology development
– Test beds, clinical effectiveness
Economic
– Direct job creation
– Uncompensated care
– Extramural funding; indirect job creation
– Intellectual property, business creation

to serve the indigent [1]. The almost 400 teaching hospitals in the U.S. account for about 6% of all hospitals, but provide almost 50% of the charity care [3]. Various funding mechanisms have been developed to help cover such expenses, including the disproportionate share hospital (DSH) and indirect medical education (IME) programs of Medicare. However, ongoing regional and national attempts to reduce healthcare costs (and reimbursement to providers), as well as the growing numbers of uninsured and under-insured populations, are creating increased pressure on the clinical operating income of AHCs. This in turn is reducing the ability of AHCs to adequately support the increasing costs of their own clinical activities, let alone to help subsidize their academic missions.

The sustainability of support for the unfunded overhead expenses of education and research, as well as the uncertain future of reimbursement for physician and hospital services, provide the basis for a potential "perfect storm" in the financial stability of many AHCs. Contributing factors exacerbated by the major economic recession of 2008–2009 include the decline in university endowments and endowment income, reduced access to capital for facilities and equipment, decreased yields in fundraising from prospective donors, and diminished ability and willingness of students and families to pay relatively high tuition costs. Likewise, potential decreases in hospital and physician reimbursement, as well as support for indigent care and resident training, may put even greater strain on clinical units of AHCs. Together, these factors are having the dichotomous impact of driving tighter internal alignment at some AHCs and wider separation at others.

2. The value of academic health centers

The mission of AHCs to serve society through healthcare, education, research, and service provides enormous value to the local community as well as society at large in many ways, as outlined in Table 1.

2.1. Healthcare delivery

The most tangible and direct benefit of AHCs is in the breadth and depth of the healthcare they provide. Unlike other healthcare providers that offer a scope of services based primarily on local market conditions and financial considerations, AHCs must also offer services that are needed to train a broad range of medical specialists and healthcare professionals, as well as compete on a national level for the best students and clinical staff. In addition, as part of their research mission, AHCs generally offer experimental treatments and clinical trials that further expand healthcare offerings locally as well as to patients referred for treatment from regional, national, and in some cases international sites. Because of the interactions of faculty and programs across AHCs in education and research, as well as healthcare, another benefit is their ability to identify and refer patients to other AHCs having specialty care that might not be available locally.

As the provider of last resort in many situations, AHCs also provide a direct community benefit through their disproportionately high level of uncompensated healthcare. It is customary for an AHC to care for a community's most severely ill patients, as well as a relatively large percentage of its poor and uninsured [28]. This care takes two forms: indigent care for patients with no insurance, and catastrophic care for people who have some insurance coverage but whose medical bills are beyond their financial means. Many of these charity patients have extremely complex and challenging illnesses that have already used up their family resources and any insurance coverage they had.

AHCs provide another healthcare community benefit through their educational mission by increasing the pool of physicians, nurses, and other healthcare professionals who often opt to remain in the community in which they trained. With the growing shortage of health professionals in many communities, the value of this benefit is substantial.

2.2. Education of health professionals

2.2.1. The next generation

Rapid advances in biomedical knowledge and technology are changing how healthcare is practiced. This means health profession students today have more to learn than those of previous generations, and often are expected to apply new knowledge instantly. This increased need for knowledge content and its application requires AHCs to develop innovative courses and curriculums that prepare students adequately – not only academically, but also in real-world experience. In many medical and other health professional schools, there is too little integration of content, too little interaction with role models, inadequate exposure to longitudinal ambulatory care, and under-use of standardized patients, simulators, and computer-assisted instruction.

Perhaps the greatest challenge facing health profession schools is the rapid move from teaching knowledge content to teaching knowledge management. The exponential increases in data, information, and knowledge on every topic make it virtually impossible to expect that what is taught today will be what is useful in practice next year. Fortunately, useful data, information, and knowledge management tools are also developing rapidly. Increasingly, these tools are providing a practical means for accessing the vast amounts of data and information available, as well as a means of converting them into useful knowledge. Teaching students about the availability and application of such tools and methods for knowledge management will ultimately become the major thrust of most education programs.

For academic health centers, this presents a unique challenge – the difficulty of changing legacy curriculums, which those trained in an analog world of knowledge content (usually the educators) may feel isn't broken, while those trained in a digital world of knowledge access and management (usually the students) feel is not relevant.

An additional factor AHCs face in educating students is a new world in which the scope and complexity of knowledge content that is relevant to many topics now comes from multiple disciplines. The historical curriculum of medical and other health professional schools was constructed by individual discipline-based departments either in sequence or parallel. In contrast, the best approach for providing complex content and concepts that span multiple disciplines to students requires an integrated approach involving multiple departments. Thus, the development of multidisciplinary, trans-disciplinary, and interdisciplinary teams (see later section) to deliver contemporary healthcare services are also needed to deliver contemporary educational services. Changing the content and manner of educating future physicians and other healthcare professionals is critical to improving healthcare delivery [3].

2.2.2. New medical specialties and health professions

The academic innovation of AHCs is not limited to new ways of teaching existing specialties, but also includes the creation of new professions and specialties as their value and need is identified. The rapid evolution of basic biomedical science disciplines such as neuroscience and clinical specialties such as emergency medicine provide good examples. Just 30 years ago, the content of neuroscience was largely distributed among numerous other disciplines and taught piecemeal in medical schools through their corresponding departments such as anatomy, physiology, pathology, pharmacology, as well as clinical units such as neurology and neurosurgery. As the content and complexity of neuroscience increased rapidly, those interested in the emerging field increasingly came together, resulting in the creation of programs and then departments as the primary home for neuroscience research and education. The academic discipline of neuroscience was born.

In an analogous manner, emergency rooms in hospitals prior to the 1990s were staffed by specialists from numerous medical and surgical clinical services, with often less than optimal care delivery. With no single existing specialty or department comprising the full range of practices needed to meet the need, several AHCs developed trans-professional interdisciplinary teams and training programs focused primarily on emergency care to improve outcomes and effectiveness. The specialty of emergency medicine rapidly emerged, with the creation of a free-standing department of Emergency Medicine at Johns Hopkins in 1995 providing the impetus for the rapid creation of similar departments across the country.

This trend continues with the development of other basic and clinical science disciplines and departments. The creation of departments of Biomedical Informatics at Ohio State and Vanderbilt in the early 2000s has set the stage for recognizing the importance of this discipline which spans activities in many basic and clinical departments.

Similarly, the past 15 years have seen a significant increase in "hospitalists" – physicians who specialize in providing care for hospitalized patients. According to the Society of Hospital Medicine, there are more jobs available for hospitalists than for any other specialty within internal medicine. Recognizing the increasing demand for specialists in this newly emerging field, many AHCs have begun to offer residencies and fellowships in hospital medicine. Hospital medicine programs now focus on the wide range of issues that face hospital physicians [50].

Similarly, clinical and corresponding educational training programs are emerging at several AHCs in critical care medicine. These programs span activities in departments and specialties such as anesthesiology, emergency medicine, pulmonary medicine, and surgery, and have developed to prepare 'intensivists" to specialize in the care of critically ill patients, usually in an intensive care unit.

The next few years will see more structure around emerging disciplines such as biomedical informatics, hospital medicine, palliative care, and critical care medicine with the creation of formal departments and centers at AHCs. Likewise, programs are evolving for new specialties that are even earlier in their evolution.

In addition to the development of academic and clinical specialties within existing health professions, AHCs continue to develop and foster the creation of new professional and para-professional health occupations. For example, the concept of the physician assistant (PA) was originated by Dr. Eugene Stead as chairman of the Department of Medicine at Duke University, with the development of the first PA training program in the mid-1960s [16]. Likewise, the educational programs of numerous other health professions have become standardized in content and training by incorporation into AHCs, while new ones such as health coaches, navigators, and informaticians are evolving. As discussed later, the development of new specialties is critical to improving the effectiveness and efficiency of healthcare, and is dependent upon the educational mission of AHCs.

2.3. Health discovery

The research activities in AHCs provide benefits to society and the community through their discoveries in basic biomedical science, the development of technology, and clinical investigation that lead to translation into new diagnostics and therapeutics. In particular, clinical trials and effectiveness research have an immediate local and ultimately global impact in improving the standards of care.

2.3.1. Clinical and translational research

The structure and function of academic health centers make them uniquely qualified to translate laboratory findings about disease into successful clinical tests and treatments. Likewise, clinical observations have a major impact in identifying research questions and models for the lab. While the value of translating basic scientific discoveries into useful clinical applications, and vice-versa, is of extraordinary value in improving healthcare, it is also time-consuming, costly, and complicated. Challenges in translating bench research to the bedside include insufficient trial participants, infrastructure, clinical investigators, and funding. Reciprocally, there are insufficient models and support for bringing clinical observations into basic research models that in turn identify solutions that can be brought back to the bedside. A recent survey of publications found that just one in five basic research articles with potential clinical applications actually led to a clinical trial, and only one in 100 that made it to clinical trial resulted in a new therapy [13].

One crucial barrier to successful translational research is the increasingly complex nature of regulatory challenges. As the number of clinical trials has increased, the regulatory environment has expanded in scope and complexity in order to ensure safe and effective patient experiences. In response, funding allocations by AHCs for infrastructure, personnel, and information technology to support clinical trials continue to grow significantly. For a one-year period, some AHCs have reported as much as a 70% increase in these expenses in order to address regulatory compliance requirements [36]. Despite these challenges, translating scientific discovery into healthcare delivery is crucial to the mission of AHCs and the health of society.

A major initiative of the NIH in the past five years has been to develop the Clinical and Translational Science Award (CTSA) as recognition and support of translational research [39]. Each AHC with such an award has a unique set of assets and priorities for successful translation of science into practice and healthcare delivery. For example, the Atlanta Clinical and Translational Science Institute (ACTSI), sponsored by the Emory University Woodruff Health Sciences Center, brings together basic, translational, and clinical investigators; community clinicians; professional societies; and industry collaborators in dynamic translational research projects [6]. The Institute directly engages multiple institutions including Emory, Georgia Institute of Technology, Morehouse School of Medicine, Children's Healthcare of Atlanta, Grady Hospital, the Atlanta VA Hospital, and others. The ACTSI focuses on accelerating the translation of laboratory discoveries into healthcare innovations by supporting researchers from all these institutions. The Institute provides regulatory support, clinical research coordinators, technology transfer assistance, and project management. It also offers funding for start-up research projects, better access to analytical tools, and training for clinical and translational investigators.

ACTSI is one of 39 such consortiums working to improve the way biomedical research is conducted across the country, and its collaborative approach is a model for AHCs nationwide in translating basic science research findings into clinical practice.

2.3.2. Healthcare technology creation, development, and application

The creation, development, and application of technology is another important means of improving healthcare and is significantly tied to the partnership of AHCs with industry. While companies (as for-profit enterprises) are focused on creating products that generate revenue for shareholders, AHCs (as public-benefit institutions) are focused on creating knowledge that generates value for society. Because they are noncompetitive and essentially complementary in mission and goals, AHCs can serve as neutral parties with industry partners, leveraging the assets held by each to more efficiently and effectively bring new technology to broad clinical use. This also allows individual companies to have multiple AHC partners and vice-versa, further facilitating technology development.

As partners to industry, AHCs can provide a unique environment for basic and clinical outcomes research, as well as patient care applications. The broad range of diverse scientific disciplines concentrated in single AHCs is not duplicated even by the largest and most complex corporations engaged in product development. Furthermore, the simultaneous presence in AHCs of the diverse healthcare sub-specialties needed to determine the effective use of technology provides a truly unique environment that spans basic mechanistic scientific discovery to the clinical delivery of new technology.

Despite the potential synergies of corporate-AHC interactions, the relationship between them is often contentious. In many cases, either or both sides view a "partnership" as only a surrogate for a vendor-client relationship. In such cases the motivation is essentially to gain as much from the other as can be negotiated, and usually involves a level of "segment arrogance" in which either partner does not value the mission or goals of the reciprocal partner, often resulting in a win-lose scenario. Moreover, in such cases the perception of the industry partner may be that the AHC does not have the understanding, ability, or desire to work effectively on product development. Reciprocally the AHC may perceive that the industry partner has no interest in the underlying innovation, science, technology or healthcare benefits of the product, and is only interested in its own marketing, sales, and revenue.

Most commonly, the corporate-AHC relationship is a limited contractual agreement with specific milestones and deliverables that effectively provide a win-win situation. In rare circumstances, a broader relationship is established that provides potential but not guaranteed mutual benefits. The manifestations of such true partnerships is a reciprocal value of the different missions, goals, and cultures of each partner; full disclosure and transparency; and aligned vision, respect, and understanding. The true test of such relationships is the ability of occasional lose-win circumstances to not destroy the relationship since the long-term overall relationship is a clear win-win.

2.4. Economic value

2.4.1. Across the missions

The healthcare, education, and research activities at AHCs have a direct benefit on the economy of communities served in many respects. In most cases, the healthcare systems of AHCs are among the largest employers in a community, creating well paying jobs across a wide spectrum of professional and support service sectors.

In fact, over the past seven years, the majority of new jobs created in the United States have been in the health sector, with AHCs representing a significant component of this growth. As examples, the Emory University Woodruff Health Sciences Center ("Emory Health") employs some 19,000 faculty and staff, making it one of the largest private employers in the state of Georgia. Likewise, according to the Columbus Chamber of Commerce, the Ohio State University Medical Center was the largest creator of new jobs in central Ohio over the past five years [11].

In addition to jobs created by healthcare delivery, research activity also creates significant jobs. Every $1 million of research funding generates an average return of $2 million and 32 jobs [31]. Since most funding for AHCs comes from extramural sources, especially the NIH, this means local jobs are created largely from federal funds. For example, Emory Health in 2008 received $389 million in sponsored research funding. This in turn generated more than $775 million in economic impact and nearly 12,500 additional jobs for the state of Georgia across a wide range of industries and services that support the research enterprise.

The intellectual property created from research often results in significant business creation and relocation to local communities, providing a significant economic benefit. Moreover, the income from technology licensing can benefit the community in job creation, especially when reinvested in program growth. For example, Emory University received $525 million in 2005 for its rights to the widely used anti-HIV drug Emtriva that was developed by its faculty. A significant portion of these funds are being used to support a range of strategic initiatives that create direct and indirect local economic benefit.

Taken together, the combined impact of AHCs in direct and downstream jobs and economic benefit is considerable. Emory Health's total economic impact to the community is more than $5.5 billion – in addition to the immeasurable value of providing help and hope to people in need – which is typical of AHCs across the country.

2.4.2. AHCs in the knowledge economy

By definition, academic health centers are embedded in the knowledge economy through their missions of research (knowledge creation), education (knowledge dissemination), and healthcare (knowledge application). One way in which AHCs stay at the leading edge of health discovery and practice is by harnessing the power of the rapidly increasing body of biomedical knowledge. Resource-intensive, technology-based knowledge management initiatives can provide information that is tailored to the needs of students and faculty and that can streamline delivery of information resources, enhance technology support, and fuel innovation.

The digital age has revolutionized research, education, and patient care through such advances as complex molecular, genomic, and proteomic maps; interactive learning; decision support; and electronic medical records. The convergence of three important elements is necessary for academic health centers to take full advantage of these and other advances:

- Data – facts and figures
- Processes – technology and context
- Understanding – people and expertise

Table 2
The value of AHCs: Innovation at interfaces

Missions
– Healthcare
– Education
– Research
– Community service
– Societal benefits
Organizations
– Medical school, other health science schools, university
– Affiliated health system, hospital, clinical practices
– Other academic, clinical partners
– Corporate, government, other partners
Academic disciplines
– Health sciences
– Physical, natural, and computational sciences
– Basic and clinical biomedical sciences
– Social, behavioral sciences
– Professional (e.g., engineering, business, law)

Together these elements constitute knowledge management, a concept with its roots in the business world, but one with important implications for academic health centers as well [9]. To assimilate and manage a wealth of information that is expanding rapidly and continuously, AHCs are the leading edge of creating new, innovative structures that tap the information, technology, and human expertise of both the health sciences library and information technology. By organizing these disparate entities into a single-point, multidimensional knowledge entity, AHCs leverage and synergize the three components of their mission:

- Knowledge creation – basic, applied, and clinical research
- Knowledge dissemination – undergraduate, graduate, professional, post-graduate, and continuing education
- Knowledge application – patient care therapies and technology development

2.5. *Innovation at interfaces*

The major characteristic of AHCs that makes them such a unique part of the healthcare delivery system is the value of working at the interface of multiple missions, organizations, and disciplines all in one enterprise (Table 2).

The synergy among missions adds significant value to each: the creation of knowledge (research) enhances the quality of education and healthcare; the dissemination of knowledge (education) enhances the impact of research; and the application of knowledge (healthcare delivery) provides the environment to educate and to conduct translational and clinical research.

Similarly, the potential synergy among the primary organizational components of the AHC (schools, hospitals, practices) can add significant value to each other, as can the interaction between AHCs and other academic, clinical, corporate, and government partners. The added value of such mission and organizational alignments are programmatically manifested in the development of interdisciplinary alignments among the health sciences and between health science disciplines and other natural, physical, computational, social, and behavioral sciences.

Much of the healthcare innovation of the last half of the 20th century was the result of research at the interface of the biomedical and physical sciences, leading to new understandings in areas such

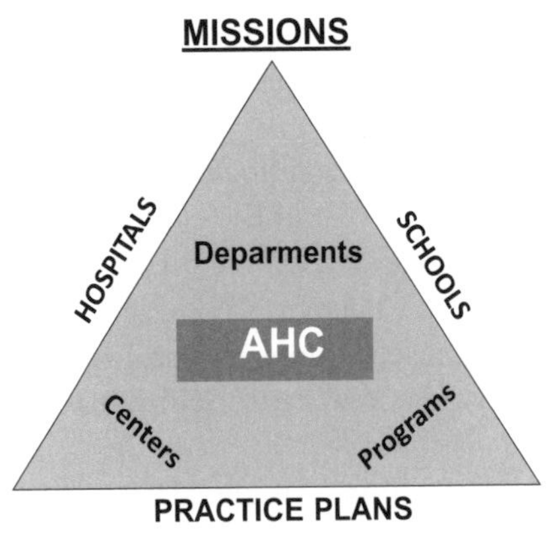

Missions	Functions	Outcomes
Healthcare	Decision-making	High Performance
Education	Strategic planning	Constructive culture
Research	Resource allocation	Workplace of choice
Community service	Goal setting	
	Programmatic priorities	
	Rewards, recognition	

Fig. 1. Academic health centers: Organizational structure-function.

as molecular genetics and new tools in areas such as imaging. The past 10 years are showing that innovation is currently most evident at the interface of the biomedical and computational sciences, leading to new understandings in areas such as systems biology and genomics, and new tools in areas such as biomedical informatics and drug design. The tremendous power of informatics provides the possibility to address healthcare delivery solutions such as predictive and personalized health (see below). Such complex applications and solutions are most likely to be made in an environment that spans the missions, organizations, and disciplines that uniquely characterize AHCs. Interdisciplinary centers and programs present in AHCs offer the comprehensive approaches needed for the innovations that will continue to improve productivity, quality and value in the complex system of healthcare delivery.

3. Organizational structure and function

3.1. Alignment of component units

A major factor in the success of the AHC in healthcare delivery, as well as in education and research, is the degree of alignment among its academic and clinical components – the schools, the health system of hospitals and clinics, and the professional practice plans (Fig. 1). Of even greater importance is the alignment of functions across the functional subcomponent entities such as departments, centers and programs.

Most people are familiar with the architectural adage, “form follows function,” which means that the design of a building should be predicated on its intended purpose. The same principle applies to AHCs. Unfortunately, in some cases structural alignment at the governance or management levels may not result in functional alignment. The converse is also true in that some AHCs have good functional alignment despite limited organization structural alignment. The key functions that best reflect good

AHC functional alignment include decision-making, strategic planning, resource allocation, goal setting, program priority, and rewards and recognition. Key outcomes of good functional alignment are high performance and constructive culture (see below).

The internal alignment of AHCs is fundamentally reflected by the degree to which mission, vision, and values are shared across its component units. Naturally, education and research missions tend to be more associated with the schools, while clinical and service missions are associated with the hospitals and practices. Thus, those AHCs with a greater balance among their missions more often have greater alignment among their component units because of more shared interests. When service and academic missions are less balanced or more tightly associated with individual units, there is less likelihood of good functional alignment.

It is not surprising that many cultures exist within a single AHC – an academic culture in the schools, a service culture in the clinical practices, and a business culture in the hospitals. While some degree of heterogeneity is to be expected within an organization with multiple missions and organizational units, the highest performance occurs when the overarching vision, values, and culture are synergistic and coherent across all units of the organization. More importantly, functional alignment is most likely when there is an overall sense of commitment by all unit leaders to each of the missions, and accountability to the AHC as well as their own unit.

Alignment within each AHC component is also important, since misaligned values and goals within one unit can result in competitive versus collaborative interactions with other component units. Within the medical school, misalignment may occur between the basic and clinical sciences and among educators, researchers, and clinicians. Within the health system, alignment issues depend on many factors including the staff model (open or closed); the authority and accountability of service chiefs (vis-à-vis department chairs); the balance of specialty and primary care; and the relationship of revenue-generating with revenue-losing specialties. Within the practice plan, alignment issues can include structure (e.g., single vs. group practices, leadership of the plan, corporate model); funding (e.g., revenue vs. cost center model; subsidy model; retained earnings); and operations (e.g., scheduling, consults, billing).

Another key to achieving an aligned structure and function is a strong synergy between the AHC and its academic partners, especially if the AHC is part of a larger university. An aligned governance and administration structure allows the AHC and its parent or partner university to leverage each other's strengths and achieve the complementary and coordinated visions of both.

3.1.1. Organizational models

Most AHCs have developed along one of two basic organizational models: an "affiliative" model or an "integrated" model. In affiliative organizational models, the academic and clinical operations of the AHC are managed by multiple leaders who report to multiple governing bodies. Therefore, no single administrative or governing entity has ultimate decision making authority over all components of an affiliated model AHC. Conversely, in the integrated organizational model, all AHC functions ultimately report to one administrative leader and to one governing board.

As competition and funding pressures across missions have driven AHCs to become more efficient and effective, they have adopted increasingly integrated organizational models. In a 2005 survey, the Association of Academic Health Centers (AAHC) found evidence of increasing integration of the academic and clinical components of many AHCs. At a majority of institutions polled, the leader of the AHC had authority over the head of the health system and school of medicine [54]. In some cases, the leader of the AHC also served as the head of the hospital or health system (e.g., Duke) or as dean of the medical school (e.g., Hopkins, Penn, UCLA). In other cases, the head of the AHC had authority over all health science schools, but not the health system (e.g., Minnesota, Cincinnati). In other cases, the AHC leader had direct authority over the health system and school of medicine, but not other health science schools (Michigan, Ohio State). In rare instances, the AHC leader had direct authority over the leaders of all health science schools as well as the health system (e.g., Emory).

The affiliative model usually represents a relationship between a university and an independent health system, each of which has its own governing boards and management leadership (e.g., Northwestern, Washington University). In most affiliative model AHCs, mutual self-interests are usually sufficient to drive alignment, although this often requires extensive negotiation, especially about program priorities and resource allocation between entities. Some affiliative model AHCs operate as multiple independent entities with different visions and goals for research, education, and healthcare. This can result in the potential loss of synergy and leverage across units, and in some cases frank competition and conflict.

Among the benefits of an integrated model cited by AAHC are decreased financial risk, more expeditious advances in scientific discovery, greater efficiency, and heightened public trust. But perhaps the most important benefit of the integrated model is a greater likelihood of alignment in mission, vision, values, goals, strategy, and therefore functionality. In most, but not all cases, the integrated model allows more cohesive strategic planning and decision making, especially regarding resource allocations and program priorities across academic and service missions [43].

3.2. Programmatic alignment

Functional organizational alignment is most important for units directly involved in executing the missions of the AHC (often referred to as "functional units") and those involved in administrative functions directly supporting these activities (i.e., "support units"). Functional units include those representing specific disciplines such as academic departments in schools, individual clinical practices, and hospital services, as well as interdisciplinary and inter-organizational units such as centers, institutes, and programs. Support units may be within or across AHC components and include activities such as finance, communications, planning, marketing, human resources, fundraising, and information services.

Functional unit alignment at a discipline or specialty level is most evident in the relationship between clinical departments in medical schools and their counterpart physician practice plans and hospital services. In some AHCs the alignment may represent ownership or integration of the practice plan in the corresponding medical school (e.g., Johns Hopkins), or of the practice plan with the corresponding hospital service (e.g., Pittsburgh, Case Western Reserve). In others, all three components are independent organizationally and are tied together under the AHC (e.g., Duke, Emory). The evidence for good alignment includes clear leadership authority by a single chair /director/chief over the corresponding medical school department/practice plan/hospital service respectively, as well as transparency and synergy of funds flow, budgeting, planning, and compensation across all three organizational units.

Alignment of centers and programs that span multiple departments, practices, and services is more difficult because of the need for shared responsibility and authority between center directors and leaders of associated units in the schools, practices, and/or hospitals. Even simple mission-specific clinical product lines, research centers, and education programs that are interdisciplinary but only span medical school, practice plan, or hospital service units are often difficult to align. Those programs that span missions as well as disciplines and organizational units are an even greater challenge in complexity of management and governance.

While the alignment of individuals and programs across disciplines, professions, and organizations is difficult, the value produced by the leverage and synergy provided is significant. The most common examples of a matrix model program that demonstrate the added value borne from the alignment of activities across AHC components and missions are National Cancer Institute (NCI) designated Comprehensive Cancer Centers. Almost all NCI designated Comprehensive Cancer Centers are at AHCs, largely because AHCs have the range of programs that, when aligned, can meet NCI criteria for clinical, research, and service excellence. The strategy and processes for aligning programs and teams is discussed in a later section.

3.2.1. Evolving management practices

Just as the organizational model of AHCs has adapted in response to the opportunities and challenges of a rapidly changing economy and environment, so too have management practices. In order to remain competitive, many AHCs are adopting management practices that are more corporate than their traditional academic and clinical management styles. One key way in which many AHCs are adopting a corporate approach is to identify a single unifying vision and organize in ways that empower individual components to work together to achieve it. In addition to creating interdisciplinary and inter-organizational functional and support units to achieve this, it also means creating expanded and complex roles for AHC leaders that often provide more influence than control. Together, the organizational and management alignments can facilitate the development of policies and practices that align key functions as listed above in Fig. 1.

The greater need for positions with multiple responsibilities and reporting relationships has increased the importance of assuring alignment of authority with responsibility and accountability for each role. Often the goal of academic and physician leaders is to have significant authority with minimal accountability, whereas the goal of corporate and administrative leaders is often the opposite; i.e., to provide others minimal authority with significant responsibility and accountability. Clarifying and aligning these expectations among the various functional and support unit leaders are critical factors for programmatic success, as are management practices that push both increased delegation of authority and centralization of accountability.

The increasing importance of organizational, programmatic, and management alignment for AHCs has increased their emphasis on collaboration and teamwork. Clinicians, researchers, and educators have conventionally worked in academically defined department structures and as individual "free agents." Much of this culture for academic faculty is the result of promotion and rewards processes that have been traditionally based on individual rather than team achievements. This narrow focus on individual achievement has been amplified by the evaluation of performance by faculty peers in their "tenure initiating units" (academic departments). For clinical faculty, individual achievement is also reinforced by the tradition that a patient's outcome has been considered to be the responsibility of the individual attending physician rather than the healthcare team.

A critical factor in driving alignment and synergy is resource allocation. Traditional budgeting processes that are tied to legacy programs, or that involve decisions sequestered to individual parts of an organization, are less likely to result in alignments across programs and organizations. Aligning revenue and expense, as well as sources and uses, across the broader enterprise is one approach to driving greater synergy and leverage. Moving from a "cost-center" model for functional units that are thought to provide services at an expense to the organization to a "revenue center" model that emphasizes value creation is another approach. As discussed in more detail below, greater engagement of those providing the services to determine resource utilization has the dual impact of driving alignment and changing culture. The ultimate characteristics of aligned resource allocation are transparency of use, budget processes that engage multiple collaborating units, and decision-making that focuses on best use to achieve overall institutional goals.

Competitive Advantage	Valuable	Rare	Costly to Imitate	Hard to Organize
Parity	√	-	-	-
Short-term	√	√	-	-
Temporary	√	√	√	-
Sustainable	√	√	√	√

Fig. 2. Organizational alignments: Sustained competitive advantage (adapted from [7]).

4. Developing effective and efficient healthcare services

4.1. Creating high performance and value

As described above, alignment of organizational components and programs is a critical factor for success across the missions of academic health centers. For many of the same reasons, the quality and value of healthcare delivery by other service providers is significantly affected by the alignment of their various component units, programs, and personnel. This is particularly true for the relationship of physicians with other constituents including hospitals; nurses, pharmacists, and other non-physician health care professionals; other physicians and consulting specialists; health plans; and most importantly with patients and their families.

The importance of alignments and relationships in creating value and performance has been well studied in business as the strategic basis for "competitive advantage" [24,42]. Moreover, the ability of an organization or program to improve its productivity and innovation in a sustainable manner (i.e., "sustained competitive advantage") is in large part based on its ability to organize in ways that others are unwilling or unable to do [7].

Because of the intrinsic difficulties for organizations, programs, and individuals to affiliate in novel and highly interactive ways, such synergistic alignments typically provide greater and longer lasting impact than simply having assets that are valuable, rare, or costly to imitate (Fig. 2). The reasons for explaining this impact are apparent in terms of the different attributes needed to obtain parity or temporary advantage versus long-term advantage. The availability of resources is the primary determinant of whether an organization or program can create comparable value or performance by simply purchasing the assets needed. In contrast, the behavioral norms of individuals and the organizational culture of component units are the primary determinants in being able to create novel programmatic alignments and relationships. In addition, they are attributes that cannot be purchased and are hard to imitate. The leadership, strategies, and processes needed to change culture and behavioral normsare clearly more difficult and costly in time and effort for an organization than simply changing resource allocations to purchase an advantage based on tangible assets.

For AHCs, simply having assets of space, technology, or even outstanding faculty and staff provide less sustainable advantage and value because they can be purchased or recruited from one institution to the next. However, the manner in which resources (i.e., people, space, funding) at individual AHCs can be organized synergistically in complex programs spanning disciplines, organizational units, and missions cannot be easily purchased or reproduced.

This concept of achieving sustainable high value and performance through organizational alignments and synergy applies particularly well to the activities of AHCs because of their complex structures and functions, as described above. In healthcare delivery, it is no coincidence that the top two hospitals in the United States for each of the past 20 years as ranked by US News & World Report (namely, Johns Hopkins and Mayo Clinic) both are organized effectively across their physician specialty practices, hospitals, and medical schools. Moreover, they both, as do the vast majority of the nation's other top hospitals, utilize various combinations of their academic and clinical disciplines and units to effectively develop unique interdisciplinary programs. For example, as mentioned earlier, most of the nation's 40 NCI designated Comprehensive Cancer Centers (35/40, 90%) are at AHCs [37], largely because AHCs have the range of programs that, when aligned, can meet the stringent NCI criteria for clinical, research, and service excellence.

Another aspect of performance innovation and excellence associated with the novel alignment and synergy of programs is the inherent flexibility provided to address complex challenges and opportunities. This applies to complicated clinical service problems, intricate educational concepts, and difficult research questions. Moreover, a high performance AHC that is able to organize complex programs around normally non-aligned and often competitive units has the advantage of being able to nimbly use its resources to create new and different programs and centers.

4.2. Teamwork and engagement

The increasing pressure on available resources, as well as the expanding opportunities for high achievement and performance resulting from interdisciplinary, team-oriented approaches, is forcing AHCs to address their organizational culture and behavioral norms. The profound transformation of healthcare and medicine 100 years ago was the result of the alignment of organizational units (i.e., schools, physician practices, and hospitals) that created the 20th-century model of the AHC. In parallel fashion, the transformation of healthcare in the 21st century is likely to be driven by the alignment of individuals into teams across disciplines, specialties, and professions (see last section of this chapter).

A wide range of professionals and non-professionals can serve complementary and synergistic roles in providingthe highest performance in delivering healthcare, educating students, and conducting research. Thus, the academic health center, with its broad range of services and disciplines, should be the natural leader in developing and implementing team-oriented healthcare that is of high performance and value [41].

Diverse healthcare teams can include physicians, nurses, social workers, pharmacists, nutritionists, and many others. Each team member may differ in their contact with the patient, level of responsibility, and scope of practice. Although the concept is not new, the expansion of the "healthcare team," especially to include patients and their families, is gaining prominence as the most effective way to manage all factors involved in a person's health.

Depending on the specific circumstances and patient need, patient care teams may significantly range in size; they may meet physically at rounds and by phone, or virtually through email, web sites, or electronic health systems; and they may either simply assess patients or provide a full range of care. Healthcare teams (as well as teams involved in education and research) are generally categorized in one of three ways.

Multidisciplinary teams are characterized by a hierarchical structure. They are led by a senior team member, although members typically work independently within their own specialty. These teams may meet occasionally but are more likely to work in parallel, with the electronic medical record as the means of communicating assessments and recommendations with other members of the team.

Transdisciplinary teams are much more closely aligned. Each team member becomes familiar with the roles and responsibilities of other team members. In some cases, their functions may even become interchangeable.

Interdisciplinary teams are the median between these two extremes. Team members work together to develop goals and recommendations, but each retains distinct responsibilities based on expertise and experience. Leadership functions are shared, and the group meets regularly to engage with and learn from each other [12].

4.2.1. Obstacles and approaches

Although teamwork and interdisciplinary care are the most effective ways to meet the comprehensive needs of the patient, they are not without obstacles. Working across units and disciplines can increase conflicts over resource allocation of space, money, and time, and often faces barriers of culture and control. As discussed earlier, resource allocation conflicts are most common when the organizational components of the AHC are more affiliated than integrated, since the ultimate decision-making authority of the former may be more focused on the goals and priorities of the individual or a component unit than the AHC or the recipient of healthcare (or education).

Barriers of culture and control are likewise associated with the alignment of the component units, and by nature often differ in both. The differences in culture and control are generally significant between academic (e.g., university, medical school, nursing school), business (e.g., hospital and clinic), and professional service (e.g., physician practice) organizations. Moreover, the differences in culture and control typically vary within units of each organization, for example between research vs. clinical faculty; general vs. specialty and acute vs. non-acute care hospitals; and so-called cognitive vs. procedural physician practices. In particular, differences in culture are often significant among different specialists in professions such as medicine, where hierarchy and specialty pride (and occasionally arrogance) has been the behavioral norm for generations.

Several models of professional behavior characterize differences in culture at the level of individual physicians and faculty members [47]. In the "independent investigator/professional" model, healthcare professionals, especially faculty physicians, demonstrate individual thought that distinguishes them from their predecessors and peers. In the "maverick" model, independent, egocentric, and often eccentric behavior by physicians and faculty is often accepted and rewarded as an indicator of brilliance or technical skill. AHCs also have the "triple threat" model, whereby faculty are expected to be outstanding clinicians, gifted researchers, and inspired educators; this model is becoming increasingly difficult as the expertise needed for success in each of these three areas is expanding rapidly.

The attributes that help overcome these barriers are collegiality, a constructive culture with shared values and goals among team members, and a common focus on the needs of those being served; i.e., patients, students, and community. From a practical standpoint, the functionality of an interdisciplinary team often mirrors that of the overall AHC leadership. A productive approach to addressing these issues is embedded in a formal or informal responsibility assignment matrix or "RACI Chart" to identify those in each component unit who are responsible, accountable, consulted, and informed [56]. A review of these responsibilities is critical in identifying and assuring that the authority of individual leaders is aligned with their responsibility and accountability, and at the organizational level, that these relationships among leaders is transparent and well understood.

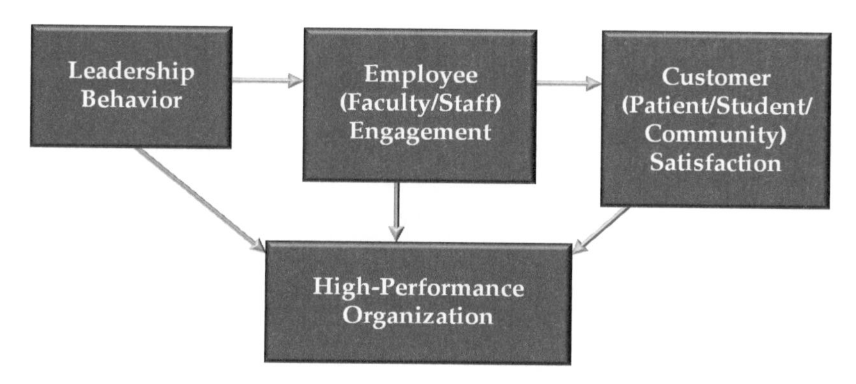

Fig. 3. The service value chain [45].

4.3. Driving change: the service value chain

To lead the transformation needed in the health delivery system, academic health centers must themselves be prepared to undergo significant changes. A critical step in this process is to reform and align their culture, goals, and strategy to drive necessary changes and high performance in the new system [29].

The service value chain (Fig. 3) [45] is based on the concept of the profit value chain [24]. It proposes that leadership behavior in pursuing organizational goals and strategy drives employee engagement, which in turn impacts customer satisfaction. Together, these factors drive an organization to high-performance and create substantial value for those it employs as well as those it serves. Developers created this model from observations of numerous service businesses where the relationships were found to exist [24,44], but had not been applied to services involving activities such as healthcare or education.

Ohio State Medical Center applied an approach using the service value chain concept from 2000 to 2007 with several interesting findings [45]. First, setting overall AHC goals and strategy through resource allocation and using decision-making to align leadership behavior resulted in statistically significant changes in the behavioral norms of the leadership. Second, the change in leadership culture was associated with increased engagement of faculty and staff. Third, these changes in leadership behavior and employee engagement were associated with statistically significant improvements in measures of student and patient customer satisfaction.

Most importantly, these changes corresponded with statistically significant improvement in the service performance of OSU Medical Center overall and each of its component units – as measured in terms of goals set for patient care, research, education, and community benefit. In particular, substantial improvements were achieved in healthcare delivery as assessed by numerous local and national benchmark measures of quality, value, and satisfaction for the OSU Health System and physician practice group. In support of the service value chain approach, these clinical achievements were in synergy rather than at the expense of similar significant achievements in research and education performance by the medical school. As expected from the profit value chain model, significant improvements also were demonstrated in operating income and financial resources.

Several aspects of the service value chain represent concepts that resonate with the importance of teamwork and alignment. Most importantly is the engagement of employees, which is essential for building aligned teams and units across the AHC. Leadership behavior is of critical importance in driving the productive engagement (or lack thereof) of employees. Leading effectively is all the more difficult and important for faculty and physician employees who provide the services of healthcare, education, research,and community service in an AHC. And the satisfaction of customers (patients, students, community), which is a key measure of quality and a high performance organization, is strongly associated with the level of leadership and staff engagement, i.e., teamwork and alignment.

5. Transformation of healthcare

5.1. Issues and opportunities

5.1.1. Defining the problems: Cost, quality, and access

As discussed throughout this book, the nation's healthcare delivery system has a wide and increasing range of problems that indicate significant and fundamental dysfunction. These concerns can be lumped or split into many categories, and essentially represent three general issues with healthcare: costs, quality, and access. Each of these issues is inter-related to the other two, each has multiple components, and each is complicated further by multiple confounding factors.

Healthcare costs present a problem from several perspectives, many of which confuse costs with expenditures. For some analysts, the problem is that the overall magnitude of expenditures in the United States at 16% of the GDP is too high; for others, it is that overall expenditures are too high for the value perceived, especially when compared to other countries; for some, it is about what costs are covered (and what costs are not); for still others, the problem lies in an inability to pay for the cost of adequate health insurance coverage; and the list goes on. Certainly, costs are an issue, but are these perspectives at the root of the real problem?

Alternative views can be considered for each of these perspectives to help get at the fundamental issues of cost. First, are total health expenditures too high? Many would argue that nothing is more important than health, so the greater the expenditures the better. Moreover, the high expenditures on healthcare have had the effect of growing a major segment of the economy over the past 20 years, which creates jobs and economic benefit, as discussed earlier. Is the core problem then that we do not receive the appropriate value for the expenditures, as suggested by comparative data from other countries that shows our expenditures are much higher but health measures are much lower?

An important confounder of healthcare costs (as well as for quality and access) is that U.S. expenditures for social services that directly impact healthcare are far below those of other benchmark countries [55]. This perspective suggests that the high cost of healthcare (really illness care) is the result of low expenditures to mitigate social determinants of health that drive up illness and the need for treatment. Inadequate funding of prevention, education, social services, and other areas clearly results in the need for more illness care.

The perspective that costs are too high because we cover too much or the wrong treatments must be considered in light of the common expectations in our society, especially the notion that each citizen is entitled to whatever is necessary to treat illness. As a result, the high percentage of expenditures in prolonging end-of-life care is ultimately more of a social-political-ethical issue that confounds the question (as it does again for quality and access), rather than a cost issue. Similarly, the issue of the high cost of health insurance to the individual must be considered from the perspective that some healthcare expenses to providers fail to be adequately covered by the under- and uninsured, as well as public payers such as Medicaid. To cover their true expenses, private insurance must be overpriced or inflated in part to make up the difference in reimbursement needed by providers to cover their expenses.

The perspectives about the quality of and access to healthcare are similarly complex and complicated by numerous factors, including those mentioned above. As measured by safety, outcomes, and satisfaction, most people in and out of healthcare see problems with all three. Likewise, most agree that the large number of uninsured and under-insured people is a major problem of access to healthcare in the United States.

Alternate perspectives on quality point to the fact that most new healthcare treatments and technology are developed and first applied in the United States. From a market perspective, those with substantial means come to the United States from around the world for specialized treatments because they perceive it to be the best. Alternate perspectives for access include the fact that those requiring care but lacking insurance ultimately find treatment, often at the local AHC. In addition, unlike other countries where some aspects of healthcare are rationed, US societal norms have not supported an approach of rationing or limiting the availability of care.

Other confounding factors that cross all three major issues include tort policy and the limited scope and scalability of specialty services. Legal practices in the United States add significant direct and indirect costs to health care compared to other countries, which often distorts the patterns of healthcare practice. In some cases, we find reduced access to some treatments for those considered more likely to sue, and in other cases, we see increased defensive practices, which can lead to increased errors, lower quality, and higher cost.

As a highly specialized service, the delivery of healthcare – especially involving technical procedures such as surgery – is dependent on individual practitioners. Therefore, it is difficult to scale comparable quality across large diverse populations. The ability to access services of the highest quality is limited because the number of highest quality service providers is limited. For example, the practices of Johns Hopkins and the Mayo Clinic are not scalable to the extent that their success is dependent, at least in part, on the specific knowledge, skills, and abilities of their staffs and the particular ways they align and deploy their personnel, technology, and facilities. This fact confounds the general perception that everyone in the United States could receive the same highest quality of care, even if they were entitled to it.

5.1.2. The solutions: AHCs can lead the way

Although there are many changes needed to improve the healthcare system in the United States, society must address each of the three fundamental issues – cost, quality, and access – if an effective and efficient healthcare delivery system is to emerge. Unfortunately, the issue presents not a set of three separate, clearly defined problems but rather a series of complex, interrelated problems, as outlined above. So solutions that only address part of the overall problem will have many unintended outcomes, some of which may create problems greater than those they seek to solve.

To effectively address these complex interrelated problems, solutions also are likely to be complex and interrelated. By focusing on increasing the value of the healthcare delivered, all three problems of cost, quality, and access must be addressed comprehensively and coordinately. Three potential solutions (Table 3) that address each of these problems include:

- Reforming financing and providing oversight by setting standards and paying for quality and value in promoting health as well as treating illness;
- Providing personalized, predictive care by engaging each individual continuously in considering the behavioral, environmental, social, and medical determinants of his/her own health;
- Restructuring the delivery model by developing a continuously interactive and easily accessible and integrative health provider team approach that permits each user to understand and consider the risks and benefits of all potentially effective options.

Table 3
Quality and value solutions for health system transformation

Reform finance and provide oversight – Pay for quality, value, and efficiency – Provide oversight and accountability
Provide personalized, predictive care – Focus on the patient – Individualize evidence-based healthcare
Change the delivery model – Create new healthcare specialties – Develop interdisciplinary teams

These three changes should not be viewed as sequential steps or independent issues but rather as interrelated parts of the underlying problems – and the solutions. Each change has several major components that are necessary but unfortunately insufficient for successful transformation. And each of these solutions presents significant opportunities that AHCs can help address and implement.

5.2. *Reforming healthcare financing and oversight*

5.2.1. *What's needed*

The most important goal in engineering an effective and efficient healthcare system is to establish a reimbursement and oversight process that ensures the system is paying for quality and value in providing overall health and is not simply driven by the costs of disease treatment per encounter. Health plans are now beginning to include simple measures of safety and outcomes in determining payment, but predominately, they are using process compliance as a common surrogate for improved outcomes and value.

Reimbursing the true value of improving both health and healing requires that their cost and quality be examined over a long period of time. This analysis has to take place in the context of safety and intended outcomes as well as in patient engagement and satisfaction. Increasing the relationship between payment and quality would be of benefit for most AHCs. After all, they provide high quality care, especially for the most complex treatments, as demonstrated by numerous measures [35] and the high demand for their services.

A second and necessary goal is establishing an objective mechanism for oversight, accountability, and alignment of expenditures among providers, health plans, insurers, employers, and state and federal governments. Many have proposed creating a public-private "U.S. Health Authority" as a way to engage all stakeholders in setting market rules for financing and competition. Such an authority would also serve as an appropriate data repository to establish standards for access, availability, scope, and effectiveness of provided services.

5.2.2. *The public/private model of a health authority in action: The Organ Procurement and Transplant Network*

Considerations of a U.S. Health Authority have relied largely on examples of non-healthcare related public-private agencies. These include such diverse entities as the Federal Reserve Board, Federal Aviation Administration (FAA), and the Securities and Exchange Commission (SEC). Major proponents of this approach to provide regulatory oversight have ranged from former Senator Tom Daschle, to the Mayo Clinic Health Policy Center, to the Blue Ridge Academic Health Group (BRAHG), each of which has proposed such a public-private model to expand access, trim waste, stabilize the system, and improve safety and quality [14,46].

Interestingly, an excellent model similar to a U.S. Health Authority has been successfully in place for more than 20 years: the Organ Procurement and Transplant Network (OPTN), administered by a private, not-for-profit organization, the United Network for Organ Sharing (UNOS) [52]. In 1984, responding to the growing national need to improve the outcomes, safety, access, and costs of organ transplantation, the federal government passed the National Organ Transplant Act (NOTA) to establish a public-private framework for a nationwide system of organ transplantation. The problems in delivering healthcare services to those receiving kidney, heart, lung, liver, pancreas, and ultimately other transplanted organs closely mirrored the current issues facing the overall healthcare system: significant variation in practices and outcomes at different delivery sites; variable patient access and satisfaction; high costs of existing and new technology and procedures; non-standardized data and information; and uneven coverage and reimbursement by multiple private and government health plans and payers, including the Centers for Medicare & Medicare Services (CMS).

NOTA established the OPTN as a private agency under contract to the Health Resources and Services Administration (HRSA) primarily to ensure the equitable distribution of donor organs and minimize their unnecessary waste. However, it also required the OPTN to address the issues of setting standards for individual local transplant center outcomes, practices, and certification. Moreover, it established the Scientific Registry of Transplant Recipients (SRTR), begun in October 1987, to provide a transparent means for the OPTN to collect and analyze data on every solid organ transplant in the United States [48]. UNOS also was awarded this contract through HRSA, and its charge was to assure the accuracy, timeliness, and completeness of data submitted (a requirement of transplant center certification). Another charge was to measure and assess pre- and post-transplant outcomes, safety, and access using sophisticated statistical methodology.

The SRTR database generates regular reports that evaluate each transplant center to compare its actual results to those predicted by multiple parameters that have been shown to be associated with outcome. The transparency of information allows patients and providers (including private insurers and CMS) to assess the performance of each provider. Moreover, as an open resource, the SRTR is available to any interested individual or organization for research in areas ranging from basic biomedical science (e.g., the role of immunogenetics in transplanted organ outcome), to clinical risk factors (e.g., diabetes, hypertension), to clinical effectiveness (e.g., the value of new technology and practices), to social determinants of health (e.g., the impact of race and environment).

5.2.3. The analog to engineering the healthcare delivery system

Since the establishment of the OPTN and SRTR more than 20 years ago, the outcomes for organ transplantation have improved dramatically, and the number of organs transplants performed annually in the United States has grown from 6,000 to more than 28,000 – thanks not only to improvements in transplant technique but also to the more effective and efficient system of organ procurement and distribution. As importantly, the system addressed the issues raised in the 1980s that created the OPTN in a way that has improved access, quality, cost, and public confidence.

Several aspects of the OPTN are noteworthy: political interference has been minimal through multiple presidential administrations and changes in congressional leadership; a mixed system of private insurer and public (CMS) funding for transplantation has been maintained; and the scope of coverage to include new organs, technology, and procedures has continued.

UNOS works so well as the OPTN because it includes a wide range of individuals representing every part of the transplant continuum – doctors, scientists, recipients, donors, coordinators, ethicists, and others who have a vested interest in creating and administering a successful system for organ transplantation. This public-private model has created specific rules, policies, and actions that are more effective and inclusive than any public or private entity would have been able to achieve alone. And it is not coincidental that AHCs have been at the core of success of the OPTN as the major sites for organ transplantation and as the predominant provider members and officers of UNOS for more than 20 years.

It is easy to imagine an analog of the OPTN and SRTR to address the parallel problems and opportunities for the national healthcare system. Academic health centers can help spearhead this reform by focusing their public policy efforts on promoting changes in financing and reimbursement to focus on quality and value, and establishing a public-private authority to regulate the appropriate aspects of insurance cost, coverage, and the quality of health care delivery.

5.3. Providing personalized and predictive healthcare

5.3.1. What's needed

A critical way to improve health system quality and value is to shift the current focus from healthcare plans and providers to the individual recipient. This change has two components. First is having payers and providers truly engage the individual in the decision-making processes of health and healing. This engagement requires clear and accurate information and communication about the risk and benefits of the entire range of potentially effective options available for health promotion as well as for disease prevention and treatment. It should include information on complementary and alternative approaches to prevention and care, which are being increasingly sought and paid out-of-pocket by those dissatisfied with or failed by current "standard of care" approaches. And it means that payers and providers will need to accept that individuals will vary in their own definition of value and therefore choice of care. They will also vary in the degree of decision-making or direction they want from different members of the provider team.

A second key component is to accurately determine the range of potentially effective options and predicted outcomes specific to each individual, based on his/her unique behavioral, environmental, social, and medical characteristics. These factors provide tremendous individual variation in the risk of and response to illness as well as in response to intervention, whether in treating illness or promoting health. Thus, the range of healthcare options and their potential consequences is overwhelming for any individual and requires sophisticated informatics decision support tools for providing truly personalized and predictive healthcare.

5.3.2. Information and communication technology

The past decade has seen a revolutionary change in the manner in which any individual can access information – immediately and at their fingertips – to help them make decisions in real time. Modern information and communication technology has been the key to this transformation and changed the way most goods and services are provided. Banking, travel, retail, and most industries operate in a completely different manner than they did just a decade ago, with improved productivity and customer reach.

All agree that a key to engineering a more effective and efficient healthcare system requires application of these technologies to transform the way services are provided. And yet, for a wide range of reasons – high cost and low acceptance by providers being two major factors – healthcare has lagged significantly in taking part in this revolution.

Once again, AHCs are leading the way. By developing ways to take advantage of information and communication technology through research, clinical application, and education of providers and recipients of healthcare, new models of healthcare delivery are being developed at many AHCs, often in partnership with industry. This process is complex and involves the creation of robust personalized health records, "warehouses" to store huge amounts of potentially relevant health data and information, high performance computing capacity to analyze associations and predict outcomes, and interactive electronic systems to provide decision support for individualized diagnosis and treatment. The goal of the models being developed is to provide relevant information about our own personal health and for our specific treatment options wherever and whenever needed, and at the convenience of the healthcare recipient – not just the insurance companies and the healthcare providers.

The potential impact of these applications already is being seen in improvements in quality – health outcomes, safety, and satisfaction – as well as cost and access. These models are demonstrating improvements in transactional aspects of care delivery, from enhancing the compliance and adherence to treatment, to the accuracy and timeliness of billing, to rapid electronic access among patients, providers, and health plans. More importantly are the improvements seen in decision-making. Better and quicker access to data and information can be converted to knowledge and impact for use by new healthcare teams that include the patient and their family regardless of time or place.

5.3.3. A new healthcare paradigm

Medicine stands at the brink of a remarkable and achievable goal to tackle the greatest opportunity facing the health of humans – the ability to predict, reduce, and in many cases eliminate the specific illnesses we each face. To do that, we must understand why each of us responds differently to specific illnesses and their various treatment options, and then use that knowledge to determine the right treatment at the right time for each individual.

That is the idea behind predictive, personalized, and integrative health, a revolutionary new way of delivering healthcare that is being pioneered at several AHCs nationwide. The nature of every person's risk and response to illness and treatment is predictable from their unique biology, behavior, and environment. To accomplish this assessment, complex information and communication systems – many of which already exist – need to be in place to translate these parameters into an effective, individualized health care strategy for each of us.

Because behavior and environment are such important factors in predicting risk and response to various treatments, social determinants of health also are important for such assessment [32]. In some cases, social determinants that impact behavior or environment can be as or even more important as genetic or metabolic factors affecting biologic responsiveness to illness or its treatment. For example, social determinants that can predict risk of non-compliance with treatment can have a stronger impact on outcome than genetic characteristics that predict responsiveness to a drug; selecting the right individualized drug is useless if the patients cannot or will not follow the treatment protocol because of socioeconomic factors that influence their lives.

Of similar importance is capturing and utilizing information about the particular unconventional means of diagnosis and treatment being used by many individuals that are not the current standard of traditional healthcare in the United States. These aspects of complementary and alternative medicine (CAM) are important as both potential predictive factors of health and healing in their own right and as confounders of the traditional measures of biology, behavior, and environment. The importance of CAM has led to the creation of a center at the National Institutes of Health that is focused specifically on the study and use of CAM [38].

An important component of predictive, personalized, integrative healthcare is to examine the effectiveness of such currently non-standard diagnostic and therapeutic measures to identify which ones will become appropriate standards in the future. For example, 20 years ago acupuncture was considered to be

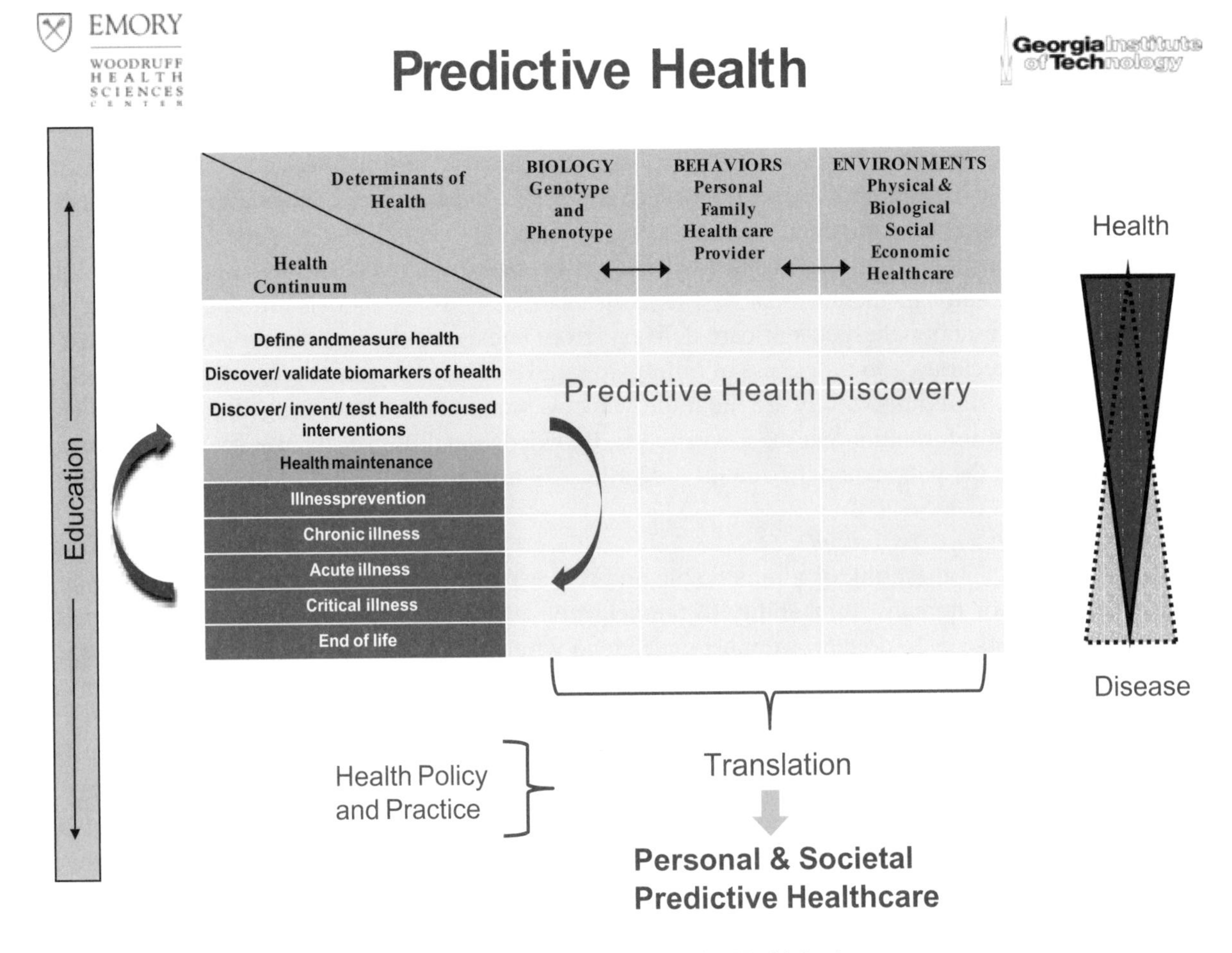

Fig. 4. Emory/Georgia Tech Predictive Health Institute.

an alternative to traditional care in the United States, whereas today it is offered as a standard of care for a variety of situations, both as a matter of choice by some patients or because other traditional treatments have failed. Likewise, many individuals use unconventional treatments that can enhance or interfere with conventional treatments; diet and diet supplements alone have a significant effect on the bioavailability and therefore effectiveness of many traditional pharmaceuticals. Knowing this information is critical in being able to accurately predict risk and response to illness and treatment. The significant use of CAM by many, even with the unreimbursed costs of such treatments, attests to the importance of careful assessment and use of these approaches.

5.3.4. Predictive, personalized, integrative health

Various initiatives in predictive, personalized, integrative health are in different phases of development and implementation at several AHCs [10,15,16,33,34,40] across the country. One such initiative, the Predictive Health Institute (Fig. 4) [18], is currently being conducted in collaboration between Emory University and the Georgia Institute of Technology as a model of how an AHC can use the opportunities of interfacing across missions, disciplines, and organizations to create new approaches to healthcare delivery.

The Emory-Georgia Tech Predictive Health Institute (PHI) is built on the premise that the most effective and efficient means of providing healthcare is by first keeping people healthy and then predicting the intervention that is most beneficial when illness occurs. The PHI is supporting more than 20 research projects that aim to advance predictive health on several fronts. One major effort involves the Center for Health Discovery and Well-Being, where patients are being enrolled in a major clinical study of the effectiveness of predictive health care [17]. Other research initiatives include large-scale genomic resequencing of an individual patient's entire genetic profile; assessing the body's immune response to threats; incorporating sociologic, epidemiologic, and behavioral risk factors into predictive health models for diabetes and Parkinson's disease; identifying the genetic conditions that lead to schizophrenia; and finding new ways to predict diseases such as Alzheimer's, drug addiction, ALS, and others.

In addition, by refocusing disease treatment to health promotion, predictive, personalized, integrative healthcare also represents a significant new role for the patient as an active partner in the healthcare process. It will be important not only to develop the data warehouses and tools that can provide decision support and determine the predictive value of various diagnostics and therapeutic interventions based on an individual's unique biology, behavior, and environment, but also to get that information into the hands of patients and providers to make real-time value judgment decisions on what suits each patient's particular best interests.

5.4. Restructuring the healthcare delivery model

5.4.1. What's needed

A necessary change in establishing an effective and efficient healthcare system is to move from sporadic and largely unconnected medical interventions to a vertically and horizontally integrated healthcare team that provides continuous care considering all potential options. Two major changes are prerequisites for this transformation. First is the need to increase the range of medical and health professions to address all potentially effective interventions regardless of derivation, as well as to create new professions that can effectively deal with the socioeconomic, behavioral, and environmental determinants of health that often trump the medical ones. Second, and even more importantly, is developing truly interdisciplinary and multi-professional health teams involving all these professions with patients and their families to provide the personalized, predictive, integrative care described above.

5.4.2. Integrative health

As discussed earlier, the tremendous increase in our understanding of the mechanisms and manifestations of disease has resulted in an expansion of the number and types of healthcare specialties, disciplines, and programs. Likewise, as discussed above, the application of information and communication technology is dramatically changing the way healthcare is being delivered. Together, these factors are converging on two corresponding aspects of what is termed "integrative" health – namely, inclusion of a broader array of treatments and healthcare providers and a change in the way these providers use information to work as a team with the patient and family to make personalized decisions.

Integrative health basically represents the alignment of an increasingly wide range of both healthcare options and healthcare professionals to provide the most effective and efficient care for the individual based on personal needs and desires. The importance of this approach is becoming increasingly understood, such that a recent summit was held at the Institute of Medicine of the National Academies to examine how best to proceed in developing integrative health [25]. Key aspects of this advance include potential use of all conventional and unconventional treatments with their corresponding providers in

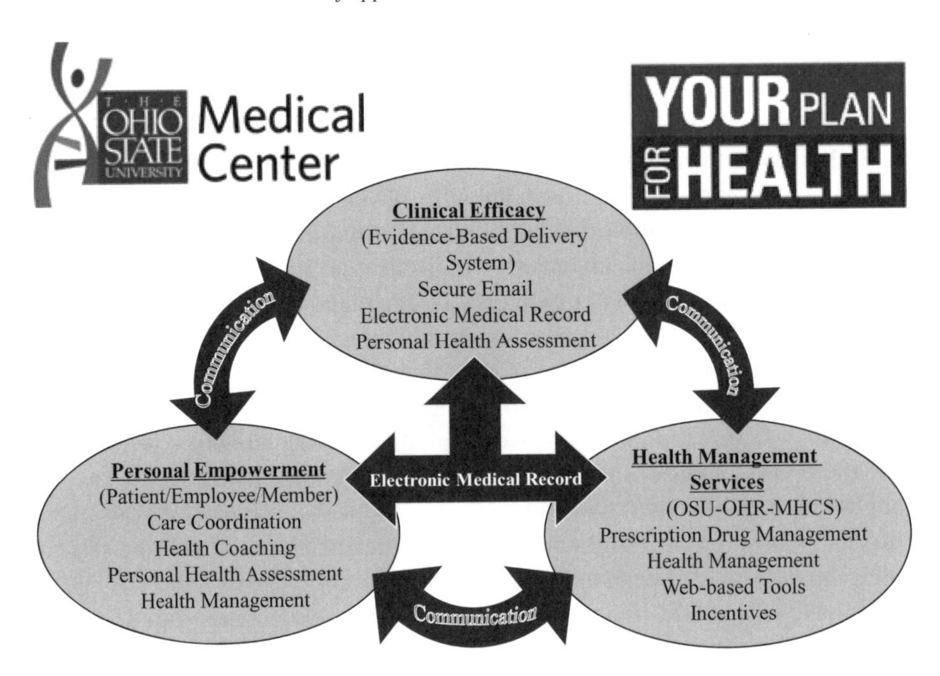

Fig. 5. Personalized Healthcare: Your Plan For Health [57].

an integrative manner that is transparent to the recipient, so each individual can have essentially one-stop, round-the-clock, comprehensive healthcare delivery to meet specific and changing needs. Here again, academic health centers are leading the way. Programs to develop and test models of integrative healthcare have been initiated at several AHCs including Duke [15], Vanderbilt [53], and Ohio State [40].

5.4.3. A model for health and healing: Your Plan for Health

To ultimately transform healthcare delivery, the development and application of predictive, personalized, and integrative healthcare models as described above must be able to scale the approach to broad practical applications. Academic health centers are leading the way in this transformation of the health system by developing and offering innovative health plans that incorporate these precepts. New health plans currently offered through the Mayo Clinic, Tufts, Geisinger, and Ohio State represent various ways to incorporate this approach [21,34,51,57].

A good example of such a new health plan is "Your Plan for Health" (YP4H) at the Ohio State University (Fig. 5). Over a two-year planning period from 2004–2006, the leadership of the OSU Office of Human Resources and the OSU Medical Center (OSUMC) developed and implemented many precepts of its pre-existing personalized, predictive, and integrative health programs into its employee health plans [10, 40]. YP4H became fully operational in January 2006, and by 2009 it has achieved many of its goals.

As an employer, healthcare provider, and administrator of its own health plans, OSU had well aligned incentives and an organizational structure that also allowed it to focus on the healthcare of its employees through all parts of the delivery system. Through discussions that included engagement of faculty and staff, administration, the university senate, and board of trustees, the university was able to align potential healthcare, research, and educational benefits across missions, along with organizational benefits across all AHC components as well as the entire university.

Many aspects of predictive, personalized, integrative healthcare were incorporated into the planning and implementation of YP4H, as outlined in Fig. 5. For example, since its onset, YP4H has offered financial incentives to encourage employees to participate in the personalized health assessment tool that OSUMC had developed. Similarly, ongoing incentives have been subsequently offered to those who maintain a health assessment and their health plan. The plan has utilized a HIPPA compliant means developed by OSUMC for allowing patients and referring physicians to access their electronic medical records and for patients to get electronic consults with physicians to improve access, timeliness, and accuracy in managing their care. Employees with chronic diseases have been provided with healthcare coordinators to help in the ongoing management of their disease. Likewise, health coaches are assigned to responsibly and proactively help other employees manage their health and prevent illness. In addition, employees have had access to 24-hour hotlines for disease management and health maintenance.

Other features developed by YP4H have included a pharmacy program, access to complementary and alternative healthcare, and a planned medical home program in fall 2009. The impact of the plan on cost, outcomes, and satisfaction were identified in developing the research aspects of the program, with some studies involving the OSU College of Public Health. Likewise, educational offerings to employees were developed through their coaches and/or care coordinators, as well as electronically.

The success to date of the program is notable from several perspectives. Healthcare costs and premiums for employees have grown far slower than at benchmark institutions; satisfaction of employees in their healthcare benefits have placed OSU in the top 5 of all university employers, with a recent survey across the entire university (with a 40% response rate) showing 88% to be highly satisfied with their healthcare; and three large local employers (public and private) have approached OSU to manage their employees' health. For the coming year, plans are to expand the financial incentives for maintaining a personal health assessment to dependents and implement disincentives by raising health premiums only for those who do not participate in the health assessment.

The YP4H at OSU and analogous plans being developed at other AHCs illustrate the special ability of AHCs to align activities across their missions, programs, and organizational units to address not only the science of predictive, personalized, integrative health but also the service delivery components of healthcare and education.

5.5. Driving change to drive performance

For the transformation of healthcare, changes in leadership behavior are a prerequisite to drive greater engagement of employees. Healthcare providers and leaders, especially at AHCs, must incentivize and reward their staff, especially physicians and administrators, who effectively engage and interact with all members of their healthcare and management team and who recognize and promote the importance of alignment and teamwork. To remain nimble and lead health system transformation, they must reinforce a culture that supports productive individuals who can lead people and inspire change. With a constructive culture, thoughtful planning, and appropriate leadership development, AHCs and other healthcare providers can significantly improve their organizational and leadership capabilities to lead the changes needed in our healthcare delivery system.

The key to successful and sustainable change is education. Medical schools, as well as other health professional and business management schools must transform content and experience to provide an integrative, relational approach to the next generation of healthcare providers and administrators. As discussed above, the functional alignment of individuals and programs is the critical measure of success that leads to innovation and high performance. Moreover, to ensure the best possible outcomes in engineering a better system, AHCs must fully engage with the many other stakeholders in testing and applying any changes under consideration. True healthcare transformation will be successful only when all sectors – public and private, state and federal, employer and employee, academic and corporate – come together for the greater good of everyone.

The magnitude of the changes that are needed (and are possible) is no less than those of 100 years ago when the Flexner report transformed the way medicine was taught and, very quickly thereafter, practiced. The challenges and opportunities of today are clearly even more complex. Yet, as was the case a century ago, they basically involve closing the gap between our current understanding of health and disease and the application of such knowledge to healthcare delivery. As the traditional homes of innovation in health and healthcare through research, and as the major drivers of change through education of healthcare professionals, AHCs have been at the forefront of improving healthcare delivery. The promise of a healthcare system that is viewed by all as our nation's greatest asset can and will be realized if academic health centers continue to lead the way.

Aknowlegements

Thanks to Drs. Leonard Schlesinger and Dennis Choi for critical review of the manuscript, Gary Teal and Rhonda Mullen for editorial advice, and Karon Schindler and Michelle Boone for help in manuscript preparation.

References

[1] AAHC, Academic health centers: creating the knowledge economy. Facts at a glance. Washington, D.C.: Association of Academic Health Centers, 2009.
[2] AAMC, AAMC statement on the physician workforce. Washington, D.C.: Association of American Medical Colleges, 2005.
[3] AAMC, Medical education costs and student debt: A report to the AAMC governance. Washington, DC: Association of American Medical Colleges, 2005.
[4] AAMC-HHMI Scientific Foundation for Future Physicians Committee, Scientific foundations for future physicians. https://services.aamc.org/publications/index.cfm?fuseaction=Product.displayForm&prd_i d=262&prv_id=321, 2009.
[5] America's Teaching Hospitals. http://www.aamc.org/teachinghospitals.htm.
[6] Atlanta Clinical & Translational Science Institute. http://www.actsi.org.
[7] J. Barney, *Gaining and Sustaining Competitive Advantage, 3rd ed.* Upper Saddle River: Prentice Hall, 2006.
[8] D. Bjorkman and L. Betz, Cutting U. of U. medical school class was tough decision to make. Salt Lake City: Salt Lake Tribune, 2009.
[9] T.J. Cain, R.L. Rodman, F. Sanfilippo and S.M. Kroll, Managing nowledge and technology to foster innovation at the Ohio State University Medical Center. *Academic Medicine* **80**(11) (2005), 1026–1031.
[10] Center for Personalized Healthcare. http://cphc.osu.edu/about/history/index.cfm.
[11] Columbus Chamber of Commerce, Columbus Chamber of Commerce 2007 Report, *Columbus CEO* **6** (4) (2008).
[12] B.S. Cooper and E. Fishman, *The interdisciplinary team in the management of chronic conditions: Has its time come?* Baltimore: Johns Hopkins University, 2003.
[13] T.P. Cripe, B. Thomson, T.F. Boat and D.A. Williams, Promoting translational research in academic health centers: navigating the roadmap. *Academic Medicine Management Series: Managing the Research Enterprise*. Washington, D.C.: Association of American Medical Colleges, 2005.
[14] T. Daschle, S.S. Greenberger and J.M. Lambrew, Critical: What we can do about the health-care crisis. New York: St. Martin's Press, 2008.
[15] Duke Integrative Medicine. http://www.dukeintegrativemedicine.org/.
[16] Duke University. Physician assistant program at Duke. http://paprogram.mc.duke.edu/s_prog_hist.asp.
[17] Emory-Georgia Tech Center for Health Discovery and Well Being. https://predictivehealth.emory.edu/chd/.
[18] Emory/Georgia Tech Predictive Health Institute. http://www.phi.emory.edu/.
[19] D. Fang and A.M. Htut, Special survey of AACN members on vacant faculty positions for the academic year 2008–2009. Washington, D.C.: *American Association of Colleges of Nursing*, 2008.

[20] A. Flexner, *Medical education in the United States and Canada: A report to the Carnegie Foundation for the Advancement of Teaching*. Boston: The Merrymount Press, 1910.
[21] Geisinger Health Plan. http://www.thehealthplan.com/employers_us/wellness.cfm.
[22] D. Giancotti and B. Walsh, Overview of research economics 2005. Washington, D.C.: National Council of University Research, 2005.
[23] C. Hannaway, Biomedicine in the twentieth century: Practices, policies, and politics. Amsterdam: IOS Press, 2008.
[24] J.L. Heskett, W.E. Sasser and L.A. Schlesinger, *The Value Profit Chain: Treat Employees Like Customers and Customers Like Employees*. New York: Simon and Schuster, 2003.
[25] A. Schultz, S. Chao and M. McGinnis, *Integrative Medicine and the Health of the Public*, Washington, Dc: The National Academics Press, 2009.
[26] Investing in clinical trial compliance top academic health center priority. (May 16, 2007).
[27] J.A. Kastor, *Governance of teaching hospitals: Turmoil at Penn and Hopkins*. Baltimore: Johns Hopkins Press, 2003.
[28] L.T. Kohn, Academic health centers: leading change in the 21st century. Washington, D.C.: Institute of Medicine of the National Academies, 2004.
[29] J.P. Kotter and J.L. Heskett, Corporate Culture and Performance: New York: Simon and Schuster, 1992.
[30] J.K. Levine, Considering alternative organizational models for academic medical centers, *Academic Clinical Practice* **14**(2) (2002).
[31] K. Makomva and D. Mahan, In your own backyard: how NIH funding helps your state's economy. Washington, D.C.: Families USA Foundation, 2008.
[32] M. Marmot and R. Wilkinson, *Social Determinants of Health (2nd ed.)*. Oxford: Oxford University Press, 2006.
[33] Mayo Clinic Health Manager. https://healthmanager.mayoclinic.com/default.aspx.
[34] Mayo Clinic Health Solutions. http://www.mayoclinichealthsolutions.com/.
[35] E. McFarlane, J. Murphy, M.G. Olmsted, E.M. Drozd and C. Hill, (2009). *2009 Methodology: America's Best Hospitals*. Washington, D.C.: U.S. News & World Report.
[36] Medical News Today. http://www.medicalnewstoday.com/articles/71023.php.
[37] National Cancer Institute. Cancer centers. http://cancercenters.cancer.gov/cancer_centers/index.html.
[38] National Center for Complementary and Alternative Medicine. http://nccam.nih.gov/health/whatiscam/.
[39] National Center for Research Resources. Clinical & Translational Science Awards. http://www.ctsaweb.org.
[40] Ohio State University Center for Integrative Medicine http://medicalcenter.osu.edu/research/centers/center_for_integrative_medicine/Pages/index.aspx.
[41] H. Pardes, Academic medical centers. Washington, D.C.: Washington Times, 2009.
[42] M.E. Porter, Competitive Advantage. New York: Free Press, 1980.
[43] P.G. Ramsey and E.D. Miller, A single mission for academic medicine: improving health, *Journal of the American Medical Association* **301**(14) (2009), 1475–1476.
[44] A.J. Rucci, S.P. Kirn and R.E. Quinn, The employee customer-profit chain at Sears, *Harvard Business Review* **76** (1998), 82–97.
[45] F. Sanfilippo, N. Bendapudi, A. Rucci and L. Schlesinger, Strong leadership and teamwork drive culture and performance change: Ohio State University Medical Center 2000–2006. *Academic Medicine* **83**(9) (2008), 845–854.
[46] J. Saxton, Blue Ridge Academic Health Group Policy Report: A United States Health Board. Atlanta: The Blue Ridge Academic Health Group, 2008.
[47] J. Saxton, Creating a value-driven culture and organization in the academic health center. Charlottesville: The Blue Ridge Academic Health Group, 2001.
[48] Scientific registry of transplant recipients. http://www.ustransplant.org/.
[49] S.W. Sedwick, Facilities and administrative issues: Paying for administration while under the cap, maximizing recovery, and communicating value, *Research Management Review* **16**(2) (2009), 1–7.
[50] Society of Hospital Medicine. Definition of a hospitalist. Hospital Medicine. http://www.hospitalmedicine.org.
[51] Tufts Health Plan. http://www.tuftshealthplan.com/employers/employers.php?sec=news&content=news_healthmgmtprgms.
[52] United Network for Organ Sharing. http://www.unos.org/whoWeAre/history.asp.
[53] Vanderbilt Center for Integrative Health. http://www.vanderbilthealth.com/integrativehealth/.
[54] S.A. Wartman, The academic health center: evolving organizational models. Washington, D.C.: Association of Academic Health Centers, 2007.
[55] WHO, (2009) Commission on Social Determinants of Health – Final Report 2009. Geneva: World Health Organization.
[56] Wikipedia. Responsibility assignment matrix. http://en.wikipedia.org/wiki/Responsibility_assignment_matrix.
[57] Your Plan for Health. https:// www.webmdhealth.com/OhioStateYP4H/default.aspx?secure=1.

Fred Sanfilippo, MD, PhD, was appointed Executive Vice President for Health Affairs, CEO of the Robert W. Woodruff Health Sciences Center at Emory University, and Chairman of Emory Healthcare in 2007. From 2000–2007, Dr. Sanfilippo led the AHC at the Ohio State University as Senior Vice President for Health Sciences and CEO of the OSU Medical Center. From

2004–2007 he was Executive Dean for Health Sciences and from 2000–2006 was Dean of the OSU College of Medicine and Public Health. From 1993–2000, Dr. Sanfilippo was the Baxley Professor and Chair of the Department of Pathology at Johns Hopkins and Pathologist-in-Chief of the Johns Hopkins Health System.

Dr. Sanfilippo received his BS and MS degrees in physics from the University of Pennsylvania, and his PhD in immunology and MD as a Medical Scientist Training Program Fellow at Duke University in 1975 and 1976 respectively. He did his residency training in Anatomic and Clinical Pathology at Duke University Hospital, and received board certification in Anatomic Pathology, Clinical Pathology, and Immunopathology. He joined the faculty at Duke in 1979, rising to Professor of Pathology, Immunology, and Experimental Surgery. With over 250 publications, $20 million in personal research grant support, and 3 patents, he has been an active leader in transplantation, pathology, and academic medicine, has served on the editorial board of 13 professional journals, has been elected president of seven academic and professional organizations, and received numerous awards for his scientific and professional activities.

Information Knowledge Systems Management 8 (2009) 415–434
DOI 10.3233/IKS-2009-0148
IOS Press

Chapter 22

Government, health and system transformation

Jonathan B. Perlin and Kelvin A. Baggett
E-mail: jonathan.perlin@hcahealthcare.com

Abstract: All levels of government have an economic and social interest in health. In the United States, Federal, state and local government are involved in the development of health policy, funding health care, and maintaining or improving public health. Federal, State and most municipalities also engage in delivery of health services. As with the private sector, government is grappling with accelerating health care costs, increasing service demands generated by an aging and more chronically ill society, and accumulating evidence that American health outcomes are not commensurate with the resources invested. Unlike the private sector, attempts to improve value in health care – whether through legislation in Congress or regulation or program design in the Executive branch – are subject to the full intensity of the partisan political process. In order to engage effectively with government in health system transformation, an understanding of both the civic processes and the political dynamics is necessary. This chapter provides an overview of the major governmental roles in health care as formally structured and identifies points of influence in the political process.

*"If we're going to have a successful democratic society,
we have to have a well educated and healthy citizenry."*
– Thomas Jefferson

1. Introduction

While the Declaration of Independence posits life, liberty and the pursuit of happiness as "unalienable rights", national policy has been more ambivalent about the right to health care. Great thinkers, like Jefferson, have noted the relationship of the health to societal success, and it is in that regard that Government has an inescapable mandate to promote the health of the citizenry.

The history of nations, including our own, is as much tied to its military successes as its experience with infectious diseases [13]. Not surprisingly, early health policy was focused on the most immediate threats. Anthropologists note the centrality of prohibitions against eating certain foods such as pork and preparing foodstuffs in a particular way in the central doctrines of both the Judeo-Christian and Islamic cultures. Through the middle ages, the ravages and fear of plagues instilled power in both religious and governmental institutions for organizing primitive preventive strategies, such as walling cities off from sick travelers, imposing quarantines, and disposing of dead animals and humans. In short, early governance responsibility included controlling diseases whose mechanisms were not known, but were understood to be transmissible in close quarters.

Against the backdrop where diseases classified today as infectious were the leading cause of mortality, and where plagues became more problematic with urbanization, the stage was set for application of the scientific tools of the Industrial Revolution. The work of Joseph Lister and Robert Koch ushered in early contemporary notions of germ theory and Pasteur introduced the concept of vaccination. Simultaneously, Rudolf Virchow advanced social theory of disease transmission and Edwin Chadwick led social reform in England through advances in public sanitation while Florence Nightingale worked to reform sanitation in health care. Given the economic link between health (or avoiding infectious disease) and societal productivity, including military capacity, increasingly organized religious and secular governmental structures had little choice but to assert interest in advancing the public health.

The contemporary American plagues include not only infectious threats such as pandemic influenza, SARS, highly drug resistant tuberculosis or HIV, but epidemics of both shortages of food and overconsumption, poverty, and lack of access to health care. And the governmental tradition of asserting an interest in the public health is in a period of rapid transformation. So, too, the capacity for effective social reform requires both an understanding of the biology of health and disease as well as a working knowledge of the social institutions and the actors through which national, state and local policy is made. This chapter focuses on the role of government and the manner in which government effects health policy, purchases or directly provides health care, and the way in which these activities are influenced.

2. Major federal governmental roles in health care

2.1. Executive and legislative branches – Policy, politics and providing care

The Federal Government serves as the major payer for health care in the United States, most notably through programs such as Medicare and Medicaid. It also organizes the national agenda for public health, funds and conducts biomedical research and operates significant health care delivery systems for rural, underserved, or otherwise disadvantaged Americans, as well as for military service personnel and eligible family members, and eligible military veterans. Thus, government's three major roles as purchaser, provider and policy-maker exert a singularly prominent influence on the direction of health care in the United States.

While judicial decisions may influence health care policy and practice substantially, such as in the case of abortion rights, eligibility for certain health services, and certainly in relation to malpractice and tort law, the Federal Government's interests in health care typically derive from the Executive and Legislative branches. In the Executive branch, health policy may be driven directly from the Office of the President through his Director of the Office of Management and Budget with input from White House Policy Advisors. Indeed, this is how the Obama Administration organized its work on health and payment reform.

A Presidential Administration also works through the major health-related Cabinet Departments and other Agencies, which are typically headed by political appointees, creating an intended alignment of interests. The Cabinet Secretaries and Agency Directors often bring new ideas related to both the specific work of their organization and government operation more generally. They are expected to be the operating executives of their organizations, but also loyal to the Administration and their political party and support the collective agenda.

Career staff work in exclusive support of their agency's mission, and support the more ephemeral "politicals" with deep knowledge of government, their respective institutions, and working within the boundaries of political influence and propriety. Indeed, there is often a constructive tension between the energy for change that a new administration brings, and a stabilizing inertia or continuity of programmatic activity that is embedded in long-standing bureaucracies. These pressures are ultimately complementary:

There is a need for evolution to meet new challenges, and there is a need for stability so that programs that citizens depend upon are sufficiently stable to operate without disruption.

Health and Human Services is the most central of the Cabinet Departments to issues of health, care and policy, however, the Department of Veterans Affairs and Department of Defense operate large Federal health care delivery systems. Virtually every agency or Department, from Treasury contemplating the Federal budget and the economy, to the Environmental Protection Agency, and the Department of Homeland Security, directly or indirectly influences issues ranging from access to health services, to environmental health and safety, to managing threats of bioterrorism, respectively. The ultimate purview of the Executive Branch is to execute or operate programs and, in this capacity, it makes "rules" in the regulatory process.

These same issues of public health, care, access to health services, and especially funding of Federal (Executive Branch) health programs are contemplated and acted upon by the Legislative Branch. In this regard, it is the role of Congress to make policy by enacting laws. Because of the rapidly escalating costs and the concomitant effect on the broader economy, as well as novel threats from bioterrorism and pandemic infection, health care is an increasingly central consideration in Congress. Major Committees in the House and Senate, such as "Ways and Means" and the "Health, Education, Labor and Pensions" committees, respectively, have direct responsibility for legislation regarding – and oversight of – major Federal health programs. Moreover, health care is a prominent consideration of the Appropriations committees of both the House and the Senate. Congressional support of programmatic activities of the Federal Government typically requires both *authorization* of those activities through bills promulgated by the policy committees, as well as *appropriation* of resources through a parallel legislative process.

2.1.1. The Department of Health and Human Services

In its role as the "United States government's principal agency for protecting the health of all Americans and providing essential human services," the Department of Health and Human Services seeks to execute its agenda through the coordination and oversight of 11 major Agencies, including:

- Centers for Medicare and Medicaid Services (CMS),
- National Institutes of Health (NIH),
- Centers for Disease Control and Prevention (CDC),
- Agency for Toxic Substances and Disease Registry,
- Food and Drug Administration (FDA),
- Indian Health Services (IHS),
- Health Resources and Services Administration (HRSA),
- Substance Abuse and Mental Health Services Administration (SAMHSA),
- Agency for Healthcare Research and Quality (AHRQ),
- Administration for Children and Families (ACF), and
- Administration on Aging (AOA).

The key leaders in the Department of Health and Human Service (HHS) include not only the Secretary, but also each of the agency heads. A full depiction of the organizational structure of HHS is shown in Fig. 1. In particular, the "Administrator" of CMS, with responsibility for operating the Medicare and Medicaid programs, has unique influence in shaping national health policy. Decisions about coverage for new treatments, diagnostic services, and levels of reimbursement growth – or payment cuts – have ramifications for the health care industry and are often "shadow priced" into the policies of commercial insurers and health plans. Similarly, programs operating in the Secretary's office, such as National Coordinator for Health Information Technology's "Strategic Plan," have the capacity to change the daily

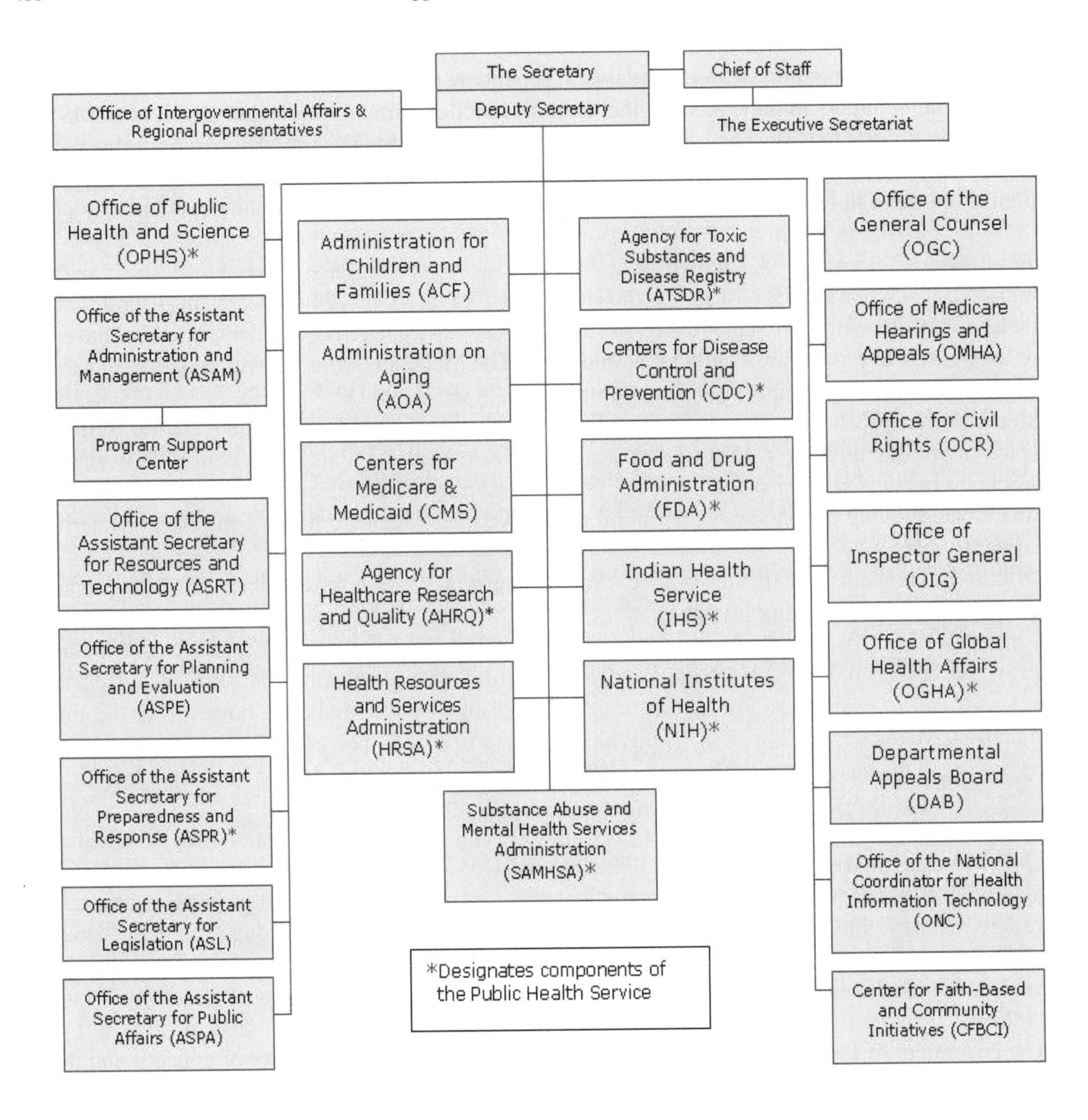

Fig. 1. Organizational chart of the U.S. Department of Health and Human Services [37].

operation of health care throughout the country, especially if they are tied to Medicare reimbursement to health care providers.

2.1.2. Medicare and Medicaid

Lyndon Johnson's "Great Society" initiative included transformative social programs that sought to eliminate poverty and racial injustice. To achieve this purpose, programs enacted or proposed as part of this social reform effort addressed medical care, education, urban problems and transportation. Two of the enduring programs of that effort, Medicare and Medicaid, were passed as part of the Social Security Act of 1965 and represent the United State's first national public health insurance programs.

Their collective purpose was to broaden access to health care among persons older than 65 years of age, children deprived of parental support, caregivers, dependent family members, the disabled and the poor. These programs today, administered by the Centers for Medicare and Medicaid Services (CMS), are providing health care to almost one-third of Americans. In short, Medicare is a more monolithic national program and is directed primarily at providing coverage for older and disabled Americans. Medicaid is administered through each of the states and is intended to enable coverage for the poor.

2.1.3. Medicare

Individuals 65 years of age or older, those less than 65 years of age with certain disabilities, and persons of any age with End Stage Renal Disease, who lawfully entered the United States and have lived here for at least five years are eligible for Medicare. The Medicare program, which is managed by the Federal Government,is comprised of four components: A, B, C and D.

Medicare Part A provides payment for inpatient care received in a hospital, skilled nursing facilities, in hospice environments and for certain home health services. Medicare Part B covers medically necessary physician services and other outpatient care. With the passage of the Balance Budget Act of 1997, Part C was created giving beneficiaries the option to receive their Medicare benefits through private health insurance plans.

Originally known as "Medicare+Choice," Part C plans today are referred to as Medicare Advantage plans. The notion of allowing private insurers and health plans to bid for operating Medicare programs was predicated on the idea that competition would foster lower costs, higher quality, and potentially improved access to preferred physicians and provider organizations. Indeed, in some instances, initial Part C *per capita* costs were lower than traditional fee-for-service Medicare, however, at the time of publication, Medicare Advantage programs are projected to cost 13 percent more than the conventional program [4]. This has invited both criticism and legislative interest in reducing Medicare Advantage to no more than parity with traditional Medicare *per capita* expenditures.

In 2003, due to concerns over soaring prescription drug costs, Congress passed the Medicare Prescription Drug, Improvement and Modernization Act (MMA), also known as Medicare Part D. This legislation's major provision created an outpatient prescription drug benefit that provides access to drug coverage for those individuals entitled to Medicare Part A or enrolled in Medicare Part B. "Dual eligibles," defined as individuals who are entitled to Medicare Part A and/or Part B and are eligible for some form of Medicaid benefit, are automatically enrolled. The coverage became effective on January 1, 2006.

The enactment of Part D is instructive in appreciating the increasing intensity of concern and debate over the affordability of American health care, the value it provides, and the tension surrounding an expanded governmental role. As such, it serves as a model for understanding many of the dynamics in the ongoing discussion of health reform and transformation. It introduced, but failed to resolve, questions of whether the Federal government should leverage its position as the largest single purchaser of prescription drugs to reduce àcquisition cost. It also required confronting questions of the social utility of particular expenditures, especially in regard to "life-style" medications, as well as questions of distributive justice that inevitably require consideration of trade-offs between the breadth and depth of coverage decisions [6,31,32].

2.1.4. Medicaid and the State Children's Health Insurance Program

Medicaid is jointly funded by the Federal Government and individual states. Eligibility is based upon both Federal and state laws, and coverage is available to certain low income individuals and families.

Criteria for coverage include age, pregnancy, disability, income, assets and resources. As a result of the flexibility given to states in the administration of the Medicaid program, there can be significant variability. Rules governing income, assets and resources vary by state. States that choose to extend coverage to other populations that are not eligible based upon existing rules are able to obtain Federal waivers to do so. Consequently, there is significant variation in enrollee demographics and the scope of benefits among the states.

In an effort to reduce the number of low income uninsured children not covered by the Medicaid program, Congress createdthe State Children's Health Insurance Program (S-CHIP) as part of the Balanced Budget Act of 1997. At the time of this publication, S- CHIP covers more than 7 million children. Unlike Medicaid, however, Federal S-CHIP funds are capped and, therefore, there is no individual entitlement.

2.1.5. The increasing cost of government sponsored health programs

At their inception, Medicare and Medicaid had a total enrollment of 19 million individuals. By 2008, Medicare alone provided health insurance for more than 44 million individuals. In that same year, Medicaid provided coverage for more than 50 million low-income persons, including more than 24 million children [36,37]. While increases in cost attributable to population growth can generally be spread over an increasing tax base, increases in the cost of Medicare and Medicaid have substantially exceeded the rate of inflation [25]. A number of factors have been identified. These include those that are endogenous to the patients themselves, such as the desirable increase in longevity. Other factors include the deteriorating health status that may be attributed to advanced age, but also the burden of chronic illness due to lifestyles of inactivity, excess consumption of food, and inaccessible or ineffective preventive health care. It has also been argued that Medicare and Medicaid, like commercial insurance, serves to overly isolate patients from the financial consequences of health-related behaviors or drives over-utilization of some services or medications, especially in the presence of direct-to-consumer advertising [5].

Factors accelerating health care costs beyond inflation that are exogenous to patients include the advent of expensive, new, and beneficial technologies. Less favorably, the inappropriate use of new technologies with no or marginal improvement over existing treatments adds cost without commensurate value. Similarly, the systematic incentives of fee-for-service reimbursement drive over-utilization of certain services (especially those that are procedurally oriented) and under-utilization of others, like preventive services [16,23,29]. The administrative inefficiencies of the third-party payment process and claims adjudication are substantial, and the absence of computerized health records, leading to redundant testing, unnecessary hospitalization, and avoidable adverse events also generate unproductive expenditure [27]. The tendency toward defensive medicine, over-testing, and over-treatment in a litigious society is also inefficient and burdensome. In aggregate, it has been estimated that almost a third of every dollar spent on health is lost to inefficiency [43].

Whatever the causes, the effect on the Federal budget is substantial. According to the Comptroller General, a non-political official, by 2015 the combination of costs attributable to Social Security, Medicare, Medicaid and the interest on the national debt will equal all revenues deposited into the Federal Treasury! [10]. Every other expenditure – defense, education, infrastructure, etc. – is "above the line." (See Fig. 2). Moreover, Medicare is no longer self-sustaining.

In 2006, for the first time ever, expenses exceeded revenues into the "Medicare Trust Fund," and the 2009 Medicare Trustees' Report indicates complete insolvency of the Trust in 2017, if the course of the program's present operating deficits does not change [17]. Moreover, the increasing cost not only jeopardizes the program's sustainability, but it exerts a pressure for increasing taxes on both citizens and

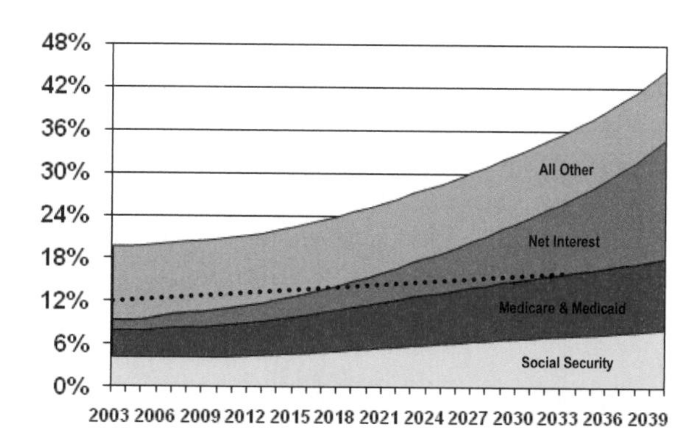

Fig. 2. Social security (lower band), medicare and medicaid spending (second band) as a percent of U. S. gross domestic product. Net interest on the national debt (third band), all other federal spending (upper band), and all federal revenues also shown by dotted line [40].

businesses, two groups that may be simultaneously contending with facing a difficult global economy and their own ability to fund the escalating costs of commercial insurance for employees and beneficiaries not specifically covered by Medicare (and Medicaid) programs.

As has been noted, Medicare and Medicaid can drive broader health policy. Importantly, then, they can also serve as large scale "labs" for understanding how to improve, safety, quality, efficiency and, ultimately, value. One area of intense interest is the management of beneficiaries who have multiple chronic conditions. Among Americans aged 65 years or older, approximately 88% have one or more chronic conditions [44]. Ninety percent of Medicare expenditures are for beneficiaries with three or more chronic conditions [1]. Improved chronic disease management and better coordination of care longitudinally, with payment reform serving as a vehicle to incentivize these activities, is an increasing focus for HHS and the Medicare program.

As value may be construed as the relationship between health outcomes and the resources used in seeking those outcomes, health and payment reform must contemplate not only the control of costs (the denominator), but the effectiveness of health services themselves (the numerator). Quality, safety, prevention, personal responsibility, and the continuity of care and health information across environments are but some of the tools being explored to improve value.

2.1.6. Mechanisms to test improving value in the Medicare and HHS programs

Through changes made to Medicare in 1972 and the subsequent MMA, the Secretary of Health and Human Services can approve demonstration projects that encourage improvement in quality and safety of care and the efficient allocation of resources. In support of the reform movement toward a payment methodology that places reward not on the volume of care but on the value of care delivered, several demonstrations have been designed to identify and to better understand ways to promote better clinical quality with increased efficiency.

Under the current Medicare Prospective Payment System (Part A), hospitals are reimbursed on an average cost associated with a diagnosis related group (DRG). On the other hand, physicians are compensated on a fee-for-service basis under Part B. If one accepts studies demonstrating variation in cost without commensurate improvement in care outcomes, then significant barriers to improved resource utilization are inappropriate or misaligned incentives [15,19].

Several demonstration projects seek to better align the incentives between physicians and hospitals. In May 2008, CMS announced the three-year Acute Care Episode (ACE) Demonstration project designed to link reimbursement of hospitals and physicians for the inpatient treatment of 28 cardiac and 9 orthopedic inpatient surgical procedures. ACE includes a global payment for an entire episode-of-care *in lieu* of all Medicare Part A and Part B payments [8].

Beyond the intention to increase quality and efficiency through better coordination between hospitals and physicians, ACE also seeks to evaluate the effect of price and quality transparency on beneficiary choice and physician referral patterns. With global payment for a diagnosis, the "lead" physician would be incentivized to refer to effective and efficient (not just familiar) consulting specialists.

2.1.7. Improving access to care through Medicare or insurance cooperatives

However vexing improving the value proposition of Medicare and Medicaid might be, the United States continues to wrestle with the reality that one-in-six Americans are uninsured at any moment and that, problematic to improving preventive services, over one-in-four Americans is without insurance at some point during the year. Among the latter, nearly half are employed full-time [6,30]. Despite the looming insolvency of Medicare, and perhaps counter-intuitively, one suggestion has been extending Medicare eligibility. If younger, presumably healthier, individuals were able to enroll, theoretically the risk pool and the balance between premium revenue and health care expenditures would improve. Perennially, the political challenge in embracing this approach has been the criticism that it sets a trajectory toward a single-payer system.

Other possible mechanisms to enfranchise the uninsured include publically-available insurance plans that may operate as a Federal, state, or other cooperative that allows (or mandates) enrollment at an affordable rate. The logic is that if the benefits were specified nationally (or for a sizeable population, such as a state), the cooperative could receive bids on that package from insurers or health plans that felt they could profitably provide services within the determined pricing of the premium.

Operating as a cooperative, some revenues would be periodically redistributed to guarantee each insurer's viability. No plan would be allowed to exclude patients with "pre-existing conditions," and because disease burden is shared among all in the cooperative, the attraction for "cherry picking" only the healthiest patients should be diminished. Incentives should exist for reducing health risks through preventive services or disease management, especially if patients are insured within the cooperative over the longer term. While conceivable that the cooperative may actually aggregate higher risk patients who lose or cannot get insurance elsewhere, some contend that the existence of a "public option" could destabilize private insurance as employers abandon subsidy of employee insurance programs, *in lieu*, contributing to the employee's public plan premium paying a tax penalty.

Whether insurance cooperatives would operate as predicted is not fully understood. There is a need for more health services research in this regard, as well as for better understanding of the data that are currently being generated from initial state-based efforts, as in Massachusetts. While alternative strategies might derive from expanding CMS programs, extending coverage without improving value would only compound financial challenges. Conversely, effective strategies for value in Medicare would likely find broader adoption. The posture that CMS takes on driving value, bundling payment for longitudinal episodes, or the use of comparative or cost-effectiveness research in defining covered services will affect not only beneficiaries of their programs, but will influence all other sectors of health care through shadow pricing and policy.

2.2. Selected Health and Human Services agencies

2.2.1. The Agency for Healthcare Research and Quality

The Agency for Healthcare Research and Quality (AHRQ) is charged with improving the quality, safety, efficiency and effectiveness of health care for all Americans. In this capacity, the agency commissions, funds, and conducts research to advance care that improves health. As reform seeks to move payment models from volume-based reimbursement to value-based payment methodologies, understanding which treatments generate the best outcomes most efficiently in a particular situation will need to be the basis for clinical practice. This is the essence of comparative effectiveness research.

Identifying ineffective, but potentially expensive, practices is not without political risk. Indeed, the agency's predecessor, known as the Agency for Health Care Policy Research, had a near-death experience that jeopardized its continuing funding from Congress for promulgating evidence-based guidelines that demonstrated limited indications for spinal fusion [12]. Despite the need for comparative effectiveness data, the capacity of a government agency to transcend politics is difficult, leading some to suggest that an entity with this mandate would need to established by government, but not be beholden to the annual Congressional funding process. Notwithstanding its history, AHRQ provides leadership in understanding what works best in areas of clinical practice, payment design and incentives, and the adoption and use of information technology in health care.

2.2.2. Food and Drug Administration

The Food and Drug Administration was created in 1906. Its charge evolved to ensure that foods, cosmetics, biological products and medical devices are safe and efficacious. According to HHS, these products represent almost one-fourth of annual consumer spending in the United States [36,37].

The FDA has been one of the most scrutinized Federal agencies. In the late 1980's, the agency was criticized for what were perceived to be lengthy delays in the approval process for new medications to treat the then little-understood and highly life-threatening disease, HIV/AIDS. In response, the FDA developed a policy for expedited drug approval. In 2004, the agency was accused of ineffectiveness in appreciating the limitation of manufacturer-sponsored studies of the risk for heart attacks associated with the use of a new class of nonsteroidal anti-inflammatory drugs, known as COX-2 inhibitors. Ironically, to obtain resources for accelerating the review process, FDA had introduced "user fees" that are paid by the pharmaceutical or device manufacturer. This situation has raised questions about the potential for conflicts-of-interest.

FDA has also been challenged on its post-marketing surveillance process which provides its ability to monitor safety issues after approved products enter the public domain [39]. Subsequently, it has been accused of failing to protect public safety for products that included surgical materials, blood thinners, and peanut butter. In January 2009, the Government Accountability Office (GAO) issued a report that questioned FDA's ability to fulfill its mission, concluding that the agency faced significant challenges that "compromise its ability to protect Americans from unsafe and ineffective products." [38]. That FDA's mission is critical is indisputable, but like AHRQ it serves as an example that the Government's role in health policy and regulation is complex, highly-politicized by multiple stakeholder interests, and requires adequate investment to be effective. Those same attributes apply to Federal health care delivery systems.

2.3. Government as health care provider

2.3.1. Indian Health Service and Heath Resources and Services Administration

The Indian Health Service (IHS) and the Health Resources and Services Administration (HRSA) are two HHS agencies that function primarily as providers of health care. IHS provides comprehensive health services to almost two million American Indians and Alaska Natives. The Indian health system is comprised of 46 hospitals, 324 health centers, 309 health stations and Alaska Native village centers, and 34 urban Indian health programs [36,37].

In 2008, it was projected that Health Resources and Service Administration (HRSA) funded health centers would provide health care services to 17 million patients at more than 4,000 sites throughout the United States. This care is provided to people who are low-income, uninsured or to those residing in underserved rural, remote or urban settings [36,37].

HRSA also administers the National Health Service Corps and the Ryan White CARE Act programs. The National Health Service Corps provides scholarships and loan repayment for health professionals that chose to serve in areas of the country with provider shortages for defined periods of time. Ryan White CARE Act programs provide assistance with medical care and other services for people with HIV/AIDS who demonstrate financial need and lack adequate health insurance to pay for necessary care.

2.3.2. Centers for Disease Control and Prevention and the Public Health Service Commissioned Corp

Founded in 1946 as the Communicable Disease Center, the Centers for Disease Control and Prevention (CDC) is one of the few Federal agencies located outside of Washington, DC. Based in Atlanta, CDC bears primary responsibility for public health, health promotion, disease prevention and emergency preparedness. The agency in coordination with the states (discussed below) provides a surveillance system to maintain national health statistics, and to prevent and respond to disease outbreaks.

The role of the CDC has come into prominence in the recent past, with the emergence of important infectious diseases like HIV/AIDS, infectious threats like SARS and avian flu, pandemic (swine) flu, and bioterrorism. The CDC operates the "strategic national stockpile" as a cache of antibiotics, antidotes, and support supplies to help respond to pandemics, natural disasters and terrorism with biological and radiological agents.

While the Public Health Service Commissioned Corp reports to the Assistant Secretary of Health and Human Services, the Corp of 6,000 uniformed public health professionals works closely with CDC and in support of the Federal Government's public health activities.

2.3.3. The Military Health System and the Veterans Health Administration

The Military Health System (MHS) is large and complex. While one might correctly imagine that a central mission is to provide health services to assure the operational readiness of troops, the MHS is also responsible for providing for the health needs of eligible family members of service personnel, civilians employed by the armed services and eligible military retirees. The MHS creates its worldwide network as both a direct care provider and as a purchaser of health services. It also stands ready to assist in humanitarian relief efforts and conducts medical research, especially related to military health issues.

MHS operates 63 hospitals and 413 clinics under the command of the Army, Navy and Air Force [35]. Each service has a Surgeon General who is the senior executive of the service's health system. The Surgeons General ultimately report to their military Service chief, but their work is coordinated by the Office of the Assistant Secretary of Defense for Health Affairs (ASDHA). The TriCare Management Activity or "TMA" also reports to the ASDHA, and is the office that coordinates the purchase and administration of health services for eligible beneficiaries, especially dependents of military personnel and military retirees. In aggregate, the majority of health services for beneficiaries of the Military Health Service are now obtained in the private sector, and providers are reimbursed by TMA. Care provided on military bases, in battle, or in support of troops deployed on missions outside of the continental United States is almost exclusively rendered by the Services directly.

Among the most notable achievements in military medicine are the extraordinary improvements in survival of battlefield injuries. Due to organization of rapid field response capabilities, improved communications and evacuation, and technology, survival from life-threatening injuries has increased from 78 percent in World War II, to 84 percent in Viet Nam, to over 92 percent in Afghanistan and Iraq [34].

While health care supports the primary mission of the Department of Defense, caring for "him who shall have borne the battle" – in Lincoln's words – is the central mission of the Department of Veterans Affairs (VA). The three operating units of VA include Memorial Affairs, operating the national network of veterans' cemeteries, the Veterans Benefits Administration, offering life insurance, pensions and educational benefits, and the Veterans Health Administration (VHA), the nation's largest integrated health system.

Of the approximately 25.5 million military veterans alive today, about 40 percent are eligible to enroll for VHA health care. Eligibility is determined by statute. In addition to an honorable discharge, criteria include such things as service in a Presidentially-declared war zone, illness or injury during service, certain catastrophic physical or mental illnesses, or impoverishment. Periodically, VHA may enroll additional veterans who agree to pay for treatment of conditions that are not "service-connected." Currently, VHA has nearly 8 million enrollees, and approximately 6 million veterans will use VHA care in any given year. In contrast to the MHS, VHA typically provides care directly to Veterans (family members or dependents are generally not eligible) in more than 1,400 sites, including 165 hospitals and more than 900 outpatient clinics.

VHA may serve as a model for some of the tenets of value-based health care. From a history of bureaucracy, inefficiency, and notoriously poor quality, VHA emerged in the late 1990's and new century as a leader in clinical performance measurement, patient safety, and implementation of electronic health records. By 2004, VHA outperformed mainstream health care across 294 metrics of preventive services and chronic disease management [2].

As preventive services became more accessible – the number of outpatient clinics increased 350 percent between 1996 and 2004 – and as disease was better managed across care settings using electronic health records and telehealth services, VHA clinical performance improved and efficiency increased. In contrast to Medicare *per capita* costs which increased 44.7 percent in nominal dollars between 1996 and 2004, VHA care increased by only 0.8 percent [14]. Adjusted for inflation, better VHA care actually became less expensive. Comprehensive measurement of quality, computerized decision-support and error-checking systems, transparent performance accountability, and a national health services research network, were tools leadership used to effect transformation [27].

While some may dismiss VHA's relevance to the broader health care challenges in the United States, an entire issue of a Canadian health services research journal was devoted to extrapolating lessons from VHA's transformation for improving the Canadian health care system [21]. Whether VHA can maintain its leadership depends less on whether it has adequate financial resources, then on whether VA and VHA leadership are permitted sufficient degrees of freedom to continue innovation.

2.4. Federal watchdog organizations

Two organizations, neither directly decisional in promulgating health policy, regulation, or delivery of care services, bear mentioning because of their influence on all aspects of health care. The Government Accountability Office (GAO) is the investigative arm of Congress. Headed by the Comptroller General, a non-political appointee with up to a 15-year term, the nonpartisan organization's central role is to ensure responsible use of Federal resources. Beyond audits and investigations to assure compliance with law and appropriate use of resources, GAO performs policy analysis and provides reports and testimony to Congress outlining alternative policy options.

The Inspector General Act of 1978 assigned a specific watchdog organization to detect "fraud, waste and abuse" to major cabinet departments and Federal agencies. Appointed by the President, it is notable that each Inspector General (IG) does not report to the cabinet secretary or agency head, though they usually try to work collaboratively. In HHS, the IG has both the general charge to assure programmatic integrity, as well as the specific mandate to operate the "Exclusions Program" which forbids HHS payment to entities including physicians, hospitals and nursing homes with convictions for violations of laws relating to fraud, patient abuse, or for health care practitioners specifically, certain adverse licensure actions. As with GAO, IG reports highlighting problems with programs are dealt with swiftly by the agency, because however significant, well-researched, or measured in tone, they can become incendiary in both partisan politics and the media.

2.5. The role of Congress in Federal health care and policy

2.5.1. Senate & house committees

While it may seem that the policy direction of Federal health-related programs would reside in the Executive Branch agencies in which they operate (e.g., Medicare in the Department of Health and Human Services), policy direction is also set through the legislative process. Not surprisingly, Congressional Representatives and Senators may exert influence with respect to the more parochial interests of their districts or states. This may include seeking special funds for hospitals or health services, vulnerable populations, research interests, business development, public health, and so forth as earmarks to health-related or other legislation. However, the organized influence on national health policy is concentrated within a number of House and Senate committees charged with oversight of particular Federal programs or appropriation of resources for those programs to operate.

2.5.2. Appropriations committees

The House Appropriations Committee's charge is to appropriate Federal funds in support of Government operations. The Subcommittee on Labor, Health and Human Services, Education and Related Agencies has jurisdiction over most units of the Department of Health and Human Services, except most notably, the Food and Drug Administration. The Subcommittee on Defense appropriates funding for military health, and the Subcommittee on Military Construction and Veterans Affairs provides appropriations for veterans' health care. The Medicare Payment Advisory Commission or "MedPAC," which advises Congress on the operation of Medicare and such issues as access, quality and setting the rates for provider reimbursement, reports to the House Appropriations Committee.

The Senate Appropriations Committee has similar jurisdiction to the House Committee. The Subcommittee structure is also nearly parallel to the House with the Subcommittee on Labor, Health and Human Services, and Education having purview over most agencies of the Department of Health and Human Services. While the appropriations process proceeds simultaneously each year in the House and the Senate, resolution of differences between appropriations agendas occurs through the bicameral conference and mark-up process. While the policy committees described below would seem to be where Congressional policy is set, what is or is not funded is a powerful and often ultimate determinant of Federal programmatic direction.

2.5.3. Health-related Congressional committees

While it may seem redundant, the Senate Finance Committee has financial policy jurisdiction over proposed legislation regarding Health programs specified under the Social Security Act and health programs financed by a specific tax or trust fund. This includes Medicare, Medicaid and the State

Children's Health Insurance Program, which are specifically considered by the Subcommittee on Health Care.

The Senates Health, Education, Labor and Pensions (or "HELP") Committee has broad policy purview over the areas suggested by its name. Topics germane to its consideration range from public health, to health education, and to health insurance and coverage. Senate Committees on Armed Services and Veterans Affairs have policy jurisdiction over military and veterans health programs, respectively.

House committees of particular relevance to health policy are also numerous. The Ways and Means Committee has specific jurisdiction for Medicare, and its Subcommittee on Health focuses on how health services and biomedical research is funded. The Energy and Commerce Committee has purview over health facility operations, public health related to imposition of quarantine, and exerts its watchdog role through its Subcommittee on Oversight and Investigations. The Subcommittee on Health has House jurisdiction for Medicaid, food and drugs and drug abuse programs. The Education and Labor Committee's interests address health professions training and workforce issues. Again, the respective Committees on Military and Veterans Affairs each have subcommittees on health for Department of Defense and Department of Veterans Affairs related health activities.

2.5.4. Influences on the legislative process

Policy development is influenced in both Appropriations and other committees by a variety of factors. At times, party policy direction may be tightly organized by the senior legislative members of each chamber. The House of Representatives leadership includes not only the Speaker, but the Majority Leader who, as second in charge' organizes daily party activities, and the Majority Whip' whose role is to influence party position on votes. Roles are parallel for the House Minority Leader and Whip, respectively. The Senate is also organized along party lines with majority and minority party Leaders and Whips. Of course, dissension within party lines does occur on particular issues, and durable coalitions may organize around shared interests or political beliefs. One such example is the fiscally conservative "Blue Dog Democratic Coalition."

At times, influence is sought from a variety of trusted advisory bodies. MedPAC is Congressionally-chartered for advice on setting Medicare reimbursement rates. The Institute of Medicine and the National Academies may be called to testify on specific issues or mandated by statute to produce a report on a topic of interest to particular legislators, Committees, or Subcommittees. The Congressional Budget Office is a Federal Agency. Its specific mandate is to provide, "... objective, nonpartisan, and timely analyses to aid in economic and budgetary decisions on the wide array of programs covered by the federal budget and (provide) information and estimates required for the Congressional budget process." [11]

The direction of legislation is also influenced by who is asked to provide input into developing legislation (a process known formally as "technical assistance"), who gains access to discuss issues with Members of Congress and their staff, and who is called to testify at hearings of relevance to health issues. The research for legislation as well as for formulation of speaking points, policy positions and position papers is done substantially by Congressional staff. Depending on the Committees that a Representative or Senator is assigned, the Member's office may have professional staff with deep, relevant subject matter expertise. At the same time, junior staff in the office, often recently graduated from college or post-graduate programs, are relied upon heavily. Their influence should not be underestimated.

In the legislative process, the interests of particular witnesses who may stand to benefit from the outcome of a legislative, investigative, or appropriations hearing may be evident. As well, appropriations bills may include mandates for consultants to research a particular issue. This may occur with the belief that the consultant's report so chartered will provide further evidence for or against a specific policy direction.

Table 1
Selected major health sector political action committees

Health sector	Sponsoring organization	PAC name
Doctors	American Medical Association	AMPAC
Health Insurers & Plans	America's Health Insurance Plans	AHIP-PAC
Hospitals	American Hospital Association,	AHAPAC
	Federation of American Hospitals	FEDPAC
Labor	Service Employees International Union	SEIU-Committee on Political Education
Nurses	American Nurses Association	ANA-PAC
Nursing Homes	Alliance for Quality Nursing Home Care	AQNHC-PAC
Pharmaceutical & Device	Pharmaceutical Research and Manufacturers of America (PhRMA)	See Text

Congressional activity is not just self-initiated. While the role of professional lobbyists, political-action committees (PACs) representing trade associations or other big and well-funded interests, and political activism among citizens themselves and grass-roots organizations may be clear, the magnitude of their influence on the political agenda is substantial.

In health care, this influence is exerted through PACs representing health care workers such as doctors and nurses, medical specialty societies, health care providers such as hospitals and nursing homes, pharmaceutical and device manufactures, health insurers, disease advocacy organizations, and organized labor. Table 1 identifies some of the major industry PACs and their relationship to particular organizations and health sector interests. Based on information reported to the Federal Election Commission, 127 health care oriented PACs made nearly $50 million in contributions to the campaigns of candidates for Federal office in the 2008 election cycle [9].

Sometimes the influence of a particular interest group is exerted more obliquely. For example, the consumer-advocacy group, Public Citizen, asserts that the Pharmaceutical Research Manufacturers Association (PhRMA), underwrites a number of non-profit, 501(c) organizations that are reported to essentially lobby in the ostensible interest of cohorts of patients, but carry a message that is conducive to pharmaceutical business growth around that cohort. The inherent tensions between a vendor's interest in liberalizing reimbursement for their product and an insurer's interest in controlling cost is but one example of the high stakes and why influence in the Congressional decision-making process and the election of particular candidates is considered valuable.

3. State and local government roles in health and care

Like politics, much of healthcare is local. It is locally delivered in hospitals and other care settings that are integral parts of the communities that they serve. While communities across the United States have strong similarities, they are not homogenous. Therefore, consideration of their uniqueness also guides decisions regarding the allocation of healthcare dollars. In their role of promoting health and minimizing disease, state and local governments bear tremendous responsibility to optimize resource use and provide infrastructure to meet the needs of their constituents.

3.1. State health officials

Each state has a Secretary of Health or a State Health Commissioner who leads in establishing and executing the state's health agenda. Typically, these positions are appointed by the Governor. In addition to serving as an advocate, liaison and regulator of healthcare within their state, they also share in the responsibility for public health. They execute their responsibility with policy, regulatory, administrative, and clinical staff, and generally work closely with a network of county and city health departments.

3.2. State and local health departments

There are thousands of local health departments within the United States. They are responsible for health assessment, tracking population health, and for the development of community health services to prevent disease and disease spread. They serve an epidemiologic function in collecting data to characterize health status, and they construct programs to influence positive changes in health, such as reducing tobacco use.

Beyond prevention and wellness programs, in many communities, primary care and specialty services are also available for mental health, pregnancy, sexually transmitted diseases and HIV/AIDS. As the number of uninsured individuals has grown, it has placed additional responsibility on public health programs, given the role of local health departments in providing safety net services for the indigent.

As noted previously, the structure of the Medicaid program gives states latitude to determine eligible beneficiaries, to define benefits and to establish the terms for provider compensation [18]. This is often influenced by the Governor's political beliefs and guided by the Health Secretary or Commissioner. In some instances, Medicaid or other state health programs are accountable for their budget to the state's Commissioner of Finance. Not surprisingly, the variables that help shape the administration of Medicaid in a particular state often include population demographics, disease prevalence, environmental conditions, socioeconomics, resource availability, and the political disposition of the majority party.

3.3. State public health roles

State public health programs provide a critical link in the nation's health infrastructure. Beyond the clinical services provided directly to individuals, state and local health departments are essential conduits of information for national health surveillance. They contribute, at a grass-roots level, to monitoring and understanding normal patterns of population health, as well as identifying variation that might suggest the occurrence of an outbreak. Through effective coordination of local and state systems with CDC, the epidemiology is available to discern when increased incidence of illness might be an isolated cluster, endemic to the area, novel, or epidemic.

States laws also govern required reporting of communicable disease, vital statistics and environmental conditions as necessary prerequisites for effective epidemiology. Communicable diseases are defined as including sexually-transmitted diseases, and certain rashes, bacterial and viral illnesses. Healthcare providers, facilities and local health departments bear the responsibility for collecting and reporting these diseases to the state. Notably, for "reportable diseases," it is not necessary to obtain the patient's consent under the Health Insurance Portability and Accountability Act of 1996 which governs virtually all other communication of a patient's health information by health professionals or institutions [24]. This provider protection is afforded to assist identification of emerging patterns of reportable diseases and, especially, to thwart additional sickness within the population when cases of communicable diseases or conditions related to environmental hazards are detected. State and local governments also bear responsibility for setting health codes,and regulating other aspects of sanitation and hygiene, such as the treatment of sewage and the quality of water.

States also serve as the repository of information regarding vital statistics. These demographic data which uniformly consist of births, deaths, marriages and divorces, help to produce information that directs research, policy and the allocation of resources. Population data can assist in understanding common causes of illness and mortality and guide decision-making about potential interventions.

State and local departments of public health have key roles in leading immunization programs. These include the administration of vaccines, the maintenance of immunization records, and efforts to determine compliance with vaccinations and rates of disease screening. State laws not only govern the immunizations of the population, but state resources often fund vaccine programs to insure that vulnerable segments of the population, such as impoverished children, are protected from vaccine-preventable diseases. In coordination with schools and places of employment, states also organize efforts to increase or require compliance.

3.4. Emergency management and preparedness

Emergency preparedness involves the creation of a structure to address emergencies when they arise and mitigate risks. This includes the capacity to manage public health emergencies resulting from bioterrorism, outbreaks of infectious disease, ionizing radiation, and mass casualties, such as might result from explosions and natural disasters [7].

Events ranging from the nuclear accident at Three Mile Island to the H1N1 "swine flu" pandemic demonstrate the importance of having systems in place for rapid situational assessment, reporting of data to national officials, and immediate local response. By having the requisite structures and support in place and practiced, local and state entities are equipped to deliver health information and services in a manner that minimizes both risk and harm to the populations they serve.

3.5. State regulatory function

States have jurisdiction for regulating many aspects of health services, and the authority for oversight of care quality. Their regulatory purview extends to the licensure of health services, allowing them to define what types of care are provided and where the services may be offered. States use the licensure of health care professionals to assure appropriate qualifications for practice, a role that entails verification of required credentials, such as professional education, passage of required examinations and years of practice. States vary in their requirements for practitioner qualification and thus obtaining a license in one state does not automatically transfer to another.

States specifically regulate health care entities, including hospitals, physician practices, laboratory testing services, ambulatory surgical centers, nursing homes, and mental health facilities. The regulatory process defines not only necessary certifications, but extends from requirements for the physical structure of health facilities and life safety to rules regarding patient payment.

A controversial approach states use in trying to balance population need with supply of health infrastructure – ranging from hospitals to CT scanners – is known as certificate-of-need (C.O.N.) programs. Currently, 36 states use C.O.N. [26] In contrast to general economic theory, by limiting supply, proponents argue, costs are reduced. In markets with excess capacity, they propose that since fixed costs must be paid even if the service is underutilized, charges are inflated. As well, it is argued that excess capacity leads to overutilization, a phenomenon known as supplier-induced demand [41]. In those states with C.O.N. programs, hospitals must apply for approval prior to new construction or purchases of major equipment.

3.6. Summary

In summary, states and municipalities have roles that are parallel to Federal Government. They are purchasers of care for their beneficiaries; they serve as insurers and payers through Medicaid, S-CHIP, and other programs; they provide care directly through state and local hospitals and health departments; and they are responsible for public health and are health service regulators. As with health care at the Federal level, there are state roles that are vested primarily in the Executive Branch, as described here, and there exist the checks-and-balances of negotiating authorization and funding with the Legislative Branch. Similarly, the ability to effect transformation at the state and local level requires an understanding of the institutions involved, the influences and the evidence, and, of course, the politics.

4. Conclusions

While recognized that the United States can offer the world's most sophisticated health care, there is also agreement that there are significant shortcomings in safety, quality, access and value. Independent of politics, the complexity and sheer number of various governmental bodies with roles determining health care financing, policy, regulation and delivery of services is itself a formidable barrier to transformation. With the overlay of partisan politics and the particular interests of specific stakeholders, one can appreciate that transformation is magnitudinally more difficult: By definition, transformation dislocates established interests.

The imperative for improving safety, quality, access and value would seem clear. However, these issues are contested on the basis of both legitimate concerns, supported by scientific evidence or other strong data, as well as parochial interests regarding aspects of reform that might determine "winners" and "losers." The proverb that "one man's waste is another man's treasure" may be no more true than in the established bureaucracy of contemporary American health care. For example, redundant laboratory testing or the use of a more expensive, but inferior or even equivalent medication or device, adds little value from a broader social perspective. However, the individual interests of the laboratory, or pharmaceutical or device manufacturer may be antithetical to reform. Moreover, the traditional orientation of American health care toward fee-for-service reimbursement incentivizes volume, not value, *per se*.

As described earlier in the chapter, value may be construed as the relationship of outcomes to resource inputs, or more specifically for health care, as the relationship of safe and effective clinical outcomes to cost. In the extreme, one could envision that value-based health care would reward better providers – those achieving consistently superior outcomes more efficiently – with favorable payment and volume growth [28]. In its simplest reduction, value-based health care would encourage "pay-for-performance." Indeed, the Medicare program has been attempting to introduce this concept for some time [33].

While changing incentives through payment reform would seem a rational policy for promoting value, the complexity at both a policy and political level is substantial. Policy this significant is not unilaterally promulgated from within CMS. Coordination with other HHS agency agendas, such as AHRQ's role in advancing quality or the National Coordinator's role for implementing health information technology, is required. The political lens of the Secretary's office weighs stakeholder sentiment with the Administration's priorities, and Federal budget impact is evaluated by White House through the Office of Management and Budget.

Significant policy changes may be implemented by regulation, but coordination with the Congressional committees of jurisdiction is required to prevent alienating legislators with responsibility for authorization, oversight or appropriations. Some changes require legislation, whether for authority or resources, and Congress may enact law that yields the tools for intended programmatic direction, modifies direction substantially, or refutes it entirely. Beyond influences and pecuniary interests in the legislative process already detailed, policy-making and legislation occurs in the glare of an information-age media cycle, in which public reaction may elicit rapidly shifting commitments.

The other central challenge that reform seeks to resolve, access, is equally problematic. Realizing that safety net care is inefficient – problems are treated, not prevented or managed – and expensive, it would seem logical that coverage of the uninsured would be more desirable than cost-shifting from the uninsured to the insured. Still, initial investments in health promotion and disease management are unlikely to provide positive returns in the short run, leading to contention over affordability in a down economy.

Others worry that "public plan" options destabilize commercial insurance. The corollary to this belief is that, for all of the shortcomings, those with acceptable coverage don't want to give up what they have. The infamous "Harry and Louise" commercials during the Clinton Administration's attempts at reform highlighted this concern [42]. Thus, the alignment of interests among commercial insurers, providers who use more lucrative commercial insurance to offset lower-paying or uninsured patient costs, and patients themselves, worried about limitations to utilization (rational or otherwise) creates a challenge for transforming access to health services. Balancing expansion of access with alignment of incentives toward value would resolve aspects of the economic argument, but not necessarily those of patients, providers, or those vendors whose business improves with increased utilization.

In conclusion, though the logic and need for improving value (and all that is implied in terms of safety, quality and cost) and access would seem self-evident, change is not without potential dislocation of interests. These range from predictable business interests in the private sector, to issues of authority and jurisdiction among Federal, state and local agencies, to political capital among the executive and legislative branch leaders, to the traditional "pork barrel" politics of "bringing home the bacon" to elected official's districts, states, or party. These challenges are formidable. Thus, factors that would traditionally predict greater success for transformative actions would include: aligning political interests across party lines to the extent possible; aligning policy intent among Federal (or state) agencies; coordinating executive branch policy with legislative branch committees of jurisdiction; understanding and anticipating stakeholder concerns and engaging stakeholders in constructive support; and limiting the scope of change so that battles are not waged on too many fronts simultaneously. Conversely, the inability to achieve alignment politically or administratively, and alienation of influential stakeholders whether on specific issues or cumulatively by virtue of the breadth of change considered, inhibits transformation.

There may, however, be moments when the broader context – typically a crisis– produces a unifying tension that, shared among stakeholders, creates a "burning platform" for change. Characterized by a desire for rapid action and ephemeral political alignments, these moments are unusually permissive for rapid and sweeping transformation. Notable examples have included war efforts, such as followed the bombing of Pearl Harbor and more recently 9/11, the development of Social Security following the Great Depression, the "stimulus programs" that followed the global economic downturn of 2008, and even VHA's transformation during the past decade. In VHA's case, the mandate was clear: Change or go out of business.

Whether health care's shortcomings produce sufficient shared pain for a burning platform for sweeping reform to be perceived is debatable. Concerns about the broader economy, viability of American businesses, and the country's global competitiveness, may be effective in fueling the fire for change. The most likely scenario for the next decade may be that sufficient pressure does exist to set forth a transformational agenda, but that the agenda is implemented with the incrementalism characteristic of more traditional policy and politics. Whichever the case, the ability to engage effectively in health system transformation requires appreciation of both the civic processes and the political dynamics.

References

[1] G. Anderson, *Chronic Conditions: Making the Case for Ongoing Care*, Retrieved on June, 29, 2009 from http://www.fightchronicdisease.org/news/pfcd/documents/ChronicCareChartbook_FINAL.pdf, 2007.

[2] S.M. Asch, E.A. McGlynn, M.M. Hogan, R.A. Hayward, P. Shekelle, L. Rubenstein et al., Comparison of the quality of care for patients in the Veterans Health Administration and patients in a national sample, *Annals of Internal Medicine* **141** (2004), 938–945.

[3] J. Avorn, Part "D" for "Defective" – The Medicare drug-benefit chaos, *New England Journal of Medicine* **354**(13) (2006), 1339–1341.

[4] B. Biles, J. Pozen and S. Guterman, The continuing cost of privatization: extra payments to medicare advantage plans jump to $11.4 billion in 2009. New York, NY: The Commonwealth Fund, 2009.

[5] P. Budetti, Market justice and U.S. health care. *Journal of the American Medical Association* **299**(1) (2008), 92–94.

[6] S.R. Collins, J.L. Kriss, M.M. Doty and S. D. Rustgi, *Losing ground: How the loss of adequate health insurance is burdening working families: Findings from the Commonwealth Fund Biennial Health Insurance Surveys, 2001–2007*, New York: The Commonwealth Fund, 2009.

[7] Centers for Disease Control and Prevention. Emergency Preparedness and Response. Retrieved on June 29, 2009 from http://www.bt.cdc.gov.

[8] Centers for Medicare and Medicaid Services.(2009). Medicare News. Retrieved on June 28, 2009 from http://www.cms.hhs.gov/DemoProjectsEvalRpts/downloads/ACEPressRelease.pdf.

[9] Center for Responsive Politics. PAC Contributions to Federal Candidates. Retrieved on June 28, 2009 from https://www.opensecrets.org/pacs/sector.php?cycle=2008&txt=H01.

[10] Congressional Budget Office. (2009). *The Budget and Economic Outlook: Fiscal Years 2009 to 2019*. Washington, DC.

[11] Congressional Budget Office. About CBO. Retrieved on June 28, 2009 from http://www.cbo.gov/aboutcbo.

[12] R. Deyo, B. Psaty, G. Simon, E. Wagner and G. Omenn, The messenger under attack – Intimidation of researchers by special-interest groups, *New England Journal of Medicine* **336**(16) (1997), 1176–1180.

[13] J. Diamond, *Guns, Germs, and Steel*, New York, NY: W. W. Norton & Company, 1997.

[14] D.C. Evans, P. Nichol and J.B. Perlin, Effect of the implementation of an enterprise-wide electronic health record on productivity in the Veterans Health Administration, *Health Economics, Policy and Law* **1** (2006), 163–169.

[15] E.S. Fisher, D.E. Wennberg, T.A. Stukel, D.J. Gottlieb, F.L. Lucas and E.L. Pinder, The implications of regional variations in Medicare spending, part 2: Health outcomes and satisfaction with care, *Annals of Internal Medicine* **138**(4) (2003), 288–322.

[16] A. Gawande, The Cost Conundrum: What a Texas town can teach us about health care, *New Yorker*, Retrieved on June 1, 2009 from http://www.newyorker.com/reporting/2009/06/01/090601fa_fact_gawande?yr ail, 2009.

[17] A. Goldstein, Alarm sounded on Social Security: Report also warns of Medicare collapse, *Washington Post*. (2009) Retrieved on June 29, 2009 from http://www.washingtonpost.com/wp-dyn/content/article/2009/05/12/AR2009051200252.html?nav=emailpage, 2009.

[18] S. Jonas and A. Kovner, Health care delivery in the United States, New York, NY: Springer Publishing Company, 2002.

[19] S. Jencks, T. Cuerdon, C. Burwen, B. Fleming, P. Houck, P. Kussmaul et al., Quality of medical care delivered to medicare beneficiaries: a profile at state and national levels, *Journal of the American Medical Association* **284**(13) (2000), 1670–1676.

[20] Kaiser Family Foundation, State Children's Health Insurance Program (CHIP): Reauthorization History. Retrieved on June 29, 2009 from http://www.kff.org/medicaid/7743.cfm, 2009.

[21] P. Leatt, ed., *HealthcarePapers* **4**(5) (2005), 1–67.

[22] T. Lincoln and N. Pattison, *Big PhRMA's stealth PACs: How the drug industry uses 501(c) non-profit groups to influence elections*. Washington, D.C.: Public Citizen, 2004.

[23] E. McGlynn, S. Asch, J. Adams, J. Keesey, J. Hicks, A. DeCristofaro and E. Kerr, The quality of health care delivered to adults in the United States, *New England Journal of Medicine* **348**(26) (2003), 2635–2645.

[24] Minnesota Dept of Public Health. Retrieved on June 28, 2009 from http://www.health.state.mn.us/divs/idepc/dtopics/reportable/rule/hipaacomm.html.

[25] M. Mitka, Growth in health care spending slows, but still outpaces rate of inflation, *Journal of the American Medical Association* **301**(8) (2009), 815–816.

[26] National Conference of State Legislatures, Retrieved on June 20, 2009 from http://www.ncsl.org/IssuesResearch/Health/CONCertificateofNeedStateLaws/tabi d/14373/Default.aspx.

[27] J.B. Perlin, Transformation of the U.S. Veterans Health Administration, *Health Economics, Policy and Law* **1** (2006), 99–105.

[28] M. Porter and E. Teisberg, *Redifining Healthcare*. Boston, MA: Harvard Business School Press, 2006.

[29] U. Reinhardt, Does the aging of the population really drive the demand for health care? *Health Affairs* **22**(6) (2003), 27–39.

[30] C. Schoen, S.R. Collins, J.L. Kriss and M.M. Doty, How many are underinsured? Trends among U.S. adults, 2003 and 2007, *Health Affairs*, Web Exclusive, (2008), w298–w309.
[31] L. Slaughter, Medicare Part D – The product of a broken process, *New England Journal of Medicine* **354**(22) (2006), 2314–2315.
[32] B. Stuart, L. Simoni-Wastila and D. Chauncey, Assessing the impact of coverage gaps in the Medicare Part D drug benefit, *Health Affairs*, Web Exclusive, 2005, W5167–W179.
[33] C. Tompkins, A. Higgins and G. Ritter, Measuring outcomes and efficiency in Medicare value-based purchasing, *Health Affairs, Web Exclusive* **28**(2) (2009), w251–w26.
[34] US Department of Defense, *Caring for America's heroes: 2008 MHS stakeholders' Report*, Retrieved on June 30, 2009 from http://www.tricare.mil/stakeholders/downloads/stakeholders_2008.pdf, 2008.
[35] U.S. Department of Defense. US Department of Defense Military Health System. Retrieved on June 28, 2009 from http://www. health.mil/.
[36] U.S. Department of Health and Human Services. What we do. Retrieved on June 28, 2009 from http://www.hhs.gov/about/whatwedo.html.
[37] U.S. Department of Health and Human Services. Retrieved on June 28, 2009 from http://www.hhs.gov/about/orgchart/index.html.
[38] U.S. Government Accountability Office (2009). High-risk series: an update. (Rep. No. GAO-GAO-09-271.). Washington, DC.
[39] U.S. Government Accountability Office (2006). Drug safety: improvement needed in FDA's postmarket decision-making and oversight process. (Rep. No. GAO-06-402). Washington, DC.
[40] U.S. Government Accountability Office. Social Security, Medicare and Medicaid spending as a percent of GDP. Retrieved on June 20, 2009 from http://www.gao.gov/cghome/townhall092905/img18.html.
[41] J. Wennberg, B. Barnes and M. Zubkoff, Professional uncertaintly and the problem of supplier-induced demand, *Social Science & Medicine* **16**(7) (1982), 811–824.
[42] D. West, D. Heith and C. Goodwin, Harry and Louise Go to Washington: Political Advertising and Health Care Reform, *Journal of Health Politics, Policy and Law* **21**(1) (1996), 35–68.
[43] S. Woolhandler, T. Campbell and D. Himmelstein, Costs of health care administration in the United States and Canada, *New England Journal of Medicine* **349**(8) (2003), 768–775.
[44] J. Wolff, B. Starfield and G. Anderson, Prevalence, expenditures, and complications of multiple chronic conditions in the elderly, *Archives of InternalMedicine* **162**(20) (2002), 2269–2276.

Dr. Jonathan B. Perlin is President, Clinical Services and Chief Medical Officer of HCA (Hospital Corporation of America). He provides leadership for clinical services, improving performance, and implementing electronic health records at HCA's 166 hospitals and 168 outpatient centers. Before joining HCA in 2006, Dr. Perlin was Under Secretary for Health in the U.S. Department of Veterans Affairs. As CEO of the Veterans Health Administration, Dr. Perlin directed care to over 5.4 million patients annually by more than 200,000 healthcare professionals at 1,400 sites with a budget of over $34 billion. A champion for implementing electronic health records, Dr. Perlin led VHA quality performance to international recognition as reported in academic literature and lay press and as evaluated by RAND, Institute of Medicine, and others. Dr. Perlin has served on numerous Boards and Commissions including the National Quality Forum, the Joint Commission, Meharry Medical College, the National eHealth Collaborative, and he chairs the HHS Health IT Standards Committee. He is a Fellow of the American College of Physicians and the American College of Medical Informatics. Dr. Perlin has a Master's of Science in Health Administration and received his Ph.D. in pharmacology (molecular neurobiology) with his M.D. as part of the Physician Scientist Training Program at the Medical College of Virginia of Virginia Commonwealth University.

Dr. Kelvin A. Baggett is Chief Operating Officer and Vice President, Clinical Services Group, HCA. He is responsible for executing strategies and coordinating activities that improve quality, safety and clinical performance throughout HCA's 166 hospitals and 168 outpatient centers. Dr. Baggett completed his training in Internal Medicine at the Yale University School of Medicine. A Robert Wood Johnson Clinical Scholar, he completed advanced training in the Department of Medicine at the Johns Hopkins University School of Medicine and as a General Internal Medicine Fellow at the Duke University School of Medicine. His major area of research interest and investigation is clinical performance improvement. He earned his M.D. from the East Carolina University School of Medicine, his M.P.H. from the Johns Hopkins Bloomberg School of Public Health and a M.B.A. from the Fuqua School of Business at Duke University.

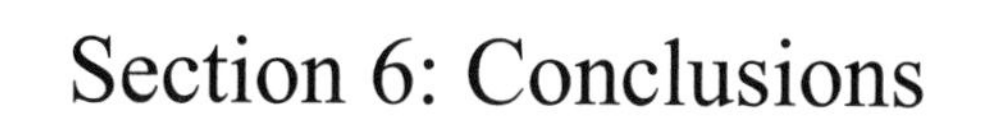

Section 6: Conclusions

Information Knowledge Systems Management 8 (2009) 437–463
DOI 10.3233/IKS-2009-0150
IOS Press

Chapter 23

Barriers to change in engineering the system of health care delivery

Jonathan F. Saxton and Michael M. E. Johns
E-mail: michael.johns@emory.edu

Abstract: Significant reform of the health care system sufficient to achieve universal coverage, a value-driven system and administrative simplification faces enormous barriers at the level of our societal ecosystem – barriers as large as any that can be faced in public policy. These barriers exist within the health system itself as a complex adaptive system, and are structured by our economic, legal, cultural and political systems. Because there are so many barriers, significant reform is a relatively rare occurrence. Yet it does happen and there are some important examples of major health care reforms.

There are a number of lessons to be learned from the successful enactment of the Medicare and Medicaid programs that appear relevant to current and future reform efforts. First, a necessary condition for achieving significant reform is the existence of large and sufficiently enduring social forces sufficient to disrupt legislative and policy stasis and drive the necessary political solutions. Second, public sentiment and electoral "mandates" might be necessary to significant reform, but they are not sufficient. Third, assuming the theoretical capacity to manage the constellation of systemic, economic, legal, cultural and legislative barriers, there remains a political "tipping point" that must be crossed and translated into a Congressional super-majority in order to enact significant nationwide reform.

1. Introduction

Reform of America's health care system has become a major domestic policy priority. There is near-consensus that the health care system is plagued by significant, systemic problems, which include underperformance on key population health outcomes indicators, endemic inefficiencies, irrational payment systems, the inability to provide universal coverage, and unsustainable overall costs. The ability to engineer a better system of health care depends upon understanding and overcoming barriers to change.

The discussion of barriers to health care reform can be framed by reference to a four-tiered interconnected architecture for health care delivery described by Rouse, which can usefully be applied to the entire health system [57].

At the micro or ground level are clinical practices, the actual interpersonal activities involved in providing care to patients. The next level up is the level of delivery operations, including the clinical processes and information systems within which clinical practices are embedded. Delivery operations, in turn, are embedded within system structures, like medical group practices, surgery departments and intensive care units, hospitals, academic health centers, and local health systems. These, in turn, are embedded within our overall healthcare ecosystem at the highest level of the architecture. The health care ecosystem includes all of the elements of the societal social system that structure and influence

1389-1995/09/$17.00

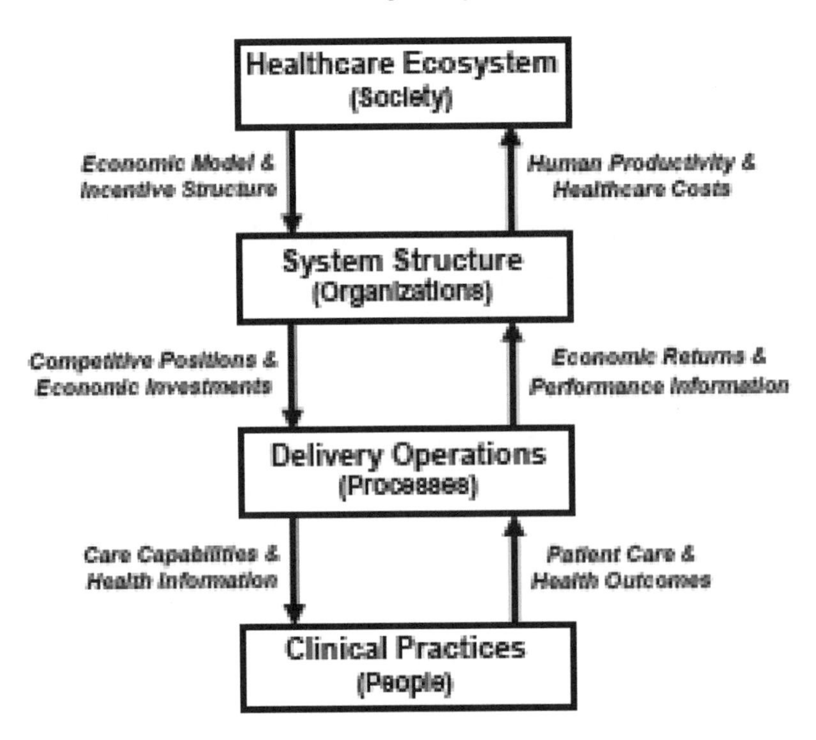

the health care delivery system, including laws and regulations, codes, and larger economic, policy and political factors. Processes and activities of each level are structured and enabled and/or limited by the characteristics of those higher-level structures and systems within which they are embedded [56].

The identification of barriers to change is an essential precondition to engineering reform. Barriers to change exist within each of the levels of the heath care delivery system architecture. This means that there are layers and layers of barriers and they come in many forms. They can be physical, technological, psychological, operational, economic, structural, cultural, ethical, and political, to name some of the most common. Certain barriers to change are generic (e.g., inertial barriers) and exist in almost all situations. Other barriers are contingent and situational (e.g., legal or political barriers). Some barriers exist or arise "naturally" because of the structure, organization or functioning of existing factors (e.g., inadequate funds available to invest in improved health information technology). Some barriers are created or erected through purposeful actions or omissions (e.g., the actions of particular interest groups to block a proposed change). Some barriers can be relatively trivial (e.g., the reluctance of any particular provider to change a particular practice) while others can be quite substantial (e.g., the costs of reform).

Any process of change that aims for significant reforms must expect to encounter and overcome significant barriers. The higher-up in the architecture one travels, the more elements of the entire heath system are implicated in any reform effort. Local reforms may affect only a single individual or episode of care. System-wide reforms will have system-wide repercussions affecting large numbers of actors, stakeholders, and/or processes.

Our focus is primarily on barriers to change at the macro level of the health care delivery system. At this level, health care reform involves change in the system-wide properties that structure the health care system and the behaviors and functions of key actors and systems. Change at this level also implicates the overall social ecology that structures and defines the role of health care in society. The health care ecosystem includes all of the elements of the societal social system that structure and influence the health care delivery system, including:

- They are *nonlinear and dynamic* and do not inherently reach fixed-equilibrium points. As a result, system behaviors may appear to be random or chaotic.
- They are composed of *independent agents* whose behavior is based on physical, psychological, or social rules rather than the demands of system dynamics.
- Because agents needs or desires, reflected in their rules, are not homogeneous, their *goals and behaviors are likely to conflict*. In response to these conflicts or competitions, agents tend to adapt to each other s behaviors.
- Agents are *intelligent*. As they experiment and gain experience, agents learn and change their behaviors accordingly. Thus overall system behavior inherently changes over time.
- Adaptation and learning tend to result in *self-organization*. Behavior patterns emerge rather than being designed into the system. The nature of emergent behaviors may range from valuable innovations to unfortunate accidents.
- There is *no single point(s) of control*. System behaviors are often unpredictable and uncontrollable, and no one is "in charge." Consequently, the behaviors of complex adaptive systems can usually be more easily influenced than controlled [55].

Fig. 1. Characteristics of complex adaptive systemsd.

– Inherent health care system characteristics
– Economic factors and interests
– Legal and regulatory frameworks
– Cultural values and ideology
– Political factors and interests

We will review how each of these elements of health care's societal ecology structures barriers to health system reform. But the discussion of barriers to health care reform must begin from an understanding the current health care system and then by identifying the goals for reform.

2. The origins of barriers: The current health care system

Since much of this volume is concerned with contextualizing and understanding the current health care system, we will only briefly discuss a fundamental characteristic of the health care system that is the source of major barriers to reform. The reader is referred to other the relevant discussions in this volume.

Perhaps the most important characteristic of our health care system, for the purposes of this discussion, is that it is a "complex adaptive system" (CAS). (See Fig. 1) As Rouse describes it, a complex adaptive system is a dynamic, adaptive, and ever-changing system populated by hundreds of thousands of relatively independent actors, including practitioners, health care provider organizations, government agencies, insurance, pharmaceutical and device manufacturing companies, and many other actors that function and interact through a multitude of modes of organization and operation, as well as contractual and relational mechanisms that include state and federal rules and regulations, and professional guidelines [56].

Perhaps the most common objective that cuts across all of these relationships and activity is the objective of ultimately providing health care products and services to individuals and populations. This goal is pursued through much creative effort and collaboration. Yet this goal is also often pursued only in episodic, uncoordinated fashion or in the context of fierce competition, where providers and payors work at cross-purposes, have conflicting interests and pursue various objectives with questionable relevance to the larger social purpose of helping people to be healthy. There is no single point of overall command, control and accountability. It is not a coherent system of structures, processes, and actors working in concert. In health care, we have not so much a system as a patchwork of systems that defies many traditional approaches to purposeful, goal-directed control [56].

As we will see, these characteristics contribute to the existence and generation of significant barriers to intentional health care reforms at the system level.

3. The origins of barriers: Reform objectives

Understanding barriers to health care reform requires not just understanding the nature of the current system of health care delivery, but must be understood with respect to the specific reform objectives and methods being pursued. While certain barriers, like inertia, are somewhat generic and non-specific, other barriers arise or become apparent only in the context of particular reform objectives and initiatives.

In these early years of the 21st Century, it has been possible to discern a growing convergence around a number of key reform objectives. This growing consensus can be seen in proposals from key stakeholder organizations at a very high level of specificity. We summarize several of these.

The Institute of Medicine (IOM): The IOM has proposed rebuilding the health system into one designed to meet two fundamental national health policy goals.

1. Our nation should provide "health insurance that will promote better overall health by providing financial access for everyone to necessary, appropriate and effective health services" [32].
2. Our nation should transform its health care system so that it will be:
   - Safe – avoiding injuries to patients from the care that is intended to help them.
   - Timely – reducing waits and harmful delays for both those who receive and those who give care.
   - Effective – Providing services based on scientific knowledge to all who could benefit and refraining from providing services to those not likely to benefit (avoiding underutilization and over-utilization, respectively).
   - Efficient – avoiding waste, including waste of equipment, supplies, ideas, and energy.
   - Equitable – proving care that does not vary in quality because of personal characteristics such as gender, ethnicity, geographic location, and socio-economic status.
   - Patient-centered – providing care that is respectful and responsive to individual patient preferences, needs and values and ensuring that patient values guide all clinical decisions [31, pp. 41–42].

In addition to calling for universal insurance and a "STEEEP" health care system, the IOM has recently called for the creation of a national capability for comparative effectiveness research. The IOM Committee on Reviewing Evidence to Identify Highly Effective Clinical Services, in January 2008, called on Congress to create a semi-private government agency that would conduct scientific reviews that compare existing and new medical treatments to determine the treatments that work best for various conditions [36].

The Commonwealth Fund (CWF): The CWF established a commission to chart a course for the reform of the U.S. health care system. The commission articulated the concept of a "High Performance Health System" [14]. A high performance health system would be designed to achieve four core goals:

– high quality, safe care;
– access to care for all people;
– efficient, high value care; and
– system capacity to improve

The mission of such a health care system would be "to help everyone, to the extent possible, lead long, healthy, and productive lives." [14].

The CWF Commission recently updated its proposals with a proposed "Path to a High Performance Health System." It identified five strategies for comprehensive reform, including:

– Affordable coverage for all.
– Align incentives with value and effective cost control.
– Accountable, accessible, patient-centered, and coordinated care.
– Aim high to improve quality, health outcomes, and efficiency.

Accountable leadership and collaboration to set and achieve national goals [15].

The National Coalition on Health Care (**NCHC**): The NCHC is comprised of more than 70 organizations, including large and small businesses, the nation's largest labor, consumer, religious and primary care provider groups, the largest health and pension funds and a number of leaders from academia, business, and government. This diverse membership supports the following principles as a framework for improving our nation's health care:

– Health care coverage for all.
– Cost management.
– Improvement of health care quality and safety.
– Equitable financing.
– Simplified administration [45].

America's Health Insurance Plans (**AHIP**): AHIP, the key insurance industry interest group, recently put forth principles for health care reform in line with those proposed by the IOM and others. These principles are "... aimed at moving the nation toward a restructured health care system in which no one falls through the cracks, all Americans have high quality, affordable coverage, and the efficiency and effectiveness of the system are greatly improved" [47]. These include:

– **Controlling costs**: A financially sustainable and affordable health care system can only be achieved by bringing underlying medical costs under control. If health care costs are allowed to continue rising at rates far exceeding economic growth, they will thwart all efforts to improve coverage and care.
– **Adding value**: The nation must create a 21st century system where quality and effectiveness are rewarded, administrative efficiency is achieved, and primary care and wellness are encouraged.
– **Helping consumers and purchasers**: Insurance market rules need to be reformed to help individuals and small businesses access affordable coverage, while avoiding duplication of administrative and regulatory responsibilities. These reforms must be coupled with initiatives to provide one-stop access to coverage options and clear, consistent information on the quality and cost of care.
– **Achieving universal coverage**: By addressing rising costs, reforming insurance market rules, strengthening the health care safety net, and enhancing value in care delivery, the nation can provide all Americans – those with and without coverage today – affordable coverage they can keep [47].

The Blue Ridge Academic Health Group (BRAHG): The BRAHG is a group of academic health center leaders and health policy thought leaders that yearly convenes to consider a high-priority health system challenge and to produce a consensus report with recommended solution or problem solving processes (See blueridgegroup.org).

The BRAHG itself has developed the concept of a "value-driven" health care system characterized by the pursuit of only necessary, appropriate and effective services with an effective information and communications infrastructure. A value-driven health system would utilize performance-based incentives and balanced competition to improve the health of both individuals and populations. The group maintains that a value-driven health system requires that our nation achieve universal access to necessary health services, whether provided by government programs or the private sector, or both [10].

More recently, the BRAHG has joined a number of other leading health policy thought leaders in proposing the establishment of an agency that would have the sort of independence from the vicissitudes of politics that the Federal Reserve Board has with respect to the financial system, that would be charged with key functions. Such a proposed US Health Board might function to:

a) Bring together leaders from across the healthcare spectrum in a private-public organizational structure buffered from political influences and conducive to long-term planning and decision-making;
b) Take-up the key challenges facing our health care system such as health insurance benefit equity, attention to mission-critical and vulnerable populations, insurance reform and pooling risk; and economic viability. This could enable a course of needed change that allows system participants to make long-term investments;
c) Standardize and simplify the capture of health information and financial data, including encounter forms and billing transactions among the government, private insurers and providers of health care services;
d) Collect and analyze encounter-level data specific to individual providers so as to enable identification of best practices and the most effective models for health services delivery and reduce practice variation; and
e) Make information available to the public and to the health care community to inform and improve health care decision-making [11].

This proposal is congruent with those of a number of organizations and thought-leaders who have suggested in some way the creation of such an independent federally chartered body that can enable the establishment of common standards for health care data and transactions, and other information and technological infrastructure reforms necessary to achieving health care reform goals [3,17].

Obama Administration Health Reform Objectives: Very important to the overall health care reform debate are the proposals that President Barack Obama advocated during his successful campaign for the presidency and that have since become the foundation for the guidance provided to the Congress and the American people about his Administration's ambitious goals for achieving significant health care reforms early in his presidency.

The Obama Administration believes that comprehensive health reform should adhere to the following set of eight principles:

- Guarantee Choice. The plan should provide Americans a choice of health plans and physicians. People will be allowed to keep their own doctor and their employer-based health plan.
- Make Health Coverage Affordable. The plan must reduce waste and fraud, high administrative costs, unnecessary tests and services, and other inefficiencies that drive up costs with no added health benefits.

- Protect Families' Financial Health. The plan must reduce the growing premiums and other costs American citizens and businesses pay for health care. People must be protected from bankruptcy due to catastrophic illness.
- Invest in Prevention and Wellness. The plan must invest in public health measures proven to reduce cost drivers in our system – such as obesity, sedentary lifestyles, and smoking – as well as guarantee access to proven preventive treatments.
- Provide Portability of Coverage. People should not be locked into their job just to secure health coverage, and no American should be denied coverage because of preexisting conditions.
- Aim for Universality. The plan must put the United States on a clear path to cover all Americans.
- Improve Patient Safety and Quality Care. The plan must ensure the implementation of proven patient safety measures and provide incentives for changes in the delivery system to reduce unnecessary variability in patient care. It must support the widespread use of health information technology with rigorous privacy protections and the development of data on the effectiveness of medical interventions to improve the quality of care delivered.
- Maintain Long-Term Fiscal Sustainability. The plan must pay for itself by reducing the level of cost growth, improving productivity, and dedicating additional sources of revenue [48].

These Obama Administration goals for health care reform track well with those of the other thought leader constituent organizations surveyed here. This selection of leading health policy reform proposals illustrates the considerable convergence around the goals and principles for a reformed health care system. These can be summarized as:

1. Achieving affordable universal coverage;
2. Creating a value-driven or "STEEEP" health system
3. Administrative simplification: Developing inter-operable health information technology (HIT) systems and common standards for health system data, transactions and records that can simplify administration, whether through the auspices of an independent, quasi-governmental entity like the Fed, or otherwise.

Understanding that these are the broad, nearly-consensus goals for health care reform, we can now proceed to identify the major barriers to achieving these goals.

4. Barriers to achieving universal coverage, value-driven health care, and simplified administration at the level of the healthcare ecosystem

The health care ecosystem includes all of the elements of the societal social system that structure and influence the health care delivery system, including:

- Inherent CAS system characteristics
- Economic factors
- Legal and regulatory frameworks
- Values and ideology
- Political and partisan interests

4.1. Barriers inherent in our health care system as a complex adaptive system

Understanding the processes of and barriers to change is difficult enough in relatively static and well-organized systems. However, healthcare is a complex adaptive system that by definition is always changing and adapting through the actions and reactions of untold individuals, groups or institutions. It contains thousands of different administrative, service, accountability, practice, safety, data and information systems. The fact that the health care system is a complex adaptive system can be one of the most significant barriers to intentional health care reform.

Rouse and others have observed that complex adaptive systems present unique challenges to intentional change or reform. Lacking traditional command and control mechanism, individual actors and institutions exercise wide latitude in managing their own affairs.

Yet Rouse has suggested that a CAS can experience significant change through the action of relatively simple mechanisms at the highest levels, suggesting that the management of complex systems is "highly influenced by the nature of the objectives adopted" [56, p. 13]. The IOM Chasm Report had likewise concluded that, "[R]elatively simple rules can lead to complex, innovative system behavior" [31, p. 8]. The key is to identify rules that can lead to desired behaviors and then to create the wherewithal to promulgate and enforce these rules and reward and otherwise reinforce the desired behaviors. But even relatively simple mechanisms can be hard to identify, define and deploy.

By analogy, if the U.S. economy is understood as a CAS, then the Federal Reserve ("the Fed") can be seen as a locus of the capacity to effectuate systemic changes and desired policy outcomes. The Fed sets the rules of monetary policy through several policy "levers," as summarized by its Board of Governors:

"The Federal Reserve implements U.S. monetary policy by affecting conditions in the market for balances that depository institutions hold at the Federal Reserve Banks... By conducting open market operations, imposing reserve requirements, permitting depository institutions to hold contractual clearing balances, and extending credit through its discount window facility, the Federal Reserve exercises considerable control over the demand for and supply of Federal Reserve balances and the federal funds rate. Through its control of the federal funds rate, the Federal Reserve is able to foster financial and monetary conditions consistent with its monetary policy objectives" [20, p. 27].

The Fed's capacity to influence the banking and other financial systems through these levers is profound, but certainly not straightforward. As the recent collapse of the credit markets both in the U.S and worldwide has demonstrated, rules and levers may not be enough to keep a CAS from developing self-destructive or counter-adaptive dynamics. Nevertheless, the Fed does demonstrate the point that relatively simple rules and mechanisms can be effective in structuring the ecosystem of a complex adaptive system as large and complex as our economy. Theoretically it should be possible to create similar mechanisms and rules by which to affect intentional changes in our health care system.

Rouse and others have suggested that changing the rules for health care payments and finding the appropriate mechanism by which to deploy and refine these new payment rules might engender important change in our health care system [56]. Existing third-party fee-for-service payment systems differentially reward particular kinds of discreet health care encounters. Fee-for-service payments do not generally provide incentives for service providers to achieve "value" for services delivered, either through efficiencies or by attaining particular health outcomes. "The fee-for-service model central to healthcare in the United States assures that provider income is linked to activities rather than outcomes" [56]. Therefore, the health care system lacks key incentives to structure actors' interactions to achieve socially desired goals of universal coverage, value and administrative simplicity.

The significant barrier here, then, is the nature of the health care system itself. The challenge is to create the capacity to systemically influence the complex adaptive health care system in the direction of desired goals. As rouse suggests:

"I suspect that recasting of "the problem" in terms of outcomes characterized by wellness and productivity may enable identification and pursuit of efficiencies that we cannot imagine within our current frame of reference" [56].

4.2. Barriers associated with economic factors

4.2.1. Costs: Impact on federal budget

A significant barrier to achieving universal coverage, a value-driven health care system, and simplified administration is the large costs involved. Current estimates range between $1 trillion and $1.5 trillion or more, over ten years [18].

The economic footprint of the health care sector is vast. In 2007, the U.S. spent $2.2 trillion on health care, an average of $7,421 per person. The health care system's share of the U.S. gross domestic product (GDP) stood at 16.2 percent having grown on average 2.4 percentage points faster than the GDP since 1970, when it consumed 7.2 percent of GDP. Projections are that health spending will be 20.3 percent (one-fifth of GDP) by the year 2018 [28,29].

This cost barrier has been made even more daunting within the current economic context. The U.S. is in a major recession, with unemployment currently at 8.9% and projected to rise to 9.5% in 2010. The Obama Administration has already spent more than $700 Billion to jump-start the rescue of the financial and automobile industries and to support small businesses, among others. Another $787 Billion has been allocated to an economic stimulus package, along with a further $410 Billion in additional spending. And many estimate that $1 Trillion will ultimately be invested in a public-private bank rescue plan. The Congress has passed a record budget resolution for FY 2010 totaling $3.56 Trillion. The Congressional Budget Office expects the economy to further contract in FY 2009 [18]. The 2009 federal deficit is expected to total $1.84 Trillion, or 12.9% of GDP. In this context, especially, there are unprecedented challenges in finding the $1 Trillion or more in savings required in order to adhere to Congressional PAYGO provisions [18].

And because of the nature of budgeting and accounting in both the Federal and in state budgets, health care spending is always viewed through the lens of costs for care rather than the lens of investments in health. This is reinforced by the fact that, as Rouse explains, "The focus on disease and restoration of health rather than wellness and productivity assures that healthcare expenditures will be viewed as costs rather than investments" [56].

4.2.2. PAYGO rules

In the current health care reform debate, President Obama has pledged that health care reform will be structured for long-term fiscal sustainability, and that therefore health care reform must pay for itself. This is in keeping with Congressional "PAYGO" rules, which, when in effect, require that any new mandatory discretionary spending be offset by savings or additional revenues [19]. This is monitored by the Congressional Budget Office (CBO), which is responsible for evaluating and "scoring" the net new costs associated with such legislative proposals. Reform plans under development in both the U.S. Senate and in the U.S. House of Representatives are attempting to meet this fiscal sustainability goal through strategies like reducing the rate of cost growth, improving productivity, and identifying additional sources of revenue. But success in defining and achieving a strategy that can finance the enormous costs of covering the uninsured has eluded past presidents and other would-be reformers.

4.2.3. Stakeholder economic interests

A third important barrier to reform of our health care system is that it consists of a wide variety of constituents with a wide array of socio-economic profiles and interests. For instance, the majority of physicians work in single or 2–3 member small group practices. These physicians are essentially small business people. They must daily navigate the difficult terrain of running a small service business and on top of that manage the especially complex regulatory and administrative processes required in this particular business.

But other physicians serve as faculty in academic health centers, where they may teach and conduct research as well as have clinical responsibilities. They are generally salaried and their careers and lives are very different from those who are primarily practitioners in small private practices. Still other physicians are members of larger physician group practices where they might be significantly incentivized around throughput; while many are on the staffs of HMOs, where they might be salaried and perhaps incentivized by quantity and/or quality metrics. Other physicians work with relatively modest resources and remuneration in rural areas or in state institutions. There are many other models and situations. The economic and practice interests of these variously situated medical professionals can differ significantly.

And beyond the physician provider community are other health care workers and professionals, including nurses and an array of allied health workers. These providers' interests are different from those of physicians and also differ among themselves. And all of these providers' interests in turn differ from those of the hospitals, health centers and health systems in and through which they work. These, in turn, differ from the interests of insurers, employers, government agencies, the pharmaceutical industry, and many more stakeholders. And all of these interests are vigorously and thoroughly represented by professional, trade and industry organizations.

Health care represents a large proportion of personal and corporate income for all of these various stakeholders in our nation. Health care is perennially one of the fastest growing employment sectors and this employment is dispersed and integrated in its many components and in significant ways in every state in the nation. As the largest industry in 2006, health care provided 13.6 million jobs for wage and salary workers and about 438,000 jobs for the self-employed. Seven of the 20 fastest growing occupations are health care related. And health care is projected to generate 3 million new wage and salary jobs between 2006 and 2016, more than any other industry [12].

One important implication of this is that any significant change has economic impacts on many individuals and corporations. One person's cost-saving reform can be another's job loss. Cost savings identified in a national health reform plan are likely to have negative income or revenue implications for certain key stakeholders. Expansion of public programs like Medicare and Medicaid inevitably implicate the need to raise addition public revenues. And, as one prominent health economist puts it, "...the fiercest political conflicts of the past three decades have concerned taxes and spending" [27]. All of these have stakeholder economic implications and, in turn, have consequences for the capacity to effect system-wide change.

4.2.4. Provider payment system barriers

The basis upon which most health care providers are paid represents a substantial barrier to health care reform. Three characteristics of our health payment system are especially relevant.

1. Most health care is paid for or reimbursed through third-party insurance. This fact means that those who actually purchase and consume health care services and products are relatively price-insensitive. This means, within some important limits, that individuals can demand more and more health services and products without considering the costs. This fact contributes to the ongoing growth in demand and intensity of health services.
2. Approximately 65–70% of persons under sixty-five years of age with insurance obtain it as an untaxed benefit through their employer. And their employers can deduct the cost of providing benefits as a business expense. As a result, employee health benefits have become a staple of employment relationships and expectations. Health benefits can represent a significant addition to salary and other forms of compensation for employed individuals and covered family members.

3. Most insurance pays providers on a "fee-for-service" (FFS) basis. FFS payments essentially pay health care providers on the basis of their charges for discreet activities. Given the open-ended, cost-plus nature of such payment arrangements, in the 1980s, the Medicare program developed a prospective payment system (PPS) that paid providers on the basis of estimates of average costs of particular services. Other forms of prospective payment include capitation and bundling of services where the provider is paid on a per-patient or per-episode of care basis, but these payment innovations and others have not been adopted widely. Providers and most payers favor payments that reimburse for discreet activities and Medicare traditionally sets the standards for these payments, including both the definition and rate of payment [32].

The predominant FFS and PPS payment systems have been widely criticized for their impacts on health care utilization and costs. Over decades of regulatory and insurance industry refinement, these payment systems have tended increasingly to reward higher utilization and intensity, to provide much higher reimbursement to specialists than to generalists, and to "... pay for care regardless of whether services are appropriate or of high quality" [44].

The result is an overall payment system that reinforces the fragmented nature of the care delivery system, while at the same time structuring consumer and provider behaviors across the entire spectrum of health care services. There have been ongoing experiments with new forms of payment, sponsored by a wide array of public and private payers and provider organizations, designed to enable better coordination of services, administrative simplification and a value-driven health system. But for policymakers or health care leaders interested in developing integrated teams and services or in redesigning systems for better efficiency, patient safety and outcomes, the FFS payment system creates enormous barriers. As a result, thought-leaders have long called for fundamental nationwide payment system reforms [34].

4.2.5. Tax system barriers

Another significant barrier to reform can be seen in the tax treatment of employer-provided health care benefits. Employers can generally deduct the cost of health care benefits provided to employees, while at the same time, these benefits are provided tax-free to employees. This makes the employer tax exclusion the largest subsidy in the tax code. The exclusion of employer-sponsored health care was worth approximately $246 billion in lost federal tax collections in 2007 [23]. These tax subsidies are a primary reason why employer-based coverage is so widespread and remains popular, particularly with large employers and with unions that have negotiated generous benefits packages for their members.

However, the employer tax exclusion is widely understood by policy analysts to be inequitable. It disproportionately benefits those with the highest incomes because people of lower income are less likely to have jobs that offer health insurance and are less likely to be able to afford their share of premiums when insurance is available.

The tax exclusion has been targeted for PAYGO savings offsets by some thought leaders and policymakers. But critics worry that modifying the exclusion could undermine employer-based insurance, which continues to be the primary source of health coverage for people of working age and their dependents. And it is not clear that even the broader public is ready to accept changes in policy that threaten employer-sponsored health care benefits [42]. Further there are advantages to employer sponsored health benefits in that employers have an incentive to focus on prevention and wellness among their employees as evidence by programs at Safeway, Johnson & Johnson among others that have demonstrated measurable improvements in the heath status of their employees and reduction in health costs to say nothing of increased productivity.

As a result, the varied economic interests of millions of individual workers and thousands of businesses and organizations, each invested in one way or another in the health care economy, serve as a major barrier to health care reform.

4.3. Barriers associated with law and regulation

The legal barriers to health care reform are quite extensive and not as clearly or widely appreciated as many of the economic and political barriers. The law pertaining to health care includes: "... statutes duly adopted by legislatures, regulations promulgated by administrative agencies; and binding precedents established by courts. But law, at least as it is understood by lawyers, also includes other authorities–guidances issued by administrative agencies that are in principle non-binding but are ignored at great peril; contracts that are crafted by private parties; even accreditation or certification standards that claim to be voluntary but that must be satisfied to participate in government programs" [38]. Each of these forms of law operates within our health care system, including the "alphabet soup" of more than 400 hundred accrediting, certifying, and licensing bodies that regulate health care providers and provider organizations [33].

Health care reforms that can achieve universal coverage, a value-driven health care system and administrative simplification would require substantial changes to a wide array of laws and regulations related to health care. At the level of the healthcare ecosystem, this includes laws that define the relationship between the respective roles of the federal and state governments in health care, laws that define health care entitlements, and laws regulating health insurance and health care markets, among others.

Jost provides a helpful overview of the legal factors to be considered in contemplating significant health care reform [38]. Our federal system makes for an extraordinarily complex framework within which to understand the role of law. As he observes, "The current health care system is one in which some Americans have rights to health care financing protected by federal law, others have rights protected by state law, and many have no rights at all; in which low-income Americans have federal rights under some sections of the Medicaid statute but not under others and rights that vary from one federal circuit to another; and where some employee benefit plans are largely regulated by state law and others largely unregulated" [7, p. 38]...

Federal law that affects the health care system starts with the U.S. Constitution where the Commerce Clause enables the Federal Government to regulate activities that cross state lines; with the spending power, which enables the government to put certain conditions on state use of federal funding; the tenth Amendment, which proscribes the government's power to force states to act or carry out federally-imposed policies; and the Due Process Clause, provides for procedural protections for individuals who are beneficiaries or providers of government programs. There are still further Constitutional implications that are beyond the scope of this chapter.

Then there is a complex body of federal legislation that has been passed over the years that structures health care. Parts of Title XVIII of the Social Security Act (SSA) commit the Medicare program to noninterference in the practice of medicine and to free choice of provider. The Health Insurance Portability and Accountability Act Privacy Regulations (HIPAA), protects the privacy of individual health information. The Employee Retirement Income Security Act of 1974 (ERISA) is a labyrinth bill that protects the ability of employers to determine the scope of health benefits offered to employees without state government interference [38, p. 2].

In addition, Congress and the Supreme Court have long recognized the primacy of state authority for licensing professionals or health care institutions, for regulating health insurance, and for protecting the public health [38, p. 5].

4.3.1. The law concerning health care entitlements

To the extent that there exists actual entitlements to health care services, this is determined and provided through federal and/or state laws. Federal law defines the entitlement to, and the benefits available, in the Medicare program, although determinations on the applicability of coverage to particular cases is delegated to Medicare contractors. In the Medicaid program, federal law establishes a list of benefits that states must provide as well as optional benefits that states can choose to provide. But the states have great discretion in determining eligibility criteria [38, p. 10].

To achieve universal coverage that is consistent and equitable, health care reform legislation will have to create national standards through federal law that can override the existing body of law defining entitlement to health care on a largely state-by-state basis. This represents a substantial legal challenge and barrier.

4.3.2. The law concerning health care markets

4.3.2.1. Insurance market

One of the most serious issues driving health care reform is the inability of many people to obtain affordable health insurance, or health insurance at any cost, because of pre-existing conditions, known risk factors and other causes. Insurers everywhere have sophisticated underwriting, rating and related practices designed to minimize their exposure to higher-risk individuals or groups. As a result, there has been a great deal of activity in some states across the nation aimed at regulating insurance underwriting and rating practices. This regulation varies considerably among jurisdictions. It is also important to note that ERISA law exempts self-insured plans from state regulation. This is the reason why so many larger employers self-insure. Moving to a health system where everyone is insured and where private insurance plays a significant role in providing this coverage will require a major overhaul and federalization of health insurance entitlement and market regulation [38, p. 15].

It appears doubtful that universal coverage will be achieved through a wholly public (single payer) insurance plan. Assuming the possibility of universal coverage being achieved primarily through expansion of private coverage with possibly a public option as well, new regulations, incentives, and subsidies for insurers will undoubtedly be required. A mandate for individuals to obtain insurance coverage would also likely be required in order to level the playing field for competition in the insurance market [38, p. 18].

4.3.2.2. Provider and "product" markets

Both federal and state laws also govern not only markets for health insurance but also the entry of professionals, providers, and products into the marketplace. The Food and Drug Administration has a leading role in regulating the introduction of drugs and devices. Federal anti-trust and anti-kickback laws regulate anti-competitive and self-dealing practices by providers [63]. State professional licensure laws determine professional qualifications and scope of practice, while thirty-six states have adopted certificate-of-need (CON) programs to regulate the supply of health care services [38, p. 19].

A reformed, value-driven health care delivery system likely would aim to be structured by laws and rules that drive coordinated and efficient delivery of care, and some standardization of provider credentialing, while allowing sufficient leeway for refinement for local, state, and regional markets and conditions. Given both constitutional constraints and the wide variety of existing state laws and practices, this presents another barrier and will be a significant challenge for lawmakers.

4.4. Barriers associated with cultural values and ideology

In the paper, "A Primer for Journalists on Reforming American Health Care," Ewe Reinhardt, one of the most respected health economists and thought-leaders in health care, suggested that judgments about the relative merits of particular health care reform proposals always rest, in the end, on one's values and ideology. "Ultimately the answer depends on one's preferred *social ethics* regarding health care, on which Americans cannot agree. Therein lies one major obstacle to effective health reform" [59, p. 20]. Reinhardt characterizes this ideological divide as between those who see health care as a private consumption good and those who view health care as a social good. Those who view health care as a private good prefer market-based solutions and believe that such markets would most efficiently and effectively allocate health care resources. Those who view health care as a public good that "... should be available to all who need it on roughly equal terms, without regard to the individual's ability to pay for the care they receive" [59, p. 20] Reinhardt identifies this basic divide, our nation's inability to resolve the place of health care in our national life, as a major barrier to significant health care reform [59, p. 20].

The extent and persistence of this ideological divide can be seen in polling on public opinion over time. One recent study of a series of polls starting in the mid 1990s shows that over 70% of Americans consistently express the sentiment that health care reform is necessary rather than just letting it remain as it is [42]. But a strong divide persists about the extent to which the government should be involved in such reform. While there has been a steady increase in the number who think government should do more, that number, as of 2007, still barely reaches over 50% [42]. There are many other polling studies that corroborate these results (See, e.g. [15]).

Based on this and additional polling specifically on the role of government in health care, the authors conclude that continuing fundamental division over the role for government, plus little clarity on the part of the public about how to best achieve needed reforms, means that significant reform is unlikely: "... the data continue to demonstrate that incremental policy tweaks are more likely to take place than any wholesale change" [42, p. 703]

4.5. Barriers associated with political and partisan interests

Both the structure of the American political system and the partisan interests of particular groups and individuals contribute mightily to the barriers to health care reform. Political scientist Grant McConnell, one of the pioneers in studying interest group politics described the challenges inherent in effectuating change through the American political system as monumental. "American institutions are studded with so many barriers to action that stalemate is the essential reality of the United States" [40, p. 377]

4.5.1. Legislative barriers

Barriers inherent in the legislative process arguably are the most difficult to overcome. Political theorists have developed conceptual frameworks for understanding the essentially conservative nature of the legislative process and how this barrier is sometimes overcome to effect significant change. Theories of legislative stasis, process and change matter because, as has been seen throughout U.S. history, and as recently as the Clinton Administration, even if the president and many influential thought-leaders and policy makers agree on the need to enact significant reform, legislative action at that level fails more often than not.

Understanding such political dynamics begins with an understanding of how structural features of our political system condition how policy is created. As one leading political scientist has observed, "The first basic fact of U.S. lawmaking is that gridlock occurs often but not always. Therefore, ... a good theory of lawmaking should identify conditions under which gridlock is broken" [39, p. 5]

In analyzing political barriers at the federal level, it has been found that super-majority partisan control of the executive and legislative branches produces significant, change-oriented legislation no more frequently than when control is more evenly divided between the two major parties. Most often, regardless of who is in power or what is the balance of political power, attempts to significantly change domestic policy either fail outright or result in small, incremental measures. But, occasionally, significant change is enacted. It has also been observed that significant pieces of legislation are rarely passed by a simple majority, but rather by supermajorities. Such supermajorities ensure, depending upon the situation, that supporters can override a possible presidential veto or put a halt to a Senate filibuster. Winning such significant change requires large, bipartisan coalitions [43].

A leading theory seeking to explain this dynamic postulates that this process depends less upon political party discipline enforced by party leaders and more upon the actions of key "pivotal" members of Congress who represent pivotal votes, whether for a broad majority of members in the political center or for a veto- or filibuster-proof supermajority [39]. Other political theorists postulate that the parties in power act like "procedural cartels" [16]. Here, the theory is that a majority party will use its control of leadership positions to determine what is voted on, and then often cobble together legislation suffused with elements designed to meet the interests of particular Members and their constituents. This manner of controlling the legislative agenda translates into assembling needed majorities but primarily for legislation that is less ambitious and coherent and more incremental [16].

4.5.2. Special interests and lobbying

Interest groups play important roles in maintaining the general stasis of the legislative system. And even at times when that stasis might be interrupted, interest groups can play a strong role in blocking reform or in blunting reform efforts. Such special interests can be a major barrier to reform.

Powerful interest groups and constituencies populate the health care sector with sizable and often competing interests. Among the major groups are: physicians, nurses and other practitioners, health care provider organizations (like hospitals, health systems, both public and private), federal and state governments and their agencies, labor unions, the insurance industry, the pharmaceutical and medical device industries, the not-for-profit academic health center and the biomedical/bioscience research community. In the normal course of legislative activity, these groups collaborate and/or vie against one another for favorable consideration and legislative or regulatory outcomes.

The role and influence of special interests and lobbying on the political process is a continual focus of attention by many concerned with integrity and fairness in the political system. Billions of dollars are spent every year by special interests for the purpose of informing legislators and affecting legislation. As a result, lobbying at the federal level is a highly regulated activity requiring lobbyist registration and the public reporting of all spending and political contributions. A number of public "watchdog" organizations monitor and track special interest and lobbyist influence (see, e.g., www.opensecrets.org). Lobbyists and special interest groups are often the focus of the press scrutiny and public discussion and can become electoral campaign issues. Yet, while often painted by the broad brush of "special interests," which has a generally negative connotation in American public life, these groups collectively function as a community of experts bringing expert information and perspective on the myriad of issues with which legislators, administrative agencies and their respective staffs must wrestle.

Lobbying activity for the most part contributes to the stasis of the legislative process and therefore to the barriers to significant change through the political system. The involvement of special interests in particular legislative issues generally contributes to the establishment of policy equilibriums around a host of issues [62]. In keeping with the tendency of the legislative system towards stasis, interest groups mostly compete and negotiate around the margins of existing policy to attain or maintain particularized outcomes. The interactive dynamic is such that lobbying interests and firms become invested in particular relationships and in normative expectations for the results of their lobbying efforts. Effectively, they work to master a particular "playing field" within which they can compete and win favorable policy outcomes.

There are some more partisan special interests that can gain or lose advantage or leverage, depending on elections that put a new party in power, or more locally, as new representatives are elected [6, pp. 5–7]. Many unions, for instance may gain leverage when a Democrat is in the White House, while the Chamber of Commerce might have more influence when there is a Republican in the White House.

However, perhaps somewhat ironically, it is not often the case that well-established special interests desire to or can effectively engineer major legislative and public policy changes. There is increasing scholarly evidence, concerning lobbying and its influence to the effect that, most often, change requires the puncturing of this lobbying equilibrium leading to a realignment of special interests around a new equilibrium. This can occur as a result of a variety of circumstances, from pressures that build within the legislative process to relatively exogenous factors, like a financial crisis, a major shift in public awareness or opinion about a particular issue, a war, or some other significant factor. In almost all of these cases, it is these new factors that disrupt the tendencies towards stasis and create the opportunities or conditions for change [5]. In such cases, the role of existing special interests becomes to attempt to manage the process so as to limit the change; or, if relatively unsuccessful in this, then they work to establish a new equilibrium within which they can once again compete and affect policy going forward.

Our complex adaptive health care system is a prime example of the legislative "sausage" that mostly results. Our health care laws and policies have been built not from a systematic plan, but have been "cobbled together" over decades of action by a variety of related and competing interests to define and enact laws and policies that enable health care products and services to be created and delivered.

4.5.3. Presidential power and executive administrative authority

The President and administrative agencies have the power to create and influence public policy, within specific legal, budgetary, and legislative constraints, both through constitutional and statutory mechanisms. This power has developed and varied over time and can manifest either as a barrier to or an enabler of significant reform.

A president can use executive orders to, "... direct the actions of agency employees and instruct them to create or implement particular policies" [13]. A presidential administration also can affect policy through administrative agencies that can issue regulations (e.g., The Centers for Medicare and Medicaid Service (CMS) has specified authority to regulate Medicare and Medicaid and other programs). Further, subregulatory guidance can be used to implement policies within an executive agency through various mechanisms, including letters, memoranda, determinations, agreements, findings, and other types of directives [13].

However, the president does not have the power to enact laws. While commanding a high-profile "bully pulpit," as we have seen historically, most presidents who have undertaken and championed significant health care reform, particularly in the direction of universal health care, have failed. This includes Presidents (F.D.) Roosevelt, Truman, Nixon, and Clinton [60]. On the other hand, the Medicare and Medicaid programs were enacted during the administration of President Johnson. This was accomplished within the context of the convergence of a number of factors reviewed earlier in this chapter, including the rise of public sentiment in favor of public policies to address poverty and inequality, public confidence in presidential leadership and support for the ideal of national sacrifice for the common good engendered by President Kennedy, and the fortuitously strong legislative skills and knowledge of both President Johnson and key leaders in the Congress [60].

For the purposes of understanding barriers to significant change, with respect to Presidential and executive administrative powers, we draw the following conclusions:

- The limited powers of the presidency and executive administrative agencies do not lend themselves to the direct attainment of significant public policy reforms.

- The political skills and influence of the president can play an important role, either positively or negatively vis a vis enacting significant legislative reforms through a variety of mechanisms, from appeals to the public, to negotiation directly with members of Congress, to the threat of a presidential veto.
- The influence of the president and administrative agencies, therefore, are largely contingent and unlikely to be determinative.

4.5.4. Public opinion

As we have seen in the earlier discussion of ideological barriers, public opinion is another variable with significant influence on the political process. Given the tendency of the policy making process towards stasis and incremental change, and the fact that the evolution of our electoral system means that Members of Congress have to run regularly for re-election and must raise millions of dollars to do so, there are many variables to be assessed by Members when significant legislation is being proposed. Among them, of course, are the views of constituents.

It is the nature of our electoral process that elections are often won based on campaign promises to make significant, sweeping changes or to lead in new and better directions. The science of polling has developed means to assess the views of the public and especially of potential voters. Polling can also assess the relative importance of particular issues and proposed solutions as well as the effectiveness of particular campaign themes and strategies. There are many other uses of polling, including not just to measure, but also to actually influence opinion, in what is known as "push-polling" [2]. Polling is regularly utilized both in formulating policy positions, in devising election strategies and in working the levers of political power and influence.

Polling in health care over the last two decades shows that our health care system has been an issue of significant ongoing concern to the general public, with large majorities often in favor of major reforms [42]. But there is ample evidence concerning how public opinion can shift in the context of any particular effort at reform. The example often cited is the extremely successful campaign engineered primarily by the health insurance industry, including the famous "Harry and Louise" ads, which helped turn public opinion against the Clinton Administration health reform plans. Given the complexities of health care reform and the difficulty the general public can have in understanding reform particulars and their implications, public opinion, like many other factors, tends to contribute to legislative stasis and the barriers to change.

The significance of the public opinion barrier may well depend upon the public's overall confidence in leadership and the integrity of the reform process. We agree with Hacker that, "The great unanswered question is whether a public disillusioned about politics can be brought to kindle some faith in their leaders and their government" [27].

5. Overcoming barriers to reform

Significant reform of the health care system sufficient to achieve universal coverage, a value-driven system and administrative simplification faces enormous barriers at the level of our societal ecosystem – barriers as large as any that can be faced in public policy.

Our health care system presents intrinsic barriers because it is a complex adaptive system. Without direct command and control mechanisms, reforms must be designed so that they can effectively and appropriately influence the behaviors and processes of the many different institutions and actors in this system so as to achieve public policy goals.

Our economic system presents enormous barriers. Health care represents one-sixth of our nation's total GDP, including approximately $2.5 Trillion in revenues, wages and tax benefits to a broad cross-section of people and institutions. System-wide reforms must be designed so as to carefully navigate the economic impact on all of these economic interests.

Our laws and constitutional system presents serious barriers. Health care reform must address a multitude of challenging legal issues implicating everything from constitutional issues of federal versus states' rights to local authority over certificates-of-need and provider regulation.

Competing ideologies and value systems create great barriers. Health care reform must bridge the ongoing cultural divide over the role of health care in American life and, especially, the role of government in the health care system.

Finally, our political structure and legislative institutions create significant barriers. Health care reform must be enacted into law through the legislative process. This requires an investment of political leadership and of legislative skill sufficient to engineer a coalition of support for significant reform large and sustained enough to overcome the historic and intrinsic tendency of the Congress towards stasis and small, incremental changes.

Because there are so many barriers, significant reform is a relatively rare occurrence. Yet it does happen and there are some important examples of major health care reforms. One is the enactment of Medicare and Medicaid in the 1960s. These programs were enacted despite profound social system barriers and the strong opposition of powerful interest groups, including the American Medical Association, representing organized medicine [60].

A number of factors contributed to puncturing the stasis that predominated in this policy area during that time. The late 1950's and early 1960's were years of significant expansion of the economy and of the economic welfare of the population as a whole. It was a time when Presidents Kennedy and then Johnson were able to galvanize popular support around a relatively liberal view of responsibility for the public good and for America as the leading laboratory for modeling liberty and equality. It was also a time when the persistence of significant pockets of poverty lent momentum to anti-poverty programs and Johnson's articulation of the goal of a "Great Society" resonated broadly. Democrats had made large gains in Congress in the 1964 elections, picking up thirty-two seats, and gaining the largest majority since the New Deal era [60, pp. 365–370]. The plight of the nation's elders and the poorest of the poor came into stark focus; and for the first time, there was a surge of popular support for a national solution to provide access to health care for the most vulnerable.

Yet, even as popular opinion surged and a strong partisan legislative majority formed, all of the major societal barriers were in play, including economic, legal, ideological and political. There was great ideological contention over both the causes and the cures for what ailed America. Opposing thought-leaders and interests regularly appealed to basic values and principles in staking out seemingly irreconcilable differences of approach to addressing the plight of the poor and underserved [60].

Despite all of the barriers, the Medicare and Medicaid programs were enacted, representing a major enlargement of the government's role in providing social supports – in this case, access to health care for vulnerable populations. Yet, while the creation of these programs was clearly a major national milestone, it is less well understood that these programs were essentially "cobbled together" from several competing legislative proposals that had been championed separately from very different ideological starting points. Part A of Medicare, the part that pays hospitals, was drawn from a relatively liberal Democratic plan for compulsory hospital insurance under Social Security. What became Part B of Medicare, the part that pays physicians, was drawn from a relatively conservative Republican proposal for government-subsidized voluntary insurance to pay physicians. And what became the Medicaid program was built from a collection of existing and demonstration programs designed to subsidize care based in poorer communities but under local and state control [60, p. 369]. In a complex process of legislative "sausage-making," legislative leaders assembled a bipartisan supermajority to win passage of this major reform.

One can easily point to many problems this legislative sausage-making created for these programs going forward and that exist to this day. Nevertheless, it is not hard to see that the result was that major reforms were enacted that continue to enable access to needed care by millions of Americans.

5.1. Lessons for reformers

There are a number of lessons to be learned from the successful enactment of the Medicare and Medicaid programs that appear relevant to current and future reform efforts.

Lesson #1: A necessary condition for achieving significant reform is the existence of large and sufficiently enduring social forces sufficient to disrupt legislative and policy stasis and drive the necessary political solutions. Assuming that economic, legal and cultural factors have developed to where reform appears at least theoretically possible, such a major social force is necessary to catalyze the extraordinary efforts required to overcome system stasis and to recast the rules that structure the myriad economic, legal and political relations and processes that characterize the existing system.

As we have discussed, most of the time, public policy issues are managed within the various societal processes designed for these purposes, whether at the local, state or national level. Public attention to these myriad issues is generally diffuse. But, there are times when an issue comes into the public spotlight in a way that fixes popular attention. As described by Baumgartner and Jones, normally, it does so in the context of a "story line" that simplifies the issue and frames it within one or more moral or other popularly compelling explanatory framework [6]. Such a major popular attention shift onto a single issue is an enormously potent force because it signals broadly that current systems are not adequately managing important problems. If the system cannot respond adequately, then a cascade of increasing popular attention can develop as all of the outlets of both expert and popular communication mobilize, including the press and media; and interest groups engage.

In the early 1960's popular sentiment became such a force. There was widespread social mobilization focused on the plight of the poor and vulnerable in the midst of growing societal prosperity. Another such force was the large Democratic Party gains in the 1964 Congressional elections – a large electoral sweep many interpreted as a popular "mandate" for significant reform to address problems and to redress grievances.

Lesson #2: Public sentiment and electoral "mandates" might be necessary to significant reform, but they are not sufficient. As was seen in the efforts of President Clinton to craft significant health care reform, partisan majorities and strong popular sentiment in favor of reform is not enough. Clinton had made health care reform an important element of his successful election effort. When he was elected a mandate for reform was invoked and a major investment was made to enact a major overhaul of the health care system.

Yet, the Administration was unable to overcome system stasis and convert this "mandate" into successful legislation. It lost traction with the public as the plan was developed in a relatively secretive process that continuously raised questions that were not easily answered. Once revealed, the bill's complexities did not lend themselves to broad public understanding and buy-in. Opponents of the bill, led by the insurance industry, were able to leverage popular uncertainty and turn public sentiment against the proposed reforms.

Lesson #3: Significant reform can be achieved where the formidable societal mechanisms that maintain stasis in current policy are overcome by strong and sustained social forces that are successfully translated into a legislative super-majority that will vote for change. The key to achieving reform is the successful engineering of the legislative process. This is an enormously complicated and high-stakes process requiring of the main proponents political leadership and skills of the highest order supported by continued public backing in the form of expectations that key system problems will be addressed and key reform goals will be met. In this regard, the examples of the cobbled-together but transformative Medicare and Medicaid programs serve as useful models.

Just as in the years prior to the enactment of Medicare and Medicaid, the environment for health care reform in 2009 developed within the context of years of growing awareness of major social problems related to lack of affordable health care. Polling shows that, for decades, the effects of high costs and inequities in access to health services have been a serious public policy concern [42]. The costs of healthcare are understood to seriously compromise the competitiveness of American companies and whole industries. More than 45 million people lack health insurance and tens of millions more have inadequate insurance, fear losing their insurance, and or are paying more to keep it. More people go into bankruptcy every year from costs incurred in health care than from any other source. Clearly, the issue of unsustainable health care costs has been widely appreciated for decades.

As we have seen, there are signs that the level of concern, and its relative importance vis a vis other concerns has grown, even among those with insurance. The Kaiser Family Fund (KFF) conducts ongoing polling across a broad spectrum of health care issues. KFF has found growing public concern with the increasingly high costs of insurance, including premiums, deductibles and co-pays. They have also found mounting concern about the inadequacy of insurance in the case of catastrophic or long-term care. And there is evidence of increased concern with higher-order social inequities in health care coverage, especially with insurance underwriting and other policies that seem unfair and unjustified, as when such policies hinder people with pre-existing conditions from procuring needed insurance coverage [29]. KFF's president recently wrote, "More than any other single factor, it is the problems the insured have paying for health care and their worries that these problems will worsen that have put health on the agenda with new political traction" [1]. The expert convergence around the health care reform agenda of affordable universal coverage, value-driven care and administrative simplicity undoubtedly reflects these worries about economic vulnerability arising from inadequate and costly health care coverage. It is not surprising that both John McCain and Barack Obama made the reform of health care a major focus of their campaigns for the presidency.

5.2. Applying the lessons

1. Harness and sustain mobilized public support. A major economic crisis struck suddenly in the last quarter of 2008. The collapse of the credit and housing markets has caused major corporate and banking failures and has led to widespread layoffs and continuing unemployment. This national financial crisis implicates the economic security of the vast majority of the American people. It has served to fix the attention of Americans on addressing the main sources of economic vulnerability. In this context, reformers would do well to continue to press their case in the court of public opinion that the reform of the health care system is necessary not only to achieving better health care but to achieving economic security.
2. Have your Sausage and Eat it Too. It is the role of the legislature to craft and pass legislation. Most legislators take that role and the legislative process very seriously. It is a role that is designed to entail engagement with a variety of points of view and interests, requiring negotiation, accommodation and the "cobbling together" of laws. Crafting legislation is intrinsically about sausage-making. Such legislative "cobbling together" characterized the successful Medicare and Medicaid legislation.

It is likely that the Clinton Administration was unsuccessful in achieving health care reform in no small part because its reform legislation was crafted primarily by carefully selected policy experts behind closed doors, shielded from input by the normal cross-section of legislators in a process designed to avoid making sausage.

In this context, as Obama Administration has done, reformers would do well to delegate to Congress the task of developing legislation consistent with the goals outlined earlier in this chapter. It bodes well that the committees with jurisdiction on health care reform issues in both the Senate and the House of Representatives have taken on this challenge and are working to coordinate their efforts. These include the Senate Finance Committee and the Health, Education, Labor, and Pensions Committee; and the House Ways and Means, Energy and Commerce, and Education and Labor committees.

3. Stay true to convergent, near-consensus goals. Thought-leadership and public opinion have achieved a remarkable convergence over the course of the last two decades around the goals of affordable universal coverage, a value-driven system, and administrative simplification.
   In this context, reformers would do well to do all they can to ensure that the legislative efforts maintain a clear focus on these goals.

6. Major barriers at other levels of the health system architecture

We began this chapter with reference to the four levels of the health system architecture described by Rouse. Our analysis of barriers to this point has been focused at the highest level of the architecture: the level of the societal ecosystem. Assuming the passage of societal-level health care reform designed to achieve affordable universal coverage, a value-driven system, and administrative simplicity, there would then be the challenge of implementing reform through every level of the system architecture.

A full accounting of the barriers throughout the rest of the health system architecture is beyond the scope of this chapter. However we point to a number of key barriers that reformers must take into account as they contemplate the design of system-wide reforms.

6.1. Barriers at the level of system structure

- Fragmentation of the health care system. Structured within a complex adaptive system, the health care system is a patchwork of organizations, providers and services that are not integrated, but instead are organized according to local contingencies and particular market needs or opportunities.

This fragmentation means that overall organizational capacity and experience in coordinating care varies tremendously among providers and provider organizations. Reforming this fragmented structure into something approaching an integrated nationwide health system will be a daunting task. Most likely as a first step, reformers will want to press for uniform standards for information systems, data and transactions, which would enable the sharing of information that would be necessary for system-wide communications. Proposals for the creation of accountable care organizations and regional insurance co-ops and other related proposals, if established, could lead to more robust local and regional health care coordination and engender new thinking on the possibilities for achieving something approaching a nation-wide system of health care.

- Problems in organizational culture. The culture of clinical medicine has changed a great deal over the last several decades, moving steadily from the traditional paternalistic model of the physician-centric practice to a more patient-centered model of the physician as a professional team member, collaborator and patient partner. Yet organizational culture remains a significant barrier in most health care settings.

Both academic and clinical medicine have long been organized according to academic and clinical specialty. This organization into "silos" is a major factor in the fragmented nature of most existing health care delivery processes. Practices organized into such silos remain rooted in a culture that prioritizes the authority and prerogatives of the autonomous professional. To achieve the public policy goals of creating a value-driven health system, it will be necessary to transition the delivery system to one based in a patient-centered culture of collaboration and teamwork. Leaders must be cultivated and developed throughout the health care delivery system who are capable of leading integrated learning organizations.

6.2. Barriers at the level of delivery operations

To be successful, health care reform must engender implementation of fundamental changes in the way delivery operations are conceived. These operations must be restructured away from existing organizing principles to new ones that will optimize care processes, including the patient-centered management of clinical operations, the development and utilization of appropriate information systems and information, and the organization of care according to performance and outcomes measures. According to the IOM, this means operations must change:

- From care that is based primarily on visits to care based on continuous healing relationships.
- From variability in care driven by professional autonomy to care customized according to patient needs and values.
- From professionals in control of care to the patient as the source of control.
- From information is a static, relatively inaccessible record to knowledge that is shared and information that flows freely.
- From decision making that is based on localized training and experience preferences to decision-making that is evidence-based.
- From do no harm as an individual responsibility to safety as a system property.
- From secrecy is necessary to transparency is necessary.
- From the care system reacting to needs to needs being anticipated.
- From seeking discreet cost reductions to systematic and continuous decrease of waste and inefficiencies.
- From clinical systems based on traditional professional hierarchies to systems designed for cooperation among clinicians [31, p. 71].

6.3. Barriers at the level of clinical practice

Barriers at the level of clinical practice are also substantial. Health care practice is extremely complex and requires many years of intensive study and training. Practitioners are trained within particular cultural and organizational contexts, often through direct mentoring that involves the attainment of particular skills and approaches to care preferred in a particular environment. While practitioners will continue to learn throughout their practice lives, there is ample evidence that much clinical practice is not well grounded in strong scientific evidence of efficacy or comparative efficacy [41]. There is also ample evidence that practitioners are often averse to changing their well-established approaches to care. In addition, changing clinical practice involves a variety of opportunity costs that can be significant, including time, financial, practice disruption, learning, productivity and other costs. Another important set of barriers at the level of clinical practice that cannot be overlooked involves the challenges of changing patient expectations and behavior.

Grol, and Wensing provide a helpful survey and typology of barriers to change at the level of clinical practice [25]. From studies on the adoption of best practices in healthcare settings, the authors suggest barriers that are likely to be found among both health care practitioners and patients. These include:

The innovation itself can have barriers with respect to both the individual professional and the patient in the form of:

- Cost
- Feasibility
- Credibility
- Accessibility
- Attractiveness

The individual professional may manifest barriers to change in the areas of:

- Awareness
- Knowledge
- Attitude
- Motivation to change
- Behavioral routines
- Cognitive and Learning styles
- Personal values/ethical issues
- The opinion of colleagues

The patient may manifest barriers to change in the areas of:

- Knowledge
- Skills
- Attitude and motivation
- Compliance
- Personal values/ethical issues [25,46]

Each of these barriers at each of these levels represents a set of challenges requiring dedicated resources, investigation and remediation. Each is structured by functions and systems at higher levels that too must be addressed either prior to or in conjunction with the changes at the lower levels. While affecting the reform of systems and practices throughout health care would be a daunting undertaking, there already exists a robust foundation of modeling and practice innovation in health care organizations and settings both nationally and internationally.

7. Conclusion

Significant health care reform depends, in the first instance, upon political leadership and skill; and in the end, upon the willingness of stakeholders throughout the health care system to follow-through and drive the changes and continuous improvement necessary to achieving public policy goals. The public policy consensus for significant change appears strong, centered on universal coverage, value and administrative simplicity. The constellation of systemic, economic, legal, cultural and political barriers are identifiable. Assuming the theoretical capacity to manage these barriers, there remains a "tipping point" political threshold that must be attained in order to enact significant reform. This tipping point may eventually be found with one or a few legislators who represent the critical "pivot" votes; or it may be found in the capacity of the dominant party "cartel" to leverage its majority status to engineer and win both the necessary allies and procedural accommodations. It is possible that the executive leadership of the President could prove decisive. All these paths and more lead to the same final and critical juncture at which point the next chapter in our nation's public policy begins.

References

[1] D. Altman, The Sleeper in Health Reform. Kaiser Family Foundation. Available: http://www.kff.org/pullingittogether/061709_altman.cfm, 2009.
[2] American Association of Public Opinion Research (AAOPR). AAPOR Statement on Push Polls. Available at: http://www.aapor.org/aaporstatementonpushpolls Accessed 6/26/09, 2007.
[3] D.L. Bartlett and J.B. Steele, Critical Condition: How Health Care in America Became Big Business and Bad Medicine, New York: Doubleday, 2004.
[4] F.R. Baumgartner, A. François and M. Foucault, Punctuated Equilibrium and French Budgeting Processes, *Journal of European Public Policy* **13** (2006), 1086–1103.
[5] F.R. Baumgartner and B.D. Jones, Agenda Dynamics and Policy Subsystems, *Journal of Politics* **53** (1991), 1044–1074.
[6] F.R. Baumgartner and B.D. Jones, *Agendas and Instability in American Politics*. Chicago: University of Chicago Press, 1993.
[7] F.R. Baumgartner and B.D. Jones, Positive and Negative Feedback in Politics, in: *Policy Dynamics*, F.R. Baumgartner and B.D. Jones, eds, Chicago: University of Chicago Press, 2002.
[8] F.R. Baumgartner, B.D. Jones and M. McLeod, The Evolution of Legislative Jurisdictions, *Journal of Politics* **62** (2000), 321–349.
[9] F.R. Baumgartner, B.D. Jones and J. Wilkerson, Studying Policy Dynamics, in: *Policy Dynamics*, F.R. Baumgartner and B.D. Jones, eds, Chicago: University of Chicago Press, 2002.
[10] Blue Ridge Academic Health Group (BRAHG). (1998). *Promoting Value and Expanded Coverage: Good Health Is Good Business*. Report 2. Washington, DC: Cap Gemini Ernst & Young US, LLC. Available: http://blueridgegroup.org/ Accessed 7/17/09.
[11] Blue Ridge Academic Health Group (BRAHG), *Fall 2008 Policy Proposal: A United States Health Board*. Atlanta: Emory University. Available: http://blueridgegroup.org/ Accessed 7/17/09, 2008.
[12] Bureau of Labor Statistics. Career Guide to Industries. U.S. Department of Labor. Washington D.C. Available: http://www.bls.gov/oco/cg/cgs035.htm, 2009.
[13] M. Chugh, Executive Authority to Reform Health: Options and Limitations The O'Neill Institute for National and Global Health Law at Georgetown Law available at: www.oneillinstitute.org Accessed 6/25/09, 2009.
[14] The Commonwealth Fund Commission on a High Performance Health System. (CWF 2006). Framework for a High Performance Health System for the United States. Washington, D.C.
[15] The Commonwealth Fund Commission on a High Performance Health System. (CWF 2008). Why not the best? Results from the national scorecard on U.S. health system performance. The Commonwealth Fund. Available: http://www.commonwealthfund.org/publications/publications_show.htm?doc_id=692682. Accessed 6/26/09.
[16] G.W. Cox and M.D. McCubbins, *Legislative Leviathan: Party Government in the House*. Berkeley: University of California Press, 1993.
[17] T. Daschle, J.M. Lambrew and S.S. Greenberger, *Critical: What We Can Do About the Health-Care Crisis*, New York: St. Martin's Press, 2008.
[18] D. Elmendorf, The Budget and Economic Outlook. Director's Blog, Congressional Budget Office Jan. 8, 2009. Available: http://cboblog.cbo.gov/?m=200901, 2009.
[19] D. Elmendorf, Statutory Pay-As-You-Go Act of 2009. Director's Blog. Congressional Budget Office. July 14, 2009 Available: http://cboblog.cbo.gov/?p=325, 2009.
[20] Federal Reserve Board of Governors, The Federal Reserve System: Purposes and Functions, Federal Reserve Board of Governors, 27, 2005.
[21] A. Gauthier and M. Serber, A Need to Transform the U.S. Health Care System: Improving Access, Quality, and Efficiency. New York: The Commonwealth Fund, 2005.
[22] A. Gauthier, S.C. Schoenbaum and I. Weinbaum, Toward a High Performance Health System for the United States. New York: The Commonwealth Fund, 2006.

[23] R. Greenstein, Statement: Robert Greenstein to Health Reform Financing Roundtable of the Senate Finance Committee. Center on Budget and Policy Priorities. Washington D.C. Available: http://www.cbpp.org/cms/index.cfm?fa=view&id=2810 Accessed 7/16/09, 2009.

[24] R. Grol, Improving the quality of medical care. Building bridges among professional pride, payer profit, and patient satisfaction, *JAMA* **286** (2001), 2578–2584.

[25] R. Grol and M. Wensing, What drives change? Barriers to and incentives for achieving evidence-based practice, *MJA* **180**(6) (2004), S57–S60.

[26] R. Grol, M. Wensing and M. Eccles, Improving Patient Care: The Implementation of Change in Clinical Practice. Oxford: Elsevier, 2004.

[27] J.S. Hacker, Perspective: Putting Politics First, *Health Affairs* **27**(3) (2008), 718–723.

[28] J. Henry, Kaiser Family Foundation (Kaiser), *Health Care Costs: A Primer Key Information On Health Care Costs And Their Impact*. Menlo Park, CA. Available: http://search.kff.org/gsaresults/search?q=Health+Care+Costs%3A+A+Primer+Key+Information+On+HealthCare+Costs+And+Their+Impact.&hl=es&site=(KFForg)&filter=0&output=xml_no_dtd&client=kff&getfields=*&sort=date%3AD%3AL%3Ad1&stylesheet=kff_middle.xslt&search_pdf=1&sp=kff, 2009.

[29] J. Henry, Kaiser Family Foundation (Kaiser Polling), Public Opinion on Health Care. Kaiser Polls. Available: http://www.kff.org/kaiserpolls/index2.cfm Accessed 7/16/09, 2009.

[30] Institute of Medicine, To err is human: Building a safer health system. Washington, DC: National Academies Press, 2000.

[31] Institute of Medicine, Crossing the quality chasm: A new health systems for the 21st century. Washington, DC: National Academies Press, 2001.

[32] Institute of Medicine, Coverage Matters. Washington DC: National Academy Press, 2001.

[33] Institute of Medicine, Health Professions Education: A Bridge to Quality. Washington DC: National Academy Press, 2003.

[34] Institute of Medicine, Insuring America's Health: Principles and Recommendations. Washington DC: National Academy Press, 2004.

[35] Institute of Medicine, Learning What Works Best: The Nation's Need for Evidence on Comparative Effectiveness in Health Care. Available at: http://www.iom.edu/ebm-effectiveness Accessed 7/16/09, 2007.

[36] Institute of Medicine, Knowing What Works in Health Care: A Roadmap for the Nation. Washington D.C. National Academies Press, 2008.

[37] T.S. Jost, Health Care at Risk: A Critique of the Consumer-Driven Movement. Duke University Press, 2007.

[38] T.S. Jost, Fresh Thinking: Legal And Regulatory Issues Presented By Health Care Reform. Washington and Lee University. Available: http://www.fresh-thinking.org/publications/LegalRegulatoryIssues.html, 2007.

[39] K. Krehbiel, Pivotal Politics: a theory of U.S. Lawmaking. Chicago: University of Chicago Press, 1998.

[40] G. McConnell, Private Power and American Democracy. New York: Knopf, 1966.

[41] E.A. McGlynn, S.M. Asch, J. Adams et al., The quality of health care delivered to adults in the United States, *N Engl J Med* **348** (2003), 2635–2645.

[42] W.D. McInturff and L. Weigel, Déjà vu All Over Again: The Similarities Between Political Debates Regarding Health Care In The Early 1990s And Today, *Health Affairs* **27**(3), (May/June 2008), 699–704.

[43] D.R. Mayhew, Divided We Govern: Party Control, Lawmaking, and Investigations, 1946–2002, Second Edition (Paperback). New Haven: Yale University Press, 2005.

[44] R.E. Mechanic and S.H. Altman, Payment Reform Options: Episode Payment is A Good Place To Start, *Health Affairs* **28**(2) (2009), w262–w271.

[45] National Coalition on Health Care (NCHC) Coalition Principles. Washington. Available: http://www.nchc.org/about/index.shtml, 2009.

[46] National Institute of Clinical Studies (NICS). Barriers and Enablers. In *Using Evidence: Using Guidelines* Symposium. Melbourne, Australia Available: http://www.nhmrc.gov.au/nics/material_resources/resources/barriers.htm, 2006.

[47] Now is the Time for Health Care Reform: A Proposal to Achieve Universal Coverage, Affordability, Quality Improvement and Market Reform, 'Board of Directors' statement December 2008. Available at: http://www.ahip.org/content/default.aspx?docid=25124.

[48] Office of Management and Budget (OMB). President Obama's Fiscal 2010 Budget. Available: http://www. whitehouse.gov/omb/fy2010_key_healthcare/ (accessed 6/12/09), 2009.

[49] M.E. Porter and E.O. Teisberg, Redefining health care: Creating valuebased competition on results. Boston: Harvard Business School Press, 2006.

[50] President's Advisory Commission on Consumer Protection and Quality in the Health Care Industry, "Quality First: Better Health Care for All Americans" (Washington, D.C.: 1998), available at http://www.hcqualitycommission.gov/press/.

[51] W.B. Rouse, Managing complexity: Disease control as a complex adaptive system, *Information · Knowledge · Systems Management* **2**(2) (2000), 143–165.

[52] W.B. Rouse, Engineering complex systems: Implications for research in systems engineering, *IEEE Transactions on Systems, Man, and Cybernetics – Part C* **33**(2) (2003), 154–156.
[53] W.B. Rouse, Agile information systems for agile decision making, in:*Agile Information Systems* (*Chap. 2*), K.C. Desouza, ed., New York: Butterworh – Heinemann, 2006.
[54] W.B. Rouse, Complex engineered, organizational & natural systems: Issues underlying the complexity of systems and fundamental research needed to address these issues, *Systems Engineering* **10**(3) (2007), 260–271.
[55] W.B. Rouse, People and organizations: Explorations of human-centered design. New York: Wiley, 2007.
[56] W.B. Rouse, Healthcare as a complex adaptive system, *The Bridge* **38**(1) (2008), 17–25.
[57] W.B. Rouse, Engineering perspectives on healthcare delivery: Can we afford technological innovation in healthcare? *Systems Research and Behavioral Science* **26** (2009), 1–10.
[58] P.P. Reid, W.D. Compton, J.H. Grossman and G. Fanjiang, Building a better delivery system: A new engineering/health care partnership. Washington, DC: National Academies Press£‹2005.
[59] E. Reinhardt, A Primer for Journalists on Reforming American Health Care: Proposals in the Presidential Campaign, September 2004.
[60] P. Starr, The Social Transformation of American Medicine: The rise of a sovereign profession and the making of a vast industry. New York: Basic Books, 1982.
[61] R.A. Stevens, C.E. Rosenberg and L.R. Burns, (eds), History & Health Policy in the United States. New Brunswick, NJ: Rutgers University Press, 2006.
[62] J.L. True, B.D. Jones and F.R. Baumgartner, Punctuated-Equilibrium Theory: Explaining Stability and Change in American Policymaking, in: *Theories of Policy Process* (*2nd ed.*), P. Sabatier, ed., Boulder: Westview Press, 1999.
[63] U.S. Department of Justice and the Federal Trade Commission (U.S. DOJ & FTC), Statements of Antitrust Enforcement Policy in Health Care Issued August 1996. Available: http://www.usdoj.gov/atr/public/guidelines/1791.htm Accessed 7/17/09, 1996.
[64] C.F. Von Gunten, Culture Eats Strategy for Lunch, *J Palliat Med* **10**(5) (Oct 2007), 1002.
[65] M. Wensing, M. Laurant, M. Hulscher and R. Grol, Methods for identifying barriers and facilitators for implementation, in:*Changing Professional Practice. Theory and Practice of Clinical Guidelines Implementation*, T. Thorsen and M. Mäkelä, eds, Copenhagen: DSI, 1999, pp. 119–132.

Jonathan F. Saxton is an expert in health policy, advocacy and leadership communication in the academic medical center. He served for eleven years as special assistant for health policy and communications to the CEO of the Woodruff Health Sciences Center of Emory University and before that as director of health policy and governmental affairs for the Johns Hopkins University School of Medicine. Most recently, he was vice president and director at Isaacson Miller, Inc, specializing in recruiting health care executive leadership. He has co-authored more than a dozen original articles and reports in health policy and has written more than 300 speeches and related public affairs materials supporting leadership and institutional advancement missions. He earned his undergraduate degree from Haverford College and his law degree with honor from the University of Maryland School of Law.

Michael Johns assumed the post of chancellor for Emory University in October 2007. Prior to that, beginning in 1996, he served as executive vice president for health affairs and CEO of the Robert W. Woodruff Health Sciences Center and chair of Emory Healthcare. As leader of the health sciences and Emory Healthcare for 11 years, Dr. Johns engineered the transformation of the Health Sciences Center into one of the nation's preeminent centers in education, research, and patient care. He previously served as dean of the Johns Hopkins School of Medicine and vice president for medicine at Johns Hopkins University from 1990 to 1996. Dr. Johns received his bachelor's degree from Wayne State University and his medical degree with distinction at the University of Michigan Medical School. From 1977 to 1984 he was a faculty member at the University of Virginia Medical Center in Charlottesville.

In addition to leading complex administrative and academic organizations to new levels of excellence and service, Dr. Johns is widely renowned as a catalyst of new thinking in many areas of health policy and health professions education. He has been a significant contributor to many of the leading organizations and policy groups in health care, including the Institute of Medicine (IOM), the Association of American Medical Colleges (AAMC), The Commonwealth Fund Task Force on Academic Health Centers, the Association of Academic Health Centers, and many others. In 1993, in response to interest from the Clinton White House, he created an ad hoc organization of medical school deans known as the "Saturday Morning Working Group," which developed policy proposals pertaining to medical schools for the Clinton Health Care Reform proposal. He is also the immediate past co-chair of the Blue Ridge Academic Health Group, which has published 12 annual reports on issues of concern for academic health centers and broader health policy thought leadership. He frequently lectures, publishes, and works with state and federal policy makers, on topics ranging from the future of health professions education to national health system reform.

Dr. Johns was elected to the IOM in 1993 and has served on many committees and as Vice Chair of the Council of the IOM. He is a Fellow of the American Association for the Advancement of Science, past co-chairman of the AAMC's Council of Teaching Hospitals and chairman of the AAMC's Board of Advisors of the Institute for the Improvement of Medical Education.

He is a past member of the Governing Board of the National Research Council, the National Governing Board of the Clinical Center of the National Institutes of Health (NIH), and the Council of the National Center for Research Resources, NIH. He has served as member of the Board of Directors and as president of the American Board of Otolaryngology, as chair of the Association of Academic Health Centers, and as Chair of the Council of Deans of the AAMC. He chairs the Journal Oversight Committee of the journal *Academic Medicine. Dr. Johns was* editor of the *Archives of Otolaryngology* from 1992–2005, and serves on the editorial board of the *Journal of the American Medical Association*.

Dr. Johns also serves on a variety of other boards, including Johnson & Johnson, the Genuine Parts Company, AMN Healthcare, the Uniformed Services University of the Health Sciences, the National Health Museum, and the Satcher Health Leadership Institute.

Information Knowledge Systems Management 8 (2009) 465–477
DOI 10.3233/IKS-2009-0151
IOS Press

Chapter 24

Prospects for change

Denis A. Cortese and William B. Rouse
E-mail: cortese.denis@mayo.edu

Abstract: This chapter addresses the prospects for change in health care delivery. The focus is on value – high quality, affordable care for everyone. We consider three domains that participate in the flow of value and the nature of the interfaces among these domains. We also discuss strategic priorities that should align in various ways with these domains. Finally, we address the business transformations needed to enable the provision of value by enterprises that are viable and successful.

1. Introduction

Most people think that the health care system in the United States is broken and that we need to get about the business of fixing it. The truth is that "the system" cannot be fixed because it does not exist in the sense that it was never engineered to provide quality, affordable health care to everyone. This chapter considers the prospects for an engineered system that will provide these benefits.

There has never been a vision or systematic design for health care in this country. Historically, physicians – as independent business owners – hung out their shingles and provided care to patients. Little thought was given to how these providers would relate to one other or to ancillary health care entities, such as medical supply and insurance companies. We should not be surprised, then, with the outputs of our "non-system": lack of insurance, widely variable outcomes, inconsistent service and low safety results – and all this at very high overall cost.

It is clear that tweaks to our home-grown approach will not work. Instead, we need to step back and design a true system of health care. Engineering clearly plays a crucial role in this process. Several universities – including Georgia Tech, University of Wisconsin – Madison, and Purdue – have begun to offer engineering programs in health care delivery science. Physicians, nurses, and engineers must become partners to design interdependent systems that will measure and produce what we want from our health care delivery system – the best outcomes, safety, and service for all citizens at the lowest possible costs. In other words, value.

2. Health care by design

A simple series of patient-centered questions can help us begin to outline the health care system of the future.

1. The first question: Who wants to be admitted to a hospital tomorrow – even if it's the best hospital in the world?

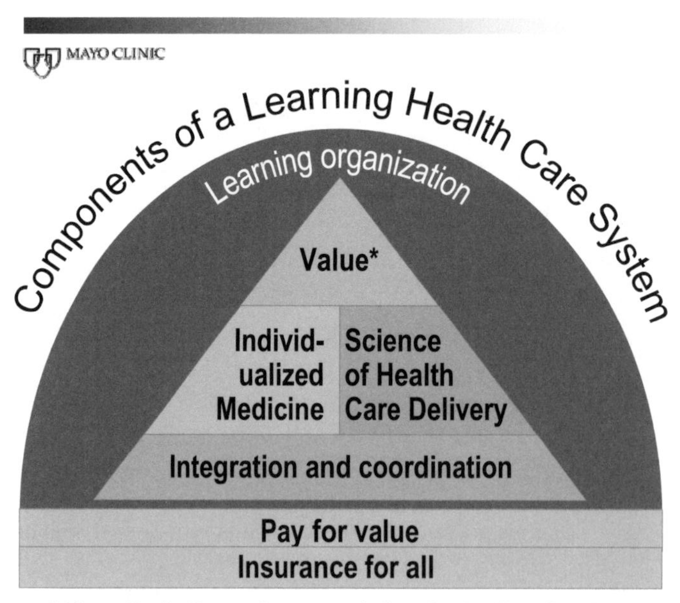

Fig. 1. Framework for the key components of a learning health care system.

2. The second question: Who would like to be sick tomorrow?
3. The last question: Who wants to be a patient, someone who long suffers and endures?

About 99 percent of people answer no to these three questions. The implications of these answers are profound, and require a new approach and design for a new health system. For instance, if we all want to stay out of hospitals for as long as possible – to stay healthy – then should we view a hospitalization as a possible failure of the system?

This short exercise points to the goal of a new health care system: health. The delivery system should strive to keep individuals as healthy and high-functioning as possible, and provide quality, affordable health care services if they do get sick – in short high value health care.

3. Provider responsibilities

The central responsibility for providers is to create a learning health care system [12]. Figure 1 summarizes the key components of a learning heath care system.

To create healthy populations, health care professionals must share information across time and space. Leaders in health care must create an environment within and among organizations in which it is natural to share successes and what we have learned from failures. For instance, when a hospital in one area of the United States finds a way to reduce the risk of administering a medication or eliminate a complication of surgery, would it not be appropriate for every other hospital to learn of this quickly? This is how we can quickly raise the quality (outcomes, safety, and service) – by creating a health care system that is a learning organization [5].

Information is key to providing safe and effecting ongoing care, and is mandatory if we are to generate knowledge. New information and knowledge will develop at ever-increasing speeds during the next few years – biotechnological discoveries in genomics, proteomics, immunology, phamacogenomics, vaccines, micromonitoring and electrical stimulation are a few examples. Therefore the role of Information Technology (IT) becomes clear, and is paramount to enable a functioning learning system for health care. Information technology is the key tool that underpins all components in Fig. 1. We must use information technology to assemble an individual's relevant data and the most up-to-date treatment recommendations, and use them to make evidence-based medical decisions. Right now, some integrated medical practices and commercial companies are building computer systems that provide point-of-service information with push technology to improve medical decision making for patients.

The learning organization concept provides the framework for a new health care system, the output of which should be quality, affordable care for all. To generate this product, providers must focus on four elements: value, integration/coordination, individualized medicine and the science of health care delivery.

3.1. Value

The sole purpose of a learning organization concept for health care is to produce high-value health care – high quality, affordable care. A proposed definition of value is to measure these parameters and express them in the following equation: Value equals Quality divided by Cost Over Time, or V = Q/C.

Quality (Q) – the numerator – includes clinical outcomes, safety and patient-reported satisfaction.

- Examples of outcome measures for hospital care, procedures and chronic conditions: hospital admissions, emergency department visits, unplanned readmissions, mortality rates, post-operative complications, days absent from school or work, measures of organ function and Short Form health survey scores
- Examples of safety measures: central line infection rates, medication errors, post-operative complications
- Examples of patient satisfaction: National Research Corporation's *Healthcare Market Guide*

Performance measurement information is currently available through a variety of respected sources, including the Agency for Healthcare Research and Quality, Ambulatory Care Quality Alliance, National Quality Foundation, Leap Frog, AQA Alliance, University HealthSystem Consortium, Medicare Provider Analysis and Review, and the Commonwealth Fund.

Cost (C) – the denominator – encompasses the cost of care *over time* (not per line item of service). Regional Medicare spending data from Medicare itself or from the Dartmouth Atlas of Healthcare could provide the information necessary to round out the equation.

Using these data, we can create a publicly displayed "value score" for different medical institutions. The value score would offer clearer information on many aspects of a medical provider's care. If one institution can diagnose and treat a patient with $10,000 worth of tests while another, for the same result, costs $15,000, there is a clear value gap. Armed with concrete data, people could choose a high-value facility over a place that charges more but delivers less. Health care providers would then begin to compete on the elements that matter most – outcomes, safety, service and cost. Providers with worse outcomes, less-satisfied patients and higher costs would lose patients, which would spur them to improve the factors that are lowering value.

3.2. Integrated, coordinated care

As our society ages, more people are living with multiple complex, chronic conditions such as diabetes and heart failure. They need an integrated, coordinated approach to their health care. Often, however, a wife or adult child takes on the complex task of coordinating care for an ailing relative, perhaps from thousands of miles away.

The new health care system should foster integrated, coordinated care for all patients. Integration – which focuses on the way that providers interact and organize themselves in order to create value for patients – is sorely lacking in American health care, in part because of the entrepreneurial spirit in which medicine is rooted. Care coordination, such as the efficient organization of patient visits, tests and procedures, should be a natural outgrowth of well-integrated care.

Moving forward, physicians, nurses, and other providers can organize themselves in a variety of ways – group practices, integrated networks of independent providers, physician hospital organizations or "virtual" groups – to better integrate and coordinate care. The point is to develop mechanisms to coordinate care among medical and surgical specialists so that patients have access to teams of providers who can effectively and efficiently meet their needs [4].

3.3. Individualized medicine

The emerging science of Individualized Medicine (IM) holds promise to drive high-value care by growing medical knowledge to facilitate prediction of disease risk, prevention, precise diagnosis, and tailored treatment and follow-up for genetically similar groups and ultimately, a single person.

For example, we used to think all breast cancer was alike. We now know that there are more than 100 types of breast cancer that can be genetically identified, and we offer combinations of eight to 10 different treatments right now. Ten years from now we may have 100 different treatments that will be specific for each woman's genetic make-up.

As the science of IM develops, trial-and-error in medical practice will be replaced by more precise diagnosis and evidence-based treatments based upon genetic and proteomic characteristics. In a *Boston Globe* editorial, Francis S. Collins, M.D., Ph.D., who led the Human Genome Project, envisions a time when patients will have their genomes sequenced for $1,000 or less, possibly through microchip or other innovative DNA sequencing technology. "That information can then be used to guide prescribing patterns and develop a lifelong plan of health maintenance customized to our unique genetic profiles," he writes [2].

IM has tremendous potential to increase the value of health care by allowing medical professionals to get it right the first time – better predicting disease risk, preventing disease development and managing disease treatment more efficiently – thereby keeping people healthier and active longer, improving outcomes, shortening hospital stays and decreasing long-term health care expenditures [3].

3.4. Science of health care delivery

Health care delivery science uses systems engineering principles to analyze outcomes and processes of care with the goal of improving quality and reducing costs.

Consider an example of this principle from a Mayo Clinic benefactor, who founded the Cutter Insect Repellant Company. He noted that when he started Cutter, the product contained 0.001 percent of the active ingredient DEET, which was dissolved in a hydrocarbon solvent. This solvent – which delivered the active ingredient – was expensive and toxic. People didn't like it because it was oily and irritated the skin. So while most of his competitors were doing basic research to improve the active ingredient, the Cutter entrepreneur set out to change the "delivery system" – the method by which the user received the active ingredient. After all, the delivery system was the most expensive and toxic component of the product. The company formed a team to set about solving the delivery system problem. Within several months, the team had completed the task. Using a new delivery method, Cutter was able to reduce their internal costs, completely eliminate the toxicity, and lower the price for their product. This is a real example of an engineering approach that increased value by focusing on the delivery system. This example illustrates how engineering thinking can improve the delivery of health care?

If we can apply the full scope of engineering sciences to the science of health care delivery, we will learn how to bring teams of people together to solve problems with the way health care is currently provided. Using the aviation industry as an example, just imagine the improvements in safety that could be accomplished by applying human-factors analysis and classification systems to medical errors, medication errors and procedural complications [13].

4. Government responsibilities

Within a reformed health care system, the government has two responsibilities: insurance for all and payment reform that rewards value.

4.1. Insurance for all

Tens of millions of Americans are uninsured or underinsured and frequently don't seek the care they need because they cannot afford it. Conversely, lack of insurance creates significant economic problems for health care providers and employers. The American Hospital Association [1] reports that hospitals provided $34 billion in uncompensated care to the uninsured and underinsured in 2007. And many companies – finding it difficult to compete globally when faced with paying billions of dollars to insure employees, retirees and dependents – are reducing or eliminating health insurance coverage.

For both humanitarian and economic reasons, we must guarantee that all Americans have access to health insurance, regardless of their ability to pay.

The current private health insurance system must be reformed to align with a proposal from Len Nichols and John Bertko [8] of the New America Foundation:

- Require Americans to purchase health insurance
- Provide sliding-scale subsidies to help those in need to buy the insurance
- Prohibit pre-existing condition exclusions
- Define a minimum health benefit package or actuarial equivalent
- Adjust risk-levels among enrollees

Within the context of a reformed insurance system, the government could create a simple coordinating mechanism for individuals to select a basic private insurance plan from several options – perhaps modeled after the Federal Employees Health Benefit Plan (FEHBP).

4.2. Pay for value

Politicians typically tell us that the United States is not getting what it pays for in health care. The reality is that we *are* – we are getting more tests, procedures and hospitalizations because the sicker the patient is, the more money providers make. There is a huge variation in Medicare spending for similar patients with similar outcomes in different parts of the country [6]. Those who do more – such as ordering more tests and procedures, for example – earn more money, even if those tests do not improve the patient's outcome.

These trends should not be surprising – they are the inevitable results of the laws of economics in a fee-for-service environment. Legislators must focus energy on creating new ways to provide fair payment to doctors and hospitals that offer high-quality, lower-cost care. The Medicare program is the lever that Congress can use to start us along this path.

Meaningful change – meaningful improvement in health care – will require that we overhaul how we pay for health care by financially rewarding providers who give patients the value that they expect and deserve – good outcomes and compassionate, coordinated care at a reasonable price over time. (See the section on "value.") Using standard performance data, we can create and base portions of payment on a simple "value score" for clinics and hospitals. Over time, we believe that basing payment on value scores will put downward pressure on the cost curve by rewarding high-quality, efficient providers with payment increases over the standard Medicare rate. When a portion of their payments are based upon value, doctors and hospitals will begin to seriously weigh the benefit of ordering more tests because additional medical spending that does not improve outcomes reduces overall value – and consequently would reduce their Medicare reimbursement.

We propose that Congress set a three-year deadline for creating and implementing new Medicare payment methods. To align the payment system with value, we recommend that Congress clearly delegate responsibility and authority to establish new Medicare payment methods to either the Secretary for Health and Human Services (who could form an advisory board, if desired) or a quasi-independent commission. The idea is to create a longer-term, problem-solving function that is outside of yet reports progress to and is accountable for results to the US government. Other issues – such as administrative simplification, safety reporting and medical-evidence dissemination – could also be under this board's purview.

5. Re-engineering to create a health care system

System engineers – who study complex interdependent functions and help them work together more effectively and efficiently – need to lend their expertise to health care design, specifically focusing on creating a learning health care system that generates value. Although no intentionally designed health care system exists in the United States, we can start the discussion of how to design a system by focusing on the three dominant domains of activity in the current milieu – see Fig. 2.

5.1. The knowledge domain

The knowledge domain is where research and development is done. In this domain, we find research institutions, academic medical centers, drug and device manufacturers, funding agencies such as the National Institutes of Health and regulatory agencies such as the Food and Drug Administration. There is some connectivity within this domain – scientists from different centers collaborate on projects; device manufacturers work with researchers to design and test products. For the most part, however, these working relationships form randomly.

5.2. The care-Delivery domain

The second domain is where the patient receives health care services. The patient should be at the center of all efforts here, where care is coordinated. People who work in this domain must provide coordinated, integrated, high-value care that is effective, efficient, timely, safe, equitable and patient

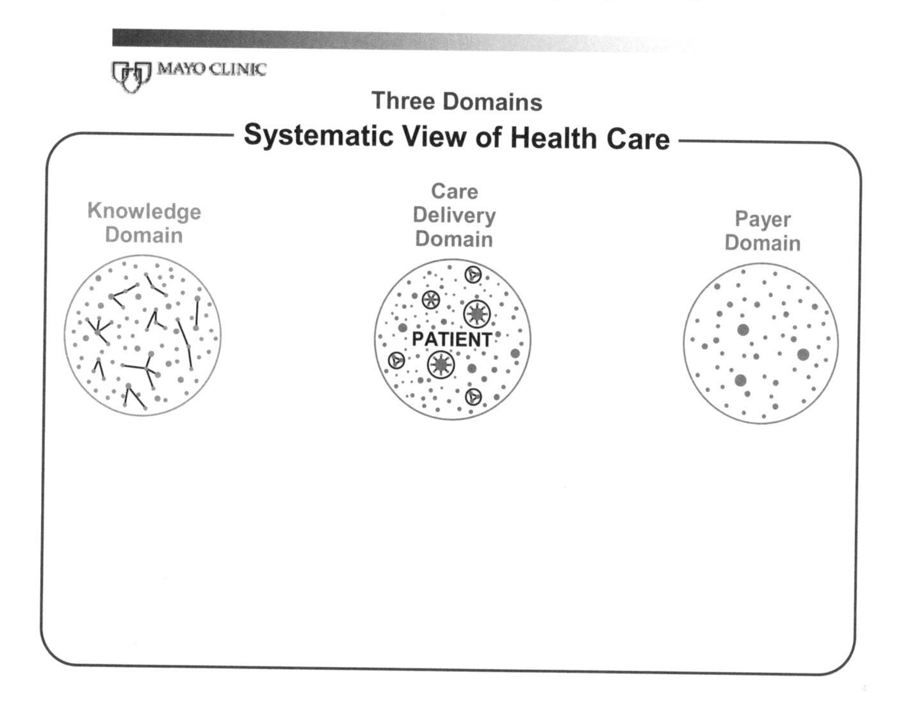

Fig. 2. A Systematic View of Health Care: Knowledge Domain, Care Delivery Domain and Payer Domain.

centered. All incentives within health care must be aimed at this "target" domain, where health and value are generated for patients.

The majority of health care providers operate as islands within this domain. As a general rule, there are few connections between and among the providers here. Granted, there are pockets of collaboration that occur in spite of current barriers. In a newly designed system, inter-institutional collaboration should be a natural output of the system.

However, some organizations – integrated group practices, academic medical centers and virtual medical associations – operate as systems. These groups organize and coordinate care for their patient base. Examples include Geisinger Medical Center, Intermountain Health, Marshfield Clinic, Gunderson Clinic, Health Partners (Minneapolis), Partners Health (Boston), Scott White Clinic, Group Health of Puget Sound and Kaiser. These institutions demonstrate the possibilities of optimizing collaboration among providers in order to deliver better care to patients. Here's another example: Staff at Mayo Health System – a network of 500 physicians, 18 hospitals and 65 delivery sites within a 200-mile radius of the main Mayo Clinic campus in Rochester, Minnesota – work together to provide patients with the right care at the right time and in the right setting.

5.3. The payer domain

Finally, we have the payer domain. This is the "group of groups" that pays for health care services. It includes individuals, private insurance companies, big and small employers, self-insured employers, the state and federal governments, the military and the Veterans Administration. In the near future, this domain must outline new rules for insuring all Americans and change incentives to drive high-value care.

From a provider's perspective, this domain appears to be in a state of chaos at the moment. It is rare that any medical payments are linked to any logical measure of outcomes, safety, service or lower spending

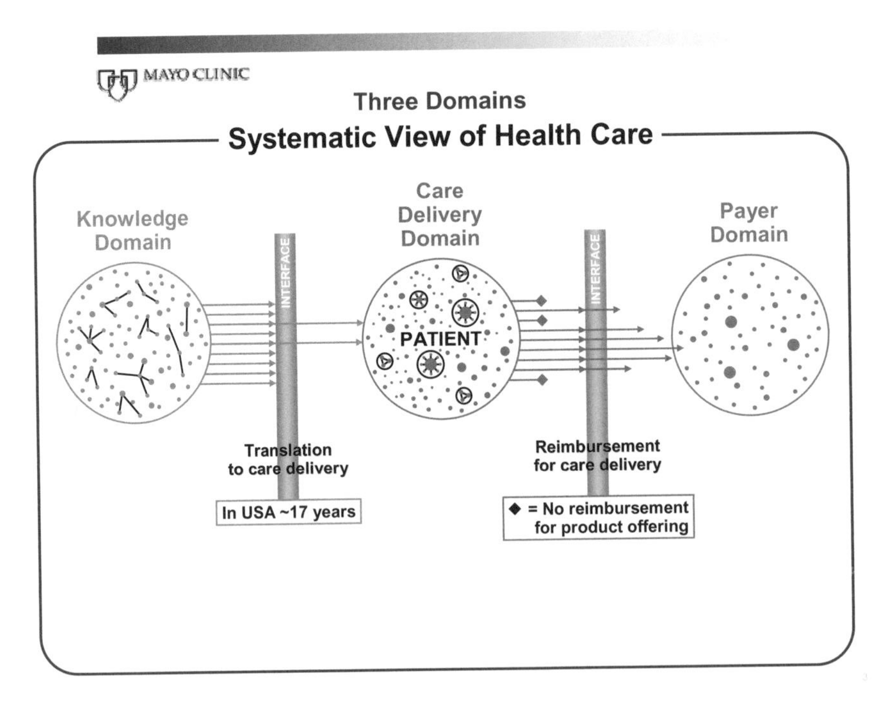

Fig. 3. The interfaces between domains are ripe for engineering solutions.

over time for patients. As a general rule the payments are not linked to patient-centered, high-value care. In fact there are few common rules guiding payment and very little data transparency. This domain also contributes significant administrative costs to the overall price tag of health care.

5.4. Interfaces between domains

Although there is much work to be done to improve function *within* these three domains, an urgent priority should be to focus attention at the interfaces, where value is seeping through the cracks. One of the major problems in this country is that no organization, person or group has managed what happens at these junctures. As indicated in Fig. 3, we continue to pay a huge price for our lack of attention.

For example, take a look at the interface between the knowledge and care-delivery domains. We have all kinds of great ideas coming out of the knowledge domain, in large part because of the huge investments that the government, benefactors and drug/device manufacturers make in science. Then those ideas hit the interface to care delivery, and what happens? A lot of waiting. The feedback loop – from bedside to bench – occurs fairly quickly, but the translation to care delivery is extremely slow.

On average, it takes about 17 years to translate a medical advancement into common practice. Even after the knowledge makes it through the interface, users apply it correctly only 50 percent of the time [7]. Instead, patients receive *their doctors'* current state of knowledge – but certainly not what the whole system knows.

In addition, there is no rationality at the interface between the care delivery and payer domains. For example, providers may offer a potentially high-value service such as an e-consult, but the government-run insurance companies (Medicare, Medicaid) and most private insurance companies deny coverage because it falls outside of the traditional realm of the office visit. Given this situation, it is no surprise that providers quickly read the feedback loop and make sure they provide care for people in a way that

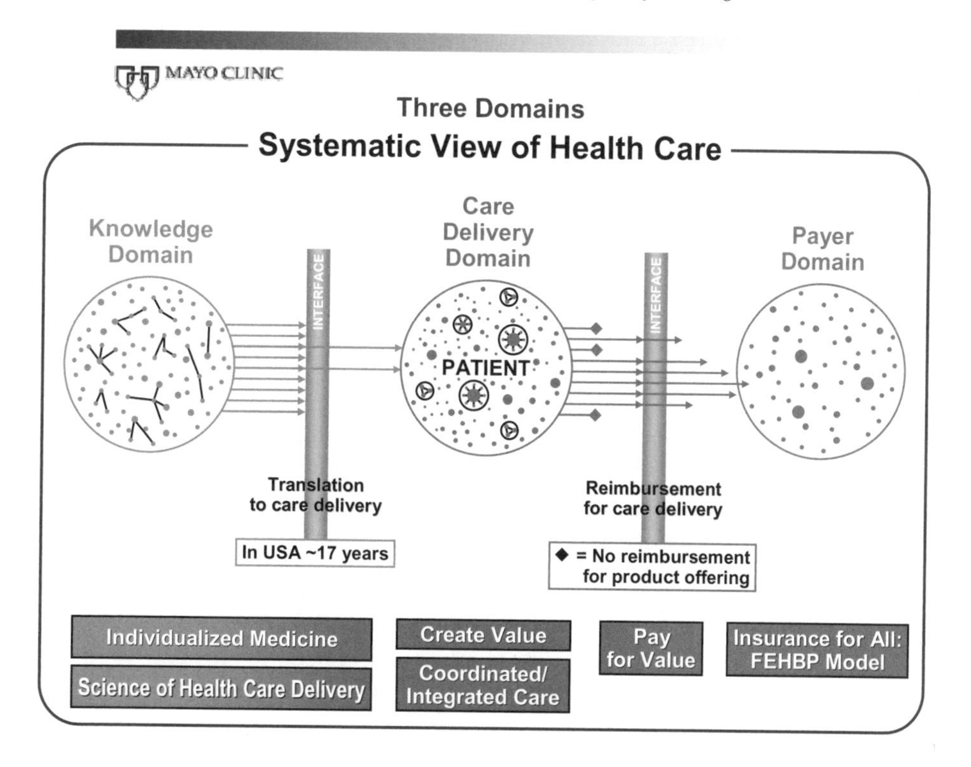

Fig. 4. Alignment of strategic priorities with three domains.

they can get paid – in the office, hospital, or worse yet, in the ER. (In fairness, some private insurers are beginning to collaborate with selected providers and experimenting with non-traditional care delivery.)

For those medical services that make it through the interface, there is little predictability about whether the payment will cover the cost. Private insurance companies rely on negotiated discounts as their predominant mechanism for establishing payments, while the government-run insurance companies set the fee with little or no negotiation with providers. The results are arbitrary. Some are underpaid, overpaid or denied, without a sensible or predictable rationale.

5.5. *Aligning six strategic priorities within the three domains*

There are six strategic priorities required to create a learning organization for health care that spans the domains and provide a starting point for managing interactions at the interfaces:

- Value
- Integrated, coordinated care
- Individualized medicine
- The science of health care delivery
- Pay for value
- Insurance for all)

Figure 4 aligns these strategic priorities with the three domains. The nature of these strategic priorities and their relationships with the domains are as follows:

- Individualized Medicine research emanates from the knowledge domain and is translated for use into the care delivery domain to increase value for patients.

- The science of health care delivery is a key concept that acts at the interface between knowledge and application in the care delivery domain, but it also plays a significant role in improving value within the care delivery domain itself.
- Value generation and integrated, coordinated care are responsibilities of the care delivery domain.
- Paying for value is key to getting the interface between the care delivery domain and the payer domain to function correctly. In order to get high-value health care, we should be certain we are paying it.
- Within the payer domain, new rules for insuring all Americans must be established.

5.6. Managing at the interfaces: Opportunities for engineering

Today and into the future, engineers have significant opportunities to collaborate with providers, scientists, patients, businesses and payers to actively manage domain intersections with the goal of creating a high-value learning organization for U.S. health care. We need to apply system, financial, software and behavioral engineering principles to address a number of important questions, including:

- Within the knowledge domain, how can we speed knowledge creation and dissemination back and forth across the interface so patients always receive the best advice?
- Within the payer domain, how can we align incentives to encourage the provision of high-value care? How can we design incentives to encourage individuals to make healthy choices?

There are no straightforward answers to these complex questions, but we should begin the journey toward solutions. That's why engineers must become an integral part of the health care team. America can no longer afford the high price associated with disorganization.

6. Business transformation

Thus far, we have focused on the transformation of healthcare delivery. Now we shift our attention to the business side of the equation. We expect healthcare businesses will transform in the process of transforming healthcare delivery, but which will be the chicken and which the egg? Fortunately, there is a rich history of enterprise transformation to draw upon [10].

Our studies of what drives fundamental change, how change is addressed, and what practices seem best – or worst – have led to a theory of enterprise transformation [9].

Enterprise transformation is driven by experienced and/or anticipated value deficiencies that result in significantly redesigned and/or new work processes as determined by management's decision making abilities, limitations, and inclinations, all in the context of the social networks of management in particular and the enterprise in general

In light of our line of reasoning advanced earlier in this chapter, the types of health care value deficiencies are quite clear. From a business perspective, enterprises that do not remediate these healthcare deficiencies will experience business deficiencies in terms of lost revenue, profits, and share prices. Innovators will transform the work they do and how they do it. This will require that the managers of these enterprises make decisions, that many will argue are too risky, while also assuring that the social networks associated with the enterprise commit to the needed changes.

To move beyond this rather abstract argument, consider the transformation of the retail industry over the past six decades. After World War II, consumer product companies like Proctor & Gamble pretty

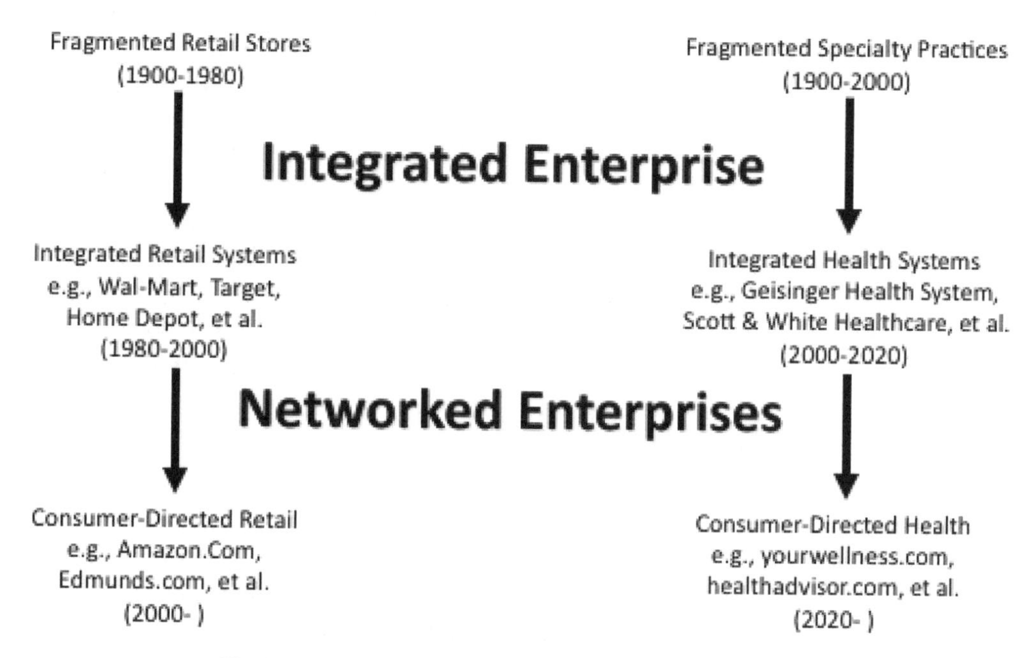

Fig. 5. Parallels between transformation of retail and healthcare.

much dictated the choices consumers had and the prices of these choices. The highly fragmented retail industry (sound familiar?) had little leverage in this process.

Wal-Mart was founded in 1962. By the late 1970s and early 1980s, Wal-Mart was transforming the retail marketplace. They led the revolution in retail that resulted in a small number of big box retailers dominating via integrated supply chain management, vendor-managed inventory, etc. The result was the retailers controlling the game and consumer product companies marching to their tunes.

With the advent of the Internet in the late 1990s, consumers came to have easy access to information on prices, quality, reliability, service and availability. They know where the best deals are and seek value in terms of price, variety, convenience, and so on. The consumer is now in charge. Both the retailers and the consumer product companies have to chase the consumers.

As shown in Fig. 5, we see healthcare evolving in a similar manner. The current craft industry will adopt the best practices of integrated health systems like Cleveland Clinic, Geisinger Health System, Gundersen Lutheran, Intermountain, Kaiser, Marshfield Clinic, Mayo Clinic, Scott & White Healthcare, and Virginia Mason. In the process, thousands of independent providers will be reduced to perhaps 40–50 integrated systems across the US This will result in dramatic cost savings as well as greatly enhanced quality of care.

This transformation will be driven by the inability of small providers to invest in the infrastructure and expertise to compete based on value. There will be many acquisitions and mergers. There also are likely to be alliances and federations to share services such as back office functions. The successful acquisitions, mergers, alliances, and federations will be those who can provide value – high quality, affordable care. Simply stitching together a number of poorly performing providers will only result in a large poorly performing provider.

In parallel with the above trend, but probably lagging a bit, will be the emergence of empowered consumers. Online resources such as personal electronic health records, personalized wellness and health advice (from vetted sources), and provider performance and cost information will empower consumers to make better decisions, possibly supported by their personal health advisor. Direct control of whatever mechanism they use to pay for healthcare will enable making these decisions. Providers will have no choice but provide the health equivalent of "everyday low prices" in the sense that consumers will know precisely what they should pay for what level of service. If these expectations are not met, they will go elsewhere.

Some health thought leaders have argued with the possible parallels between healthcare and retail. Our retort has been, "If retail operated like you operate, three months after you bought a toaster at Wal-Mart you would get 12 invoices from all the suppliers to the toaster manufacturer, many for things that you never would have imagined were in a toaster." The point is that retail is a huge success story. Sure, healthcare is much more complicated than toasters; that's why you will have a health advisor but not an appliance advisor.

7. Conclusions

This chapter has addressed the prospects for change in health care delivery. The focus was on value – high quality, affordable care for everyone. We considered three domains that participate in the flow of value and the nature of the interfaces among these domains. We also discussed strategic priorities that should align in various ways with these domains. Finally, we addressed the business transformations needed to enable the provision of value by enterprises that are viable and successful.

The resulting vision is both profound and compelling. It also involves enormous change by a wide variety of stakeholders, many of whom have made substantial investments in the business models that must be displaced [11]. The needed changes are likely to be quite disruptive. Fortunately, the worsening crisis in financing health care for an aging population with a steadily increasing prevalence of chronic disease will force fundamental change. This book has outlined a wealth of best practices and success stories. We know much of what is needed to engineer the system of healthcare delivery. We need to collectively embrace the many good ideas in this book and get going.

References

[1] American Hospital Association, Uncompensated Hospital Care Cost. http://www.aha.org/aha/content/2008/pdf/08-uncompensated-care.pdf, 2008.

[2] F.S. Collins, Personalized medicine, A new approach to staying well, *The Boston Globe* (17 July 2005).

[3] D.A. Cortese, A Vision of Individualized Medicine in the Context of Global Health, *Clinical Pharmacology & Therapeutics* **82** (2007), 491–493.

[4] D.A. Cortese and J.O. Korsmo, Getting American Health Care on the Right Track, *New England Journal of Medicine*, In press, 2009.

[5] D.A. Cortese and R. Smoldt, Healing America's Ailing Health Care System, *Mayo Clinic Proceedings* **81**(4) (2006), 492–496.

[6] Dartmouth, Atlas of Healthcare. http://www.dartmouthatlas.org/, 2009.

[7] E.A. McGlynn, S.M. Asch, J. Adams et al., The quality of health care delivered to adults in the United States, *New England Journal of Medicine* **348** (2003), 2635–2645.

[8] L. Nichols and J.M. Bertko, A Modest Proposal for a Competing Public Health Plan, *New America Foundation* (11 March 2009).

[9] W.B. Rouse, A Theory of Enterprise Transformation, *Systems Engineering* **8**(4) (2005), 279–295.

[10] W.B. Rouse, ed., Enterprise Transformation: Understanding and Enabling Fundamental Change. New York: Wiley, 2006.
[11] W.B. Rouse, Healthcare as a complex adaptive system, *The Bridge* **38**(1) (2007), 17–25.
[12] P. Senge, The Fifth Discipline: The Art and Practice of The Learning Organization. New York: Doubleday, 1990.
[13] D.A. Wiegmann and S.A. Shappell, A Human Error Approach to Aviation Accident Analysis. Ashgate Publishing, 2003.

Denis A. Cortese, MD, is President and CEO of Mayo Clinic. He is a graduate of Temple University Medical School, and completed Internal Medicine and Pulmonary Diseases training at Mayo Clinic. Dr. Cortese is a professor of medicine and former director of pulmonary disease training program. He served in US Navy Medical Corp during 1974–1976. His major research interests focus on interventional bronchoscopy including appropriate use of photodynamic therapy, endobronchial laser therapy and endobronchial stents. He is a former president of the International Photodynamic Association. Cortese's memberships include The Institute of Medicine of the National Academies (US) and chair of the Roundtable on Evidence Based Medicine; Healthcare Leadership Council, chair for 2007–2009; Harvard/Kennedy Healthcare Policy Group; Academia Nacional de Medicina (Mexico); the Royal College of Physicians (London); Division on Engineering and Physical Science (DEPS), and National Research Council. He received the 2007 Ellis Island Award, the Medal of Merit Award in 2008, and the National Healthcare Leadership Award in November, 2009.

William B. Rouse, is the Executive Director of the Tennenbaum Institute at the Georgia Institute of Technology. He is also a professor in the College of Computing and School of Industrial and Systems Engineering. His research focuses on understanding and managing complex public-private systems such as healthcare and defense, with emphasis on mathematical and computational modeling of these systems for the purpose of policy design and analysis. Rouse has written hundreds of articles and book chapters, and has authored many books, including most recently *People and Organizations: Explorations of Human-Centered Design* (Wiley, 2007), *Essential Challenges of Strategic Management* (Wiley, 2001) and the award-winning *Don't Jump to Solutions* (Jossey-Bass, 1998). He is editor of *Enterprise Transformation: Understanding and Enabling Fundamental Change* (Wiley, 2006), co-editor of *Organizational Simulation: From Modeling & Simulation to Games & Entertainment* (Wiley, 2005), co-editor of the best-selling *Handbook of Systems Engineering and Management* (Wiley, 1999, 2009), and editor of the eight-volume series *Human/Technology Interaction in Complex Systems* (Elsevier). Among many advisory roles, he has served as Chair of the Committee on Human Factors of the National Research Council, a member of the US Air Force Scientific Advisory Board, and a member of the DoD Senior Advisory Group on Modeling and Simulation. Rouse is a member of the National Academy of Engineering, as well as a fellow of four professional societies – Institute of Electrical and Electronics Engineers (IEEE), the International Council on Systems Engineering (INCOSE), the Institute for Operations Research and Management Science (INFORMS), and the Human Factors and Ergonomics Society (HFES).

Information Knowledge Systems Management 8 (2009) 479–480
DOI 10.3233/IKS-2009-0154
IOS Press

Epilogue

Healthcare Costs or Investments?

We are currently embroiled in two debates involving healthcare. One debate involves how the costs of making healthcare available to everyone should be apportioned among individuals, employers, and the government. The second debate concerns how to achieve reductions in the high costs of healthcare to provide the best value. Both debates have to be resolved effectively to achieve our goals. Only addressing one – by, for example, solely making everyone insured – may worsen our cost problems by having many more people demanding very expensive, and sometimes marginally effective care.

Of course, both of these endeavors will require money. How much are we willing to spend to have a healthy, educated, and productive population? There is an underlying subtlety to this question. Is healthcare an expense or an investment? One could argue that it is an investment in human capital that will provide future returns in terms of a productive, competitive workforce and income tax revenues, as well as reduced healthcare costs.

As a savvy investor, we would like the value of this human capital to exceed its cost. As noted above, we have been vigorously debating costs. What about the value of human capital investments? There are data, methods, and tools for estimating the economic value of investments in people's training, education, safety, health, and productivity. We know how to estimate the savings in future healthcare costs that can be achieved by investing now in prevention and early treatments of chronic disease for example.

The difficulty is not our inability to estimate the economic value of investing in healthcare. The problem is that there is no place to put the numbers once we have them. The costs of these investments appear on the national Income Statement, but the value of these investments do not appear on the national Balance Sheet. The reason is simple – we do not maintain a Balance Sheet. Congress has a checkbook, but not a full set of financial statements.

Consequently, in these two ongoing debates, no one at the table owns the future. No one feels responsible for assuring that we have the human capital assets we need to be competitive in Tom Friedman's hot, flat and crowded world. As a result, there is no felt need for a Balance Sheet on which to tally the value of these human capital assets. Our inadequate accounting system is keeping us from making the investments we need to make to assure the standard of living to which we aspire.

We believe that some combination of the Office of Management of the Budget, Congressional Budget Office, and General Accountability Office should take the lead in adding a Balance Sheet to the national Income Statement. It could begin as an oversight scorecard and then, with experience, become an element of the decision making process. This would result in healthcare investments having much greater asset values than "bridges to nowhere."

We are all better off if everyone is healthy, educated, and productive. The fact that we send our children to school, exercise and try to eat a healthy diet, and pursue advanced education all attest to this philosophy. We know how to balance the near-term and long-term. For instance, how much are you willing to spend on your monthly utility bill? Less the better is our response. How much are you willing to "spend" on your 401(k)? More the better is our answer.

The healthcare debates need to shift from minimizing the costs of our utility bills to maximizing the value of our 401(k)s. These debates also need to broaden to include education. While productivity may primarily involve private sector investments, an educated populace will make it easier to have a healthy populace. We need human capital that is both well and smart.

William B. Rouse
Executive Director of the Tennenbaum Institute at Georgia Institute of Technology
E-mail: bill.rouse@ti.gatech.edu

Michael E. Johns
Chancellor of Emory University and former CEO of Emory Health Sciences
E-mail: mmejohns@emory.edu

Denis A. Cortese
President and CEO of Mayo Clinic
E-mail: cortese.denis@mayo.edu

Author Index